Board Review Series

Pediatrics

Board Review Series

Pediatrics

Lloyd J. Brown, MD, FAAP
Associate Director, Pediatric Residency Training Program
Cedars-Sinai Medical Center
Course Chair, Pediatric Clerkship
Associate Professor of Pediatrics
David Geffen School of Medicine at UCLA

Lee Todd Miller, MD, FAAP
Director, Pediatric Residency Training Program
Cedars-Sinai Medical Center
Professor of Pediatrics
David Geffen School of Medicine at UCLA

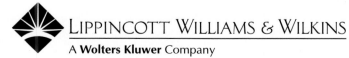

LIPPINCOTT WILLIAMS & WILKINS
A **Wolters Kluwer** Company
Philadelphia · Baltimore · New York · London
Buenos Aires · Hong Kong · Sydney · Tokyo

Editor: Neil Marquardt
Managing Editor: Elena Coler
Senior Project Editor: Karen Ruppert
Marketing Manager: Scott Lavine
Designer: Risa Clow
Compositor: Peirce Graphic Services
Printer: C&C

Printed in China

Library of Congress Cataloging-in-Publication Data

Pediatrics / [edited by] Lloyd J. Brown, Lee Todd Miller.
    p. ; cm.—(Board review series)
  Includes index.
  ISBN 13: 978-0-7817-2129-5
  ISBN 10: 0-7817-2129-6
    1. Pediatrics—Examinations, questions, etc. I. Brown, Lloyd J. II. Miller, Lee T. (Lee Todd) III. Series.
  [DNLM: 1. Pediatrics—Examination Questions. WS 18.2 P37051 2004]
  RJ48.2.P385 2004
  618.92′00076—dc22

                  2004048308

15 16

Dedication

To Bobbie, my love, for her friendship, support, and laughter, and for being a truly wonderful mother to our son; and to Danny—I thank God every day you are here—you are the sweetness of my life.

Lloyd Brown

To my family, my dear friends, and to Kai, for their unwavering support and encouragement and love; and to my father, who was excited and very proud of this project, but who did not make it to see its completion, with much love from Lee.

Lee Miller

Preface

We created this text to provide medical students and physicians with a comprehensive, yet hopefully very manageable, overview of the basic principles of pediatric medicine.

It is our great hope that junior medical students on their core pediatric clerkships, senior students on pediatric subinternships and pediatric subspecialty rotations, and students or physicians studying for the USMLE Step 2 examination will gain a strong foundation in pediatrics on which to build their subsequent learning in both primary care and subspecialty pediatrics.

We have created a case-based review test (simulating USMLE Step 2 questions) at the end of each chapter to emphasize key take-home points and to help the reader to assess his or her understanding of each chapter's contents. The review questions are followed by answers and detailed explanations for both the correct and incorrect choices. Cross references to the text appear in square brackets.

There is also a comprehensive 100-question examination at the end of the text to provide the reader with a comprehensive self-assessment tool and additional review of the primary care and subspecialty areas covered in this text. Similar to the chapter review tests, the comprehensive examination includes detailed explanations for both the correct and incorrect choices.

Acknowledgments

We would both like to recognize individuals who have made tremendous impacts on our medical education and on our professional growth and development.

I have been so privileged to learn from some outstanding teachers and mentors, both at UCLA and at Cedars-Sinai. Lee Miller, the coeditor of this book, is perhaps the most effective teacher I have known and has influenced my career immeasurably. I would not have discovered my love for teaching without his mentorship and encouragement. I am also grateful to friends and colleagues who are role model educators and clinicians, including Dr. Kate Perkins and Dr. Neal Kaufman.

Lloyd J. Brown

I will be forever grateful for the mentorship, teaching, encouragement, and friendship of Mrs. Sylvia Civin of New York City and of Dr. Leigh Grossman, Dr. Dick Kesler, and Dr. Frank Saulsbury of the University of Virginia School of Medicine.

Lee T. Miller

We would not have been able to undertake and complete this text without the professional encouragement, great mentorship, and wonderful support of Dr. David Rimoin, our Chair of the Department of Pediatrics at Cedars-Sinai Medical Center, and Professor of Pediatrics and Internal Medicine of the David Geffen School of Medicine at UCLA.

We would also like to thank our colleagues within the Division of Academic Primary Care Pediatrics at Cedars-Sinai Medical Center for their great support, and for being the wonderful colleagues and dear friends that they are to both of us.

We owe much gratitude as well to Lisa Payne and Lois Kuperman in the Department of Pediatrics at Cedars-Sinai Medical Center, whose technical support, friendship, hard work, warm spirits, and endless cups of coffee were so tremendously appreciated.

And lastly, we owe so much to our present and past pediatric and medicine-pediatric housestaff with whom we feel very close, and to the hundreds of medical students from all across the country, but most especially those from the David Geffen School of Medicine at UCLA, who have stimulated us, energized us, and taught us so much along the way.

Lloyd J. Brown
Lee T. Miller

Contributors

Lloyd J. Brown, MD, FAAP
Associate Director, Pediatric Residency
  Training Program
Cedars-Sinai Medical Center
Los Angeles, California
Course Chair, Pediatric Clerkship
Associate Professor of Pediatrics
David Geffen School of Medicine at UCLA
Los Angeles, California

Lee Todd Miller, MD, FAAP
Director, Pediatric Residency Training
  Program
Cedars-Sinai Medical Center
Los Angeles, California
Professor of Pediatrics
David Geffen School of Medicine at UCLA
Los Angeles, California

Tiffany Merrill Becker, MD
Division of Academic Primary Care
  Pediatrics
Cedars-Sinai Medical Center
Los Angeles, California

Peter A. Blasco, MD, FAAP
Director, Neurodevelopmental Program
Child Development and Rehabilitation
  Center
Portland, Oregon
Associate Professor of Pediatrics
Oregon Health and Science University
Portland, Oregon

David Seung Chun, MD
Fellow, Pediatric Cardiology
James Whitcomb Riley Hospital for
  Children
Indiana University School of Medicine
Indianapolis, Indiana

David A. Ferry, MD, FAAP, FACC
Director, Pediatric Cardiology
Cedars-Sinai Medical Center
Los Angeles, California
Clinical Associate Professor of Pediatrics
David Geffen School of Medicine at UCLA
Los Angeles, California

Carole Hurvitz, MD, FAAP
Director, Pediatric Hematology-Oncology
Cedars-Sinai Medical Center
Los Angeles, California
Professor of Pediatrics
David Geffen School of Medicine at UCLA
Los Angeles, California

Elaine S. Kamil, MD
Clinical Director, Pediatric Nephrology
Program Director, Pediatric Nephrology
  Fellowship Program
Cedars-Sinai Medical Center
Los Angeles, California
Professor of Pediatrics
David Geffen School of Medicine at UCLA
Los Angeles, California

Deborah Lehman, MD, FAAP
Associate Director, Pediatric Infectious
  Diseases
Cedars-Sinai Medical Center
Los Angeles, California
Assistant Professor of Pediatrics
David Geffen School of Medicine at UCLA
Los Angeles, California

Calvin G. Lowe, MD, FAAP
Medical Director, Children's Emergency
  Transport
Attending Physician
Division of Emergency and Transport
  Medicine
Childrens Hospital Los Angeles
Los Angeles, California
Assistant Professor of Pediatrics
Keck School of Medicine at the
  University of Southern California
Los Angeles, California

Elizabeth Mumper, MD, FAAP
President and CEO, Advocates for Children
Lynchburg, Virginia
Associate Professor of Clinical Pediatrics
University of Virginia School of Medicine
Charlottesville, Virginia

Ronald A. Nagel, MD, FAAP
Clinical Assistant Professor of Pediatrics
David Geffen School of Medicine at UCLA
Los Angeles, California

Charles E. Niesen, MD, FRCPC
Division of Pediatric Neurology
Cedars-Sinai Medical Center
Los Angeles, California
Assistant Professor of Pediatrics and
  Neurology
David Geffen School of Medicine at UCLA
Los Angeles, California

Kathy L. Perkins, MD, PhD, FAAP
Vice Chair, Pediatric Clinical Services
Cedars-Sinai Medical Center
Los Angeles, California
Associate Professor of Pediatrics
David Geffen School of Medicine at UCLA
Los Angeles, California

Robert K. Rhee, MD
Pediatric Ophthalmologist
Departments of Pediatrics and Surgery
Associate Professor of Ophthalmology
Medical College of Ohio
Toledo, Ohio

Marta R. Rogido, MD, FAAP
Division of Neonatal-Perinatal Medicine
Assistant Professor of Pediatrics
Emory University School of Medicine
Atlanta, Georgia

Annette B. Salinger, MD, FAAP
Palo Alto Medical Foundation
Palo Alto, California
Clinical Instructor
Stanford University School of Medicine
Stanford, California

Srinath Sanda, MD
Division of General Internal Medicine
Division of Academic Primary Care
  Pediatrics
Cedars-Sinai Medical Center
Los Angeles, California

Margaret Sanford, MD
Associate Pediatric Hematologist-
  Oncologist
Cedars-Sinai Medical Center
Los Angeles, California
Clinical Assistant Professor of Pediatrics
David Geffen School of Medicine at UCLA
Los Angeles, California

Harry W. Saperstein, MD
Director, Pediatric Dermatology
Cedars-Sinai Medical Center
Los Angeles, California
Clinical Associate Professor of Pediatrics
  and Medicine
David Geffen School of Medicine at UCLA
Los Angeles, California

Frank T. Saulsbury, MD
Head, Division of Immunology and
  Rheumatology
Department of Pediatrics
University of Virginia Health Systems
Charlottesville, Virginia
Professor of Pediatrics
University of Virginia School of Medicine
Charlottesville, Virginia

Nirali P. Singh, MD, FAAP
Fellow, Pediatric Infectious Diseases
Cedars-Sinai Medical Center
Los Angeles, California

Liliana Sloninsky, MD
Associate Pediatric Hematologist-
    Oncologist
Cedars-Sinai Medical Center
Los Angeles, California
Clinical Assistant Professor of Pediatrics
David Geffen School of Medicine at UCLA
Los Angeles, California

Augusto Sola, MD, FAAP
Director, Neonatal-Perinatal Medicine
Professor of Pediatrics and Obstetrics
    and Gynecology
Emory University School of Medicine
Atlanta, Georgia

Jerome K. Wang, MD, FAAP
Associate Director, Internal
    Medicine–Pediatrics Residency
    Training Program
Cedars-Sinai Medical Center
Los Angeles, California
Assistant Professor of Pediatrics
David Geffen School of Medicine at UCLA
Los Angeles, California

Frederick D. Watanabe, MD, FAAP
Pediatric Liver and Intestinal
    Transplantation
Childrens Hospital Los Angeles
Los Angeles, California
Associate Professor of Pediatrics
David Geffen School of Medicine at UCLA
Los Angeles, California

Lauren J. Witcoff, MD
Division of Pediatric Pulmonary Medicine
Lucile Packard Children's Hospital
Palo Alto, California
Clinical Associate Professor of Pediatrics
Stanford University School of Medicine
Stanford, California

Kenneth W. Wright, MD, FAAP
Director, Wright Foundation for
    Pediatric Ophthalmology
Director, Pediatric Ophthalmology
    Research and Education
Cedars-Sinai Medical Center
Los Angeles, California
Clinical Professor of Ophthalmology
Keck School of Medicine at the
    University of Southern California
Los Angeles, California

Sharon L. Young, MD
Associate Medical Director, Children's
    Health Clinic
Cedars-Sinai Medical Center
Los Angeles, California
Assistant Professor of Pediatrics
David Geffen School of Medicine at UCLA
Los Angeles, California

Table of Contents

Part 2 Specific Problems

Part 1

General Concepts

Part 1

General Concepts

1

Pediatric Health Supervision

Kathy L. Perkins, M.D., Ph.D.

I. Well Child Care—General Concepts

A. **The purpose of routine well child care** is to provide for the longitudinal health care needs of children from birth through adolescence. Components of well child care include:

1. **Anticipatory guidance** (e.g., diet, healthy lifestyle promotion)

2. Specific **preventive** measures (e.g., immunizations)

3. **Screening tests** to detect asymptomatic diseases (e.g., vision, hearing, newborn metabolic screening, tuberculosis screening)

4. **Early detection and treatment** of symptomatic acute illness to prevent complications

5. **Prevention** of disability in chronic disease

6. Assessment of **growth and development**

B. **Content of the well child visit**

1. **History** provides an opportunity to obtain diagnostic information and to form a doctor–patient–family alliance. The interview is shaped by family and patient concerns and by **age-specific trigger questions** about common problems (e.g., sleep, nutrition, behavior).

2. **Developmental surveillance** is gathered through age-specific questioning, developmental questionnaires, observations during the visit, screening tests, and review of academic school performance.

3. **Observation of parent–child interaction**

4. **Physical examination** should be comprehensive and also should focus on **growth** (i.e., length/height, weight, head circumference, and body mass index).

5. **Additional screening tests** depend on the age of the child and may include lead level, hemoglobin, and urinalysis screens and at 4 years of age, blood pressure and hearing and vision assessment.

6. **Immunizations**

7. **Anticipatory guidance** includes a discussion of safety issues, and upcoming developmental issues.

II. Growth

A. **Normal Growth**

1. **Weight, height, head circumference** (until 2 years of age), and **sexual maturity** are routinely monitored during well child care to assess for adequacy of growth and development.

2. **Standardized growth curves** represent normal values for age for 95% of children and are used to plot weight, height, body mass index, and head circumference. Special growth curves exist for children with particular genetic conditions (e.g., Down syndrome, achondroplasia).

3. **Tables 1-1, 1-2, and 1-3** detail general "rules of thumb" for expected gains in weight, height, and head circumference. **Sexual maturity rating scales are found in Chapter 3, Figures 3-1 and 3-3.**

B. **Growth disturbances** are defined as growth outside of the usual pattern. Two common types of growth disturbance include **failure to thrive** and **head growth abnormalities.**

1. **Failure to thrive (FTT)**

a. **Definition.** FTT is a term used to describe a growth rate of less than expected for a child, and is of particular concern when a child's weight crosses two major percentile isobars on National Health Statistics charts.

b. FTT may involve all growth parameters although weight gain is generally the most abnormal. This should be distinguished from isolated short stature, in which height is the most abnormal growth parameter (see Chapter 6, section I).

c. In children with FTT, weight is usually affected before length, which is usually affected before head circumference (head circumference is initially spared in FTT).

Table 1-1. Rules of Thumb for Expected Increase in Weight

Age	Expected Weight Increase
Birth–3 months	30 g/day Regain birth weight by 2 weeks
3–6 months	20 g/day Double birth weight by 4–6 months
6–12 months	10 g/day Triple birth weight by 12 months
1–2 years	250 g/month
2 years–adolescence	2.3 kg/year

30 g = 1 ounce body weight.

Table 1-2. Rules of Thumb for Expected Increase in Height

Age	Expected Height Increase
0–12 months	25 cm/year Birth length increases by 50% at 12 months
13–24 months	12.5 cm/year
2 years–adolescence	6.25 cm/year Birth length doubles by age 4 years Birth length triples by age 13 years

   d. Etiologies of FTT are outlined in Figures 1-1 and 1-2, which include both **inorganic or psychosocial causes** and **organic etiologies.**

   (1) The **most common cause of FTT** is **inorganic FTT** (i.e., a disturbed parent–child bond that results in inadequate caloric intake or retention).

   (2) Organic etiologies suggest underlying organ system pathology, infection, chromosomal disorders, or systemic illness.

   e. Evaluation of FTT requires a careful history and physical examination, a complete dietary history, and observation of the parent–child interaction.

   (1) Routine screening tests are usually not useful, and laboratory evaluation should therefore be focused and directed by clues from the history and physical examination.

   (2) Evaluation of potential organic etiologies will be directed by the timing or onset of FTT, i.e., prenatal onset of inadequate weight gain (as in intrauterine growth retardation) should be distinguished from postnatal onset of inadequate weight gain.

   2. Head growth abnormalities include microcephaly, craniosynostosis, deformational plagiocephaly, and macrocephaly.

   a. General concepts. Almost all head growth occurs prenatally and during the first 2 years of life.

   (1) Head circumference at birth is 25% of the normal adult head size, and it increases to 75% of the normal adult head size by 1 year of age.

   (2) Scalp edema or **cephalohematoma** (subperiosteal hemorrhage of the newborn cranium after a traumatic delivery) may interfere with accurate head circumference measurements.

Table 1-3. Rules of Thumb for Expected Increase in Head Circumference

Age	Expected Head Circumference Increase
0–2 months	0.5 cm/week
2–6 months	0.25 cm/week
By 12 months	Total increase = 12 cm since birth

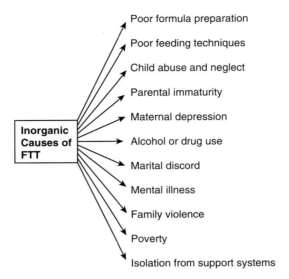

Figure 1-1. Causes of inorganic failure to thrive (FTT).

b. Microcephaly

    (1) Definition. Head circumference is 2–3 standard deviations below the mean for age.

    (2) Incidence is **1–2/1000** children.

    (3) Etiologies are classified as either **congenital** or **acquired** (**Table 1-4**).

        (a) Congenital microcephaly is associated with abnormal induction and migration of brain tissue.

        (b) Acquired microcephaly is caused by a cerebral insult in the late third trimester, perinatal period, or first year of life. Affected children are born with a normal head circumference that does not grow after the cerebral insult.

    (4) Clinical features

        (a) Because head size generally reflects brain size, **microcephaly is always associated with a small brain.**

        (b) Microcephaly is usually associated with **developmental delay** and **intellectual impairment.**

        (c) Microcephaly may be associated with **cerebral palsy** or **seizures.**

c. Craniosynostosis

    (1) Definition. Premature closure of one or more of the cranial sutures.

    (2) Etiology is often unknown. 80 to 90% of cases are **sporadic** and 10 to 20% are familial or a part of a genetic syndrome (e.g., Crouzon and Apert syndromes). Known etiologies or risk factors include intrauterine constraint or crowding and metabolic abnormalities, including hyperthyroidism and hypercalcemia.

    (3) Clinical features

        (a) Cranial sutures remain open until cessation of brain growth, which is **90% completed by age 2** and complete by age 5.

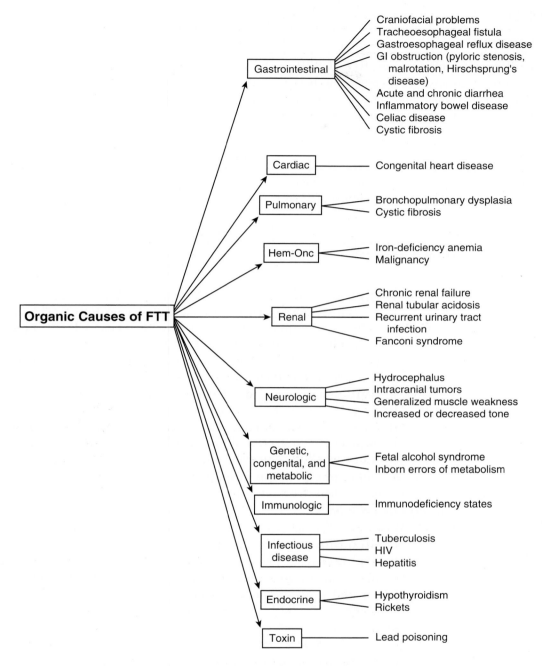

Figure 1-2. Organic causes of failure to thrive (FTT).

(b) Head shape in craniosynostosis is based on which suture closes prematurely.

    (i) Premature closure of the **sagittal suture** results in an **elongated skull** (termed **dolichocephaly or scaphocephaly**) and is the **most common form of craniosynostosis.**

Table 1-4. Causes of Microcephaly

Congenital

Early prenatal infection (e.g., HIV, TORCH)
Maternal exposure to drugs and toxins (e.g., fetal alcohol syndrome)
Chromosomal abnormality (e.g., trisomy 13, 18, or 21)
Familial microcephaly (autosomal dominant or autosomal recessive inheritance)
Maternal phenylketonuria

Acquired

Late third trimester or perinatal infections
Meningitis or meningoencephalitis during first year of life
Hypoxic or ischemic cerebral insult
Metabolic derangements (e.g., hypothyroidism, inborn errors of metabolism)

TORCH = toxoplasmosis, other (syphilis), rubella, cytomegalovirus, herpes simplex virus.

        (ii) Premature closure of the **coronal suture** results in a **shortened skull** (termed **brachycephaly**). This is more common in boys and may be associated with **neurologic complications** such as optic nerve atrophy.
        (iii) Premature closure of the metopic suture leads to a triangular-shaped head (termed **trigonocephaly**).
        (iv) Premature closure of multiple sutures is rare but is associated with severe neurologic compromise.
    (4) **Diagnosis** is made by physical examination of the head. Craniosynostosis is usually noted by 6 months of age. The diagnosis is confirmed by skull radiographs and head CT scan.
    (5) **Management** is **surgical repair,** most often indicated when cosmetic concerns are significant.
  d. **Plagiocephaly**
    (1) **Definition.** Asymmetry of the infant head shape usually **not associated** with premature suture closure.
    (2) **Clinical features.** The **most common type of plagiocephaly is positional plagiocephaly,** associated with flattening of the occiput and prominence of the ipsilateral frontal area. Viewed from the top, the skull is shaped like a parallelogram.
        (a) May be associated with **congenital muscular torticollis** (see Chapter 17, section II.A.1)
        (b) Incidence has increased as a result of current recommendations that infants sleep on their backs to prevent sudden infant death syndrome.
        (c) **Management** may include range of motion exercises for associated torticollis, repositioning the head during sleep, helmet therapy, and increased time in the prone position when awake ("tummy time").
  e. **Macrocephaly**
    (1) **Definition**. Head circumference > 95% for age.

(2) **Unlike microcephaly, the size of the head in patients with macrocephaly does not necessarily reflect brain size.**

(3) **Etiologies**

    (a) **Familial,** associated with an otherwise normal physical examination and a family history of large heads

    (b) **Overgrowth syndromes** (e.g., Sotos syndrome), in which all growth parameters are enlarged

    (c) **Metabolic storage disorders** (e.g., Canavan syndrome, gangliosidoses)

    (d) **Neurofibromatosis** (see Chapter 19, Table 19-3)

    (e) **Achondroplasia** (see Chapter 5, section III.D.2)

    (f) **Hydrocephalus** (see Chapter 12, section II)

    (g) Space-occupying lesions (e.g., cysts, tumors)

(4) **Evaluation** includes measurement of parental head circumferences and a careful physical examination that includes observation for split cranial sutures, bulging anterior fontanelle, irritability, or vomiting, all of which may suggest **elevated intracranial pressure.** Head ultrasound or CT scan is performed to rule out **hydrocephalus,** if suggested by physical examination. Genetic evaluation may be useful if a genetic syndrome is suspected.

III. Immunizations

A. Immunizations are one of the most important components of well child care and are the cornerstone of pediatric preventive care.

B. Types of Immunizations

1. **Active immunization** involves induction of long-term immunity through exposure to live attenuated or killed (inactivated) infectious agents.

    a. **Live vaccines** are more likely to induce long-lasting immunity, but carry the risk of vaccine-associated disease in the recipient or secondary host. As a result, live vaccines should generally be **avoided in patients with compromised immunity** (e.g., cancer, congenital or drug-induced immunodeficiencies). Examples of live vaccines include oral polio (OPV); varicella; and measles, mumps, and rubella (MMR) vaccines.

    b. **Non-live vaccines** are not infectious and tend to induce immunity for shorter periods, thus requiring booster immunizations. Examples include diphtheria, tetanus, and acellular pertussis (DTaP); hepatitis A and B; inactivated polio (IPV); *Haemophilus influenzae* type b (HIB); influenza; pneumococcal and meningococcal vaccines.

2. **Passive immunization** involves delivery of preformed antibodies to individuals who have no active immunity against a particular disease but who have either been exposed to or are at high risk for exposure to the infectious agent. Examples include:

    a. Varicella zoster immune globulin (VZIG) for immunocompromised patients who have been exposed to varicella and are at high risk for severe varicella infection.

b. Newborns born to hepatitis B–positive mothers receive hepatitis B immune globulin at birth.

c. Visitors to high-risk areas may receive hepatitis A immune globulin before travel.

C. Specific Immunizations

1. Hepatitis B vaccine (HBV)

a. Rationale for vaccine: hepatitis B infects 300 million worldwide.

b. Type of vaccine: HBV in the United States is a **recombinant vaccine** with particles of hepatitis B surface antigen (HBsAg).

c. Timing of vaccination: HBV is given as a three-shot series within the first year of life.

2. Diphtheria, tetanus, and acellular pertussis vaccine (DTaP)

a. Rationale for vaccine: Diphtheria, tetanus, and pertussis all may cause serious disease, especially in young infants.

b. Type of vaccine

    (1) Vaccine is inactivated.

    (2) **DTP,** which contained **whole-cell,** killed *Bordetella pertussis* and had a high rate of side effects, has now been replaced with **DTaP,** a vaccine that contains purified components (**acellular**) of *B. pertussis* and has lower rates of vaccine-associated fever, seizures, and local reactions.

c. Timing of vaccination

    (1) **DTaP** is recommended at 2, 4, and 6 months with boosters at 12–18 months and 4–6 years.

    (2) **dT** (diphtheria and tetanus combined) contains one tenth the dose of diphtheria toxoid and is recommended at age 11–12 and every 10 years thereafter. Note that dT rather than DTaP is given to children $\geq$ 7 years of age.

3. Oral and inactivated polio vaccines (OPV/IPV)

a. Rationale for vaccine: Poliovirus is an enterovirus with propensity for the central nervous system, causing transient or permanent paresis of the extremities and meningoencephalitis. Polio has been eradicated from the Western hemisphere and South Pacific but remains in isolated pockets throughout the world.

b. There are two types of vaccines.

    (1) **Live attenuated (OPV),** administered orally

        (a) **Advantages** include induction of both host immunity and secondary immunity because it is excreted in the stool of the recipient and may infect, and thus immunize, close contacts (i.e., herd immunity).

        (b) **Disadvantages** include the possibility of vaccine-related polio. In recent years, the only cases of polio in the United States have been associated with OPV.

    (2) **Non-live or inactivated (IPV),** administered subcutaneously or intramuscularly, has the advantage of no vaccine-related polio but the disadvantage of not inducing secondary immunity.

    c. Timing of vaccination: In the United States, **only IPV is now recommended** and is given at 2 and 4 months, with boosters at 6–18 months and at 4–6 years.

4. *Haemophilus influenzae* **type b vaccine (HIB)**

    a. Rationale for vaccine: *H. influenzae* type b was a serious cause of invasive bacterial infection, including meningitis, epiglottitis, and sepsis, before vaccine licensure in 1985. Since licensure it has become a rare cause of such infections.

    b. Type of vaccine: HIB is a **conjugate vaccine** with *H. influenzae* polysaccharide linked to various protein antigens, including diphtheria or tetanus toxoids, to augment immunogenicity.

    c. Timing of vaccination: HIB is recommended either at 2, 4, and 6 months with a booster at 12–15 months or at 2, 4, and 12 months, depending on the type of vaccine conjugate.

5. Measles, mumps, and rubella vaccine (MMR)

    a. Rationale for vaccine: immunizes against three viral diseases:

        (1) Measles is a severe illness with complications that include pneumonia associated with significant mortality.

        (2) Mumps is most commonly associated with parotitis but may also cause meningoencephalitis and orchitis.

        (3) Rubella causes a mild viral syndrome in children but may cause severe birth defects in offspring of susceptible women infected during pregnancy.

    b. Type of vaccine: **live attenuated vaccine**

    c. Timing of vaccination: MMR is recommended at 12–15 months with a booster at either 4–6 years or 11–12 years of age.

6. Varicella vaccine

    a. Rationale for vaccine: Varicella is the virus responsible for chicken pox and zoster. Varicella often causes uncomplicated illness but may cause severe disease in very young and in older patients.

    b. Type of vaccine: **live attenuated vaccine**

    c. Timing of vaccination: Vaccine is recommended at 12–18 months.

7. Hepatitis A vaccine (Hep A)

    a. Rationale for vaccine: **Hepatitis A is the most common viral cause of hepatitis worldwide,** although it is asymptomatic in up to 70% of infected children younger than 6 years of age. More severe disease is seen in older children and adults, although it is rarely associated with fulminant hepatitis.

    b. Type of vaccine: **inactivated**

    c. Timing of vaccination and recommendations: Hep A vaccine is recommended at 2 years of age or older, with a booster 6 months later for the following groups:

        (1) Susceptible children living in communities with high hepatitis A rates (i.e., incidence twice the national rate) and those traveling to endemic areas.

        (2) Individuals in other groups with high hepatitis A rates, including those with chronic liver disease, homosexual and bisexual men, users of illicit drugs, patients with clotting factor disorders receiving blood products, and patients at high risk for occupational exposure.

8. **Pneumococcal vaccines (Pneumovax and Prevnar)**
   a. Rationale for vaccine: Pneumococcus (*Streptococcus pneumoniae*) is the **most common** cause of acute otitis media and invasive bacterial infections in children younger than 3 years of age.
   b. There are two types of vaccines.
      (1) **Pneumovax** is composed of polysaccharide capsular antigens from 23 pneumococcal serotypes.
         (a) **Major advantage** is that the vaccine contains antigens from pneumococcal strains causing **almost all** cases of bacteremia and meningitis during childhood.
         (b) **Major disadvantage** is that the vaccine has **little immunogenicity** in children younger than 2 years.
         (c) **Indications.** Vaccine is used primarily for older children and adults at high risk for pneumococcal disease (e.g., patients with sickle cell anemia who are functionally asplenic, immunodeficiency, chronic liver disease and nephrotic syndrome, and patients with anatomic asplenia).
      (2) **Prevnar** is composed of seven pneumococcal serotypes.
         (a) **Major advantages** include **immunogenicity and efficacy** in preventing meningitis, pneumonia, bacteremia, and otitis media from the most common pneumococcal strains in children **younger than 2 years of age.**
         (b) **Major disadvantage** is that it does not confer as broad coverage against pneumococcal strains as Pneumovax.
         (c) **Indication.** Vaccine is recommended for all children younger than 2 years of age and for selected children older than 2 years of age who are at high risk for pneumococcal disease. Prevnar is recommended at 2, 4, and 6 months with a booster at 12–15 months.

D. **Adverse Effects of Immunization**
   1. Most vaccine side effects are mild to moderate in severity and occur within the first 24 hours after administration (e.g., local inflammation and low-grade fever).
   2. Because **MMR** and **varicella** vaccines are live attenuated vaccines, fever and rash may occur **1–2 weeks after immunization** (i.e., after the incubation period of the virus).
   3. Serious side effects that may result in permanent disability or be life-threatening are rare (e.g., vaccine-related polio after OPV).

E. **Contraindications and precautions to immunization**
   1. **Contraindications** to immunization include:
      a. **Anaphylaxis** to a vaccine or its constituents
      b. **Encephalopathy** within 7 days after **DTaP** vaccine

    c. Patients with progressive neurologic disorders, including uncontrolled epilepsy, should not receive the DTaP vaccine until neurologic status is stabilized.

    d. Immunodeficient patients should not receive OPV, MMR, and varicella vaccines. Household contacts of immunodeficient patients should not receive OPV vaccine as it is shed in the stool.

    e. Pregnant patients should not receive live vaccines.

2. Precautions (i.e., caution should be exercised) to immunization include:

    a. For all vaccines, **moderate to severe illness** (with or without fever). Note that mild illnesses, including febrile illnesses, are **not** contraindications to immunization.

    b. DTaP vaccine
        (1) Temperature of 40.5°C within 48 hours after prior vaccination
        (2) Collapse or shocklike state within 48 hours after prior vaccination
        (3) Seizures within 3 days after prior vaccination
        (4) Persistent, inconsolable crying lasting $\geq$ 3 hours occurring within 48 hours after prior vaccination

    c. MMR and varicella vaccines: Immunoglobulin (IVIG) administration within the preceding 3–11 months, which might interfere with the patient's immune response to these vaccines.

IV. Well Child Screening

A. The focus of each well child visit is to identify undetected problems and to identify the risks of such problems.

B. Screening assessments include a complete history and physical examination, **growth measurements,** blood pressure measurements, strabismus and vision screening, hearing screening, tuberculosis screening, and laboratory screening.

C. Vision screening for ophthalmologic disorders begins after birth and is detailed in Chapter 18.

D. Hearing Screening

1. Until recently, healthy children without risk factors had formal audiometric testing beginning at 4–5 years of age, as most types of screening require the patient's participation. However, **universal newborn hearing screening,** preferably before hospital discharge, is now recommended because of evidence that moderate-to-profound hearing loss in early infancy is associated with **impaired language development.** Early detection and intervention for hearing loss may improve speech and language acquisition.

2. Two types of audiometric tests are used.

    a. Brainstem auditory evoked response (BAER) measures electroencephalographic (EEG) waves generated in response to clicks via electrodes pasted to the infant's scalp. BAER is the **most accurate test**, but it requires costly equipment and trained operators.

    b. Evoked otoacoustic emission (EOE) measures sounds generated by normal cochlear hair cells that are detected by a microphone placed into the external auditory canal. EOE accuracy may be affected by debris or fluid within the external or middle ear. It requires less expensive equipment and less operator training.

    3. The **most effective screening** is thought to be use of both of the above tests in combination.

E. Neonatal Metabolic (State) Screening

    1. Many metabolic diseases can be diagnosed and treated in the newborn period.

    2. Although there is variability from state to state in which conditions are screened, **all states** screen for **congenital hypothyroidism** and **phenylketonuria (PKU),** and the majority of states also screen for **galactosemia.** Each of these conditions is treatable and, if not detected early, each leads to irreversible brain injury.

    3. The majority of states screen for **sickle cell anemia** and other hemoglobinopathies because early intervention in a comprehensive treatment program (e.g., penicillin prophylaxis) significantly decreases morbidity and mortality.

    4. Newborn screening tests for additional metabolic disorders (e.g., congenital adrenal hyperplasia) are in use in some states.

F. Cholesterol and Lipid Screening

    1. **Routine screening** of cholesterol and lipid panels is **not recommended** because of the lack of information about the risks and benefits of treating hyperlipidemia during childhood and because of the costs and limitations of currently available screening tests.

    2. Screening **is recommended** for children > age 2 with a **family history of hypercholesterolemia, hyperlipidemia, or early myocardial infarction** as follows:

        a. Screening cholesterol if either parent has a history of hypercholesterolemia

        b. Screening fasting lipid panel if either parents or grandparents have a history of cardiovascular disease or sudden death at ≤ 55 years of age

    3. Children with **elevated cholesterol** levels (75th–90th percentile) should have a **fasting lipid panel** that includes total cholesterol, triglycerides, high-density lipoprotein (HDL), and low-density lipoprotein (LDL).

G. Iron-Deficiency Anemia Screening

    1. Iron-deficiency anemia occurs most commonly in children < 6 years of age, peaking between 9 and 15 months of age.

    2. **Risk factors** for iron-deficiency anemia include:

        a. Prematurity

        b. Low birth weight

        c. Early introduction of cow's milk (before 9 months of age)

        d. Insufficient dietary intake of iron

        e. Low socioeconomic status

3. **Universal screening** of hemoglobin levels is recommended between 9 and 15 months of age and between 4 and 6 years of age.

H. **Urinalysis screening** has been recommended by some physicians, although there is little evidence that routine surveillance of urinalysis or routine urine cultures are efficacious or cost effective. Urine studies are recommended only when clinically warranted or when required for school entry or by local health departments.

I. **Tuberculosis Screening**

1. Tuberculin skin testing with intradermal injection of purified protein derivative (PPD, Mantoux skin test) is recommended for children at risk for tuberculosis, including:

   a. **Contacts** of persons with **confirmed or suspected infectious tuberculosis**

   b. Children in contact with **high-risk groups,** including adults incarcerated or institutionalized during the preceding 5 years, HIV-infected household members, homeless persons, users of illicit drugs, and migrant farm workers

   c. Children with **radiographic or clinical findings suggestive of tuberculosis**

   d. Children who have immigrated from endemic areas, those with a history of travel to endemic areas, or those with significant contact with indigenous persons from endemic areas (e.g., Asia, Africa, Middle East, Latin America)

   e. Children with HIV

   f. Children without specific risk factors who reside in high prevalence areas

2. **Skin tests** are analyzed at **48–72 hours** after placement and are interpreted on the basis of the level of risk for tuberculosis in the particular child (see also Chapter 7, section XVII.C.6).

J. **Lead Screening**

1. **Lead intoxication (plumbism)** is a public health risk among children < age 5. Up to 4% of all children in the United States have evidence of increased lead absorption, including up to 20% of inner city children.

2. **Risk factors** for lead intoxication include:

   a. **Ingestion of lead-containing paint** or putty from homes built before 1978

   b. Drinking water from **lead pipes** or pipes with lead-containing solder

   c. Exposure to lead smelters or lead-painted commercial structures during demolition

   d. Use of **lead-glazed pottery** in food preparation

   e. Use of **lead-containing folk remedies**

3. **Clinical features** of lead intoxication

   a. **Children < age 6 are most susceptible to the effects of lead.**

   b. **Acute lead intoxication** may lead to the acute onset of anorexia, apathy, lethargy, anemia, irritability, and vomiting. These symptoms may progress to encephalopathy (see also Chapter 20, section VIII.D.4).

    c. Chronic lead intoxication is most commonly **asymptomatic;** however, even patients with very low levels of lead may suffer **neurologic sequelae,** including **developmental delay, learning problems, and mental retardation.**

4. Because lead intoxication may be asymptomatic, **lead screening** is recommended for the following groups:

    a. All children 9 months–6 years of age living in older, dilapidated housing.

    b. All children 9 months–6 years of age who are siblings, visitors, or playmates of children with lead intoxication.

    c. All children 9 months–6 years of age living near lead smelters or lead-processing plants or whose parents or family members have a lead-related occupation or hobby.

    d. Children of any age living in older housing where renovation is occurring.

    e. All children of any age living in areas in which the percentage of 1- to 2-year-olds with elevated lead levels exceeds 12%.

5. Although no threshold for the toxic effects of lead has been identified, even blood lead levels ≤ 10 µg/dL have been associated with effects on cognition in young children.

6. **Management** of lead poisoning is based on serum lead levels after repeat testing and generally includes education to decrease exposure and chelation for very high lead levels.

V. Circumcision

A. Approximately 60% of male infants in the United States are circumcised.

B. Medical benefits of circumcision are **controversial.**

1. Although there is a slightly increased incidence of **penile cancer** in uncircumcised adult men (possibly associated with human papilloma virus) and a possible increased incidence of **cervical cancer** in the female sexual partners of uncircumcised men, these associations may be influenced by other factors.

2. Circumcision for medical reasons is **not** recommended by the American Academy of Pediatrics.

3. **Urinary tract infections** (UTIs) are 10 times more common in uncircumcised male infants. However, there is insufficient evidence that circumcision decreases the risk of UTIs in male infants.

4. **Ten percent** of uncircumcised males ultimately require circumcision for any of the following conditions:

    a. Phimosis is an inability to retract the foreskin. Phimosis is normal up to age 6 but is always abnormal if ballooning of the foreskin occurs during urination.

    b. Paraphimosis occurs when the retracted foreskin cannot be returned to its normal position and acts as a tourniquet, resulting in obstruction to lymphatic flow and edema. Surgery is required emergently should venous return also become obstructed.

      c. **Balanitis** is inflammation of the glans of the penis. It may be associated with *Candida* spp. or Gram-negative infections in infants and with sexually transmitted infections in adults.

  C. Anesthesia and analgesia are strongly recommended during circumcision.

  D. Complications from circumcision include bleeding, infection, poor cosmesis, phimosis (secondary to insufficient foreskin removal), urinary retention, and injury to the glans or urethra. Repeat circumcision is needed in 10%.

  E. Contraindications to circumcision include **penile abnormalities** (e.g., hypospadias), prematurity, and bleeding diatheses.

VI. Pediatric Dental Care

  A. Counseling about dental care issues is an important component of anticipatory guidance.

  B. Tooth Eruption
    1. **Range for initial tooth eruption is between 3 and 16 months, with an average of 6 months.**
    2. The first tooth is generally a **lower central incisor.**
    3. **Primary teeth** (20 teeth in total) are generally established by 2 years of age.
    4. **Secondary tooth eruption** also begins with the lower central incisor between 6 and 8 years of age. There are 32 secondary or permanent teeth.
    5. **Tooth eruption may be delayed or early.**
      a. **Delayed dental eruption** is defined as primary eruption occuring **after 16 months of age.** Causes include **familial, hypothyroidism,** hypopituitarism, and genetic syndromes such as **Down syndrome** and **ectodermal dysplasia** (associated with conical-shaped teeth, dysmorphic facial features, decreased numbers of sweat glands, and alopecia).
      b. **Early dental eruption** is defined as primary eruption **before 3 months of age.** Causes include **familial, hyperthyroidism,** precocious puberty, and growth hormone excess.

  C. Dental Hygiene
    1. **Tooth brushing** should begin **as soon as teeth erupt.** A moist washcloth or gauze pad may be used initially, and a soft toothbrush may be used as early as tolerated. Once children are 2–3 years of age, they are often able to assist in brushing their own teeth. A fluoride toothpaste may be used at this time.
    2. **Dental floss** to remove plaque from between teeth should be initiated when tight contact exists between teeth.
    3. **Fluoride**
      a. Children who consume optimal amounts of fluoride from birth until adolescence have 50–75% less dental decay than expected.

    b. Sources of fluoride include fluoridated water, fluoride supplements, and fluoride toothpaste. Note that water is not fluoridated at a uniform level in the United States.

    c. Excess fluoride can lead to **fluorosis.**

        (1) Fluorosis affects permanent teeth and leads to abnormalities in dental enamel and dentin.

        (2) Effects are cosmetic only and include white streaks, pitting, or brown-gray staining.

        (3) The most **critical time for dental vulnerability to excess fluoride is between 2 and 4 years of age.**

    d. Although care must be taken to prevent fluorosis, fluoride supplementation remains important for the following children:

        (1) Exclusively breastfed children older than 6 months, as breast milk contains little fluoride.

        (2) Children who live in areas where tap water contains < 0.3 ppm fluoride.

D. Dental Abnormalities

    1. Neonatal and natal teeth. Occasionally infants are born with teeth or have teeth that erupt within the first month of life.

    a. Definitions

        (1) Natal teeth are those that are present at birth.

        (2) Neonatal teeth are those that emerge during the first month of life.

    b. Teeth most commonly present early are **mandibular central incisors.** More than 90% are primary teeth that erupt early and < 10% are supernumerary teeth (teeth in excess of usual number).

    c. Etiology is often unknown but may be caused by exposure to environmental toxins or may be familial.

    d. Management. No intervention is needed unless the teeth are **hypermobile,** cause breastfeeding difficulty, or cause trauma to the infant's lip or tongue. Aspiration of a natal or neonatal tooth is feared but is very unlikely.

    2. Nursing or bottle caries

    a. Epidemiology. Occurs in 3–6% of children and is most often seen in the child at 24–30 months of age

    b. Etiology

        (1) Most frequently associated with a history of **falling asleep with a nipple** (breast or bottle) **in the mouth** or in children who breastfeed excessively or who carry around a bottle as a habit.

        (2) Any liquid, other than water, that is retained around the teeth may serve as a substrate for bacteria capable of causing caries (including human and cow's milk).

        (3) *Streptococcus mutans* is the **most common bacterial agent.** It does not appear in the oral cavity until teeth erupt, and children acquire this bacteria from colonized parents or siblings.

    c. Clinical features. Caries involve the **maxillary incisors, canines,**

and primary first molars. The lower teeth are spared initially because they are covered by the tongue.

  d. **Management** may include placement of dental crowns or extraction.

E. **Dental Trauma**

  1. **A permanent tooth** that has been traumatically avulsed **may be re-implanted** if the avulsed tooth is placed into the socket rapidly.

  a. **Extraoral time** is the **most important factor** affecting the prognosis for successfully re-implanting a tooth.

  b. **Prognosis is highest if the avulsed tooth is stored in liquids,** especially milk.

  c. A **dry-stored tooth** has a poor prognosis for re-implantation, even after only 30 minutes.

  2. **Management** includes gentle rinsing of an avulsed tooth with saline, placement into the socket, and referral to a dentist.

  3. Avulsed primary teeth do not require re-implantation.

VII. Developmental Screening.

One of the most important preventive measures of well child care is assessment of developmental milestones. Development is therefore assessed at each well child visit from infancy through school age. School performance substitutes for formal developmental assessment in developmentally normal children older than 5–6 years of age. Development is discussed in depth in Chapter 2.

VIII. Anticipatory Guidance

A. **Anticipatory guidance** is **patient and parent education** and is provided during each well child visit. It is tailored to the child's current developmental level and to anticipated changes in the child's development in the interim before the next scheduled well child visit.

B. **Topics covered by anticipatory guidance include:**

  1. **Health habits,** including counseling about tobacco, drugs, and alcohol

  2. **Prevention of illness and injury** (e.g., safety counseling)

  3. **Nutrition**

  4. **Dental care**

  5. **Social development and family relationships**

  6. **Sexuality**

  7. **Parental health**

  8. **Self responsibility**

  9. **School and vocational achievement**

C. **Age-appropriate anticipatory guidance** topics for children from birth to 5 years of age are detailed in **Table 1-5.**

Table 1-5. Age-Appropriate Anticipatory Guidance Topics for Discussion for Children from Birth to Age 5

Age	Healthy Habits	Injury and Illness Prevention	Nutrition	Parent–Child Interaction
Newborn	Cord care Circumcision care Skin and nail care Normal vaginal discharge and bleeding Normal sneezing and hiccups Stools change from meconium to transitional Amount of clothing needed, temperature regulation	Rear-facing car seat until 1 year and 20 lb Sleep on back Hot water heater < 120° F Never leave alone Early signs of illness: fever, failure to eat, vomiting, diarrhea, dehydration, irritability or lethargy, jaundice, rash Use of thermometer	Breastfeeding Feeding schedule for breast or formula on demand (8–12 times/day) for 4–6 weeks If no sunlight exposure, supplement with vitamin D during the first year of life to prevent rickets Instruct regarding preparation of formula with iron	Approach to crying Burping and spitting up Thumb sucking and pacifiers Normal sleep patterns, sleeping arangements Never shake a baby Screen for maternal depression
1 month	Sleeping 18–20 hours/day, 3–4 hours at a stretch Stooling decreasing in frequency and changes to brown and more formed Some infants strain with stool	Same as newborn	Same as newborn No cereal No solids No honey until age 1 Relief bottle for breast-feeding moms	Colic may begin at 3–4 weeks
2 months	Sleep 4–8 hours at a stretch Feed every 3–4 hours Stooling qod to 3–4 times/day	Risk of aspiration of small objects	Same as 1 month old	Establish bedtime routine Encourage vocalizations Most working mothers return to work by 4 months
4 months	Feeding every 4–5 hours Sleeping 6–8 hours at a stretch	Aspiration risk No infant walkers	Milk continues to be primary source of nutrition through 1 year of age Iron-fortified infant cereal and solids introduced	Encourage vocalizations—talking, singing, and reading to infant Introduce transitional object (e.g., toy, stuffed animal, blanket)

Age	Feeding/Sleep	Safety	Nutrition	Anticipatory Guidance
6 months	Feedings spaced out Sleeping through night for many	Baby-proof home Pool and water safety Weapons and pet safety Child gates on stairs Aspiration risk Sunscreen use No infant walker	More solids introduced Continue breast or bottle feeds plus solids Avoid foods with aspiration risk or choking risk (e.g., peanuts, popcorn, hot dogs, carrots, celery sticks, whole grapes, raisins, corn) Avoid egg whites, fish, citrus, chocolate, nuts, wheat until 1 year	Provide opportunities for exploration Establish nighttime routine, transitional object To discipline, use distraction and routines Discuss separation anxiety Encourage reading
9 months	Drinks from cup Eats appropriate finger foods	Same as 6 months	Same as 6 months	Observe increasing independence and autonomy Anticipate separation anxiety and sleep disturbances
12 months	Feeding 3 times/day plus 2–3 snacks Establish sleep hygiene—transitional objects, bedtime routine, sleeping through night Begin weaning from bottle	Child-proof house Switch to toddler car seat and face front	Switch to whole milk Drink from cup Table food—watch aspiration risk Weight gain slows down, intake decreases	Praise good behavior Encourage language development—read to toddler Encourage exploration and initiative Discipline with distraction, gentle restraint, "time out" Limit TV to 1 hour/day
15 months	Feeds self Naps 1–2 times/day	Same as 12 months	Same as 12 months	Begin discussion of toilet training readiness; do not push; be patient
18 months	Feeds self May begin toilet training Naps 1–2 times/day	Same as 12 months	Avoid cookies and sweets as bribe to eat Whole milk < 24 oz/day	View negativism as budding independence Encourage language development by reading, singing, talking Make discipline brief and specific Anticipate night terrors, nightmares, night fears Don't expect toddler to share

(continues)

Table 1.5. Age-Appropriate Anticipatory Guidance Topics for Discussion for Children from Birth to Age 5 (*continued*)

Age	Healthy Habits	Injury and Illness Prevention	Nutrition	Parent–Child Interaction
2 years	Change to bed from crib Initiate toilet training if not prior	Same as above	Food struggles are common Change to 2% milk Never force child to eat Offer nutritious foods	Anticipate new fears, indecision—provide reassurance Anticipate parallel play, sibling rivalry if new baby expected Acknowledge conflict but don't allow behavior; biting and hitting are common
3 years	90% bowel trained 85% bladder (day) 65% bladder (night)	Bicycle helmets Street safety Stranger danger Firearm safety Tricycle safety Pet and water safety	Continue healthy food choices	Use correct terms for genitalia Introduce notion that some areas of the body are private Anticipate preschool Observe beginning of sharing during play
4 years	95% bowel trained 90% bladder (day) 75% bladder (night)	Child booster seat (4 years and 40 lb) Swimming lessons Scissor and pencil use Firearm safety Bicycle helmets	Continue healthy food choices Anticipate imitating peers in eating choices	Provide opportunities for socialization with other children Establish and enforce consistent, explicit rules for safe behavior Observe beginning of imaginative play Observe discovery of sexual identity
5 years	Sleeps 10–12 hours/night Teach personal care and hygiene	Bicycle helmets Stranger danger Firearm safety Phone number memorized Booster seat	Continue healthy food choices, including school lunch	Library cards, learning to read Rules for bedtime, TV watching Age-appropriate chores School participation encouraged

Review Test

1. A 6-month-old girl has been noted to fall off her growth curve and now is < 5% for her age. You suspect failure to thrive (FTT) and consider the most common causes. Which one of the following is the most common cause of FTT?

(A) A disturbed parent–child bond that results in inadequate caloric intake or retention
(B) Prenatal onset of inadequate weight gain that persists in the postnatal period
(C) A skeletal abnormality resulting in short stature with associated poor weight gain
(D) Malabsorption, or the inability to completely absorb ingested calories and nutrients
(E) Endocrinologic abnormalities, such as growth hormone deficiency or hypothyroidism

2. A 2-month-old male infant is seen for routine well child evaluation. At birth, his head circumference was < 5% for age. His head circumference has increased 1 cm in size since birth. Which one of the following is the most likely cause of the infant's condition?

(A) Intraventricular hemorrhage
(B) Perinatal asphyxia
(C) Third trimester infection with cytomegalovirus
(D) Craniosynostosis
(E) First trimester infection with Toxoplasmosis

3. A 4-week-old boy is evaluated for macrocephaly. In addition to a head circumference > 95%, his coronal and sagittal sutures are split 1 cm and his fontanelle is bulging. Both of his parents' head circumferences are > 95%. Which one of the following is the most likely explanation for the infant's macrocephaly?

(A) Familial
(B) Achondroplasia
(C) Hydrocephalus
(D) Metabolic storage disorder
(E) Neurofibromatosis

4. A 9-month-old girl is diagnosed with iron-deficiency anemia. Her past medical history includes an uncomplicated delivery at 38 weeks. The infant was fed with formula until 6 months, at which time she was switched to baby foods and whole milk. Which one of the following is correct regarding her iron-deficiency anemia?

(A) Her age is atypical for the presentation of iron-deficiency anemia.
(B) Her early birth at 38 weeks gestation has led to the anemia.
(C) Early introduction of cow's milk is the likely cause of her anemia.
(D) Insufficient dietary intake of iron is the likely cause of her anemia.
(E) The patient's early introduction of solids is the likely cause of her anemia.

5. An asymptomatic 12-month-old girl is screened for lead exposure. Which one of the following is correct regarding lead screening and lead intoxication?

(A) Most patients exposed to lead are asymptomatic.
(B) Children between 5 and 10 years of age are at highest risk for lead effects.
(C) Low lead levels on screening indicate that a child is at no risk for the neurologic sequelae of lead exposure.
(D) Chelation has not been shown to be effective for patients with high lead levels.
(E) Ingestion of paint from a home built in 1990 would place a child at risk for lead poisoning.

6. At a prenatal visit, the expectant parents of a first-born male child ask you to summarize the benefits, risks, and contraindications to performing a circumcision on their son. Which one of the following statements is correct?

(A) Circumcision has been demonstrated definitively to decrease the risk of urinary tract infection.
(B) Because of the young age at which circumcision is performed, analgesia is generally not required, thus decreasing the risks of the procedure when performed in the newborn period.
(C) If their child is not circumcised in the newborn period, he may require circumcision at 9 months of age if he is subsequently diagnosed with phimosis.
(D) The American Academy of Pediatrics recommends routine circumcision for medical benefit.
(E) Hypospadias is a contraindication to circumcision.

7. A 20-month-old boy is seen for routine well child care. Physical examination reveals caries involving the maxillary incisors. Which one of the following is most likely to have contributed to this condition?

(A) The use of both fluoride drops and fluoride toothpaste simultaneously, which has caused fluorosis
(B) Falling asleep with a water-filled bottle in the mouth
(C) Falling asleep while breastfeeding
(D) Oral colonization with *Staphylococcus aureus*
(E) Living in an area in which tap water contains < .2 ppm fluoride

8. A 1-year-old child living in an apartment with old chipping paint is suspected of being at high risk for lead intoxication. Which of the following findings on a routine health maintenance visit would support this diagnosis?

(A) Failure to thrive
(B) Anemia
(C) Fluorosis
(D) Microcephaly
(E) Impaired hearing

9. On a routine health maintenance visit, a 9-month-old infant is noted to have normal growth and development, and an unremarkable physical examination. Which of the following should be included in your counseling of the parents at this time?

(A) Vitamin D supplementation should be initiated if the patient has minimal exposure to sunlight.
(B) The patient should be encouraged to begin using a walker to stimulate gross motor development.
(C) The infant should now be placed in a forward-facing car seat.
(D) Toilet training should be initiated.
(E) Eggs and fish may now be introduced into the infant's diet.

10. You receive a telephone call from the parents of a 10-month-old infant, who are concerned that their baby does not yet have any teeth. A review of the infant's growth chart reveals that the patient's weight, length, and head circumference are at the 50th, 25th, and 25th percentiles, respectively. The infant's developmental milestones are normal. Which of the following would be the most appropriate course of action?

(A) Refer the patient to a pediatric dentist.
(B) Refer the patient to a geneticist.
(C) Reassure the parents that their infant's pattern of dental eruption is within the normal range.
(D) Order radiographs to assess the patient's bone age.
(E) Order radiographs of the patient's oral cavity.

The response options for statements 11–13 are the same. You will be required to select one answer for each statement in the set.

(A) Immunization with a non-live vaccine is indicated.
(B) Immunization with a live vaccine is indicated.
(C) Immunization is indicated, and both live and non-live vaccine options are available.
(D) Passive immunization is indicated.
(E) No immunization is indicated at this time.

For each patient, select the appropriate type of immunization indicated at this time, if any.

11. A 2-year-old child living in a region of the country at high risk for hepatitis A exposure presents for a routine health maintenance visit. His immunizations are up-to-date through 18 months of age.

12. A 5-year-old child with otherwise up-to-date immunization status presents with no known history of chicken pox exposure and no record of having received the varicella vaccine.

13. An HIV-positive patient presents 24 hours after being exposed to varicella, with no prior history of chicken pox, nor any record of having received the varicella vaccine.

14. The diagnosis of plagiocephaly is made at a 4-month routine health maintenance visit. Parents report the child has a preference for looking to the right side. Which of the following would be the most appropriate course of action at this time?

(A) Obtain a head ultrasound if the patient's anterior fontanelle is still open, or a head CT scan if the anterior fontanelle is closed.

(B) Obtain skull radiographs to better delineate which cranial sutures may have fused prematurely.

(C) Reassure the parents that this is a normal variant that will resolve spontaneously during the subsequent 6–8 months.

(D) Reassure the parents that this is likely positional plagiocephaly, and recommend stretching exercises, repositioning the head during sleep, and increased time in the prone position when awake.

(E) Counsel the parents that this condition may be associated with a genetic syndrome and refer the patient for a consultation with a geneticist.

Answers and Explanations

1. The answer is A [II.B.1]. The most common etiology of failure to thrive (FTT) is inorganic FTT, in which there is a problem with the parent–child bond that interferes with either food intake or retention. Underlying biomedical causes of FTT, including malabsorption, endocrinologic abnormalities, and intrauterine growth retardation are much less common causes of FTT. Short stature should be distinguished from FTT. Those with FTT have primary failure of weight gain (and subsequent poor linear growth and poor head circumference growth), whereas those with short stature have primary failure of linear growth.

2. The answer is E [Table 1.4; II.B.2.b]. Given his small head circumference at birth, this patient's microcephaly is congenital. Causes of congenital microcephaly include TORCH (**t**oxoplasmosis, **o**ther-syphilis, **r**ubella, **c**ytomegalovirus, **h**erpes simplex virus) infections during the first trimester, in utero exposure to drugs and toxins, and chromosomal abnormalities. In addition, congenital microcephaly may be familial. Perinatal asphyxia, intraventricular hemorrhage, craniosynostosis, and late prenatal and perinatal infections may all cause acquired microcephaly. Patients with acquired microcephaly are born with a normal head circumference.

3. The answer is C [II.B.2.e]. This patient has signs of increased intracranial pressure, which includes split sutures and a bulging fontanelle. Other symptoms of intracranial pressure include irritability and vomiting. Hydrocephalus is the only option that is associated with increased intracranial pressure. Metabolic storage disorders, neurofibromatosis, achondroplasia, and familial macrocephaly are associated with enlarged head circumference but are not associated with increased intracranial pressure in a patient of this age.

4. The answer is C [IV.G]. The introduction of cow's milk should occur only after 9 months of age, as its early introduction (in this case at 6 months) is a known risk factor for iron-deficiency anemia and is the likely cause in this case. This is because whole cow's milk offers less bioavailable iron and may also result in stool blood loss. Although insufficient dietary intake of iron is a possible cause, this patient received iron-fortified formula for at least 6 months, making this cause less likely. Prematurity (defined as < 37 weeks) may result in lower iron stores with resultant anemia. Iron-deficiency anemia classically peaks between 9 and 15 months of age. Finally, solids were introduced at an appropriate time in this patient (6 months) and are not a risk factor for anemia.

5. The answer is A [IV.J]. The majority of patients with elevated lead levels are asymptomatic. Children younger than 6 years of age are at highest risk for the effects of lead, and risk factors for intoxication include ingestion of lead-containing paint from homes built before 1978, drinking water from lead pipes, use of lead-glazed pottery in food preparation, and use of lead-containing folk remedies. Even patients with very low lead levels may suffer from developmental delay and learning problems. Chelation is sometimes required and is effective for very high lead levels.

6. The answer is E [V.B, C, D, and E]. Contraindications to circumcision include hypospadias, bleeding diathesis, and prematurity. Although phimosis is an indication for circumcision in some patients, it is considered normal up until 6 years of age. Other indications for circumcision include balanitis and paraphimosis; however, the American Academy of Pediatrics does not recommend routine circumcision for medical benefit. Circumcision has also not been conclusively demonstrated to decrease the incidence of urinary tract infections. No matter the patient's age, circumcision requires analgesia and anesthesia.

7. The answer is C [VI.D.2 and VI.C.3.c]. Because of the patient's age and involvement of the maxillary incisors, this patient likely has nursing or bottle caries. Nursing or bottle caries are found in 3–6% of children and are associated with falling asleep with a bottle or a nipple in the mouth. Any liquid other than water can serve as a substrate for infection, including breast milk. *Streptococcal mutans* is the most common bacterial agent. Those who live in areas of low fluoride (< 0.3 ppm) are at higher risk for caries. Excess fluoride may cause cosmetic abnormalities to the enamel, but the risk of caries is not increased.

8. The answer is B [IV.J.3]. Lead intoxication may cause a variety of clinical manifestations, including neurocognitive impairment, lethargy, anemia, vomiting, and irritability. Most patients exposed to lead, however, are asymptomatic. Fluorosis is not associated with lead exposure, and lead exposure has not been known to result in microcephaly, failure to thrive, or hearing impairment.

9. The answer is A [Table 1.5]. Oral vitamin D supplementation is recommended to prevent the development of rickets in patients who are exposed to minimal sunlight during the first year of life. Infant walkers are not recommended because of the risk of injury associated with their use. Infants should be placed in a rear-facing car seat until they are 12 months of age and weigh 20 pounds. Toilet training is generally initiated between 1 and 2 years of age. Because of the risk of allergy, fish, egg whites, wheat, citrus fruits, nuts, and chocolate are avoided until at least 1 year of age.

10. The answer is C [VI.B]. Although the average age of initial tooth eruption is 6 months, there is a wide range of normal variability, ranging from 3 months to 16 months. Delayed dental eruption is defined as primary eruption after 16 months of age and may be related to endocrine disorders (hypothyroidism and hypopituitarism) or to genetic syndromes (Down syndrome and ectodermal dysplasia) or may be familial.

11, 12, and 13. The answers are A, B, and D, respectively [III.B. and III.C]. Immunizations are categorized as active (live or non-live) or passive. Active immunizations stimulate an immune response in the patient, whereas passive immunization involves the delivery of preformed antibodies to those who previously had no immunity to a particular disease. Examples of live vaccines include the varicella and the measles, mumps, and rubella vaccines. Examples of non-live vaccines include *Haemophilus influenzae* type b, diphtheria, tetanus, and acellular pertussis, and hepatitis A and B vaccines. Note that polio vaccines are available in both live (OPV) and non-live or killed (IPV) forms. Children living in regions of the country with a high incidence of hepatitis A infection should receive the hepatitis A vaccine (a non-live vaccine) at 2 years of age, with a booster 6 months later. An immunologically intact child with no immunity to varicella may receive the varicella vaccine (a live vaccine) at any age ≥ 12 months. An immunocompromised patient, such as a child with HIV, exposed to varicella, would be at high risk for acquiring a severe varicella infection and should therefore receive varicella zoster immune globulin (an example of passive immunization), ideally within 96 hours of exposure to the disease.

14. The answer is D [II.B.2]. Plagiocephaly is defined as asymmetry of the infant head shape and is usually not associated with premature closure of a cranial suture. The most common type of plagiocephaly is positional plagiocephaly, and it is often associated with congenital muscular torticollis. The initial management of this patient should include range of motion stretching exercises for associated torticollis (the likely cause of the gaze preference), repositioning the head during sleep, and increased time in the prone position when awake ("tummy time"). Radiographic studies are not indicated, and there is no association between positional plagiocephaly and underlying genetic syndromes, In contrast, the diagnosis of craniosynostosis, or premature closure of one or more cranial sutures, may require radiographic confirmation (either with skull radiographs or CT scan) and may be associated with underlying genetic syndromes.

2

Behavioral and Developmental Pediatrics

Elizabeth Mumper, M.D., and Peter Blasco, M.D.

I. Normal Developmental Milestones

A. General Principles

1. **Developmental assessment and surveillance** are central components of health maintenance.

2. **Developmental domains include motor development, language development, problem solving, and psychosocial skills.**

3. **It is essential to understand normal development** and acceptable developmental variations to recognize pathologic patterns. In addition, it is **important to monitor the attainment of developmental milestones in each domain to accurately diagnose children with developmental disabilities** who may benefit from referral to early intervention programs.

4. **Development occurs in an orderly, predictable, intrinsic manner.**

   a. Development proceeds from **head to toe** in a **proximal to distal fashion.**

   b. **Generalized reactions to stimuli develop into more specific, goal-directed reactions** that become increasingly precise.

   c. **Development progresses from total dependence to independence.**

5. **Infants normally vary in their attainment of milestones.**

6. **Development may be influenced by both intrinsic factors** (e.g., child's physical characteristics, state of health, temperament, and genetic attributes) and **extrinsic factors** (e.g., personalities of family members, economic status, depression or mental illness in caregivers, availability of learning experiences in the environment, cultural setting into which the child is born).

B. **Developmental Assessment**

1. **Developmental milestones** provide a **systematic way to assess an infant's progress.**

   a. **Attainment of a particular skill depends on the achievement of earlier skills** (only rarely are skills skipped).

   b. **Delays in one developmental domain may impair development in another domain** (e.g., deficits caused by neuromuscular disorders may affect a child's ability to explore the environment, which in turn affects cognitive development).

   c. **A deficit in one developmental domain may compromise the assessment of skills in another domain** (e.g., it may be difficult to assess problem-solving skills in the child with cerebral palsy who understands the concept of matching geometric forms but lacks the physical ability to demonstrate that knowledge).

2. **Developmental screening tests provide structured methods of assessing developmental progress. Because many developmental screening tests lack sensitivity, parental concern should not be disregarded,** even if the initial screen is normal.

3. **Developmental quotients** are used to determine whether a child's development is delayed and to measure the extent of delay. The quotient may be calculated as follows:

   $$\text{Development quotient (DQ)} = \frac{\text{developmental age}}{\text{chronologic age}} \times 100$$

   a. DQ > 85: normal

   b. DQ < 70: abnormal

   c. DQ 70–85: close follow-up is warranted

C. **Developmental domains** include **motor development, language skills, cognitive development, and social skills.**

1. **Motor development.** Information about motor milestones should be obtained from the history as well as from observation during the physical examination.

   a. **Gross motor development evaluation** includes an assessment of milestones and neuromaturational markers. **Milestones of gross motor development** are listed in **Table 2-1. Neuromaturational markers** should also be assessed; these include **primitive reflexes and postural reactions, as described in Table 2-2.**

   (1) **Primitive reflexes,** such as the **Moro reflex,** develop during gestation and are **present at birth.** They usually disappear between 3 and 6 months of age. Each primitive reflex requires a specific sensory stimulus to generate the stereotypical motor response. **Infants with central nervous system (CNS) injuries show stronger and more-sustained primitive reflexes.**

   (2) **Postural reactions,** such as the **parachute reaction, are not present at birth (i.e., they are acquired).** These reactions, which help facilitate the orientation of the body in space, require a complex interplay of cerebral and cerebellar cortical adjustments to proprioceptive, visual, and vestibular input. **Infants**

Table 2-1. Gross Motor Milestones*

Age	Milestone
Birth	Turns head side to side
2 months	Lifts head when lying prone Head lag when pulled from supine position
4 months	Rolls over No head lag when pulled from supine position Pushes chest up with arms
6 months	Sits alone Leads with head when pulled from supine position
9 months	Pulls to stand Cruises
12 months	Walks

*Normal infants exhibit significant variation in the attainment of these milestones.

> with CNS damage may have delayed development of postural reactions.

b. **Fine motor skills** involve the use of the small muscles of the hands. An infant's fine motor skills progress from control over proximal muscles to control over distal muscles. **Fine motor milestones** are listed in **Table 2-3.**

(1) During the first year of life, as balance in sitting and ambulatory positions improves, the hands become more available for the manipulation of objects. As control over distal muscles improves, reaching and manipulative skills are enhanced.

Table 2-2. Primitive Reflexes and Postural Reactions*

Description of Reflex/Reaction	Appears	Disappears
PRIMITIVE REFLEXES		
Moro reflex: Symmetric abduction and extension of arms with trunk extension, followed by adduction of upper extremities	Birth	4 months
Hand grasp: Reflex grasp of any object placed in palm	Birth	1–3 months
Atonic neck reflex: If head is turned to one side, arms and legs extend on same side and flex on the opposite; "fencer position"	2–4 weeks	6 months
Rooting reflex: Turning of head toward same side as stimulus when corner of infant's mouth is stimulated	Birth	6 months
POSTURAL REACTIONS		
Head righting: Ability to keep head vertical despite body being tilted	4–6 months	Persists
Parachute: Outstretched arms and legs when body is abruptly moved head first in a downward direction	8–9 months	Persists

*Different sources may vary on the precise timing of the appearance and disappearance of the listed primitive and postural responses.

Table 2-3. Fine Motor Milestones*

Age	Milestone
Birth	Keeps hands tightly fisted
3–4 months	Brings hands together to midline and then to mouth
4–5 months	Reaches for objects
6–7 months	Rakes objects with whole hand
	Transfers object from hand to hand
9 months	Uses immature pincer (ability to hold small object between thumb and index finger)
12 months	Uses mature pincer (ability to hold small object between thumb and tip of index finger)

*Normal infants show significant variation in the attainment of these milestones.

         (2) During the second year of life, the infant learns to use objects as tools (e.g., building blocks).

   c. Red flags in motor development

       (1) Persistent fisting beyond 3 months of age is often the earliest sign of neuromotor problems.

       (2) Early rolling over, early pulling to a stand instead of sitting, and persistent toe walking may all indicate spasticity.

       (3) Spontaneous postures, such as scissoring in a child with spasticity or a frog-leg position in a hypotonic infant, are important visual clues to motor abnormalities.

       (4) Early hand dominance (before 18 months of age) may be a sign of weakness of the opposite upper extremity associated with a hemiparesis.

   d. Differential diagnosis of motor delay includes CNS injury, spinal cord dysfunction, peripheral nerve pathology, motor endplate dysfunction, muscular disorders, metabolic disorders, and neurodegenerative conditions.

  2. Language skills

   a. General principles

       (1) Delays in language development are more common than delays in other domains.

       (2) Receptive language is always more advanced than expressive language (i.e., a child can usually understand 10 times as many words as he or she can speak).

       (3) Language and speech are not synonymous. Language refers to the ability to communicate with symbols (i.e., in addition to speech, this includes sign language, gestures, writing, and "body language"). **Speech** is the vocal expression of language.

       (4) A window of opportunity for optimal language acquisition occurs during the first 2 years of life.

       (5) Basic speech and language milestones are listed in Table 2-4.

   b. Periods of speech development

Table 2-4. Basic Language Milestones

Age	Milestone
Birth	Attunes to human voice Develops differential recognition of parents' voices
2–3 months	Cooing (runs of vowels), musical sounds (e.g., *ooh-ooh, aah-aah*)
6 months	Babbling (mixing vowels and consonants together) [e.g., *ba-ba-ba, da-da-da*]
9–12 months	Jargoning (e.g., babbling with mixed consonants, inflection, and cadence) Begins using *mama, dada* (nonspecific)
12 months	1–3 words, *mama and dada* (specific)
18 months	20–50 words Beginning to use two-word phrases
2 years	Two-word telegraphic sentences (e.g., *mommy come*) 25–50% of child's speech should be intelligible
3 years	Three-word sentences More than 75% of the child's speech should be intelligible

      (1) Prespeech period (0–10 months): Expressive language consists of musical-like vowel sounds (**cooing**) and adding consonants to the vowel sounds (**babbling**). Receptive language is characterized by an increasing ability to localize sounds.

      (2) Naming period (10–18 months) is characterized by the infant's understanding that people have names and objects have labels.

      (3) Word combination period (18–24 months): Early word combinations are "telegraphic" (e.g., without prepositions, pronouns, and articles). Typically, children begin to combine words 6–8 months after they say their first word.

   c. Differential diagnosis of speech or language delay

      (1) Global developmental delay or mental retardation

      (2) Hearing impairment

      (3) Environmental deprivation

      (4) Pervasive developmental disorders, including autism spectrum disorders

  3. Cognitive development involves skills in thinking, memory, learning, and problem solving.

   a. General principles

      (1) Intellectual development depends on attention, information processing, and memory.

      (2) Infant intelligence can be estimated by evaluating problem solving and language milestones. **Language is the single best indicator of intellectual potential.** Gross motor skills correlate poorly with cognitive potential.

      (3) In the school-age child, standardized intelligence tests measure both verbal skills and performance (nonverbal) skills. Significant discrepancies between verbal and nonverbal abilities suggest possible learning disabilities.

b. **Stages in cognitive development**

  (1) The **sensorimotor period** (birth to age 2 years) is a time during which the infant explores the environment through **physical manipulation of objects.** At first, the infant brings objects to the mouth for oral exploration. As peripheral motor skills improve, the infant's ability for precise manual-visual manipulation improves, leading to true inspection of objects. **The infant therefore progresses from "learning to manipulate" to "manipulating to learn."**

  (2) The **stage of functional play begins at about 1 year of age when the child recognizes objects and associates them with their function** (e.g., a 15-month-old boy puts a toy telephone to his ear and vocalizes).

  (3) The **stage of imaginative play begins when the child is able to use symbols** (24–30 months; e.g., a young child uses blocks to build forts or uses sticks as eating utensils or guns).

  (4) **Concrete thinking** (i.e., interpreting things literally) evolves during the preschool and early elementary school years.

  (5) **Abstract thinking** (i.e., manipulating concepts and contingencies) evolves during the adolescent years.

c. **Cognitive concepts that evolve over time**

  (1) **Object permanence,** developing at about **9 months,** is the concept that people and objects continue to exist even when an infant cannot see them. As a result of this ability to maintain an image of a person, **separation anxiety (common at 6–18 months)** develops when a loved one leaves the room.

  (2) **Cause and effect** is understanding which actions cause certain results (e.g., learning that dropping toys over the high chair tray makes them fall to the floor). Infants typically explore this concept **at 9–15 months.**

  (3) **Magical thinking** is a normal state of mind during the **preschool toddler years** when a child assumes that inanimate objects are alive and have feelings.

d. **Red flags in cognitive development.** Language development estimates verbal intelligence, whereas problem-solving skills estimate nonverbal intelligence.

  (1) If skills are delayed significantly in both language and problem-solving domains, **mental retardation** should be considered.

  (2) If only language skills are delayed, **hearing impairment or a communication disorder** should be considered.

  (3) If only problem-solving skills are delayed, **visual or fine motor problems** that interfere with manipulative tasks may be present.

  (4) If there is a significant discrepancy between language and problem-solving skills, the child is at high risk for **learning disabilities.**

4. **Social skills** are the ability to interact with other people and the environment. Development of social skills is dependent on cultural and environmental factors. **Milestones**, in order, include developing:

a. **Attachment.** Bonding with a primary caregiver begins at birth. Developing empathy is critical during the first 3 years of life.

b. **A sense of self and independence.** The process of separation and individuation begins at about 15 months of age.

c. **Social play.** Toddlers exhibit parallel play during the first 2 years of life. They learn to play together and share at about 3 years of age.

II. Disorders of Development

A. Motor Deficits

1. **Cerebral palsy**

   a. **Definition. Cerebral palsy** is a group of **static (i.e., nonprogressive) encephalopathies** caused by injury to the developing brain in which **motor function is primarily affected. Intelligence may be normal, but injuries to the brain that cause cerebral palsy often lead to other neurologic effects, including seizures, cognitive deficits, mental retardation, learning disabilities, sensory loss, and visual and auditory deficits.**

   b. **Epidemiology and etiology. Risk factors** are listed in **Table 2-5.** The **timing of the injury** may be prenatal or perinatal, or occur during the first few years of life. **Prevalence of cerebral palsy is 0.2–0.5%.** Five to fifteen percent of surviving infants with birth weight < 1500 g have cerebral palsy.

   c. **Diagnosis.** The basis of diagnosis is **repeated neurodevelopmental examinations** showing increasing tone or spasticity, hypotonia, asymmetric reflexes or movement disorder, or abnormal patterns in the disappearance of primitive reflexes or emergence of postural responses.

   d. **Classification of cerebral palsy** (Table 2-6)

      (1) **Spastic cerebral palsy.** Affected patients have increased tone. This type of cerebral palsy may be subclassified into three groups.

Table 2-5. Risk Factors for Cerebral Palsy

Risk Category	Specific Risk Factor
Maternal	Multiple gestation Preterm labor
Prenatal	Intrauterine growth retardation Congenital malformations Congenital infections (e.g., TORCH infections)
Perinatal	Prolonged, precipitous, or traumatic delivery Apgar score < 3 at 15 minutes Premature (< 37 weeks) or postdates (> 42 weeks) birth
Postnatal factors	Hypoxic-ischemic encephalopathy Intraventricular hemorrhage Trauma Kernicterus

TORCH = *t*oxoplasmosis, *o*ther infections (syphilis), *r*ubella, *c*ytomegalovirus, *h*erpes simplex.

Table 2-6. Classification and Characteristics of Types of Cerebral Palsy

Type and Description	Clinical Clues	Risk Factors
Spastic cerebral palsy		
Spastic diplegia		
Weakness that involves the lower extremities more than the upper extremities or face	History of early rolling over Increased tone **"Scissoring"** (extension and crossing of the lower extremities with standing or vertical suspension; a sign of spasticity)	Prematurity
Spastic hemiplegia		
Unilateral spastic motor weakness	Upper extremity involvement is typically greater than lower extremities Early hand preference (unusual in normal infants before 18 months of age) Attempts at grasping always on the same side and fisting or absent pincer on one side	Perinatal vascular insults, postnatal trauma, CNS malformations
Spastic quadriplegia		
Motor involvement of head, neck, and all four limbs	Seizures Scoliosis Weakness of face and pharyngeal muscles, dysphagia Gastroesophageal reflux or aspiration pneumonia, failure to thrive Speech problems and sensory impairments	Hypoxic-ischemia encephalopathy CNS infections, trauma, malformations
Extrapyramidal (nonspastic) cerebral palsy		
Involvement of extrapyramidal motor system, resulting in **athetoid** movements Problems involve modulating control of the face, neck, trunk, and limbs Arms are usually more affected than legs Oral motor involvement may be prominent	Marked hypotonia of neck and trunk, limiting child's ability to explore the environment Movement disorder consisting of intermittent posturing or movement of head, neck, and limbs Problems with feeding, speech, and drooling because oral motor function is impaired	Full-term infant with hypoxia-ischemia Kernicterus leading to basal ganglia damage

CNS = central nervous system.

    (a) Spastic diplegia involves the lower extremities more than the upper extremities or face.

    (b) Spastic hemiplegia is characterized by unilateral spastic motor weakness.

    (c) Spastic quadriplegia is characterized by motor involvement of the head, neck, and all four limbs.

  (2) Extrapyramidal cerebral palsy (commonly referred to as **athetoid cerebral palsy**). These patients have problems modulating the control of the face, trunk, and extremities, often writhing. Significant oral motor involvement often occurs.

2. Other causes of motor deficits include **metabolic abnormalities** (see Chapter 5, section IV), **chromosomal abnormalities** (see Chapter 5, section III) **motor neuron diseases, degenerative diseases, spinal cord injury, congenital myopathies, leukodystrophies, and CNS structural defects.**

B. **Cognitive deficits include mental retardation and learning disabilities.**

1. **Mental retardation** is defined as **significantly subaverage general intellectual functioning** associated with **deficits in adaptive behavior,** such as self-care, social skills, work, and leisure. It is **manifested before 18 years of age.**

a. **Etiology. Causes** are listed in **Table 2-7.**

b. **Classification and diagnosis.** Using the **Wechsler Intelligence Scale for Children** or another appropriate psychometric measure of the **intelligence quotient (IQ),** the degree of mental retardation can be classified as:

   (1) **Mild** (IQ = 55–69)

   (2) **Moderate** (IQ = 40–54)

   (3) **Severe** (IQ = 25–39)

   (4) **Profound** (IQ < 25)

c. **Management**

   (1) Early intervention programs promote optimal development.

   (2) Behavior management strategies are used to teach activities of daily living.

   (3) Community resources and parent support groups are helpful.

Table 2-7. Causes of Mental Retardation

Etiologic Category	Specific Etiologic Factor
IDIOPATHIC	
Genetic causes	Chromosome abnormalities (e.g., Down syndrome, fragile X syndrome)
	Inborn errors of metabolism (e.g., Hurler syndrome)
	Single gene abnormalities (e.g., tuberous sclerosis)
Prenatal and perinatal problems	Fetal malnutrition
	Placental insufficiency
	Maternal drug and alcohol use
	Brain malformations (e.g., hydrocephalus)
	Perinatal hypoxia or asphyxia
	Infection (e.g., herpes simplex, rubella, cytomegalovirus, toxoplasmosis)
Environmental problems	Psychosocial deprivation
	Parental mental illness
Postnatal acquired insults	Infection (e.g., meningitis, encephalitis)
	Head trauma
	Near drowning

(4) There is a trend away from institutionalization of mentally retarded individuals. Many live in foster care or group homes and work in sheltered or supported environments.

2. **Learning disabilities** are defined as a significant discrepancy between a child's academic achievement and the level expected on the basis of age and intelligence.

   a. **Etiology.** Causes include **CNS insults** (e.g., prematurity, closed head injury, lead poisoning, fetal alcohol syndrome), **genetic disorders** (e.g., fragile X syndrome), and **metabolic disorders** (e.g., galactosemia). The **most common cause is idiopathic.**

   b. **Types. Learning disabilities** may involve **deficiencies in specific academic subjects** (e.g., developmental disorders of reading, mathematics, or written expression) and **defects in processing of information** (e.g., visual or auditory processing disorders).

   c. **Management.** Classroom accommodations, special education, individualized instruction, and bypass strategies (e.g., presenting information visually for the child with an auditory processing disorder) may be used to help compensate for the learning disability.

C. **Pervasive developmental disorder (PDD).** This spectrum of **developmental disabilities affects multiple developmental areas, especially behavior and learning, with a wide range of severity.**

   1. **Autism. This condition is the prototypical PDD.**
      a. **Epidemiology**
         (1) **Incidence** is subject to debate.
         (2) **Onset is prior to age 3 years.**
         (3) **Autism is more common in boys.**
      b. **Clinical features**
         (1) **Difficulty using language to communicate with others.** Speech may be absent or limited and may have atypical intonation, cadence, and inflection. Children may use **echolalia** (i.e., repetitive words and phrases). At one extreme, there is no verbal language. At the other extreme, there are mild deviations in social language that may not be obvious to the casual observer.
         (2) **Unusual ways of relating** to people, objects, and events. Infants and toddlers may show decreased eye contact or may be difficult to console.
         (3) **Unusual or restrictive ranges of interests,** play, and responses to sensations
         (4) **Unusual perseverative behavior or stereotypic movement rituals.** Young children may have **preoccupations** with ideas, spinning objects, or shiny surfaces, whereas older children may develop more symbolic preoccupations, such as with train or bus schedules.
         (5) **Self-injurious behaviors** such as head banging, hand flapping, or body slapping
      c. **Associated clinical features.** Other findings may include seizures, mental retardation, chronic diarrhea, constipation, difficulty toilet

training, multiple ear infections, sensitivity to sensory input, or unusual pain thresholds.

2. Asperger syndrome

   a. This syndrome is also more common in boys.

   b. Clinical features

     (1) Qualitative impairment in peer relationships and social interactions

     (2) Repetitive, restricted, and stereotyped patterns of behavior, activities, and interests

     (3) No clinically significant language delay. Language, in fact, may be advanced.

III. Dysfunctions of Attention (Attention Deficit/Hyperactivity Disorder, ADHD)

A. Definition

  1. Characteristics of ADHD include poor selective attention, difficulty focusing, or distractibility. Hyperactivity may or may not be present.

  2. Children with disorders of attention may show **impulsivity, distractibility, disinhibition, and general behavioral immaturity.**

B. Epidemiology and etiology

  1. ADHD is **more common in boys.**

  2. The **cause of ADHD is unknown.**

   a. Genetic factors play a large role; 30–50% of affected children have a first-degree relative with ADHD.

   b. Abnormalities in neurotransmitter function, especially dopamine and norepinephrine, also lead to symptoms.

C. Differential Diagnosis (Table 2-8)

D. Clinical Features. Specific criteria must be present, including:

  1. Symptoms before 7 years of age

  2. Symptoms in more than one environment (e.g., school and home)

  3. Impairment in functioning in school or in personal relationships

  4. Symptoms of **inattention,** including not being able to focus during classroom instruction, difficulty with organization, and forgetfulness

  5. Symptoms of **hyperactivity,** which may include fidgeting, acting as if driven by a motor, excessive talking, and difficulty remaining seated in the classroom

  6. Symptoms of **impulsivity,** which may include behavior such as blurting out answers before a question is completed

E. Effect of attention problems on the child with ADHD

  1. Difficulty conforming to classroom routine

Table 2-8. Differential Diagnosis of Attention Deficit/Hyperactivity Disorder

Hearing or vision deficits
Sleep disorders, including obstructive sleep apnea
Food reactions
Thyroid disease
Anemia
Toxins or heavy metal exposure (e.g., lead poisoning)
Anxiety
Depression
Bipolar disorder
Mental retardation
Specific learning disabilities
Medication side effects (e.g., albuterol, methylphenidate, anticonvulsants, decongestants, antihistamines)
Family dysfunction
Normal child, but parents have unreasonable expectations for age or developmental stage
Caffeinated beverages

    2. **Social adjustment problems**

    3. **Damage to self-esteem**

    4. **Impaired relationships with parents and peers**

    5. **Difficulty learning**

    6. Possible comorbidities: anxiety, conduct disorder, oppositional-defiant disorder, and obsessive-compulsive disorder

 F. Assessment and diagnosis of ADHD

    1. **Methods** include parent and teacher questionnaires, psychoeducational testing, direct observation, a complete physical examination, and hearing and vision testing.

    2. Most valid, reliable assessments use **several sources** (teachers, parents, and counselors) and combine several methods. Direct and specific observations are most useful.

    3. **The key focus** of assessments should be to **identify the child's strengths and coping strategies.**

 G. Management. Therapy is multifaceted and includes:

    1. **Demystification.** This vital process **explains ADHD** to the child and family.

    2. **Classroom modifications.** Preferential seating and elimination of distractions may be useful.

    3. **Educational assistance.** Help should be tailored to the individual needs of the student. Strategies include placement in small groups or one-on-one teaching, help with organizational skills, and strategies to bypass weak areas (e.g., keyboarding if handwriting is a problem).

   4. **Counseling.** Topics to address may include self-esteem enhancement, depression, anxiety, behavioral modification, and social skills training. Parents also need support, education, and training.

   5. **Medications**
      a. **Stimulants** are **first-line pharmacologic treatment.** These drugs may **improve attention, impulsivity, and hyperactivity.**
         (1) **Mechanism of action. Stimulants appear to enhance catecholamine transmission** in the CNS. Higher levels of dopamine and norepinephrine improve ADHD symptoms.
         (2) **Dosage. The dosage needed to control symptoms varies among patients.**
         (3) **Side effects (Table 2-9). Medication effects should be monitored** using side effect diaries and behavior rating scales.
         (4) **Useful stimulants. Options** include **methylphenidate (Ritalin)** and **amphetamines (e.g., dextroamphetamine, dextroamphetamine-amphetamine combination [Adderall]).**
      b. **Nonstimulant medications** may be considered as **second-line** therapy. These drugs include tricyclic antidepressants and adrenergic agents such as clonidine. Clonidine may be especially useful at bedtime to counter stimulant effects or in combination with a stimulant for patients who have comorbid aggression or tic disorders. The treatment of comorbid depression or anxiety with selective serotonin reuptake inhibitors or bupropion may improve attention problems.

IV. Specific Sensory Impairments

   A. **Hearing Impairment**
      1. **Epidemiology. Permanent hearing loss** occurs in at least 1:600 new-

Table 2-9. Common Side Effects of Stimulants

Anorexia
Weight changes minimal but frequent

Insomnia
Common

Gastrointestinal
Nausea and abdominal pain

Headache

Irritability
Common as the stimulant is wearing off

Cardiovascular
Palpitations and hypertension

Effect on stature
Methylphenidate may decrease growth velocity but ultimately stature is not affected significantly

Tics
Tourette's syndrome and attention deficit/hyperactivity disorder may be genetically related
Transient tics occur in 9% of children treated with stimulants

borns. Half these infants are normal newborns who have no obvious evidence of suspected hearing impairment.

2. **Early identification** of the hearing-impaired child is vital because **outcome** is demonstrably better if intervention occurs before 6 months of age. **Sequelae of late identification include delayed speech and language skills and academic and behavior problems.**

3. **Etiology**

a. **Genetic factors** account for at least **80%** of childhood hearing impairment; 80% of genetic transmission occurs by **autosomal recessive** inheritance.

b. About 20% of childhood hearing loss is caused by perinatal, prenatal, or postnatal factors (e.g., congenital infections, prematurity, bacterial meningitis, middle ear anomalies).

4. **Prognostic factors. Variables influencing impact** of hearing loss on function and development include:

a. **Degree of loss**

b. **Etiology.** Children who inherit deafness usually fare better than those with acquired deafness. Children with acquired deafness are at higher risk for other neurologic impairment.

c. **Family atmosphere.** Family willingness and ability to use sign language have a major impact on the child.

d. **Age at onset** of acquired deafness. Children who become deaf before 2 years of age are at a disadvantage compared with those who are able to incorporate language structure before deafness.

e. **Timing of amplification** and educational interventions. The earlier this occurs, the better.

f. **Cochlear implants.** Although these may lead to dramatic improvements in hearing, their use is controversial in some deaf communities.

5. **Medical evaluation** for hearing loss

a. **Complete history (including history of perinatal infections and antibiotic exposure) and physical examination, focused on a thorough ear examination**

b. **Genetics evaluation** and chromosome studies if there are suspicious clinical findings or family history

c. **Creatinine level,** because of the association between kidney disease and ear abnormalities (Alport syndrome; see Chapter 11, section VII. B)

d. **Viral serologies** if clinically indicated, looking for toxoplasmosis, rubella, cytomegalovirus, herpes, and other viruses that can cause deafness (i.e., TORCH infections)

e. Consider a computed tomography scan of the inner ear if etiology is undetermined.

6. **Hearing screening recommendations** are given in Chapter 1, section IV.D.

B. **Visual Impairment**

1. **Incidence** is 1:1600 children.

2. **Classification of blindness** uses measures of corrected acuity in the

better eye as determined by Snellen chart testing and by determination of visual fields.

3. **Leading causes** of blindness in children
    a. **Trachoma infection** is common in developing nations and is the **primary cause of blindness worldwide.**
    b. **Retinopathy of prematurity** (see Chapter 18, section VII)
    c. **Congenital cataracts** (see Chapter 18, section VIII.A)
4. **Effects of blindness on development** include delayed locomotion, decreased fine motor skills, and difficulties with attachment.
5. **Adaptive skills**
    a. **Developing auditory perception skills**
    b. **Using haptic perception,** (e.g., feeling someone's face to form a mental image of them by combining kinesthetic spatial feedback and input from tactile sensation)
6. **Vision screening** is described in Chapter 18, section I.

V. Common Behavioral Concerns

A. **Colic. Colic is significant because it has the potential to disrupt attachment** between infant and parents, and it can be a **source of family stress.**
1. **Definition. Colic is crying that lasts > 3 hours per day and occurs > 3 days per week.** (Normal crying usually lasts up to 2 hours/day at 2 weeks of age and increases to 3 hours/day at 3 months.)
2. **Epidemiology.** Colic occurs in approximately **10% of newborns.**
3. **Etiology. Colic has an unknown basis and may have many causes.**
4. **Characteristic features**
    a. **Occurs in healthy, well-fed infants**
    b. **Begins at 2–4 weeks of age and resolves by 3–4 months of age**
    c. **Involves periods of irritability,** which typically begin in late afternoon or early evening
5. **Differential diagnosis.** Sources of pain and discomfort that may be confused with colic include intestinal gas, milk protein intolerance, food allergy, corneal abrasion, otitis media, testicular torsion, inguinal hernia, and digital ligature (i.e., hair wrapped around finger or toe).
6. **Management**
    a. **Treat any identified conditions.**
    b. **Reassure parents** that their infant is healthy and that the colic is not the parents' fault.
    c. **Recommend comfort measures,** which may include decreased sensory stimulation (e.g., placing in front of a blank wall), increased sensory stimulation by movement or vibration (e.g., automobile rides, rocking, stroller rides), or positioning (e.g., swaddling or placing infant on side or stomach while awake).

B. Enuresis

1. **Definition.** Enuresis is urinary incontinence beyond the age when the child is developmentally capable of continence.

2. **Classification** is based on the timing and history.

   a. **Nocturnal** (occurs only during sleep) **versus diurnal** (daytime)

   b. **Primary** (never been consistently dry) **versus secondary** (at least 6 months of prior consecutive dryness)

3. **Epidemiology**

   a. **Nocturnal enuresis is more common in boys.**

   b. **Incidence is based on age.** Bed-wetting occurs at least monthly in:

      (1) 30% of 4 year olds

      (2) 15–20% of 5 year olds

      (3) 10% of 6 year olds

      (4) 3% of 12 year olds

   c. Fifteen to twenty percent of those with nocturnal enuresis also have diurnal enuresis.

4. **Etiology. Causes may include:**

   a. **Genetics. Strong familial tendency for nocturnal primary enuresis** is supported by a gene identified on **chromosome 13.**

   b. **Psychosocial. Secondary enuresis** is often associated with stressful situations, such as the birth of a sibling, death of a family member, or the separation of parents.

   c. **Chaotic social situation** at home may contribute to poor voiding habits and daytime enuresis.

   d. **Sleep–arousal mechanisms** play an elusive role. Although not proven, parents frequently report children with nocturnal enuresis have deeper sleep and are more difficult to arouse than dry siblings.

   e. **Urine volume.** Some patients may produce **large volumes of dilute urine,** which may be caused by lack of normal diurnal variation in **vasopressin release.**

   f. **Bladder capacity.** Some children may have a small bladder capacity.

   g. **Organic causes** of secondary enuresis. Etiologic factors include urinary tract infections, child abuse, and diabetes mellitus.

   h. **Constipation is a comorbid or etiologic factor** in some patients. Hard stool can impinge on the bladder. **Symptoms of encopresis** may be present.

5. **Evaluation**

   a. **History** should include questions about family history, pattern of enuresis, associated symptoms, time of onset, and parental interventions or attempts at therapy.

   b. **Physical examination** should be complete and evaluate the abdomen, genitals, perineal sensation, anal wink reflex, and lower spine. A neurologic examination should be performed.

   c. **Laboratory evaluation**

      (1) **Urinalysis and urine culture**

(2) Additional laboratory or imaging studies should be tailored to the history and physical examination. Imaging of the kidney and bladder or magnetic resonance imaging of the spine or other studies may be appropriate.

6. **Management of uncomplicated nocturnal enuresis**
    a. **Education–demystification.** It may help to uncover misconceptions, **remove blame from the child,** and explain anatomy and physiology.
    b. **Conditioning alarms.** An alarm sounds every time urine is produced, and the child learns to respond in anticipation. This technique is successful in two thirds of cases, but it **requires patient motivation and parental support.** This therapy must be used for a minimum of 3–5 months.
    c. **Pharmacotherapy. Medications, if used alone, result in frequent relapses.** Best efficacy uses a combination of alarms, medications, and behavioral modification.
        (1) **Desmopressin acetate (DDAVP),** which decreases urine volume, is used because the child with enuresis may have no normal circadian rhythm for release of arginine vasopressin. Although a child may achieve complete dryness with DDAVP, relapse after termination of medication is common.
        (2) **Tricyclic antidepressants** have limited efficacy to decrease the frequency of nighttime wetting. **Imipramine is the most widely used agent.** Patients often relapse after medication is discontinued, and there is a **danger of fatal cardiac dysrhythmias with an overdose.**
    d. **Other management options. Behavioral modification** (e.g., star charts, praise for dry nights, limited fluids before bed, voiding before bed), hypnotherapy, and treating coexisting constipation may be useful.
7. **Management of diurnal enuresis.** Bladder stretching exercises, if small bladder capacity is suggested; schedule timed voiding every 90–120 minutes; and treatment of any coexisting constipation may be effective.

C. **Encopresis** (see Chapter 10, section VII)

D. **Sleep Problems**

1. **Epidemiology.** It is estimated that more than half of infants experience sleep problems as perceived by parents.
2. **Normal sleep patterns**
    a. **Day–night reversals are common** in the first weeks of life. The normal pattern is random sleep for 4 weeks, after which clustering of sleep time occurs.
    b. **Sleeping through the night** is defined as sleeping more than 5 hours after midnight for a 4-week period. Fifty percent of infants sleep through the night at 3 months of age.
3. **Abnormal sleep patterns**
    a. **Trained night waking** occurs between 4 and 8 months of age when the infant **does not resettle without parental intervention** (e.g.,

feedings, rocking, attention) during normal night stirrings and awakenings. **Management** includes establishing routines and placing the infant in bed while drowsy but awake.

b. **Trained night feeding** occurs when the infant continues to wake to eat because the parents keep responding with a feeding. **Management** includes lengthening intervals of daytime feeding and teaching parents not to respond with a feeding every time the infant stirs.

4. **Common sleep problems**

a. **Nightmares** are common after 3 years of age, although they may occur as early as 6 months of age. These frightening dreams tend to have themes of threats to security, separation, self-esteem, or survival. They occur during **rapid eye movement (REM) sleep.**

(1) **History. The child is able to give a detailed recall** of extended and frightening dreams. The child rapidly becomes alert and oriented after awakening.

(2) **Management.** Reassurance by the parents and comforting measures are helpful. It is important to address the child's needs for security and to promote regular sleep patterns and good sleep habits. Any inciting causes (e.g., frightening movies) should be identified and eliminated. Nightmares are usually transient and not very disruptive.

b. **Night terrors** are common at 3–5 years of age but have a pattern distinct from ordinary nightmares. Night terrors occur 90–120 minutes after sleep onset during **non-REM stage 4 sleep.**

(1) **History.** Parents describe a child who suddenly arouses screaming and thrashing with signs of autonomic arousal such as tachypnea, tachycardia, and diaphoresis. The child does not respond to visual or verbal cues, and parents report the child stares "glassy-eyed" without seeing. **The child does not remember the incident the next day.**

(2) **Management.** Reassuring parents and telling them that the episodes usually terminate spontaneously and will resolve over time is helpful.

E. **Eating Problems**

1. **Overfeeding during infancy is common.** Parents may equate food with love and enjoy seeing their infant grow and thrive.

2. **Toddler feeding.** Parents may report problems such as food refusal, food gorging, and a perception that the toddler does not eat enough.

a. **Appetite normally decreases after 1 year of age.**

b. **Control is the major issue in toddler feeding problems.** Autonomy is more important than hunger to the child at this stage.

c. **Management** includes **avoiding power struggles,** offering food without comment, and counseling parents to avoid bribes, pressuring, or forcing the child to eat.

F. **School Phobia**

1. **Definition.** The typical child with school phobia is a healthy-appearing child who misses school because of vague physical complaints.

2. **Etiology**
    a. Child is usually fearful of leaving the home and caregiver.
    b. Although it is unusual for the child to be fearful of anything in particular at school, the potential impact of bullies, learning problems, and fear of violence must be considered.

3. **Symptoms.** Complaints such as abdominal pain, diarrhea, fatigue, and headache **typically occur in the morning** and worsen on departure for school. They often begin in September or October and **frequently disappear on the weekends** and during summer vacation.

4. **Management**
    a. It is necessary to perform a thorough history and physical examination to ensure the child is healthy.
    b. The child must be returned to school; however, if the child insists on staying home, a visit to a physician should be scheduled. Peer relationships should be encouraged.

G. **Temper Tantrums.** These expressions of emotions (usually anger) are beyond the child's ability to control.

1. **Epidemiology.** Temper tantrums are **common** between **1 and 3 years of age.**

2. **Etiology. Frustration or fatigue** may cause tantrums. Children with poor fine motor skills or expressive language delays are likely to have more tantrums because of frustration. **Tantrums are not necessarily manipulative** or willful.

3. **Management**
    a. **Tantrums that demand something should be ignored.**
    b. **The ability to verbalize feelings** (learned by 3 years of age) **decreases tantrums.**
    c. Children having rage attacks or harmful tantrums may need to be held by a parent, who can provide a sense of calm and control.

H. **Breath-holding spells**

1. **Definition.** Breath-holding spells are benign episodes in which children hold their breath long enough to cause parental concern. **The spells are involuntary in nature, harmless,** and always stop by themselves.

2. **Epidemiology.** Breath-holding spells occur in 5% of young children, usually starting between 6 and 18 months of age and disappearing by 5 years of age.

3. **Types**
    a. **Cyanotic spells** are most common and are usually precipitated by an event that makes the child frustrated or angry. The child cries and becomes cyanotic, and in some cases becomes apneic and unconscious, or may have a seizure.
    b. **Pallid spells** are often provoked by an unexpected event that frightens the child, resulting in a hypervasovagal response, in which the child becomes pale and limp.

4. **Management**
   a. **Reassure** the parents that the episodes will resolve without harm.
   b. **Counsel parents** not to undertake potentially harmful resuscitation efforts.
   c. **Iron** has been reported to help some patients, but the mechanism is not clear.
   d. If the spells are precipitated by exercise or excitement rather than by frustration or fright, an **electrocardiogram** may be indicated to rule out a dysrhythmia (e.g., prolonged QT syndrome or supraventricular tachycardia).

I. Sibling Rivalry

1. **Manifestations** include bids for attention, regressive symptoms (e.g., wanting a bottle or going back to diapers), and aggression toward a new sibling. **The arrival of a newborn** is especially stressful for children younger than 3 years of age. Jealousy is frequently demonstrated up to 5 years of age.

2. **Management**
   a. **Before arrival of newborn. Methods for prevention** include talking about the arrival of the new baby and praising the child for mature behavior. Mastery of new skills (e.g., toilet training) should not be demanded during this stressful time.
   b. **In older children.** Children should be encouraged to settle their own arguments without hitting, name calling, or property damage. Parents should try to keep out of arguments, teach children how to listen to one another, protect each child's personal possessions, and praise children for good behavior.

J. Toilet Training

1. **Age normals.** The average child achieves **bowel control** by 29 months of age, with a wide range of normal of 16–48 months. The average child achieves **bladder control** by 32 months, with a wide range of normal of 18–60 months.

2. **Prerequisites**
   a. Understand meaning of words such as *wet, dry, pee, poop, clean, messy,* and *potty*
   b. Prefer being dry to being wet or soiled
   c. Recognize the sensation of bladder fullness and the urge to defecate, be able to hold urine and stool, and have the ability to tell the caregiver

3. **Method. Stress encouragement, praise, and patience.** Avoid shaming or blaming the child. Parents should:
   a. Allow multiple practice tries with praise for cooperation. It may be necessary to give small treats, but social reinforcement is best.
   b. **Avoid pressure or force,** which tends to make the child uncooperative. **Resistance to toilet training** symbolizes a **power struggle** between child and parents.
   c. **Point out that autonomy issues are important** in toilet training, which proceeds optimally when parents appreciate the child's need for mastery.

K. Discipline Issues

1. The basic premise of discipline is teaching the child limits. Parents must teach the child to respect the rights of others and control his or her behavior. Parents must provide external controls over the child's behavior, beginning at about 6 months of age. **Child should start developing internal controls (self-control) between 3 and 4 years of age.**

2. **Discipline techniques** are **most effective** when they are **based on the developmental needs and stages of the child.**
   a. Before age 6 months, **no discipline is indicated.**
   b. As the infant becomes more mobile, **distraction and redirection** can be used to ensure the child's safety.
   c. From 18 months to 3 years of age, **ignoring, time-out, and disapproval** (both verbal and nonverbal) may be effective.
   d. In preschool children, **logical consequences** (e.g., losing a toy that is used to hurt another child) may be effective.
   e. After 5 years of age, **negotiation and restriction of privileges** are used.

3. **Rules must be clear, concrete, and consistent.** Parents should state explicitly what the desired behaviors are and ignore unimportant misbehavior.

4. **Guidelines for using punishment.** Apply consequences and make the punishment brief and immediate. Follow the consequence with love and trust. Direct the punishment toward the behavior, not the person.

5. **Time-out is a highly effective** form of discipline when used appropriately and consistently, but it is **frequently used inappropriately and inconsistently by parents.**
   a. **Definition.** The caregiver interrupts misbehavior by isolating the child from social interactions for a brief period of time.
   b. **Purpose.** The child has time to think about the misbehavior and what acceptable behavior could be.
   c. **Length.** A time-out should be 1 minute per year of age (maximum 5 minutes, even in the older child).

Review Test

1. The parents bring a 13-month-old child to the office for a routine health maintenance visit. The child has been well since the last health maintenance visit, and the parents have no concerns today. The parents report he is sleeping through the night in his own crib and has a balanced diet and normal elimination patterns. During your physical examination, you perform a screening developmental evaluation. Which of the following findings on your developmental assessment would be most likely to merit a referral for a more thorough developmental evaluation?

(A) The child cruises but is not walking independently.
(B) The child's only words are *mama, dada, dog,* and *ball.*
(C) The child is afraid of strangers.
(D) The child neither eats with a spoon nor drinks from a cup.
(E) The child appears to be left-handed.

2. You are seeing a 1-month-old male infant in your office for a routine health maintenance visit. He was born at 32 weeks' gestation and had Apgar scores of 3 at 1 minute and 8 at 5 minutes. His hospital course was unremarkable, and he has been feeding and growing well since going home. His mother is now concerned that he is at a higher risk for cerebral palsy because of his prematurity. It would be most appropriate to make which of the following comments?

(A) It is unlikely that the child has cerebral palsy because his growth and development so far is normal.
(B) If cerebral palsy does develop, it will cause loss of developmental milestones.
(C) The child is at high risk for cerebral palsy because of his prematurity.
(D) Repeated examinations will be necessary to assess for cerebral palsy.
(E) Laboratory testing can determine whether the child has cerebral palsy.

3. At a routine health maintenance visit, the parents of a 1-year-old child would like to learn more about toilet training. Which of the following information is most appropriate to give the parents?

(A) It is important that toilet training begin now.
(B) Toileting is a skill to be learned just like any other and depends on the interests and readiness of the child.
(C) It is important that the parents establish control over toileting now or the pattern will be set for losing power struggles later.
(D) Toilet training should be finished as soon as possible for the good of caregivers and the environment.
(E) Whatever the parents and grandparents agree on is appropriate.

4. The parents of a 3-year-old child are concerned that their child may have autism based on the ways in which their child interacts socially. Which of the following might suggest the diagnosis of Asperger's syndrome rather than autism?

(A) The parents report that their child does not enjoy playing with other children and prefers to play alone.
(B) The parents report that their child is clumsy.
(C) The parents describe that their child engages in repetitive and stereotyped patterns of behavior.
(D) The child is a boy.
(E) Your developmental assessment reveals no clinically significant language delay.

5. The parents of a 7-year-old boy bring him to see you because of secondary enuresis. He achieved daytime dryness when he was 2.5 years of age and was dry at night by 3 years of age. Recently, he has developed dribbling incontinence, which embarrasses him at school. The parents do not report any recent psychosocial stress, but they are concerned that he trips often when he runs or walks quickly. Examination is normal, except you cannot elicit an anal wink reflex. Urinalysis and urine culture are both normal. Which of the following would be the most appropriate next management step?

(A) Neuroimaging studies of the brain and spine
(B) Bladder stretching exercises
(C) Trial of desmopressin (DDAVP)
(D) Trial of imipramine
(E) Psychological counseling

6. You are evaluating a toddler during a routine health maintenance visit, which includes a thorough developmental assessment. The parents report that their son is able to point to three to five body parts, uses 20–30 words that his parents understand, and is beginning to put together two-word phrases. Assuming his language skills are normal for age, how old is this child?

(A) 13 months
(B) 15 months
(C) 18 months
(D) 24 months
(E) 30 months

7. On screening in the newborn nursery, an infant has an abnormal hearing screen. His examination is otherwise normal. Which of the following etiologic factors most likely explains the hearing loss in this infant?

(A) Prenatal factors, such as maternal substance abuse
(B) Perinatal factors associated with a traumatic or preterm delivery
(C) Postnatal infection, such as meningitis
(D) Autosomal recessive genetic defect
(E) Autosomal dominant genetic defect

8. The mother of a 9-year-old boy brings him to the pediatrician because her son is exhibiting hyperactivity and inattention in school. Before this year, the boy has performed well in school and has shown no signs of hyperactivity or inattention. His teacher reports that the boy is restless in the classroom and frequently leaves his seat. His mind seems to wander during the teacher's lectures. On questionnaires, the teacher confirms the inattention and hyperactivity. The boy shows no symptoms at home, and he does well at church school and at camp. The most appropriate first step in managing this patient would be:

(A) Explaining to the parents that he meets criteria for attention deficit/hyperactivity disorder and what that diagnosis means.
(B) Looking for other causes of the hyperactivity and inattention in the differential diagnosis.
(C) Beginning an empiric trial of stimulant medication to see whether his symptoms improve with pharmacologic intervention.
(D) Working with the school to modify the boy's assignments and the classroom setting.
(E) Referring to a counselor for self-esteem enhancement, social skills training, and behavior modification.

9. The parents of a 3.5-year-old boy are concerned that their son is experiencing nightmares. On further questioning, you make the diagnosis of night terrors. Which of the following factors would most support your diagnosis of night terrors and not nightmares?

(A) This child's events occur approximately 30 minutes after sleep onset.
(B) Nightmares tend to decrease in frequency after age 3 years.
(C) The child responds to the parent's attempts to comfort him during the events.
(D) The child becomes alert and oriented immediately after the event.
(E) The child does not remember the event the next day.

10. A 2-month-old male infant is brought to your office with concerns about excessive crying. Based on the history, you suspect colic. Which of the following findings on your evaluation best supports this diagnosis?

(A) The crying spells usually occur in the morning hours, lasting 2 hours every day, 5 days every week.

(B) The infant's weight has decreased by two growth isobars since birth.

(C) The parents have noticed an intermittent bulge in the infant's right inguinal region associated with crying spells lasting anywhere from 2 to 6 hours.

(D) The infant has been growing at the 10th percentile consistently since birth, with 3–4 hours per day of crying, 4 days every week.

(E) The infant appears to be thriving but cries for 2 hours every day of the week, more commonly in the early afternoon or evening hours.

11. The parents of an 18-month-old boy are very concerned because he has had several episodes in which he became frustrated and angry, held his breath, and turned blue. Which of the following is appropriate information for parents about breath-holding spells?

(A) The spells are voluntary, and the boy is very likely deliberately trying to gain attention from the parents.

(B) The age of onset for these spells is unusual.

(C) The boy is unlikely to lose consciousness during a spell.

(D) An electrocardiogram is indicated if the spells are associated with physical activity.

(E) The spells may eventually cause learning disabilities and poor attention if they are allowed to continue.

12. A child is still in the sensorimotor stage of development. He is beginning to look over the high chair to see where a dropped object has gone and is starting to use a brush and comb on his hair. He has not yet started building forts with blocks. Assuming he is normal cognitively, his age is most likely to be:

(A) 6–9 months
(B) 10–14 months
(C) 15–18 months
(D) 18–24 months
(E) 24–27 months

The response options for statements 13–14 are the same. You will be required to select one answer for each statement in the set.

(A) 4 months
(B) 6 months
(C) 8 months
(D) 10 months
(E) 12 months

For each of the following infants, select the most likely age of the infant based on the infant's developmental milestones.

13. While playing with blocks with an infant, the infant becomes upset when you hide the blocks out of view. The infant is only able to say *mama* and becomes upset when his mother leaves the room. He is able to hold a small object between his thumb and his index finger.

14. An infant is able to transfer objects from hand to hand and to sit alone. He is also able to mix both vowel and consonant sounds, although he is not yet saying *mama* and *dada*. You are not able to elicit a parachute reaction.

Answers and Explanations

1. The answer is E [I.C.1.c]. An early hand preference may indicate weakness or spasticity of the contralateral upper extremity. It is unusual to see a hand preference in an infant younger than 18 months of age. Infants walk at a mean age of 12 months, and the range of normal (two standard deviations) is 9–15 months. Using two words in addition to *mama* and *dada* is appropriate for a 13-month-old child. Stranger anxiety is both common and normal between 6 and 18 months. A 13-month-old child may play with household objects but may not use them appropriately in imitation until 15–18 months of age.

2. The answer is D [II.A.1.c]. Periodic developmental evaluations and physical examinations are necessary to monitor for signs of cerebral palsy. Although it is important to evaluate this infant's tone and reflexes, abnormalities of the motor examination are frequently not appreciated until the infant is older than 6 months of age. Cerebral palsy is a nonprogressive encephalopathy and should not lead to loss of milestones. Only a minority of extremely low birth weight premature infants (≤ 1000 g) develop cerebral palsy (15–25% incidence). No specific laboratory testing is available to diagnose or predict the course of the disease.

3. The answer is B [V.J]. The age of toilet training coincides with the psychological stage of developing autonomy and mastering new skills. The basic principles of rewarding appropriate behaviors apply to toileting as well as to the achievement of other new skills. One year of age is too early to begin toilet training and is likely to lead to frustration and power struggles. Although environmental issues and caregiver convenience are important considerations, they are not paramount issues. Harmony between generations is desirable, but overly coercive training by controlling parents is associated with later encopresis.

4. The answer is E [II.C.2]. Children with Asperger's syndrome do not have language delay. In fact, they often speak like "little professors," using words that are more advanced than the language of their peers. The impairment in social relationships and peer interactions is the hallmark of Asperger's syndrome; however, it is also seen in autism. Clumsiness is not associated with either condition. Children with Asperger's syndrome have many autistic-like behaviors, including repetitive and stereotyped patterns of behavior and interests. Difficulty using language to communicate with others is the hallmark of autism, although the spectrum ranges from no verbal language to subtle deviations. People with autism may have difficulty "reading" facial expressions and hand gestures. Both Asperger's syndrome and autism are more common in males.

5. The answer is A [V.B.5]. This child's history is concerning for a potential neurologic abnormality because of the reported tripping. The abnormal anal wink reflex on examination suggests spinal cord compression or spinal nerve entrapment and the need for neuroimaging studies. Bladder stretching exercises may be appropriate for the child who wets when his functional bladder capacity is exceeded, but the history here does not suggest that small bladder capacity is the problem. Conditioning alarms, desmopressin (DDAVP), and imipramine have all been used for nocturnal enuresis, whereas this child has daytime enuresis. Secondary enuresis is usually associated with an identified stress such as the birth of a sibling, divorce in the family, or a recent move. Psychological counseling can sometimes be useful in such situations.

6. The answer is C [Table 2-4]. The language milestones described are usually achieved around the age of 18 months. At 13 months, most children use about three words that the parents understand, and they are also able to play peek-a-boo and patty-cake. At 15 months, children may understand more than 20–30 words receptively but are usually only able to express between 12 and 15 words. At 24 months, children should be using multiple telegraphic two-word sentences. At 30 months, children begin to use adjectives and adverbs, ask questions, and use sentences longer than two words.

7. The answer is D [IV.A.3]. Eighty percent of childhood hearing impairment is caused by genetic factors. The inheritance of most of these genetic defects is autosomal recessive. Maternal substance abuse, traumatic deliveries, and prematurity are less frequent causes of isolated hearing impairments. Although meningitis and prenatal congenital infections are also potential causes of hearing impairment, they are among the nongenetic factors that account for about 20% of hearing loss in infants.

8. The answer is B [III.D]. It is important to establish the correct diagnosis before beginning therapeutic interventions. This child does not meet the criteria for the diagnosis of attention deficit/hyperactivity disorder (ADHD) because his symptoms appeared after 7 years of age and are present in only one setting (school). It would be important to assess whether factors such as the teacher's expectations, classroom dynamics, or peer issues are impacting his classroom behavior and performance. If a child meets the criteria for ADHD, all of the other management options become reasonable parts of a therapeutic plan.

9. The answer is E [V.D.4]. Children with night terrors do not respond to their parents' attempts to comfort them, do not become oriented during their arousals from sleep, and do not remember the event the next day. In contrast, children with nightmares rapidly become alert and oriented, recall details of the frightening dreams on awakening, and often recall the next day that they had a bad dream during the night. Nightmares occur in REM (rapid eye movement) sleep, whereas night terrors occur in stage 4 non-REM sleep 90–120 minutes after sleep onset. The peak incidence for night terrors is between 3 and 5 years of age; nightmares are common after age 3.

10. The answer is D [V.A]. To qualify for a diagnosis of colic, the infant must be between the ages of 2 weeks and 4 months, be healthy and well-fed, and cry for more than 3 hours a day more than 3 days a week. Periods of crying with colic typically increase in the late afternoon or early evening hours. Known causes of pain must be excluded to make the diagnosis of colic, including corneal abrasion, hair tourniquet wrapped around a digit, and inguinal hernia that may be intermittently incarcerated. Infants who have concurrent failure to thrive must be evaluated for other etiologic factors.

11. The answer is D [V.H]. Breath-holding spells are common, occurring in as many as 5% of children. These spells generally begin in children at 6–18 months of age and may continue up until 5 years of age. They are harmless and involuntary in nature. Even if they produce a loss of consciousness, which may occur in some children, learning problems or other long-term sequelae do not result. Spells that are associated with exercise or physical activity should be evaluated with an electrocardiogram to look for an underlying dysrhythmia.

12. The answer is B [I.C]. Knowing that this child is still in the sensorimotor stage places his age at less than 2 years. This child is old enough to start using tools for their function, which would not be seen in a typical infant who is 6–9 months of age. He is not using symbolic play, which begins at about 24–30 months. He is beginning to process the concept of cause-and-effect; infants usually start looking over the high chair for dropped objects at about 9 months of age. This developmental clue places him at the early stage of functional play, making an age of 10–14 months more likely than ages older than 15 months.

13. The answers are D [I.C.3.c; Tables 2-3 and 2-4] **and C** [Tables 2-2, 2-3, and 2-4], **respectively.** Infants develop "object permanence," an understanding that objects continue to exist even when the infant cannot see them, at about 9 months of age. Infants usually begin saying *mama* and *dada* between 9 and 12 months of age and usually have between one and three additional words in their vocabulary by 12 months of age (1 year). Separation anxiety may develop anytime between 6 and 18 months of age when a loved one leaves the infant's vision. An immature pincer, or the ability to hold a small object between the thumb and the index finger, usually develops about 9 months of age. Based on the choices provided, this infant is most likely to be 10 months of age.

Infants are able to transfer objects and to sit alone at about 6 months of age. In addition, a 6-month-old infant would be expected to mix vowel and consonant sounds but will not begin saying *mama* or *dada* until 9–12 months of age. The parachute reaction is one of the postural reactions that help facilitate the orientation of the body in space and usually develops at approximately 8 months of age. Based on the choices provided, this infant is most likely 6 months of age.

3

Adolescent Medicine

Lloyd J. Brown, MD

I. Adolescent Growth and Development

A. **Growth.** Adolescence is a time of substantial physical growth and pubertal maturation.

1. **Changes in physical growth**
   a. **The average duration of the growth spurt is 2–3 years.**
   b. **Growth** is predominantly controlled by **growth hormone,** although insulin, thyroid hormone, and sex steroids also influence growth.
   c. **Nearly 50%** of ideal adult body weight and **25%** of final adult height are gained during the pubertal growth spurt.
   d. **The growth spurt** occurs **18–24 months earlier** in females than in males.

2. **Development of genitalia and secondary sexual characteristics.**
   a. **The average duration of puberty is 3–4 years.**
   b. **Endocrinologic changes during puberty.** The factor responsible for the initiation of puberty is unknown.
      (1) **Adrenarche,** the onset of adrenal androgen steroidogenesis, occurs 2 years before the maturation of the hypothalamic-pituitary-gonadal axis.
      (2) **True puberty** is said to occur when gonadotropins, such as luteinizing hormone (LH), follicle-stimulating hormone (FSH), and gonadal sex steroids (e.g., estrogen and testosterone), increase.
      (3) **Table 3-1** lists the actions of hormones in males and females.
   c. **Physical changes during puberty**
      (1) **Males.** Puberty begins **6–12** months later in males than in females.
         (a) **Testicular enlargement** begins between ages 11 and 12 years and is the **first sign of puberty.**
         (b) **Facial and axillary hair** growth begins approximately 2 years after the growth of pubic hair begins.

Table 3-1. Actions of Sex Hormones in Both Males and Females

Hormone	Action in Males	Action in Females
Follicle-stimulating hormone	Induces spermatogenesis	Stimulates development of ovarian follicles Stimulates ovarian granulosa cells to produce estrogen
Luteinizing hormone	Induces testicular Leydig cells to produce testosterone	Stimulates ovarian theca cells to produce androgens Stimulates corpus luteum to produce progesterone Midcycle surge results in ovulation
Testosterone	Increases linear growth and muscle mass Induces development of penis, scrotum, prostate, and seminal vesicles Induces growth of pubic, axillary, and facial hair Deepens voice Increases libido	Stimulates linear growth Stimulates growth of pubic and axillary hair
Estradiol	Increases rate of epiphyseal fusion	Stimulates breast development Triggers midcycle luteinizing hormone surge Stimulates labial, vaginal, and uterine development Stimulates growth of a proliferative endometrium Low level stimulates linear growth High level increases rate of epiphyseal fusion
Progesterone		Converts endometrium to a secretory endometrium
Adrenal androgens	Stimulates growth of pubic hair Stimulates linear growth	Stimulates growth of pubic hair Stimulates linear growth

(Adapted from Neinstein LS. Adolescent Health Care, A Practical Guide. 3rd Ed. Baltimore: Williams & Wilkins, 1996.)

    (c) Figure 3-1 shows the five stages of development of male genitalia and pubic hair as described by Tanner **(Tanner staging or sexual maturity rating)**.

  (2) Females. Puberty begins with the development of breast buds **(thelarche)** at a mean age of **9.5 years.**

    (a) Pubic hair generally follows thelarche.

    (b) Menarche, the onset of the first menstrual cycle, occurs at a mean age of **12.5 years** and occurs **2–3 years after thelarche.**

    (c) Figures 3-2 and **3-3** show the development of breasts and pubic hair, respectively, as described by Tanner.

B. Psychosocial development. Adolescent development may be classified into three stages: **early, middle,** and **late.** As an adolescent passes through the stages of psychosocial development, he or she develops a sense of self,

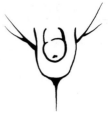

Stage 1   Preadolescent
             No pubic hair
             Prepubertal testes

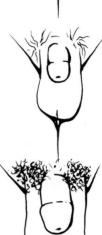

Stage 2   Testes larger
             Sparse, long, downy hair

Stage 3   Testes further enlarged
             Penis length enlarged
             Darker, coarser, and curlier hair

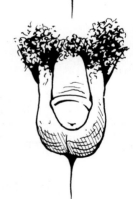

Stage 4   Darkening of scrotal skin
             Penis length and width increased;
              glans develops
             Coarse and curly pubic hair
              extending over symphysis pubis

Stage 5   Testes and penis adult in size and shape
             Adult-type pubic hair that spreads to
              medial surface of thighs

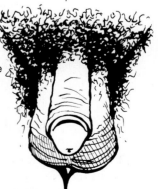

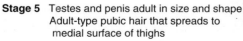

Figure 3-1. Sexual maturity ratings for male genitalia and pubic hair development.

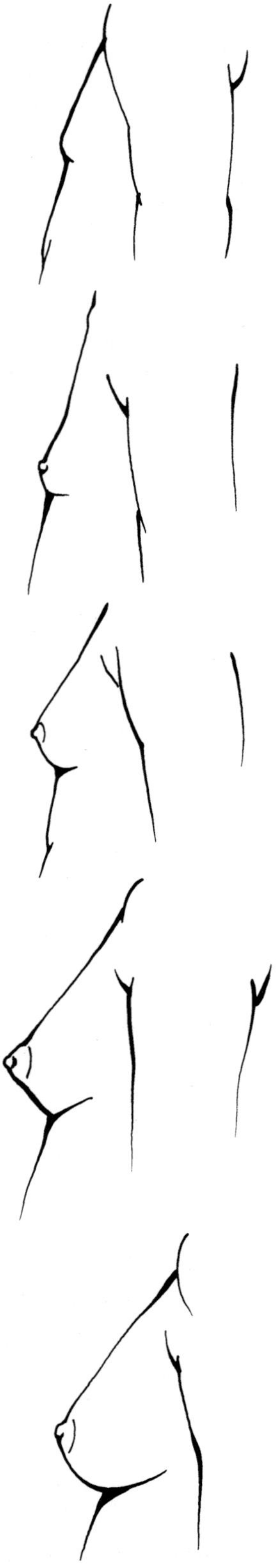

Stage 1   Preadolescent

Stage 2   Elevation of breast and nipple
          as small projections

Stage 3   Enlargement of breast
          No separation of areola and breast
          Areola enlarges

Stage 4   Areola and nipple project
          to form secondary mound above
          level of breast

Stage 5   Only nipple projects
          Areola usually recedes to
          contour of breast
          Adult breast size

Figure 3-2. Sexual maturity ratings for female breast development.

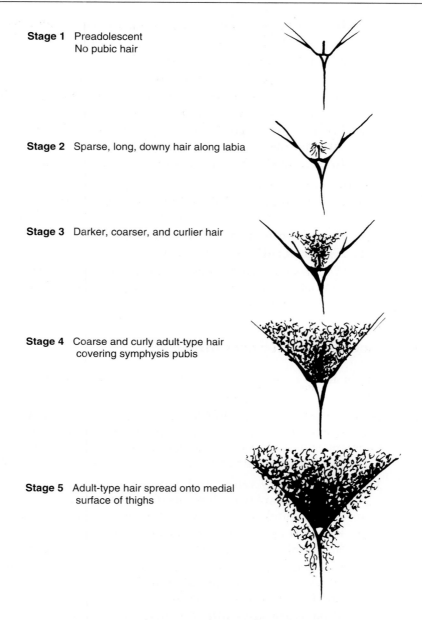

Stage 1 Preadolescent
No pubic hair

Stage 2 Sparse, long, downy hair along labia

Stage 3 Darker, coarser, and curlier hair

Stage 4 Coarse and curly adult-type hair
covering symphysis pubis

Stage 5 Adult-type hair spread onto medial
surface of thighs

Figure 3-3. Sexual maturity ratings for female pubic hair development.

achieves increasing independence from his or her parents, increases his or her involvement with peer groups, and develops a healthy body image.

1. **Early adolescence** (10–13 years of age)
   a. **Early shift to independence** from parents, with declining interest in family activities, beginnings of conflicts with parents, and the presence of mood and behavior changes
   b. Preoccupation with pubertal body changes
   c. **Same-sex peer relationships**

     d. Beginnings of abstract thinking and lack of impulse control, with **risk-taking** behaviors

  2. **Middle adolescence** (14–17 years of age)

     a. Increased conflicts with parents

     b. Diminished preoccupation with pubertal changes but increased preoccupation with methods to improve one's own physical attractiveness

     c. Intense peer group involvement and initiation of **romantic relationships**

     d. Increasingly abstract reasoning and **risk-taking**

  3. **Late adolescence** (18–21 years of age)

     a. Development of self as distinct from parents. Adolescents are better able to take and more likely to seek advice from parents.

     b. Being comfortable with own body image

     c. A shared intimate relationship with at least one partner

     d. Well-developed **abstract thought processes,** with **fewer risk-taking** behaviors. Adolescents are able to articulate future educational and vocational goals.

II. Adolescent Health Screening

  A. Goals are to promote optimal physical and psychosocial growth and development.

  B. History. Information should be obtained directly from the adolescent alone. However, the family can also be an important source of additional information. Practitioners may choose to interview the family together with the adolescent, either before or after interviewing the adolescent alone.

    1. **Confidentiality, trust, and rapport** are important to establish to provide effective care to adolescents. Confidentiality encourages adolescents to seek care and protects them from embarrassment and discrimination.

     a. Rapport can be best established by beginning the history with nonthreatening subjects such as favorite hobbies, interests, or activities.

     b. Information provided by the adolescent should remain confidential, although **sexual or physical abuse** and **suicidal or homicidal intention must be reported.**

     c. Most state laws allow adolescents to consent without parent approval for pregnancy-related care, diagnosis and treatment of sexually transmitted diseases (STDs), reproductive health care, counseling and treatment of drug or alcohol problems, and mental health treatment.

    2. **Components of the history** include present illness or concerns, past medical and family histories, and a psychosocial history using the **HEADSS** assessment (<u>h</u>ome, <u>e</u>ducation and <u>e</u>mployment, <u>a</u>ctivities, <u>d</u>rugs, <u>s</u>exual activity, <u>s</u>uicide and depression; **Table 3-2**).

  C. Physical examination. The physician should pay special attention to physical growth and pubertal development, detection of disease, and specific adolescent concerns.

Table 3-2. HEADSS Questionnaire Used in Psychosocial Assessment of Adolescents

Home	Where, and with whom, does teen live? Has teen ever run away or been arrested? How does teen interact with parents? Is there a firearm at home?
Education and employment	Is teen in school? What is teen's academic performance? What classes does teen enjoy? Dislike? Has teen ever been suspended? Dropped out? What are teen's career goals? Does teen have a job?
Activities	What are teen's hobbies? What does teen enjoy doing after school? On weekends? With whom does teen spend free time?
Drugs	Has teen tried any drugs? If yes, how much? How often? Has teen used tobacco? Alcohol? Steroids? Do teen's friends use drugs?
Sexual activity	Is teen currently sexually active? If yes, what type of contraception is used? Does teen use condoms? How many sexual partners? Any STDs? What is teen's sexual orientation? Does teen have any history of sexual or physical abuse?
Suicide and depression	Is teen ever sad or depressed? Has teen ever considered or attempted suicide?

STD = sexually transmitted disease.

1. **Height and weight** should be measured and plotted on age-appropriate growth charts.
2. **Blood pressure, pulse, and vision and hearing** assessments should be performed.
3. **Skin** should be examined for acne and fungal infections.
4. **Teeth** should be examined for malocclusion and hygiene.
5. **Thyroid** should be palpated for enlargement or nodules.
6. **Back** should be evaluated for scoliosis or kyphosis.
7. **Pubertal development** should be assessed, and a Tanner rating should be assigned (**see Figures 3-1, 3-2, and 3-3**).
8. **Male genitalia** should be examined for scrotal masses and inguinal hernias. Instruction should be given on the performance of a proper **testicular self-examination.**
9. **Female genitalia** should be examined. A **complete pelvic examination** should be performed **annually if the patient is sexually active;** if she has a history of **pelvic pain, vaginal discharge, or abnormal bleeding;** or if she is **18 years** of age or older. In addition, instruction should be given on the performance of a proper **breast self-examination.**

   D. **Immunizations**

1. **Tetanus and diphtheria booster (Td)** should be given between 11 and 12 years of age and every 10 years thereafter.
2. **Measles, mumps, and rubella booster (MMR)** and the **hepatitis B vaccine series** should be given if not given before adolescence. Hepati-

tis A vaccine should be given to those adolescents who reside in endemic areas.

3. **Varicella vaccine** should be considered if the adolescent has not had chickenpox and has not received vaccination against the disease.

E. **Laboratory Studies**

1. **Hemoglobin and hematocrit** to screen for anemia.

2. **Urinalysis** to screen for proteinuria and hematuria.

3. **Cholesterol level or fasting lipid panel** (see Chapter 1, section IV for guidelines).

4. **Human immunodeficiency virus (HIV) testing** is not routinely indicated, but it should be offered if indicated by history or if requested. Counseling must be given regarding the benefits of testing and consequences of the results.

5. **Mantoux skin test (PPD)** for tuberculosis (TB) should be administered at least once during adolescence. PPD may be necessary more often if the adolescent is at high risk of exposure to TB.

6. **Sexually active adolescent females** should be screened for the following STDs:

   a. **Cervical culture for *Neisseria gonorrhoeae***

   b. **Immunofluorescent antibody test or culture of cervical fluid, or urine ligase test, for *Chlamydia trachomatis***

   c. **Serologic test for syphilis**

   d. **Papanicolaou (Pap) smear for cervical cancer screening** and detection of **human papillomavirus (HPV)**

   e. **Vaginal wet mount for *Trichomonas vaginalis***

7. **Sexually active adolescent males** should have annual syphilis serology, routine urinalysis for pyuria, and a urine ligase test for *C. trachomatis*.

F. **Health guidance.** Counseling should be provided annually.

1. **Injury prevention.** Education should include counseling about alcohol and drug avoidance, firearm safety, and the use of seat belts and motorcycle and bicycle helmets.

2. **Benefits of a healthy diet and physical exercise**

3. **Education regarding responsible sexual behaviors**

III. Depression and Suicide

A. **Epidemiology**

1. **Suicide** is the **third leading cause of death** in adolescents 15–19 years of age, after unintentional injuries and homicide.

2. **Episodes of sadness or depressed mood** occur monthly in the majority of adolescents, and **5%** of teens are clinically depressed.

3. **Girls** are depressed two times as often as boys.

4. **Risk factors** for suicide or depression
   a. **Family or peer conflicts**
   b. **Substance abuse**
   c. **Significant loss,** including death of a loved one
   d. **Divorce or separation** of parents
   e. **Poor school performance or learning disability**
   f. **Physical or sexual abuse**
   g. **Family history of depression or suicide**
   h. **Previous suicide attempt**
   i. **Physical illness**

B. **Clinical features** of **depression**
   1. **Teens with depression** can have a wide range of behavioral, physical, and psychological symptoms.
      a. **Behavioral signs of depression** include missing school, change in school performance, acting out (e.g., arguing with family and friends, stealing, destruction of property), lack of interest in activities that previously were pleasurable, desire to be alone or being withdrawn, and substance abuse.
      b. **Physical signs of depression** include abdominal pain, headaches, weight loss, overeating, insomnia, anxiousness, diminished appetite, and fatigue.
      c. **Psychological signs of depression** include sadness, feelings of hopelessness, low self-esteem, excessive self-criticism, and feeling worthless.
   2. The following are the *Diagnostic and Statistical Manual of Mental Disorders,* **4th edition (DSM-IV) criteria for major depression: Five of nine** symptoms must be present **almost every day for at least 2 weeks** and must **impair ability to function normally.**
      a. **Depressed or irritable mood**
      b. **Diminished interest or pleasure in activities**
      c. **Weight gain or loss**
      d. **Insomnia or hypersomnia**
      e. **Psychomotor agitation or retardation**
      f. **Fatigue or energy loss**
      g. **Feelings of worthlessness**
      h. **Diminished ability to concentrate**
      i. **Recurrent thoughts of death or suicide**

C. **Clinical features** of **dysthymic disorder.** Dysthymia is a more chronic mood disturbance that lasts at least 1 year. The symptoms of dysthymia are milder than those of depression. The following are the DSM-IV criteria for dysthymia:
   1. **While depressed, two of five** of the following symptoms must be present:
      a. **Poor appetite or overeating**
      b. **Insomnia or hypersomnia**

  c. **Diminished energy**

  d. **Difficulty concentrating**

  e. **Feelings of hopelessness**

 2. **Symptoms must last for at least 1 year.**

IV. Substance Abuse

A. **Epidemiology. Ninety percent** of high school seniors have tried **alcohol, 50%** have tried an **illegal drug,** and **60%** have tried **cigarettes.**

B. **Etiology. Use by family or peers, experimentation, stress relief, poor self-esteem, boredom, social acceptance, enhancement of ability to act socially, and acting-out behavior against authority figures** are all reasons adolescents may use illegal drugs, alcohol, or tobacco.

C. **Diagnosis. Substance abuse should be considered** if the following factors are present: mood or sleep disturbances, truancy, decline in school performance, changes in friends and family relationships, diminished appetite or weight loss, depression, and diminished participation in school or household responsibilities.

D. **Most commonly used substances: alcohol, tobacco, and marijuana**

 1. **Alcohol is the most commonly used substance.**

  a. **Problem drinking** is defined as having been intoxicated six or more times within 1 year or having **problems** in areas attributable to drinking, such as missing classes at school, arguing with teachers, classmates, or friends, or driving intoxicated.

  b. **Binge drinking** is defined as five or more consecutive drinks at one sitting. As many as 50% of all college students report binge drinking, and binge drinkers are more likely to fight, drive drunk, and have unplanned sexual intercourse.

  c. **Alcoholism** is defined as a preoccupation with and impaired control over drinking, despite adverse consequences.

  d. The **CAGE questionnaire** may be used to screen for alcoholism.

   (1) Have you ever felt you had to **<u>c</u>ut** down on drinking?

   (2) Have people **<u>a</u>nnoyed** you by criticizing your drinking?

   (3) Have you ever felt **<u>g</u>uilty** about drinking?

   (4) Have you ever had a drink first thing in the morning (**<u>e</u>ye opener**)?

 2. **Tobacco**

  a. **Teens who smoke tobacco** are more likely to try other drugs and have lower academic performance.

  b. **Nicotine is highly addictive.** Most adult smokers begin smoking in their teenage years.

  c. **Health risks of smoking**

   (1) **Coronary artery disease and stroke**

   (2) **Cancers** of the lungs, mouth, esophagus, stomach, larynx, and urinary tract

        (3) Chronic lung disease and asthma

        (4) Peptic ulcer disease

        (5) Pregnancy complications, such as stillbirth, low birth weight, and higher-than-normal infant mortality

    d. More than 3 million teens chew smokeless tobacco. Smokeless tobacco is associated with oral cancers, gingival recession, and low birth weight and premature delivery in mothers who use smokeless tobacco during pregnancy.

  3. Marijuana is the most widely used illicit drug. It is derived from the plant *Cannabis sativa.* The **active ingredient** is tetrahydrocannabinol (THC).

    a. Physical effects typically include tachycardia, mydriasis, sleepiness, conjunctival erythema, dry mouth, auditory and visual hallucinations, increased appetite, and impaired cognition.

    b. Long-term consequences of heavy marijuana use may include asthma, impaired memory and learning, truancy, diminished interpersonal interactions, and depression.

V. Obesity and Eating Disorders

  A. Obesity is one of the most common chronic illnesses among adolescents.

    1. Definition. Obesity is a **body weight 20% greater than ideal body weight.**

      a. Body-mass index (body weight in kilograms divided by height in meters squared) greater than 95% for age and sex is considered obese.

      b. Body fat content may also be determined by measuring skin-fold thickness at the triceps and subscapular areas.

    2. Etiology. Causes are often multifactorial. Obesity is commonly the result of the interaction among genetic factors, increased caloric intake, diminished energy expenditure, and poor eating behaviors. Underlying endocrinologic or genetic causes (e.g., hypothyroidism, Cushing disease, hypogonadism, Prader-Willi syndrome) are found in only 5% of patients.

    3. Health effects associated with obesity

      a. Earlier pubertal development

      b. Hypertension and cardiovascular disease

      c. Hypercholesterolemia and elevated triglycerides

      d. Type 2 diabetes mellitus

      e. Gallbladder disease

      f. Orthopedic problems such as back pain and tibia vara (bowlegs)

      g. Poor body image, depression, and low self-esteem

    4. Management. Treatment is challenging and must be multifaceted. Therapies include modification of eating behaviors, promotion of healthy nutrition, a balanced weight reduction program, exercise, and psychological support.

B. Anorexia nervosa and bulimia nervosa typically occur in females 13–18 years of age.

1. **Epidemiology. Anorexia nervosa** occurs in approximately 0.5–1% of adolescents, and **bulimia nervosa** occurs in approximately 1–5% of adolescents.

2. **Diagnostic criteria for anorexia nervosa**

   a. **Caloric intake is insufficient** to maintain weight or growth.

   b. **Adolescent** has a **delusion of being fat** and an **obsession to become thin.**

   c. Specific criteria

      (1) **Refusal to maintain body weight** at normal weight for age and height. Body weight is **15% below ideal body weight for age.**

      (2) **Intense fear of weight gain** and denial of the seriousness of low weight or weight loss

      (3) **Disturbed body image**

      (4) **Absence** of **three consecutive menstrual cycles**

   d. **Excessive exercise, fluctuating emotions, withdrawal from peers and family, and a preoccupation with food** are often present.

3. **Diagnostic criteria for bulimia nervosa**

   a. **Eating pattern** includes **binge eating,** in which a large volume of food is consumed in a short period of time.

   b. Specific criteria

      (1) **Recurrent episodes of binge eating at least twice weekly for 3 months**

      (2) **Lack of control over eating** during binging. **Anxiety, guilt, or sadness** often occur after each binge.

      (3) **Purging** using vomiting, laxatives, diuretics, or enemas to prevent weight gain

      (4) **Fasting, rigorous exercise, or diet pills** may be used to prevent weight gain.

      (5) **Disturbed body image**

4. **Physical examination and laboratory findings** are described in **Table 3-3.**

5. **Management. Treatment** of an adolescent with anorexia nervosa or bulimia nervosa is challenging and often requires a team approach, including **involvement of the family.**

   a. **Normal nutrition** must be established, anorexic or bulimic behaviors must be relinquished, and the adolescent must gain insight into the reasons behind the disorder. Nutritional guidance and psychological counseling are often required.

   b. **Hospitalization** is necessary if the adolescent has evidence of severe weight loss, electrolyte abnormalities, dehydration, abnormal vital signs, suicidal thoughts, medical complications (such as seizures, cardiac arrhythmias, or pancreatitis), or failure of outpatient medical management (including food refusal).

Table 3-3. Physical Examination and Laboratory Abnormalities in Anorexia Nervosa and Bulimia Nervosa

Eating Disorder	Examination Findings	Laboratory Findings
Anorexia nervosa	Weight ≥ 15% below ideal level Hypothermia Hypotension Bradycardia Delayed growth and puberty Malnourished (wasted, hypoactive bowel sounds, dependent edema, fine lanugo hair) Evidence of dehydration	Anemia Leukopenia Low thyroxine Low glucose Low calcium Low magnesium Low phosphorus Low sex steroids High blood urea nitrogen High liver transaminases
Bulimia nervosa	Less ill-appearing Normal weight (usually) Hypothermia, hypotension, and bradycardia if excessive purging Sequelae of vomiting (trauma to palate and hands, loss of dental enamel, parotid swelling)	Low chloride, low potassium, and high blood urea nitrogen if excessive vomiting

VI. Female Reproductive Health Issues. One half of adolescents are sexually active by the end of high school.

A. Pregnancy

1. **Epidemiology. One million** adolescent females (one of every nine) become pregnant every year in the United States.

   a. **One fifth** of adolescent pregnancies occur within the first month after the teen first commences sexual intercourse.

   b. **Most (80%)** adolescent pregnancies are **unintentional.**

   c. **One half** of adolescent pregnancies result in delivery, **one third** result in abortion, and **one sixth** result in miscarriage.

2. **Associated conditions. Adolescent pregnancy** is a **high-risk pregnancy** associated with increased incidence of:

   a. **Infant health problems,** including **low birth weight** and **higher-than-usual infant mortality**

   b. **Maternal health problems,** including **anemia, hypertension, and preterm labor**

   c. **Dropping out of school**

   d. **Unemployment and need for public assistance**

B. Contraception

1. **One half** of all sexually active adolescents do not use any contraception for one or more of the following reasons:

   a. **Ignorance** of the contraceptive methods available

   b. **Denial** of the risk of pregnancy

   c. **Barriers** toward obtaining contraception, including issues of confidentiality and cost

     d. **Refusal** by partner to use contraception

     e. **Religious beliefs**

     f. **Ambivalence to, or desire for, pregnancy**

  2. **Contraceptive methods**

     a. **Abstinence** offers the greatest protection and should always be discussed as a reasonable option to sexual intercourse.

     b. **Barrier methods** include the male condom, female condom, vaginal diaphragm, and cervical cap.

        (1) **Male condom** is a sheath placed onto the erect penis to prevent passage of sperm into the vagina.

           (a) **Condoms are very important as a barrier against STDs.** Only condoms made of **latex** protect against transmission of the HIV virus.

           (b) **Advantages** include low cost and safety.

           (c) **Disadvantages** include interference with spontaneity and rare allergic reactions.

        (2) **Female condom** is a polyurethane sheath placed **into the vagina** to prevent the passage of sperm.

           (a) **Advantages** include **protection against STDs.**

           (b) **Disadvantages** include vaginal irritation or allergy and awkwardness of placement.

        (3) **Vaginal diaphragm** is a mechanical barrier placed **against the cervix** and used in combination with spermicide.

           (a) **Advantages** include spontaneity. It may be inserted as many as 6 hours before intercourse.

           (b) **Disadvantages** include need for individual fitting by a trained health care professional, awkwardness of placement, and increased risk of urinary tract infection (UTI).

        (4) **Cervical cap** is a cuplike diaphragm placed **tightly over the cervix.**

           (a) **Advantages** include the ability to leave the cap in place for up to 48 hours.

           (b) **Disadvantages** include need for individual fitting, increased risk of UTIs, and need for follow-up Pap smear to screen for cervical dysplasia, which has been associated with the cap.

     c. **Intrauterine devices (IUDs)** can be safe, effective methods of birth control for selected adolescents. Two types of IUDs, the T38A copper-bearing and the progesterone-releasing IUDs, are available.

        (1) **Mechanisms of action** include interference with sperm transport and motility (copper IUD) and induction of endometrial atrophy (progesterone IUD).

        (2) **Advantages** include convenience and privacy.

        (3) **Disadvantages** include lack of protection against STDs, uterine bleeding and cramping, need for insertion by a professional, initial higher cost, and possible increased risk of pelvic inflammatory disease (PID).

   d. **Oral contraceptives** are either a combination of estrogen and pro-
      gesterone or progesterone only.

      (1) **Mechanisms of action** include inhibition of ovulation and thick-
          ening of cervical mucus, which interferes with passage of sperm.

      (2) **Advantages** include decreased dysmenorrhea, regulation of
          menstrual bleeding, possible protection against endometrial and
          ovarian cancer, improved acne, and spontaneity.

      (3) **Disadvantages** include headache, weight gain, amenorrhea,
          breakthrough bleeding, mood changes, nausea, lack of protection
          against STDs, and the need to remember to take the pill daily.

      (4) **Absolute contraindications** to taking oral contraceptives in-
          clude pregnancy, breast or endometrial cancer, stroke, coronary
          artery disease, and liver disease. **Relative contraindications**
          include hypertension, migraine headaches, diabetes, sickle cell
          anemia, elevated lipids, and smoking.

   e. **Contraceptive injections** involve the slow release of the progestin
      depomedroxyprogesterone acetate (Depo-Provera).

      (1) **Advantages** include contraceptive protection for **3 months** after
          each injection.

      (2) **Disadvantages** include need for an intramuscular injection
          every 3 months, irregular bleeding, weight gain, and lack of pro-
          tection against STDs.

   f. **Table 3-4** lists the failure rate for each of the contraceptive methods.

VII. Sexually Transmitted Diseases (STDs). Herpes simplex virus, human papilloma virus (HPV), and *C. trachomatis* are the three most common STDs in the United States.

   A. **Epidemiology**

      1. **STDs** occur most commonly in adolescents and young adults. **Diagnosis
         of one STD** is **strongly associated** with the likelihood of having an-
         other STD.

Table 3-4. Contraceptive Effectiveness

Method	Failure Rate (%)*
Chance	85
Female condom	21–26
Spermicide alone	21
Withdrawal	19
Diaphragm with spermicide	16–18
Cervical cap	17
Male condom	12
Oral contraceptives	3–10
Intrauterine device	< 1–2
Depo-Provera	< 1

*Failure rate is percent accidental pregnancy during first year of typical use.
(Adapted from Neinstein LS. Adolescent Health Care, A Practical Guide. 3rd Ed. Baltimore: Williams &
Wilkins, 1996:678.)

2. **Risk factors** for STDs
   a. **Lack of barrier contraception**
   b. **Young age** at initiation of sexual intercourse
   c. **Spontaneous** sexual encounters
   d. **Multiple sexual partners**
   e. **Concurrent substance abuse**
   f. **Perceived lack of risk**
   g. **Incarceration**
   h. **Teen pregnancy**
   i. **Teens who are homosexual or bisexual**
   j. **Cervical ectopy in adolescent females.** In general, these individuals are at a higher risk because of the presence of cervical ectopy (the presence of cervical columnar epithelium) to which *C. trachomatis* and *N. gonorrhoeae* preferentially attach.

B. **Clinical features**

1. **Vaginitis.** This disorder may be sexually transmitted, in the case of *Trichomonas vaginalis*, or may be caused by bacterial vaginosis or candidal infection, diseases not associated with sexual transmission.
   a. ***T. vaginalis,*** a protozoan, accounts for **15–20%** of cases of adolescent vaginitis.
      (1) **Clinical findings**
         (a) **Malodorous, profuse, yellow-green discharge**
         (b) **Cervix may be friable and covered with petechiae (strawberry cervix).**
         (c) **Vulvar inflammation and itching**
         (d) **Dyspareunia** (pain during sexual intercourse)
         (e) *T. vaginalis* is **asymptomatic** in 50% of males and females.
      (2) **Diagnosis**
         (a) **Wet-mount saline microscopy** is usually sufficient for diagnosis. It demonstrates motile flagellated protozoa.
         (b) **Positive culture** for *T. vaginalis*
         (c) **Vaginal pH > 4.5**
      (3) **Management** includes oral metronidazole. Alcohol ingestion while taking this medication may result in an Antabuse-type reaction with severe vomiting. **Partners should also be treated.**
   b. **Bacterial vaginosis** is the **most common cause** of vaginitis in adolescents and is caused by a change in the vaginal flora because of a reduction of lactobacilli, which are normally present. Fewer lactobacilli result in increased concentration of *Gardnerella vaginalis*, *Mycoplasma hominis,* and anaerobic Gram-negative rods.
      (1) **Clinical findings**
         (a) **Gray-white thin vaginal discharge** that may adhere to the vaginal wall
         (b) **Pungent "fishy" odor**
         (c) **Little vaginal or vulvar inflammation**

(2) Diagnosis

    (a) Positive "whiff test" in which the "fishy" odor is enhanced on addition of 10% potassium hydroxide solution to vaginal secretions

    (b) Presence of "clue cells" on wet-mount saline microscopy (vaginal epithelial cells covered with adherent bacteria, which results in a hazy, granular appearance to the cell borders)

    (c) Typical vaginal discharge

    (d) Vaginal pH > 4.5

(3) Management includes oral metronidazole or topical intravaginal therapy with 2% clindamycin or 0.75% metronidazole gel. **Partners do not require treatment.**

  c. Candidal vulvovaginitis is usually caused by *Candida albicans.*

    (1) Clinical findings

      (a) Severe itching and a **white, curdlike** discharge

      (b) Vulvar and vaginal inflammation

    (2) Diagnosis

      (a) Clinical signs and symptoms

      (b) Fungal hyphae seen on wet-mount saline or potassium hydroxide microscopy

      (c) Normal vaginal pH (< 4.5)

      (d) Positive culture for yeast

    (3) Management includes oral fluconazole or topical intravaginal antiyeast therapies. **Partners do not require treatment.**

2. Cervicitis. This inflammation of the mucous membranes of the endocervix is most commonly caused by *C. trachomatis* or *N. gonorrhoeae.* Other causes include herpes simplex virus and syphilis.

  a. *C. trachomatis* is an intracellular bacterium that infects the cervical columnar epithelium.

    (1) Clinical findings

      (a) Purulent endocervical discharge

      (b) Friable, edematous, erythematous cervix

      (c) Dysuria and urinary frequency

      (d) Fifty percent of males and as many as seventy-five percent of females are asymptomatic.

    (2) Diagnosis

      (a) Culture of the endocervix is the **"gold standard."**

      (b) Nonculture tests, including **rapid antigen detection by direct fluorescent antibody staining** or **enzyme immunoassay,** are very sensitive but have high false-positive rates.

      (c) Newer highly sensitive and specific noninvasive tests, such as polymerase chain reaction (PCR), ligase chain reaction, and nucleic acid hybridization, may be performed on urine or cervical specimens.

    (3) Complications include PID, tuboovarian abscess (TOA), infertility, ectopic pregnancy, chronic pelvic pain, Fitz-Hugh-Curtis syndrome (perihepatitis), and neonatal conjunctivitis and pneumonia.

(4) Management of uncomplicated *C. trachomatis* cervicitis includes oral doxycycline, erythromycin, or azithromycin. **Partners should also be treated.**

b. ***N. gonorrhoeae*** is a Gram-negative intracellular diplococcus that infects the cervical columnar epithelium.

(1) Clinical findings

(a) Mucopurulent endocervical discharge, sometimes with vaginal bleeding

(b) Dysuria and urinary frequency

(c) Dyspareunia

(d) Asymptomatic infection in females is common, and males may also be asymptomatic.

(2) Diagnosis

(a) Culture of endocervical discharge inoculated immediately onto modified Thayer-Martin media is the **"gold standard."**

(b) Gram stain demonstrating intracellular Gram-negative diplococci may be considered evidence of infection in symptomatic patients.

(c) Nonculture tests such as urine PCR, or cervical or urethral nucleic acid hybridization, may also be useful.

(3) Complications include PID, TOA, chronic pelvic pain, neonatal conjunctivitis, Fitz-Hugh-Curtis syndrome, and infertility. Disseminated infection may occur in up to 3% of patients and is characterized by asymmetric polyarthritis, papular and pustular skin lesions, and, rarely, meningitis, endocarditis, and septicemia.

(4) Management of uncomplicated cervicitis caused by *N. gonorrhoeae* includes intramuscular ceftriaxone or single-dose oral therapy with ofloxacin, cefixime, or ciprofloxacin, and treatment for presumptive co-infection with *C. trachomatis* [see VII.B.2.a.(4)]. **Partners should also be treated.**

3. **Pelvic inflammatory disease** (PID). This STD is an ascending infection in which pathogens from the cervix spread to the uterus and fallopian tubes.

a. **Epidemiology**

(1) PID is polymicrobial and may be caused by *N. gonorrhoeae*, *C. trachomatis,* and nongonococcal, nonchlamydial aerobes and anaerobes.

(2) PID is more common in the first half of the menstrual cycle, because menstruation enhances the spread of infection from the lower genital tract.

b. **Clinical findings and diagnosis.** The occurrence of particular signs and symptoms confirms the diagnosis.

(1) All of the following must be present:

(a) Lower abdominal pain and tenderness

 (b) Uterine or cervical motion tenderness

 (c) Unilateral or bilateral adnexal tenderness

(2) One of the following should also be present:

 (a) Fever

 (b) White blood cell (WBC) count > 10,500 cells/mm³

 (c) Inflammatory pelvic mass on bimanual examination or ultrasound

 (d) Elevated erythrocyte sedimentation rate or C-reactive protein

 (e) Laboratory evidence of *N. gonorrhoeae* or *C. trachomatis* in the endocervix

c. Management

(1) Indications for hospitalization include presence of an adnexal mass, uncertainty regarding diagnosis or compliance, pregnancy, or failed outpatient therapy.

(2) Inpatient treatment includes intravenous cefoxitin plus oral doxycycline, or intravenous clindamycin plus intravenous gentamicin.

(3) Outpatient treatment includes 14-day therapy with ofloxacin and clindamycin or single-dose intramuscular ceftriaxone and 14 days of doxycycline.

4. Urethritis. This condition, which is defined as inflammation of the urethra, occurs more commonly in males. Females with urethritis typically have associated cervicitis.

a. Epidemiology. Urethritis is characterized as gonococcal (caused by *N. gonorrhoeae*) or nongonococcal (most commonly caused by *C. trachomatis*). Other causes of nongonococcal urethritis include *Ureaplasma urealyticum, Mycoplasma genitalium,* herpes simplex virus, and *T. vaginalis.*

b. Clinical findings

(1) Dysuria and increased urinary frequency

(2) Mucopurulent urethral discharge

(3) Asymptomatic infections are common.

c. Presumptive diagnosis

(1) Mucopurulent urethral discharge

(2) Greater than five WBCs per high-power field on Gram stain of urethral secretions

(3) Greater than 10 WBCs per high-power field on first-void urine specimen

(4) Positive leukocyte esterase on first-void urine specimen

d. Definitive diagnosis (*C. trachomatis* or *N. gonorrhoeae*). Analysis of material obtained by swabbing the urethra or by examination of discharge or urine using methods described in sections VII.B.2.a.(2) or VII.B.2.b.(2) confirms the diagnosis.

e. Management. Treatment is the same as described in sections VII.B.2.a.(4) or VII.B.2.b.(4).

    5. Genital ulcers. These lesions are most commonly caused by **herpes simplex virus types 1 and 2**, *Treponema pallidum* **(syphilis)**, or *Haemophilus ducreyi* **(chancroid)**. Clinical features, diagnosis, and management are described in **Table 3-5**.

    6. Genital warts

        a. Epidemiology. Genital warts are the **most common STD.**

            (1) Genital warts are caused by **HPV** and are transmitted by direct contact.

            (2) HPV strains 16 and 18 may cause cervical carcinoma but often do not cause visible warts.

            (3) External genital warts are also termed **condylomata acuminata.**

        b. Clinical findings

            (1) Itching, pain, and dyspareunia

            (2) Possibly visible on external genitalia

            (3) May be asymptomatic

        c. Diagnosis

            (1) Warts are diagnosed on direct visual inspection.

            (2) Cervical cancer–causing HPV is detected by **Pap smear** and by **3% acetic acid wash** during colposcopy, which colors HPV lesions white.

        d. Management. Treatment is often difficult, and recurrence is common. Therapies include topical podophyllin and trichloroacetic

Table 3-5. Genital Ulcers: Clinical Features, Diagnosis, and Management

	HSV-1 and -2	Primary Syphilis	Chancroid
Clinical features	Painful, multiple shallow ulcers Constitutional symptoms Inguinal adenopathy	Painless, single ulcer with well-demarcated border and clean base (chancre) Painless inguinal adenopathy	Painful, multiple ulcers with red, irregular borders and purulent bases Painful inguinal adenopathy; nodes may be fluctuant
Diagnosis	Typical lesions and one of the following: Positive Tzanck smear Positive HSV culture from lesion Positive DFA for HSV from lesion Elevated HSV-1 or -2 antibodies HSV on Pap smear	Typical lesion and one of the following: Reactive nontreponemal tests (VDRL or RPR) Reactive treponemal test (FTA-ABS) *Treponema pallidum* on darkfield microscopy, biopsy, or DFA of exudate or tissue	Typical lesions and positive culture for *Haemophilus ducreyi*
Management	Oral acyclovir until resolution Severe infection with disseminated disease requires intravenous acyclovir	Intramuscular penicillin or oral doxycycline if allergic to penicillin	Oral azithromycin, erythromycin, or intramuscular ceftriaxone

HSV = herpes simplex virus; *DFA* = direct fluorescent antibody; *Pap* = Papanicolaou; *VDRL* = Venereal Disease Research Laboratory; *RPR* = rapid plasma reagin; *FTA-ABS* = fluorescent treponemal antibody absorption.

acid, cryotherapy, and surgical and laser removal. Twenty-five percent of genital warts spontaneously disappear within 3 months.

VIII. Menstrual Disorders

A. Normal Menstrual Cycle

1. Characteristics of the normal menstrual cycle.

a. Length of menstrual cycle: 21–35 days

b. Duration of menstrual flow: 2–8 days

c. Blood loss during menstruation: 30–80 mL

2. Three phases of menstrual cycle (Figure 3-4)

a. Follicular (proliferative) phase begins with the onset of menstrual flow and ends with ovulation. This phase lasts 7–22 days.

(1) This phase **begins** with the pulsatile release of gonadotropin-releasing hormone (GnRH) from the hypothalamus, which in turn causes release of LH and FSH from the pituitary.

(2) **FSH** induces maturation of ovarian follicles, which produce increasing amounts of estradiol, which in turn causes endometrial thickening (proliferation).

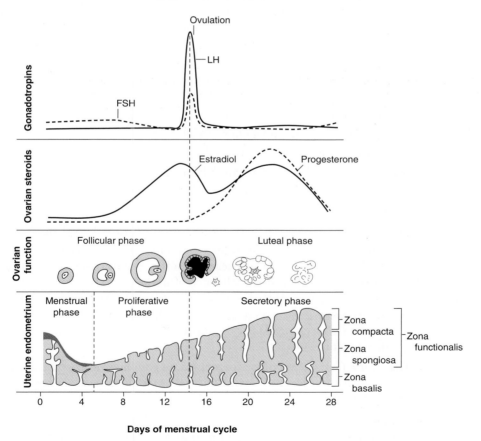

Figure 3-4. The menstrual cycle: pituitary, ovarian, and endometrial correlations. *FSH* = follicle-stimulating hormone; *LH* = luteinizing hormone. (Reprinted with permission from Sakala PE. Obstetrics and Gynecology (Board Review Series). Baltimore: Williams & Wilkins, 1997, p. 9)

b. **Ovulation phase** occurs at midcycle after a **surge** in **LH release** secondary to peaking estradiol levels. The ruptured ovarian follicle develops into a functioning **corpus luteum.**

c. **Luteal (secretory) phase** begins after ovulation and ends with menstrual flow. This phase lasts 12–16 days.

    (1) **Progesterone,** produced by the functioning corpus luteum, creates a secretory endometrium.

    (2) Without fertilization, the corpus luteum involutes. This leads to diminished progesterone and estradiol production, which in turn causes endometrial sloughing and GnRH release from the hypothalamus to start the cycle again.

3. **Menstrual cycles** are usually **irregular for 1–2 years after menarche** because of the lack of consistent ovulation.

B. **Dysmenorrhea.** This condition is the **most common menstrual disorder.**

1. **Definitions.** Dysmenorrhea is defined as **pain associated with menstrual flow.**

a. **Primary dysmenorrhea** refers to **pain that is not associated with any pelvic abnormality.** It is the **most common type of dysmenorrhea** during adolescence.

b. **Secondary dysmenorrhea** refers to **pain associated with a pelvic abnormality,** such as endometriosis, PID, uterine polyps or fibroids, or a bicornuate uterus with obstruction of menstrual flow.

2. **Etiology.** Primary dysmenorrhea is caused by **increased production of prostaglandins** by the endometrium, which results in excessive uterine contractions and systemic effects.

3. **Clinical findings**

a. **Spasms of pain** in the lower abdomen

b. **Nausea,** vomiting, diarrhea, headache, or fatigue

4. **Management.** Prostaglandin inhibitors, such as nonsteroidal anti-inflammatory agents, or oral contraceptives may be useful.

C. **Amenorrhea**

1. **Definitions.** Amenorrhea is the **absence of menstrual flow.**

a. **Primary amenorrhea** refers to the absence of any menstrual bleeding by **age 16** in an adolescent **with normal secondary sexual characteristics,** or the absence of menstrual bleeding by **age 14** in an adolescent **without secondary sexual characteristics.**

b. **Secondary amenorrhea** refers to the absence of menses for either three menstrual cycles or 6 months **after regular menstrual cycles have occurred.**

2. **Etiology.** Causes may be categorized on the basis of the presence or absence of normal genitalia and normal secondary sexual characteristics (Table 3-6).

3. **Clinical evaluation**

a. **Thorough history and physical examination,** including a pelvic examination

Table 3-6. Causes of Amenorrhea

Cause	Findings
Primary amenorrhea with normal genitalia and pubertal delay	
Turner syndrome (46, XO)	Ovarian failure caused by gonadal dysgenesis **High FSH and LH**
Ovarian failure before puberty caused by radiation, chemotherapy, or infection	**High FSH and LH**
Hypothalamic or pituitary failure before puberty	**Low FSH and LH**
Primary amenorrhea with absent uterus and normal pubertal development	
Testicular feminization syndrome (46, XY) X-linked defect in androgen receptor leading to inability to respond to testosterone	Female genital appearance; vagina ends in blind pouch; inguinal or intra-abdominal testes **Low FSH and LH**
Mayer-Rokitansky-Küster-Hauser syndrome (46, XX)	Vagina and uterus are congenitally absent **Normal FSH and LH**
Primary or secondary amenorrhea with normal genitalia and normal pubertal development	
Hypothalamic suppression Medications and drug abuse Stress and chronic illness Exercise or weight loss	**Low FSH and LH**
Polycystic ovary syndrome	**High LH and high LH/FSH ratio** Obesity, hirsutism, and acne
Pituitary infarction (Sheehan's syndrome) or pituitary failure	**Low FSH and LH**
Prolactinoma	**Low FSH and LH, high prolactin;** prolactin inhibits GnRH release Headache, visual field defect
Outflow tract obstruction Imperforate hymen Transverse vaginal septum Uterine adhesions	**Normal FSH and LH**
Premature ovarian failure Pregnancy Endocrine disorders Thyroid disease Diabetes mellitus	**High FSH and LH**

FSH = follicle-stimulating hormone; *LH* = luteinizing hormone; *GnRH* = gonadotropin-releasing hormone.

      b. Pregnancy test to confirm or rule out pregnancy

      c. Thyroid-stimulating hormone and **thyroxine levels** to confirm or rule out thyroid disorders

      d. Fasting prolactin level to identify a **prolactinoma.** If the prolactin level is high, neuroimaging is necessary to exclude a tumor of the sella turcica.

      e. FSH and LH levels

        (1) High FSH and LH levels indicate ovarian failure. Chromosomal analysis should be performed to evaluate for Turner syndrome.

        (2) Low FSH and LH levels indicate hypothalamic or pituitary suppression or failure. Visual fields and neuroimaging of the sella turcica should be performed to exclude tumor.

D. Abnormal Vaginal Bleeding

1. Definitions

  a. Dysfunctional uterine bleeding (DUB) causes **90%** of abnormal vaginal bleeding in adolescents. **DUB** describes a syndrome of **frequent, irregular menstrual periods,** often associated with **prolonged, painless bleeding.**

  b. Polymenorrhea is uterine bleeding that occurs at **regular intervals of < 21 days.**

  c. Menorrhagia is **prolonged or excessive** uterine bleeding that occurs at **regular intervals.**

  d. Metrorrhagia is uterine bleeding that occurs at **irregular intervals.**

  e. Menometrorrhagia is **prolonged or excessive** uterine bleeding that occurs at **irregular intervals.**

  f. Oligomenorrhea is uterine bleeding that occurs at **regular intervals** but **no more often than every 35 days.**

2. Etiology

  a. DUB may result from **anovulatory cycles.**

    (1) The endometrium becomes excessively thickened and unstable because of unopposed estrogen production.

    (2) Ovulation does not occur, so progesterone is not available to stabilize the endometrium.

    (3) Bleeding occurs spontaneously and frequently, and it is often prolonged because of weaker-than-usual uterine and vascular contractions.

    (4) Many conditions that cause amenorrhea, such as stress, drug abuse, chronic illness, thyroid disease, weight loss, excessive exercise, and polycystic ovary syndrome, may also cause DUB.

  b. Complications of pregnancy, including threatened or incomplete abortion, and ectopic pregnancy

  c. Infections such as PID and cervicitis

  d. Blood dyscrasias such as **von Willebrand disease** and immune thrombocytopenic purpura

  e. Cervical or vaginal polyps and hemangiomas

  f. Uterine abnormalities, including leiomyoma and endometriosis

  g. Medications, including salicylates, oral contraceptives, and anabolic steroids

  h. Foreign bodies such as IUDs or retained condoms or tampons

  i. Trauma or sexual assault

3. Clinical evaluation

  a. History should document the dates of the last three menstrual cycles, age at menarche, prior menstrual patterns, presence or absence of pain, and amount of bleeding.

b. **Physical examination** should include a pelvic examination if bleeding is painful, prolonged, or associated with anemia, or if the adolescent is sexually active.

c. **Laboratory testing,** in most cases, should include a complete blood count, pregnancy test, evaluation for *N. gonorrhoeae* and *C. trachomatis*, and evaluation for a blood dyscrasia if very heavy bleeding is present.

4. **Management. Treatment of DUB** involves cessation of bleeding and prevention of endometrial hyperplasia.

a. **Hormonal therapy should be used for all bleeding associated with anemia.** Combination oral contraceptives or progestin-only contraceptives are used to stabilize the endometrium and convert it to a secretory form. Intravenous hormonal therapy may be required for severe bleeding.

b. **Iron** should be prescribed for patients with anemia.

c. **Dilation and curettage** is also effective but should only be used if hormonal therapies fail.

IX. Reproductive Health Issues in Males

A. **Gynecomastia** is a bilateral or unilateral increase in the glandular and stromal breast tissue normally found in up to **60% of male adolescents.**

1. **Etiology is unknown.** However, gynecomastia is probably caused by increased sensitivity to estrogen or increased peripheral conversion of adrenal androgens to estrogen.

2. **Although gynecomastia is usually normal, the differential diagnosis** includes side effects of medications, testicular tumors, and thyroid and liver disease.

3. **Laboratory studies are not necessary** if growth is normal, the adolescent is healthy, and puberty has begun.

4. **Management** involves **reassurance.** Gynecomastia usually resolves within 12–15 months.

B. **Painful Scrotal Masses**

1. **Torsion of the spermatic cord** is the **most common** and **most serious cause** of acute painful scrotal swelling.

a. **Clinical findings**

(1) **Sudden onset** of scrotal, inguinal, or suprapubic pain, often accompanied by nausea and vomiting

(2) **Swollen, tender testicle** and scrotal edema with **absent cremasteric reflex on the affected side**

(3) **Pain relief** on elevation of twisted testicle, although this is often unreliable

b. **Diagnosis** is usually made by history and physical examination alone, although torsion may be confirmed by **decreased uptake** on **technetium 99m pertechnetate radionuclide scan** or **absent pulsations** on **Doppler ultrasound** of the scrotum.

   c. **Management** includes **surgical detorsion** of the involved testicle and **fixation of both testes** within the scrotum (the opposite testicle also has a high likelihood of torsion). Detorsion is a **urologic emergency that must be performed within 6 hours to reliably preserve testicular function.**

  2. Torsion of testicular appendage may be confused with torsion of the spermatic cord.

   a. **Clinical findings**

    (1) **Acute or gradual onset** of pain in testicular, inguinal, or suprapubic areas. Tenderness is most pronounced at the upper pole of the testicle.

    (2) **"Blue dot sign"** on examination of the scrotum. This represents the cyanotic appendage visible through the skin of the scrotum.

   b. **Diagnosis** is usually made by history and physical examination alone. Doppler ultrasound and radionuclide scans are **normal** or show increased flow or uptake.

   c. **Management** includes rest and analgesia. Pain usually resolves within 2–12 days.

  3. Epididymitis is infection and inflammation of the epididymis, occurring most commonly in sexually active males.

   a. **Etiology.** Epididymitis is most commonly secondary to infection with *N. gonorrhoeae* or *C. trachomatis*.

   b. **Clinical findings**

    (1) **Acute onset** of scrotal pain and swelling associated with urinary frequency, dysuria, or urethral discharge.

    (2) **Swollen, tender** epididymis

   c. **Diagnosis** is made by urinalysis demonstrating increased WBCs, a positive Gram stain, and a positive culture of urethral discharge. Doppler ultrasound shows **increased flow,** and a radionuclide scan demonstrates **increased uptake.**

   d. **Management** is similar to that for cervicitis [see VII.B.2.a.(4) and VII.B.2.b.(4)]. In addition, analgesics and bed rest are appropriate.

C. Painless Scrotal Masses

  1. Testicular neoplasms originate from germ cells within the testicle and are **one of the most common malignant solid tumors** in males 15–35 years of age. Cryptorchidism refers to testes that fail to descend into the scrotum. This condition is associated with a higher risk of malignancy.

   a. **Clinical findings**

    (1) **Firm, irregular, painless** nodule on testicle

    (2) **Solid mass** seen on scrotal transillumination

   b. **Diagnosis and evaluation**

    (1) **Doppler ultrasound** of scrotum

   (2) Evaluation for serum tumor markers human chorionic go-nadotropin and **α-fetoprotein**

   (3) Evaluation for distant metastasis

   c. **Management** includes surgery, radiation, and chemotherapy.

2. **Indirect inguinal hernia** occurs when the processus vaginalis fails to obliterate. This results in a defect within the abdominal wall that allows bowel to extend through the internal inguinal ring.

   a. **Clinical findings** include a **painless inguinal swelling.** Bowel sounds may be present on auscultation of the scrotum.

   b. **Diagnosis** is based on history and physical examination.

   c. **Management** includes referral for elective repair. Emergent referral is necessary if evidence of bowel incarceration is noted (erythema of overlying skin, pain, and tenderness).

3. **Hydroceles.** These are collections of fluid within the tunica vaginalis.

   a. **Clinical findings** include the presence of a **painless, soft, cystic** scrotal mass that may be smaller in the morning and larger in the evening.

   b. **Diagnosis** is based on history and physical examination. **Transillumination** of scrotum reveals a cystic mass.

   c. **Management** includes reassurance. If the hydrocele is very large or painful, referral for surgical repair is indicated.

4. **Varicoceles** result from dilation and tortuosity of veins in the pampiniform plexus. Varicoceles occur in **10–20%** of male adolescents.

   a. **Clinical findings**

   (1) Most commonly found in the left half of the scrotum

   (2) Characterized as a "bag of worms" appreciated on palpation, which diminishes in size when the patient is supine and enlarges with standing and with the Valsalva maneuver.

   b. **Diagnosis** is based on history and physical examination.

   c. **Management** includes reassurance. If the varicocele is painful or very distended, or is associated with a small testicle (indicative of diminished blood flow), a urology referral is indicated.

Review Test

1. A 12-year-old boy has been brought to your office by his mother, who is concerned that her son has not developed any signs of puberty. She recalls that her older daughter began pubertal development when she was younger than her son is now. Which of the following is correct regarding the normal sequence of pubertal development in males and females?

(A) Pubic hair growth is the first sign of puberty in females.
(B) Pubic hair growth is the first sign of puberty in males.
(C) Puberty begins in males 6–12 months later than in females.
(D) Facial hair growth in males begins at the same time as pubic hair growth.
(E) Menarche occurs at the same time as thelarche.

2. A 15-year-old girl presents for a routine health care visit. During your HEADSS assessment (home, education and employment, activities, drugs, sexual activity, suicide and depression), she reveals that she has been sexually active with one partner (her current boyfriend). You emphasize the importance of effective contraception. Which one of the following methods of contraception is associated with the highest failure rate with typical use?

(A) Oral contraceptive
(B) Intrauterine device
(C) Depomedroxyprogesterone acetate
(D) Vaginal diaphragm
(E) Male condom

3. A healthy-appearing short 15-year-old girl presents with primary amenorrhea, normal genitalia, and delayed pubertal development. Follicle-stimulating hormone and luteinizing hormone levels are high. Which of the following tests is most useful in diagnosing the most likely cause of her amenorrhea?

(A) Karyotype
(B) Prolactin level
(C) Thyroid function tests
(D) Pregnancy test
(E) Computed tomography scan of her sella turcica

4. A 15-year-old boy has had worsening left scrotal pain for the past 24 hours, a tender left testicle, and a bluish discoloration visible through his scrotal skin. Which of the following is correct regarding the evaluation and management of his scrotal pain?

(A) Urinalysis will demonstrate increased white blood cells.
(B) Cremasteric reflex will be absent on the affected side.
(C) Pain medication should be prescribed and bed rest recommended because this condition will resolve without surgical intervention.
(D) Immediate surgical intervention is indicated.
(E) Technetium 99m pertechnetate scan will show decreased uptake.

5. You are evaluating a 16-year-old girl who has had vaginal discharge for 5 days. Examination reveals purulent endocervical discharge. Her abdomen is nontender, she is afebrile, and she denies abdominal pain. Gram stain of the discharge reveals intracellular Gram-negative diplococci. Which of the following is the most appropriate treatment?

(A) Oral azithromycin
(B) Intramuscular ceftriaxone
(C) Hospitalization and treatment with intravenous clindamycin and intravenous gentamicin
(D) Intramuscular ceftriaxone plus oral azithromycin
(E) Oral penicillin plus oral doxycycline

6. A 15-year-old boy presents for a routine health maintenance visit. On examination you note bilateral breast enlargement and Tanner stage 5 pubertal development. The remainder of the examination is unremarkable. Which of the following is the most appropriate next step in management?

(A) Order chromosomal analysis.
(B) Order studies of thyroid function.
(C) Order studies of hepatic function.
(D) Order a serum estrogen level.
(E) Order no tests and provide reassurance that the condition will resolve spontaneously.

7. A sexually inactive 14-year-old girl presents with concerns that her current menstrual period, which is painless, has lasted 13 days and is associated with a moderate amount of bleeding. This menstrual period began 2 weeks after her previous period stopped; it lasted 15 days. A complete blood count reveals moderate anemia. Which of the following statements is correct regarding the management of this problem?

(A) Reassure her that her menstrual cycle is normal for her age and prescribe an iron supplement.
(B) Perform a complete pelvic examination, and if it is normal, reassure her that her condition is normal and no treatment is required.
(C) Perform a complete pelvic examination, and if it is normal, prescribe a progestin-only contraceptive.
(D) Prescribe combination oral contraceptives. (A pelvic examination is not necessary.)
(E) Perform a dilation and curettage.

8. A 15-year-old girl is 9 weeks pregnant with her first child. She does not want to terminate the pregnancy and would like advice and pregnancy-related care. Which of the following statements regarding her pregnancy is correct?

(A) She is at no higher risk than other teens to eventually require public assistance.
(B) She would be expected to have a lower-than-usual risk of having a sexually transmitted disease.
(C) Her parents must be informed and provide consent for medical management of her pregnancy.
(D) Her infant would not be expected to have a higher-than-usual risk of neonatal problems.
(E) Despite her young age, she is at higher-than-usual risk of hypertension and preterm labor.

9. A 17-year-old girl is brought to your office at her parents' request. They are worried because she has had diminished interest in family activities, has been fighting more often with her parents, and is spending more time alone in her room. During the past 6 months, her school performance has worsened, and her school principal recently telephoned her parents about school absenteeism. In addition, parents have noticed that she is hanging out with a new group of friends and that her appetite seems diminished. Which of the following statements regarding the management of this adolescent is most likely to be correct?

(A) She has major depressive disorder and should be seen urgently by a psychiatrist.
(B) Reassurance should be provided; her behavior is normal for age and psychosocial development.
(C) She should see a nutritionist with expertise in eating disorders.
(D) She should be evaluated for possible substance abuse.
(E) She and her parents should be interviewed together to uncover the cause of her problems.

10. A 16-year-old runaway adolescent presents to the free clinic with complaints of diffuse abdominal pain, fever, and nausea. She denies dysuria or vaginal discharge. On further questioning, she indicates she has had five sexual partners during the past year and most of the time uses condoms for protection. Pelvic examination reveals moderate lower abdominal tenderness and tenderness on palpation of her cervix and right ovary. No adnexal mass is appreciated. Which of the following statements regarding diagnosis and management is correct?

(A) Hospitalization and treatment with intravenous cefoxitin and oral doxycycline are warranted.
(B) Wet-mount saline microscopy will demonstrate motile protozoa, and oral metronidazole should be prescribed.
(C) Outpatient treatment with oral doxycycline for 2 weeks, along with one dose of intramuscular ceftriaxone, is indicated.
(D) Oral azithromycin alone should be prescribed for presumptive diagnosis of Fitz-Hugh-Curtis syndrome.
(E) Outpatient treatment with single-dose oral ofloxacin and oral azithromycin is warranted after attempts are made to obtain parental consent.

11. A 14-year-old girl is brought to the office for a routine health maintenance visit. She appears very thin, yet believes she is overweight and needs to lose 15–20 pounds. Her mother is concerned that her daughter frequently skips breakfast and eats only a small portion of her dinner, usually alone in her bedroom. She argues often with her parents, and she immediately goes to her room on coming home from school or the gym. You believe that she may have an eating disorder. Which of the following is correct regarding the expected diagnosis?

(A) Her menstrual cycles would be unaffected and normal.
(B) Physical examination would demonstrate a lower-than-normal sexual maturity rating for age.
(C) Withdrawal from friends would not occur because she will use them for support.
(D) With further discussion at a subsequent medical visit, it is likely she will gain insight into her illness and will seek treatment.
(E) Her weight is likely to be 10% below her ideal body weight for age.

The response options for statements 12 and 13 are the same. You will be required to select one answer for each statement in the set.

(A) *Haemophilus ducreyi*
(B) *Treponema pallidum*
(C) Herpes simplex virus type 2
(D) Human papillomavirus
(E) None of the above

For each patient, select the most likely causative organism.

12. An 18-year-old adolescent female with a single painless genital ulcer with a well-demarcated border, and painless inguinal adenopathy.

13. A 16-year-old adolescent female with multiple painful ulcers with a purulent-appearing base and irregular borders as well as painful inguinal adenopathy.

Answers and Explanations

1. The answer is C [I.A.2]. Both puberty and somatic growth begin earlier in females. Puberty occurs 6–12 months later in males and begins with testicular enlargement. Puberty in females begins with breast development. Pubic hair begins to grow after the beginnings of breast development in females and testicular enlargement in males. Facial and axillary hair growth begins in males 18–24 months after pubic hair. Menarche, the start of menstrual cycles, occurs an average of 2–3 years after thelarche, the beginnings of breast development.

2. The answer is D [VI.B.2.b and Table 3-4]. The vaginal diaphragm has the highest rate of failure with typical use among the methods listed. Failure is often related to lack of use during each episode of intercourse, lack of knowledge regarding proper placement, lack of use of spermicide, and improper fit. Depomedroxyprogesterone acetate and oral contraceptives are very effective contraceptive agents with low failure rates. Intrauterine devices and male condoms have a higher failure rate than hormonal contraception but are usually more effective in practice than the vaginal diaphragm.

3. The answer is A [VIII.C and Table 3-6]. This girl has primary amenorrhea, which is defined as the absence of menstrual bleeding either after age 16 in a girl with normal secondary sexual characteristics or, as in this case, after age 14 in a girl with delayed pubertal development. Disorders characterized by primary amenorrhea, normal genitalia, and delayed puberty include Turner syndrome, ovarian failure, and hypothalamic or pituitary failure. In this healthy-appearing, short girl, Turner syndrome (46,XO) is most likely, and thus a karyotype would be most useful for diagnosis. A prolactinoma and thyroid disease may result in either primary or secondary amenorrhea, but the follicle-stimulating hormone (FSH) level would be decreased or normal. A pituitary lesion would also usually result in normal or low FSH, and thus computed tomography or magnetic resonance imaging of the brain would be less useful. Pregnancy would be unlikely given the presence of pubertal delay.

4. The answer is C [IX.B.2]. This boy presents with classic findings of torsion of the left testicular appendage, which is characterized by acute or gradual onset of scrotal pain, tenderness at the upper pole of the testicle, and a "blue dot sign" reflecting the cyanosis and torsion of the testicular appendage. This condition normally resolves without surgery, and rest and pain medication are indicated. Urinalysis is normal, and the cremasteric reflex is still present. Doppler ultrasound demonstrates normal or increased blood flow, and radionuclide imaging demonstrates normal or increased uptake on the affected side, unlike torsion of the spermatic cord.

5. The answer is D [VII.B.2.b]. The presence of Gram-negative intracellular diplococci confirms the diagnosis of *Neisseria gonorrhoeae* cervicitis. The correct treatment for uncomplicated cervicitis caused by *N. gonorrhoeae* includes intramuscular ceftriaxone, oral ofloxacin, oral ciprofloxacin, or oral cefixime. However, any patient with *N. gonorrhoeae* also requires treatment for *Chlamydia trachomatis* because coinfection is very common. Thus, the most appropriate treatment includes therapy against *N. gonorrhoeae* and either oral azithromycin, erythromycin, or doxycycline for the treatment of presumptive *C. trachomatis*. Hospitalization is not indicated for uncomplicated cervicitis. The absence of abdominal pain or tenderness excludes pelvic inflammatory disease. Because of drug resistance, oral penicillin is inadequate for the treatment of *N. gonorrhoeae*.

6. The answer is E [IX.A]. Gynecomastia, the development of breast tissue, occurs in up to 60% of males during adolescence. If a male adolescent is healthy and has progressed normally through puberty, as in this case, no laboratory tests are necessary, and reassurance alone is sufficient management. Neither an estrogen level nor a karyotype would be useful in light of a male sexual maturity rating of Tanner stage 5. Although thyroid and liver disorders may result in breast enlargement, other signs or symptoms suggesting a systemic disease would likely be apparent on physical examination.

7. The answer is C [VIII.D.3 and VIII.D.4]. This girl likely has dysfunctional uterine bleeding (DUB), the cause of 90% of abnormal vaginal bleeding in adolescence. She also is anemic and, as a result, needs hormonal therapy to regulate her menstrual cycles. Because of her moderate anemia, a pelvic examination should be performed to rule out other causes of abnormal vaginal bleeding before prescribing hormonal therapy. Either a daily progestin-only contraceptive or combination oral contraceptives would be effective in stopping her bleeding. Dilation and curettage is only performed when other therapies fail.

8. The answer is E [VI.A.2]. Adolescent pregnancy dramatically affects both mother and infant. Teens who are pregnant are at higher-than-usual risk of hypertension, anemia, and preterm labor. In addition, adolescent mothers have a high rate of not completing high school, have a higher-than-normal rate of unemployment, and often need welfare assistance. Adolescents who are pregnant are also at a higher risk for sexually transmitted disease. In the majority of states, adolescents are entitled to seek pregnancy-related care without parental consent. Their infants are at higher-than-usual risk for health problems, such as low birth weight.

9. The answer is D [IV.C]. The signs and symptoms of substance abuse include disturbance in mood or sleep, decline in school performance, truancy, alterations in family relationships and peer groups, and diminished appetite. These behaviors are not normal at any age. This adolescent does not meet the criteria for major depressive disorder, although depression can occur with, and result from, substance abuse. Decreased appetite alone is insufficient to diagnose anorexia nervosa or bulimia nervosa. Although both the adolescent and her parents may be interviewed jointly, she should also be interviewed independently to facilitate rapport and discussion of confidential issues.

10. The answer is A [VII.B.3]. The constellation of clinical findings, including lower abdominal pain and tenderness, adnexal tenderness, and cervical motion tenderness, are sufficient to make a diagnosis of pelvic inflammatory disease (PID). Although many cases of PID can be effectively treated as an outpatient with oral medications, hospitalization is indicated for situations in which compliance with therapy may be problematic, as in a homeless or runaway adolescent. In addition, hospitalization is warranted for pregnant teens with PID, for those who have an adnexal mass suggesting a tuboovarian abscess, or for those who fail outpatient management. This patient's clinical findings are not consistent with *Trichomonas vaginalis,* which is diagnosed by a wet-mount saline preparation, nor with Fitz-Hugh-Curtis syndrome (perihepatitis), which presents with right upper quadrant pain.

11. The answer is B [Table 3-3 and V.B]. This girl's history of low body weight, disturbed body image, and withdrawal from her family are consistent with anorexia nervosa. In addition to these characteristics, patients with anorexia nervosa also have amenorrhea, a weight 15% below ideal body weight for age, an intense fear of gaining weight, delays in puberty and growth, and a preoccupation with food and sometimes with exercise in order to burn calories. In addition to withdrawal from family, teens with anorexia nervosa often withdraw from friends. Insight into the illness is lacking, and management of eating disorders is very challenging. Input from nutritionists and therapists and the involvement of a supportive family are essential.

12, 13. The answers are B and A, respectively [Table 3-5]. Genital ulcers may be caused by chancroid (infection with *Haemophilus ducreyi*), syphilis (infection with *Treponema pallidum*), or herpes simplex virus types 1 and 2. Syphilis is characterized by a single painless ulcer that has a well-demarcated border and a nonpurulent base (a chancre). In contrast, chancroid is characterized by painful ulcers that have irregular borders and a purulent base. Inguinal adenopathy is present in both diseases; however, it tends to be painful in chancroid and painless in syphilis. Herpes simplex virus also causes multiple painful shallow ulcers, but the base is nonpurulent. Human papillomavirus causes genital warts, not ulcers.

Part 2

Specific Problems

4

Neonatology

Marta Rogido, M.D., Augusto Sola, M.D and Lee Todd Miller, M.D.

I. **Evaluation of the Newborn.** Features of the newborn examination that differ from those of children and adolescents include:

    A. **General Appearance**

        1. Careful observation is necessary to assess spontaneous activity, passive muscle tone, respirations, and abnormal signs, such as cyanosis, intercostal muscle retractions, or meconium staining.

        2. **Apgar scores** are a simple, systematic assessment of intrapartum stress and neurologic depression at birth, conducted at 1 and 5 minutes after birth (**Table 4-1**). A persistently very low Apgar score indicates the need for resuscitation, and scoring should be continued every 5 minutes until a final score of 7 or more is reached.

    B. **Skin Examination.** Texture differs with gestational age; skin is softer and thinner in premature infants.

        1. **Lanugo** is the thin hair that covers the skin of preterm infants. It is minimally present in term infants.

Table 4-1. Apgar Scoring System*

Score	0	1	2
Heart rate	Absent	< 100/min	> 100/min
Respirations	Absent	Slow, irregular	Good, crying
Muscle tone	Limp	Some flexion	Active motion
Reflex irritability (response to catheter in nose)	No response	Grimace	Cough, sneeze, cry
Color	Blue, pale	Body pink, blue extremities	Completely pink

*Five variables are evaluated at 1 and 5 minutes after birth, and each one is scored from 0 to 2. The final score is the sum of the five individual scores, with 10 representing the optimal score. A persistently very low score indicates the need for resuscitation, and scoring should be continued every 5 minutes until a final score of 7 or more is reached.

2. **Vernix caseosa** is a thick, white, creamy material found in term infants; it covers large areas of the skin in preterm infants. It is usually absent in postterm infants.

3. **Color** is pink a few hours after birth, but **acrocyanosis** (cyanosis of the hands and feet) is very frequent during the first 48–72 hours, and in some infants it can last throughout the first month of life, particularly when the infant is cold. Acrocyanosis and **cutis marmorata** (mottling of the skin with venous prominence) are frequent intermittent signs of the vasomotor instability characteristic of some infants.

4. **Pallor** may be a sign of neonatal asphyxia, shock, sepsis, or anemia.

5. **Jaundice** is **always abnormal if detected within the first 24 hours of birth.** Subsequently, it is frequently seen during the first few days after birth but usually is not associated with serious disease (see section X).

6. **Milia** are very small cysts formed around the pilosebaceous follicles, which appear as tiny, whitish papules that are seen over the nose, cheeks, forehead, and chin. They usually disappear within a few weeks and do not require treatment.

7. **Mongolian spots** are dark blue hyperpigmented macules over the lumbosacral area and buttocks of no pathologic significance. These areas of pigmentation are most frequently seen in Hispanic, Asian, and African American infants.

8. **Pustular melanosis** is a benign transient rash characterized by small, dry superficial vesicles over a dark macular base. This rash is more frequently seen in African American infants. Pustular melanosis must be differentiated from viral infections, such as herpes simplex, and from bacterial infections, such as impetigo.

9. **Erythema toxicum neonatorum** is a benign rash seen most frequently in the first 72 hours after birth, characterized by erythematous macules, papules, and pustules (resembling "flea bites") on the trunk and extremities but not on the palms and soles. The rash occurs in about 50% of full-term infants and is found much less frequently in preterm infants. Lesions are filled with **eosinophils.** No treatment is required.

10. **Nevus simplex** (or **"salmon patch"** or telangiectatic nevus) is the **most common vascular lesion of infancy,** occurring in 30–40% of newborns and appearing as a pink macular lesion on the nape of the neck (**"stork bite"**), upper eyelids, glabella, or nasolabial region. It is often transient.

11. **Nevus flammeus,** or **"port wine stain,"** is a congenital vascular malformation composed of dilated capillary-like vessels (a form of capillary hemangioma) that may be located over the face or trunk and may become darker with increasing postnatal age. Those located in the area of the ophthalmic branch of the trigeminal nerve (cranial nerve V-1) may be associated with intracranial or spinal vascular malformations, seizures, and intracranial calcifications (**Sturge-Weber syndrome**).

12. **Strawberry hemangiomas** are benign proliferative vascular tumors occurring in approximately 10% of infants. Often first noticed a few days after birth, they increase in size after birth and usually resolve within

18–24 months. Hemangiomas that compromise the airway or vision require intervention.

13. **Neonatal acne** occurs in approximately 20% of newborns. It appears after 1–2 weeks of life and is virtually never present at birth. Typically, the lesions are comedones, but inflammatory pustules and papules may be present. No treatment is necessary.

C. Craniofacial Examination

1. **Head**

   a. **Microcephaly,** or head circumference below the 10th percentile, may be familial but may also be caused by structural brain malformations, chromosomal and malformation syndromes, congenital infections (e.g., cytomegalovirus, toxoplasmosis), or fetal alcohol syndrome.

   b. **Caput succedaneum** is diffuse edema or swelling of the soft tissue of the scalp that **crosses the cranial sutures** and usually the midline.

   c. **Cephalohematomas** are subperiosteal hemorrhages secondary to birth trauma **confined and limited by the cranial sutures,** usually involving the parietal or occipital bones.

   d. **Craniosynostosis** is premature fusion of the cranial sutures, which may result in abnormal shape and size of the skull.

   e. **Craniotabes** are soft areas of the skull with a "Ping-Pong ball" feel. They may occur in the parietal bones and are not related to rickets. They usually disappear within weeks or months.

2. **Ears** should be examined to assess maturity. By term, the ears are firm and have assumed their characteristic shape. The ears should also be inspected for preauricular tags or sinuses and for appropriate shape and location.

3. **Eyes.** An abnormal **red reflex** of the retina may be caused by cataracts, glaucoma, retinoblastoma, or severe chorioretinitis.

4. **Nose.** The nose should be examined immediately to rule out unilateral or bilateral **choanal atresia.** If this is suspected, it can be excluded by passing a nasogastric tube through each nostril.

5. **Mouth**

   a. **Clefts** of the lip and of the soft and hard palates are easily noted by inspection, but submucous clefts in the soft portion of the palate should be ruled out by digital palpation. These clefts may be isolated or associated with other dysmorphic features.

   b. **Micrognathia,** a small chin, should be noted. Micrognathia, together with cleft palate, glossoptosis (downward displacement or retraction of the tongue), and obstruction of the upper airway, can be found in **Pierre Robin syndrome.**

   c. **Macroglossia** may suggest Beckwith-Wiedemann syndrome (hemihypertrophy, visceromegaly, macroglossia), hypothyroidism, or a mucopolysaccharidosis.

   d. **Neonatal teeth** may be seen rarely, usually in the area of the lower incisors.

e. **Epstein pearls** are small, white epidermoid-mucoid cysts found on the hard palate, which usually disappear within a few weeks.

D. **Neck and Clavicle Examination**

1. **Lateral neck** cysts or sinuses include **branchial cleft cysts** and **cystic hygromas.**

2. **Midline clefts or masses** may be caused by cysts of the **thyroglossal duct** or by goiter secondary to maternal antithyroid medication or transplacental passage of long-acting thyroid-stimulating antibodies.

3. **Neonatal torticollis,** or asymmetric shortening of the sternocleidomastoid muscle, may result from being in a fixed position in utero or from a postnatal hematoma resulting from birth injury.

4. **Edema and webbing** of the neck suggest **Turner syndrome.**

5. **Clavicles** should be examined to rule out fractures, which may occur during delivery, most commonly of large neonates.

E. **Chest Examination**

1. **Accessory nipples**, which may be present along the anterior axillary or midclavicular lines, may later grow because of the presence of glandular tissue in these areas.

2. **Congenital deformities,** such as **pectus carinatum** (prominent and bulging sternum) and **pectus excavatum** (depressed sternum), are generally benign. **Chest asymmetry**, as a result of absence of the formation of ribs or agenesis of the pectoralis muscle (**Poland syndrome**), may be more serious.

F. **Respiratory Examination.** Respiratory distress is diagnosed if **tachypnea** (respiratory rate > 60 breaths/min), deep respirations, cyanosis, expiratory grunting, or intercostal or sternal retractions are present. Preterm infants breathe irregularly with short, apneic bursts that last less than 5–10 seconds and have no clinical significance (**periodic breathing**).

G. **Cardiac Examination.** Evaluation should include heart rate (normal is 95–180 beats/min and varies during feeding, sleep, or crying), rhythm, and assessments for murmurs and peripheral pulses.

1. **Diminished femoral pulses.** Consider coarctation of the aorta.

2. **Increased femoral pulses.** Consider patent ductus arteriosus.

H. **Abdominal Examination**

1. **Umbilicus.** The umbilical cord should be inspected to confirm the presence of **two arteries and one vein** and the absence of a urachus (see section I.H.5). The presence of only one umbilical artery may suggest congenital renal anomalies.

2. **Diastasis recti** is the separation of the left and right side of the rectus abdominis at the midline of the abdomen. It is a common condition in newborns, especially in premature and African American infants. No treatment is necessary because the diastasis recti gradually disappears as the infant develops and as the rectus abdominis muscles grow.

3. An **umbilical hernia** is caused by the incomplete closure of the umbilical ring. The hernia is noticed as a soft swelling beneath the skin around the umbilicus that often protrudes during crying or straining. Umbilical hernias occur slightly more frequently in African American children. Most close spontaneously and usually no treatment is required. Those that persist beyond 4–5 years of age and those that cause symptoms may require surgical treatment.

4. **Omphalocele and Gastroschisis**—see sections XII.C.1 and XII.C.2.

5. **Persistent urachus** is the complete failure of the urachal duct to close. This results in a fistula between the bladder and the umbilicus and may present with urine draining from the umbilicus, especially when pressure is applied over the bladder.

6. **Meconium plug** is obstruction of the left colon and rectum caused by dense dehydrated meconium. **Meconium ileus** is the occlusion of the distal ileum caused by inspissated (thickened and dried) and viscid meconium, usually secondary to a deficiency of pancreatic enzymes and the resulting abnormally high protein content of intestinal secretions. Meconium plug and meconium ileus, which can be the first manifestations of **cystic fibrosis,** cause delay in the elimination of meconium, resulting in abdominal distension. Normally, meconium stool is passed within 24 hours after birth in 90% of term infants and within 48 hours in 99%.

7. **Abdominal masses** in the neonate may be caused by **hydronephrosis** (most common), multicystic kidneys, ovarian cysts, or other lesions. If the liver can be palpated on the left side, situs inversus, asplenia, or polysplenia syndrome may be present.

8. The **anus** should be examined for patency. On rare occasions, an imperforate anus may not be visible. Anal patency can be confirmed with careful introduction of either a soft rubber catheter or a rectal thermometer into the anus.

I. **Genitalia Examination.** The genitalia should be examined to assess gestational age and to exclude anomalies.

1. **Female genitalia**

   a. A **hypertrophied clitoris** may result from virilization from androgen excess associated with virilizing adrenal hyperplasia (see Chapter 6, section III.E). This condition may also be seen in premature infants.

   b. **Hydrometrocolpos** is caused by an imperforate hymen with retention of vaginal secretions. It presents as a small cyst between the labia at the time of birth or as a lower midline abdominal mass during childhood.

2. **Male genitalia**

   a. **Hypospadias** describes the urethral meatus located not in its normal position at the tip of the penis but rather on the ventral surface of the penis in varying locations along the shaft. It is **not associated** with an increased incidence of associated urinary malformations.

   b. **Epispadias** describes the urethral meatus located on the dorsal surface of the penis. Epispadias **is often associated** with bladder extrophy (bladder protrusion from the abdominal wall with exposure of its mucosa).

    c. Hydrocele is a scrotal swelling caused by fluid accumulation in the tunica vaginalis adjacent to the testis. Although isolated hydroceles usually cause no clinical problems and often resolve spontaneously within a few weeks, some hydroceles are associated with inguinal hernias (see Chapter 3, section IX.C.3).

    d. Cryptorchidism, or undescended testes, may be associated with inguinal hernia, genitourinary malformations, hypospadias, and genetic syndromes. In most males with cryptorchidism, the testes descend spontaneously before 12 months of age. Cryptorchid testes that do not descend by this age are predisposed to future malignancy.

J. Extremity Examination. The extremities should be examined to detect anatomic and functional abnormalities. The lack of spontaneous movements in the upper extremities may suggest fractures, infection, or brachial plexus injury.

    1. Absence or hypoplasia of the radius may be associated with **TAR syndrome** (*t*hrombocytopenia *a*bsent *r*adii), Fanconi anemia, and Holt-Oram syndrome.

    2. Polydactyly may occur as an isolated anomaly or as part of a genetic syndrome.

    3. Edema of the feet with hypoplastic nails is characteristic of **Turner** and **Noonan** syndromes.

    4. Rocker bottom feet is frequently seen in **trisomy 18.**

    5. The **hips** should be examined for **developmental dysplasia of the hips** (see Chapter 17, section III.A).

K. Spine Examination. The spine should be examined for the presence of **hair tufts,** lipomas, or dimples in the lumbosacral area, which may suggest the presence of **spina bifida.** If a sacrococcygeal pilonidal dimple is present, a careful attempt to identify the base should be made to rule out a neurocutaneous sinus tract. A myelomeningocele (hernial protrusion of the cord and its meninges through a defect in the vertebral canal) may be present anywhere along the spine and is usually obvious at the time of birth.

L. Neurologic Examination. Evaluation of muscle tone, level of alertness, and primitive reflexes should be performed (see Chapter 2, Table 2-2).

II. Abnormalities of Maturity

A. Preterm Delivery

    1. Definition. A **preterm** delivery occurs less than 37 completed weeks from the first day of the last menstrual period.

    2. Incidence. Preterm delivery occurs in approximately 7% of all births, but this figure varies widely across the United States and throughout the world. The incidence is higher in lower socioeconomic populations and in women who do not receive prenatal care.

Table 4-2. Frequent Problems of Preterm Infants

Disrupted mother–father–infant interaction
Perinatal asphyxia
Hypothermia
Hypoglycemia
Hypocalcemia
Respiratory distress syndrome (hyaline membrane disease; surfactant deficiency syndrome)
Fluid and electrolyte abnormalities
Indirect hyperbilirubinemia
Patent ductus arteriosus
Intracranial hemorrhage
Necrotizing enterocolitis
Infections
Retinopathy of prematurity
Bronchopulmonary dysplasia
Anemia

3. **Complications. Premature infants** may have complications from the time of birth to the first several weeks of life, as presented in **Table 4-2.**

B. **Post-term Delivery**

1. **Definition.** A **post-term** delivery occurs 42 weeks or more from the first day of the last menstrual period.

2. **Complications** include increased incidence of fetal and neonatal morbidity and death from the consequences of placental insufficiency, including severe intrauterine asphyxia, meconium aspiration syndrome, and polycythemia.

III. Growth Abnormalities

A. **Small-for-gestational-age (SGA) infants and intrauterine growth retardation (IUGR)**

1. **Definition.** Infants that are born weighing below the fifth percentile for corresponding gestational age as a result of **IUGR** are considered **SGA.**

2. **Significance.** SGA is a sign that intrauterine growth has either stopped or slowed significantly some time during pregnancy.

3. **Etiology.** Causes of **IUGR** are listed in **Table 4-3.**

4. **Clinical features. Clinical problems** of SGA infants are listed in **Table 4-4.**

B. **Large-for-gestational-age (LGA) infants**

1. **Definition.** Newborns are considered **LGA** if their birth weight is > 90th percentile for their gestational age at birth. These infants should be distinguished from those infants born with **high birth weight** (birth weight > 4,000 g). A newborn may be LGA with a birth weight > 90th per-

Table 4-3. Causes of Intrauterine Growth Retardation

Type I: Early interference with fetal growth from conception to 24 weeks gestation
Chromosomal anomalies (trisomy 21, 13–15, 18, and so forth)
Fetal infections (TORCH)
Maternal drugs (chronic alcoholism, heroin)
Maternal chronic illness (hypertension, severe diabetes mellitus)

Type II: Intrauterine malnutrition from 24 to 32 weeks gestation
Inadequate intrauterine space (multiple pregnancies, uterine tumors, uterine anomalies)
Placental insufficiency from maternal vascular disease (renal failure, chronic essential hypertension, collagen vascular diseases, pregnancy-induced hypertension)
Small placenta with abnormal cellularity

Type III: Late intrauterine malnutrition after 32 weeks gestation
Placental infarct or fibrosis
Maternal malnutrition
Pregnancy-induced hypertension
Maternal hypoxemia (lung disease, smoking)

TORCH = *t*oxoplasmosis, *o*ther (syphilis), *r*ubella, *c*ytomegalovirus, *h*erpes simplex virus.

Table 4-4. Clinical Problems of Small-for-Gestational-Age Infants

Perinatal asphyxia
Hypothermia
Hypoglycemia
Polycythemia
Thrombocytopenia
Hypocalcemia
Meconium aspiration syndrome
Intrauterine fetal death
Hypermagnesemia (if mother is treated with magnesium for hypertension or preterm labor)

centile for the gestational age at birth, without having an absolute birth weight above 4,000 g.

2. **Etiology. Common causes** of increased weight and LGA include maternal diabetes, Beckwith-Wiedemann syndrome, Prader-Willi syndrome (see Chapter 5, section III.A.2), and nesidioblastosis (diffuse proliferation of pancreatic islet cells).

3. **Complications.** LGA infants, with or without high birth weight, frequently have hypoglycemia and polycythemia. Inappropriately increased weight for gestational age is often associated with congenital malformations.

IV. Cyanosis

A. **Definition.** Cyanosis is bluish discoloration of the skin and mucous membranes that is directly related to the absolute concentration of unoxygenated or reduced hemoglobin (more than 3 g/dL of reduced Hgb in arterial blood, or more than 5 g/dL in capillary blood).

B. Clinical significance. In the neonate, **cyanosis always constitutes an emergency,** requiring immediate diagnosis and treatment.

C. Etiology. Causes are extensive and include respiratory pathology (e.g., pneumothorax); the "5 T's" of cyanotic congenital heart disease (*t*etralogy of Fallot, *t*ransposition of the great vessels, *t*runcus arteriosus, *t*ricuspid atresia, and *t*otal anomalous pulmonary venous connection—see also Chapter 8, section IV); central nervous system pathology (e.g., intraventricular hemorrhage); hematologic disorders (e.g., polycythemia); and metabolic disorders (e.g., hypoglycemia, hypocalcemia, hypothyroidism, and hypothermia).

D. Evaluation

1. **Initial steps.** Evaluation includes a detailed history and physical examination, serum electrolytes with serum glucose, arterial blood gas (ABG; ± 100% oxygen test), complete blood count (CBC), and chest radiograph (CXR). At times, cultures, pre- and postductal PaO_2 measurements, electrocardiogram, and echocardiogram may be warranted.

2. **100% oxygen test.** ABG is performed after administration of 100% oxygen. The 100% oxygen test helps evaluate whether cyanosis is caused by cardiac or respiratory disease.

   a. **Oxygen test in infants with heart disease.** In infants with cyanotic congenital heart disease with reduced pulmonary blood flow (e.g., tetralogy of Fallot), administering 100% oxygen increases the PaO_2 only slightly, usually less than 10–15 mm Hg. However, in infants with cyanotic congenital heart disease associated with normal or increased pulmonary blood flow (e.g., truncus arteriosus), PaO_2 usually increases more than 15–20 mm Hg with 100% oxygen, but levels above 150 mm Hg are unusual.

   b. **Oxygen test in infants with lung disease.** The PaO_2 **usually increases considerably** when 100% oxygen is given, often reaching levels greater than 150 mm Hg. The exception to this rule is that some infants with severe lung disease or with persistent pulmonary hypertension of the newborn (see section VII) may have large right-to-left shunts through the foramen ovale or ductus arteriosus. Therefore, the PaO_2 may not increase by more than 10–15 mm Hg with 100% oxygen.

E. Management. Immediate treatment of cyanosis may be necessary and often includes administration of oxygen and rapid correction of abnormalities of temperature, hematocrit, and glucose and calcium levels. In severely cyanotic infants, intubation and mechanical ventilation may be necessary until a final diagnosis is made and definitive treatment is initiated.

V. Respiratory Distress

A. General Concepts. Respiratory problems are among the most significant causes of morbidity and mortality during the neonatal period. **Respiratory distress syndrome (RDS; also termed hyaline membrane disease and surfactant deficiency syndrome)** in preterm infants and **meconium aspiration syndrome** (MAS) and **persistent pulmonary hypertension of**

the **newborn** (PPHN) in full-term infants are the more common pulmonary causes of respiratory distress.

B. Clinical features. Manifestations include tachypnea, decreased air entry or gas exchange, retractions (intercostal, subcostal, or suprasternal), grunting, stridor, flaring of the alae nasi, and cyanosis. Many of these signs are nonspecific responses of the newborn to serious illness.

C. Etiology. Causes are extensive and involve multiple organ systems because many conditions that produce neonatal respiratory distress are not primary diseases of the lungs (**Figure 4-1**).

VI. Respiratory Distress Syndrome (RDS)

A. Definition. RDS is the respiratory distress or respiratory insufficiency caused by a lack of surfactant, most frequently in preterm infants.

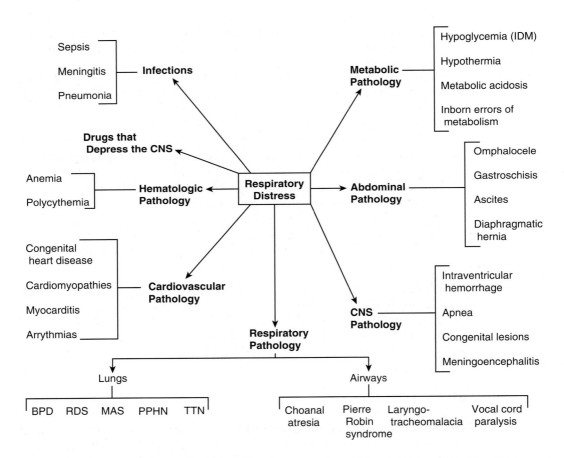

Figure 4-1. Differential diagnosis of respiratory distress in neonates. *CNS* = central nervous system; *RDS* = respiratory distress syndrome; *BPD* = bronchopulmonary dysplasia; *MAS* = meconium aspiration syndrome; *PPHN* = persistent pulmonary hypertension of the newborn; *TTN* = transient tachypnea of the newborn; *IDM* = infant of diabetic mother.

B. Pathophysiology

1. **Pulmonary surfactant** is the surface-active material that decreases alveolar surface tension and prevents atelectasis. Although surfactant is first noted at approximately 23–24 weeks gestation, a sufficient quantity is produced only after 30–32 weeks gestation; after this period, the incidence of RDS decreases significantly.

2. **Assessment of fetal lung maturity** can be made by determining the presence of surfactant in amniotic fluid obtained by amniocentesis. A lecithin-to-sphingomyelin (**L:S**) **ratio** greater than 2:1 and the presence of **phosphatidylglycerol** (a minor phospholipid in surfactant) are indicators of fetal lung maturity.

C. Epidemiology

1. **Incidence.** RDS affects approximately 0.5% of all neonates and is the **most frequent cause of respiratory distress in preterm infants.** The incidence is higher in **white individuals** and in **males.** Risk is higher the younger the gestational age (e.g., 50% have RDS if born before 30 weeks gestation, but only 10% have RDS if born at 35–36 weeks).

2. **Risk factors.** The risk of RDS increases with a low L:S ratio, prematurity, a mother with a previous preterm infant with RDS, a mother with diabetes mellitus, neonatal hypothermia, and neonatal asphyxia.

D. Clinical Features. Infants show increasing respiratory distress during the first 24–48 hours of life, with tachypnea, retractions, expiratory grunting, and cyanosis. Clinical features are more severe and prolonged in preterm infants of less than 31 weeks gestation.

E. Evaluation. A **CXR** is diagnostic and shows diffuse atelectasis with an increased density in both lungs and a fine, granular, **ground-glass** appearance of the lungs. The small airways are filled with air and are clearly seen surrounded by the increased density of the pulmonary field, creating **air bronchograms.**

F. Management

1. **Supplemental oxygen** is necessary.

2. **Continuous positive airway pressure (CPAP),** a technique for maintaining end-expiratory airway pressure greater than atmospheric pressure for the spontaneously breathing infant, promotes air exchange. CPAP may be applied via nasal prongs or nasopharyngeal tubes.

3. **Mechanical** ventilation may be indicated if hypercarbia and respiratory acidosis develop.

4. **Exogenous surfactant** administered into the trachea is often curative.

G. Complications

1. **Acute complications** include air leaks (e.g., pneumothorax and pulmonary interstitial emphysema), intraventricular hemorrhage, sepsis, and right-to-left shunt across a patent ductus arteriosus (PDA).

2. **Chronic complications**
   a. **Bronchopulmonary dysplasia** (BPD). This term is often used to describe chronic lung disease (CLD). BPD is defined as progressive

pathologic changes in the immature lung affecting both the parenchyma and airways, altering normal lung growth. The diagnosis is based on clinical and radiographic criteria:

   (1) Mechanical ventilation during the first 2 weeks of life

   (2) Clinical signs of respiratory compromise persisting beyond 28 days of life

   (3) Need for supplemental **oxygen** beyond 28 days of life

   (4) Characteristic CXR

  b. Retinopathy of prematurity (see Chapter 18, section VII.)

H. Prognosis. With aggressive treatment in an intensive care nursery, > 90% of infants with RDS survive.

VII. Persistent Pulmonary Hypertension of the Newborn (PPHN)

A. Definition. PPHN is any condition, other than congenital heart disease, associated with low blood flow to the lungs after birth. It occurs most frequently in near-term, full-term, or post-term infants.

B. Etiology. Causes are extensive, but **perinatal asphyxia** and **MAS** are most common. The perinatal history is often remarkable for fetal distress.

C. Pathophysiology. Increased pulmonary vascular resistance results in significant right-to-left shunting through the foramen ovale or ductus arteriosus with resulting hypoxemia.

D. Clinical Features. Severity is variable, ranging from cyanosis to respiratory failure. PaO_2 is often significantly decreased in response to minimal inspired oxygen changes or stimulation, and pre- and postductal PaO_2 are notably different.

E. Evaluation

  1. CXR findings are variable because of the many causes of this syndrome. Usually, pulmonary vascular markings are decreased initially in infants with idiopathic PPHN not caused by MAS or perinatal asphyxia.

  2. Echocardiogram is important to rule out congenital heart disease and to assess the degree of pulmonary hypertension and right-to-left shunting.

F. Management

  1. Prevention of hypoxemia is the cornerstone of therapy because hypoxemia is a potent pulmonary vasoconstrictor. **Oxygen** is the most potent pulmonary vasodilator.

  2. Mechanical ventilation must be started early if oxygen alone is insufficient.

  3. In severe cases, and for infants who do not respond to usual measures, high-frequency ventilation and extracorporeal membrane oxygenation **(ECMO)** are generally needed.

  4. Inhaled **nitric oxide** may also be of value as a potent pulmonary vasodilator.

VIII. Meconium Aspiration Syndrome (MAS)

A. Definition

1. **Meconium** (first stools) is a material in the fetal gut that consists of water, mucopolysaccharides, desquamated skin and gastrointestinal mucosal epithelial cells, vernix, bile salts, and amniotic fluid.

2. **MAS** describes an acute respiratory disorder caused by the aspiration of meconium into the airways of the fetus or neonate.

B. Pathophysiology.
Meconium is often passed as a consequence of distress (i.e., hypoxemia) in the fetus at term and becomes more frequent after 42 weeks gestation. The degree of meconium-stained amniotic fluid (MSAF) varies from slightly green to dark green and thick consistency (pea-soup). The MSAF may reach the distal airways and alveoli in utero if the fetus becomes hypoxic and develops gasping or deep respiratory movements, or may occur at the time of birth with the first inspirations.

C. Clinical Features.
Patients with MAS present with signs and symptoms of mild or moderate respiratory distress. Some eventually develop severe respiratory failure with severe hypoxemia and cyanosis.

D. Evaluation.
MAS is suggested by a history of meconium noted at, or before, delivery and the presence of respiratory distress. **CXR** reveals increased lung volume with diffuse patchy areas of atelectasis and parenchymal infiltrates alternating with hyperinflation. Pneumothorax or pneumomediastinum may occur.

E. Management.
Prevention is of paramount importance. The best approach to MSAF is a combined obstetric and pediatric approach and may include suctioning on the perineum and direct suctioning of the trachea via endotracheal intubation. Generally oxygen is required, and if the MAS is severe, mechanical ventilation or ECMO may be necessary. Complications include PPHN, bacterial pneumonia, and long-term reactive airway disease.

IX. Apnea of Prematurity

A. Definition.
Apnea of prematurity is a respiratory pause without airflow lasting more than 15–20 seconds, or a respiratory pause of any duration if accompanied by bradycardia and cyanosis or oxygen desaturation, as evidenced by pulse oximetry monitoring.

B. Categories of Apnea

1. **Central apnea** describes a complete cessation of chest wall movements and no airflow.

2. **Apnea secondary to airway obstruction** describes chest wall movements or respiratory efforts but without airflow. Commonly available apnea monitors do not record obstructive apnea because they continue to detect chest wall movements.

3. **Mixed apnea** is a combination of central and obstructive apnea and constitutes the **most frequent type** encountered in preterm infants.

C. **Etiology. Causes of apnea in preterm infants** include neonatal infections, lung disease, hypothermia, hyperthermia, hypoglycemia, seizures, maternal drugs, drug withdrawal, anemia, and gastroesophageal reflux, in addition to idiopathic apnea of prematurity.

D. **Idiopathic Apnea of Prematurity**

1. **Incidence.** Frequency increases with decreasing gestational age. Incidence is as high as 85% in infants < 28 weeks gestation, and 25% in infants 33–34 weeks gestation.

2. **Clinical features.** Idiopathic apnea of prematurity occurs in the absence of any identifiable cause, usually appearing 24 hours after birth and during the first week of life. It usually resolves by postconceptional age of 38–44 weeks (gestational age at birth plus number of weeks of postnatal age).

3. **Management.** Idiopathic apnea of prematurity is a diagnosis of exclusion, and therefore a search for underlying causes must be undertaken. Management principles include:

   a. Maintenance of a neutral thermal environment, treatment of hypoxia, and proprioceptive stimulation

   b. **Respiratory stimulant medications** as needed (**caffeine** or **theophylline**)

   c. Ventilation as needed (bag and mask as initial management for a severe apneic episode)

   d. CPAP or mechanical ventilation

X. Neonatal Jaundice

A. **Definition.** Jaundice is yellowish discoloration of mucous membranes and skin as a result of increased bilirubin levels. It usually occurs during the first week of life and is most frequently caused by indirect (unconjugated) hyperbilirubinemia that is **physiologic** in nature. **Visible jaundice** occurs in the neonate when serum bilirubin levels exceed 5 mg/dL.

B. **Classification of Jaundice**

1. **Physiologic jaundice**

   a. **Definition.** This term describes the benign and self-limited **indirect hyperbilirubinemia** that typically resolves by the end of the first week of life and requires no treatment.

   b. **Causes of physiologic jaundice**

      (1) Increased bilirubin load on hepatocytes

      (2) Delayed activity of the hepatic enzyme glucuronyl transferase

   c. **Clinical features.** Manifestations include jaundice in well-appearing infants and elevated indirect bilirubin levels. Peak serum concentrations in normal full-term infants reach 5–16 mg/dL at around 3–4 days of life and then start to decrease before the first week of life. In preterm infants, the peak bilirubin is reached after 5–7 days and may take 10–20 days before decreasing.

2. Nonphysiologic jaundice. This term describes jaundice that is secondary to a pathophysiologic cause and it may be further classified as follows:

    a. Indirect hyperbilirubinemia is an elevated bilirubin in which the conjugated or direct component is < 15% of the total bilirubin level.

    b. Direct hyperbilirubinemia is a conjugated or direct bilirubin level that is > 15% of the total bilirubin level. This is **always pathologic in neonates.**

C. Differential Diagnosis of Indirect Hyperbilirubinemia. Possible diagnoses include physiologic jaundice, causes of excessive bilirubin production, causes of impaired clearance of bilirubin from the blood, and causes of defective conjugation of bilirubin by the liver (**Figure 4-2**). Breastfeeding is associated with higher peak bilirubin levels as compared with formula feeding, and the resulting indirect hyperbilirubinemia is of two types:

    1. Breastfeeding jaundice typically occurs during the **first week** of life with increased bilirubin levels and is usually related to suboptimal milk intake. Poor intake leads to weight loss, dehydration, and decreased passage of stool, with resultant decreased excretion of bilirubin in the stool.

    2. Breast milk jaundice typically occurs **after the first week of life** and is likely related to breast milk's high levels of β-glucuronidase and high

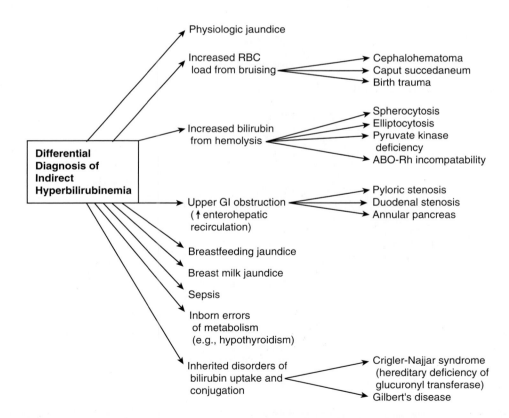

Figure 4-2. Differential diagnosis of indirect hyperbilirubinemia. *RBC* = red blood cell; *GI* = gastrointestinal.

lipase content. Elevated bilirubin is highest in the second and third weeks of life, and lower levels of bilirubin may persist until 10 weeks of life.

D. Differential Diagnosis of Direct Hyperbilirubinemia. Possible diagnoses include obstruction of the hepatobiliary tree, neonatal infection, and metabolic disorders (**Figure 4-3**).

E. Evaluation of Hyperbilirubinemia

1. **Jaundice should always be evaluated under the following circumstances:**

   a. Jaundice appears at < 24 hours of age.

   b. Bilirubin rises > 5–8 mg/dL in a 24-hour period.

   c. The rate of rise of bilirubin exceeds 0.5 mg/dL per hour (suggestive of hemolysis).

2. To evaluate **indirect hyperbilirubinemia,** CBC, reticulocyte count, and smear (for hemolysis) are necessary. Evaluation for sepsis may be indicated.

3. To evaluate **direct hyperbilirubinemia,** hepatic ultrasound (to evaluate for choledochal cyst), serologies for viral hepatitis, and radioisotope scans of the hepatobiliary tree are necessary. Evaluation for sepsis may be indicated.

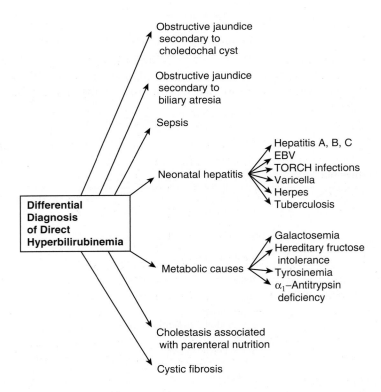

Figure 4-3. Differential diagnosis of direct hyperbilirubinemia. *EBV* = Epstein-Barr virus; *TORCH* = *t*oxoplasmosis, *o*ther (syphilis), *r*ubella, *c*ytomegalovirus, *h*erpes simplex virus.

F. Management

1. **Serial bilirubin assessments, observation, and reassurance** are appropriate for **physiologic jaundice.**

2. **Phototherapy,** which creates water-soluble photoisomers of indirect bilirubin that are more readily excreted, may be indicated depending on the infant's gestational maturity, age, bilirubin levels, and risk factors, if present (e.g., blood group incompatibility and suspected sepsis).

3. **Exchange transfusion** is performed for rapidly rising bilirubin levels secondary to hemolytic disease.

G. Complications include **kernicterus and bilirubin encephalopathy.**

1. Indirect bilirubin at sufficiently high concentrations can pass through the blood-brain barrier and produce irreversible damage.

2. Bilirubin most frequently localizes in the **basal ganglia**, hippocampus, and some brainstem nuclei.

3. **Clinical features** include **choreoathetoid cerebral palsy, hearing loss, opisthotonus,** seizures, and oculomotor paralysis.

XI. Infants of Drug-Abusing Mothers

A. Epidemiology

1. **Incidence.** In approximately 10–15% of pregnancies in the United States, fetuses are exposed to illicit drugs while in utero.

2. **Drugs used.** Most women who use illicit drugs take multiple drugs. Use of alcohol, cocaine, amphetamines, phencyclidine (PCP), and narcotics may compound the fetal risk in women already using tobacco, caffeine, or prescribed drugs.

3. **Risk factors**
   a. **Maternal risk factors** include inadequate prenatal care, anemia, endocarditis, hepatitis, tuberculosis, HIV, sexually transmitted diseases, low self-esteem, and depression.
   b. **Obstetric complications** associated with maternal drugs include abruptio placentae, precipitous delivery, and preterm labor and delivery.

B. Clinical Features. Manifestations vary with the specific drug, some of which cause both intoxication and a withdrawal syndrome. The most common signs are **jitteriness** and **hyperreflexia,** together with **irritability, tremulousness, feeding intolerance,** and **excessive wakefulness.** Their presence in a neonate should alert the clinician to the possibility of drug exposure, which may be identified by toxicology screens of urine or meconium. Infants born to women using drugs should be identified early in the neonatal period and observed for complications and withdrawal effects.

C. Mortality rates range from 3 to 10%, and fetal demise can occur in utero from withdrawal. Causes of mortality include perinatal asphyxia, congenital anomalies, child abuse, and sudden infant death syndrome.

XII. Surgical Conditions of the Newborn

A. Esophageal Atresia with Tracheoesophageal Fistula

1. **Epidemiology.** This condition occurs in 1:2,000–3,000 infants and is often associated with polyhydramnios. The **most common type** of esophageal atresia (> 90% of cases) involves atresia of the esophagus (proximal pouch) with a distal tracheoesophageal fistula.

2. **Clinical features**
   a. History of polyhydramnios
   b. Copious oropharyngeal secretions with increased risk of choking and aspiration pneumonia, particularly if feeding is attempted
   c. **Associated malformations** are found in 50% of patients with esophageal atresia and may include congenital heart disease, anorectal, skeletal, or renal malformations, or the VACTERL association (see Chapter 5, section III.A.8).

3. **Evaluation and diagnosis.** An oral gastric tube is inserted until it meets resistance. Radiographs show the tube in the upper part of the thorax. In type III, air that has crossed through the distal fistula from the trachea is seen in the stomach.

4. **Management. Surgical repair** consists of closure of the fistula and anastomosis of the two esophageal segments.

B. Congenital Diaphragmatic Hernia

1. **Overview.** The diaphragm develops between the fifth and eighth weeks of gestation. Abnormalities in the development of the diaphragm may allow herniation of the abdominal contents into the thorax, which in turn impairs appropriate growth and maturation of the lungs. Most cases involve the **left** diaphragm in the posterior and lateral area.

2. **Epidemiology.** The **incidence** is 1:4,000–5,000 live births.

3. **Clinical features.** The diagnosis may be made by ultrasound in utero (especially when there is a history of polyhydramnios). Newborns present with a **scaphoid abdomen** (with abdominal contents in the thorax). Severe **respiratory insufficiency** from pulmonary hypoplasia (abdominal contents within the chest prevents adequate development of the lungs) with severe hypoxemia and acidosis may occur. Breath sounds are decreased, and bowel sounds may be heard in the chest. The condition has a wide spectrum of clinical severity.

4. **Evaluation. Chest radiographs** reveal little or no gas in the abdomen, absence of the diaphragmatic dome, significant mediastinal shift to the contralateral side (usually to the right), and bowel loops in the thorax (usually on the left side).

5. **Management.** Bag-and-mask ventilation should **not** be used because this may distend the bowel and increase compression of the lung. Intubation and mechanical ventilation with 100% oxygen should be initiated immediately. Correction of acidosis, hypoxemia, and hypercarbia are paramount. Once the infant is stabilized, management includes surgical reduction of

the hernia and closure of the diaphragmatic defect. Fetal surgery is now being performed at some centers for defects identified by prenatal ultrasound.

6. **Complications.** PPHN, pneumothorax, and gastrointestinal complications may develop.

7. **Prognosis** is related to the size of the defect, the volume of the hernia inside the thorax, and the duration of the hernia in utero. These factors are associated with the degree of pulmonary hypoplasia and the severity of the clinical presentation. Fetal and neonatal mortality is still high (50% or greater) in infants in whom the condition is diagnosed before 25 weeks gestation.

C. **Abdominal Wall Defects.** By the 10th week of gestation, the midgut enters the abdomen. If this process is disturbed, the result is an abdominal wall defect associated with a decrease in intra-abdominal volume. **Omphalocele** and **gastroschisis** are the more common defects, both of which require surgical treatment.

1. **Omphalocele** occurs in approximately 1:6,000–8,000 live births. The defect is localized **centrally** in the abdomen (i.e., through the umbilical ring area), and there is a true hernia sac (abdominal organs are **covered with a peritoneal sac**). Omphaloceles are frequently associated with other congenital anomalies, including congenital heart defects (most commonly tetralogy of Fallot and atrial septal defects), Beckwith-Wiedemann syndrome, and some chromosomal disorders (trisomy 13 or, less frequently, trisomy 18; see also Chapter 5, section III.B).

2. **Gastroschisis** is a congenital fissure of the anterior abdominal wall, usually located in the **right paraumbilical area** (i.e., **not in the midline**). There is no true hernia sac (**no peritoneal sac covering**), and the bowel is usually the only viscera that herniates. There is no increased association with other congenital anomalies, but there is an increased risk of bowel damage (e.g., ischemia) from exposure of the abdominal contents to the amniotic fluid.

D. **Intestinal Obstruction.** Intestinal obstruction may be functional or mechanical, and if mechanical, may be acquired or congenital (see **Figure 4-4** for a complete differential diagnosis).

1. **Intestinal atresia** is the **most common cause of obstruction in the neonatal period**. It can occur in the small or large bowel. Intestinal atresias are discussed in Chapter 10, section IV.C.

2. **Meconium ileus** is a manifestation of cystic fibrosis during the neonatal period. Abnormal accumulation of intestinal secretions and deficiency of pancreatic enzymes presumably cause increased viscosity of meconium, leading to occlusion of the distal ileum.

   a. **Clinical features** include abdominal distension, lack of meconium passage, and vomiting.

   b. **Diagnosis** is by abdominal radiographs that reveal intestinal distension with minimal air-fluid levels. Air remains trapped in the meconium; thus, there is no definite air-fluid interface. Fine gas bubbles may be seen mixed within meconium, producing a characteristic **soap-bubble** appearance.

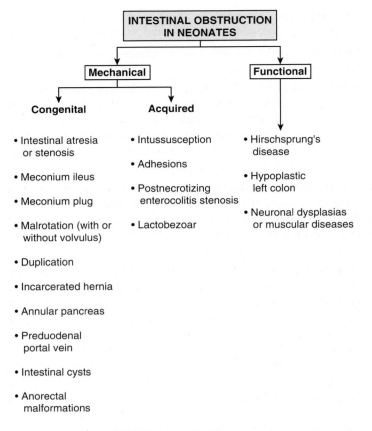

Figure 4-4. Differential diagnosis of intestinal obstruction in neonates.

    c. Management often includes enemas to relieve the obstruction. Early diagnosis and treatment are important to avoid intestinal perforation, meconium peritonitis, and volvulus.

3. Intestinal malrotation may be caused by a **volvulus** (loops of intestine twist if attached to a narrow band of mesentery) with restricted circulation to the rotated (or obstructed) segment, leading to intestinal gangrene. Malrotation and volvulus are discussed in Chapter 10, section IV.B.

4. Hirschsprung disease. Hirschsprung disease, or congenital aganglionic bowel disease, is caused by a lack of caudal migration of the ganglion cells from the neural crest. It produces contraction of a distal segment of colon, causing obstruction with proximal dilatation.

    a. Incidence is approximately 1:5,000 live births. Hirschsprung disease is five times more frequent in **male** infants, and in 80% of cases there is a family history.

    b. Clinical features include constipation, vomiting, and abdominal distension.

    c. Diagnosis is by rectal biopsy, revealing absence or paucity of ganglion cells.

    d. Management includes resection of the affected segment or colostomy.

E. **Necrotizing Enterocolitis (NEC)**

1. **Epidemiology.** NEC is one of the most common surgical conditions in neonates. It is most frequent in preterm infants, with an incidence as high as 8–10% in infants < 30 weeks gestation.

2. **Clinical features.** Manifestations include abdominal distension, abdominal tenderness, residual gastric contents, bilious aspirate, bloody stools, and abdominal erythema. Metabolic acidosis and oliguria may be present, and NEC may lead to thrombocytopenia, disseminated intravascular coagulation, and death.

3. **Diagnosis.** Classic radiographic findings include abdominal distension, air-fluid levels, thickened bowel walls, **pneumatosis intestinalis** (air in the bowel wall), and venous portal gas. Pneumoperitoneum is suggestive of perforation.

4. **Management**
   a. **Medical treatment** includes bowel rest, no oral feeds, gastric decompression, antibiotics, and parenteral fluids and nutrition. If shock is present, volume infusions and pressors are indicated.
   b. **Surgical management** with exploratory laparotomy is indicated for pneumoperitoneum, presence of a fixed loop on serial radiographs, or a positive paracentesis. Treatment may include resection of necrotic bowel.

5. **Late complications.** Intestinal obstruction (e.g., adhesions, strictures), nutritional deficiencies (e.g., malabsorption, short gut syndrome), and cholestasis may occur.

XIII. Hypoglycemia

A. **Definition.** Hypoglycemia is serum glucose concentration below 40 mg/dL.

B. **Etiology. Causes** are extensive and include:

1. **Conditions that result in insulin excess. Infants of diabetic mothers (IDMs) commonly have transient hypoglycemia.** Persistent hypoglycemia may result from insulin-producing tumors or islet cell hyperplasia (**nesidioblastosis**).

2. **Conditions that result in diminished glucose production or substrate supply** include IUGR and preterm infants with limited hepatic glycogen stores and poorly developed gluconeogenesis; stressed infants who have been asphyxiated or with sepsis; infants with inborn errors of metabolism such as galactosemia, hereditary fructose intolerance, and aminoacidopathies; and infants with endocrinopathies such as growth hormone deficiency and panhypopituitarism.

C. **Clinical Features.** The neonate may be asymptomatic or may present with diaphoresis, jitteriness, feeding problems, tachycardia, hypothermia, hypotonia, seizures, and, rarely, myocardial infarction.

D. **Management.** Treatment is directed at increasing oral feeding, if possible, and if necessary, intravenous glucose.

XIV. Infants of Diabetic Mothers (IDMs)

A. **Pathophysiology.** Maternal hyperglycemia causes fetal hyperglycemia and fetal hyperinsulinemia. This causes increased hepatic glucose uptake and glycogen synthesis, accelerated lipogenesis, augmented protein synthesis, and macrosomia.

B. **Clinical Features**

1. IDMs are large because of increased body fat and **visceromegaly,** primarily of the liver, adrenals, and heart.

2. The skeletal length is increased in proportion to weight, but the head and face appear disproportionately small. The umbilical cord and placenta are also enlarged.

3. IDMs appear plethoric with round facies.

4. Although IDMs are usually LGA, they may be SGA secondary to placental insufficiency in women with severe diabetic-induced vascular complications.

C. **Complications**

1. IDMs are at considerable risk for the perinatal difficulties summarized in **Table 4-5.**

2. **Congenital anomalies,** such as congenital heart disease, are two to four times more frequent in IDMs than in normal infants.

3. **Small left colon syndrome** is a condition occurring exclusively in IDMs, in which infants present with abdominal distension and failure to pass meconium secondary to the decreased caliber of their left colon.

Table 4-5. Clinical Problems of Infants of Diabetic Mothers

Increased risk before and at delivery
Sudden intrauterine death
Large for gestational age
Increased rate of birth trauma
Increased rate of cesarean section
Increased risk of asphyxia

Increased risk of common neonatal problems
Hypoglycemia
Polycythemia
Hypocalcemia
Hypertrophic cardiomyopathy
Persistent pulmonary hypertension of the newborn
Respiratory distress syndrome
Renal vein thrombosis

Increased risk of developing congenital malformations
Structural heart disease
Central nervous system
Musculoskeletal
Small left colon syndrome
Caudal regression syndrome (hypoplasia of the sacrum and lower extremities)

XV. Polycythemia

A. **Definition.** Polycythemia is a central venous hematocrit greater than 65%.

B. **Epidemiology.** Polycythemia occurs in 2–4% of infants born at sea level.

C. **Etiology.** Causes include increased erythropoietin secretion secondary to placental insufficiency, increased red blood cell production by the fetus in response to hypoxemia, or increased placental transfusion from delayed cord clamping.

D. **Clinical features.** Manifestations include plethora, poor perfusion, cyanosis, poor feeding, respiratory distress, lethargy, jitteriness, seizures, renal vein thrombosis, and metabolic acidosis. There is an increased risk of NEC.

E. **Management.** Treatment includes **partial exchange transfusion,** in which blood is removed and replaced by the same volume of plasma substitute (normal saline) in a stepwise manner.

Review Test

1. Soon after birth, a term newborn infant presents with increased oral secretions and mild respiratory distress. Which of the following is the most likely diagnosis?

(A) Persistent pulmonary hypertension of the newborn
(B) Pneumonia
(C) Esophageal atresia
(D) Respiratory distress syndrome (surfactant deficiency syndrome)
(E) Diaphragmatic hernia

2. An abdominal mass is detected on examination of a 2-day-old infant in the newborn nursery. Which of the following is the most likely cause of this abdominal mass?

(A) Ovarian cyst
(B) Hydronephrosis
(C) Wilms' tumor
(D) Multicystic kidney
(E) Hydrometrocolpos

3. The parents of a 5-day-old term infant notice that he is jaundiced. Your physical examination is remarkable only for scleral icterus and jaundice. The infant's total bilirubin level is 15 mg/dL, with a direct component of 0.4 mg/dL. Which of the following is the most likely diagnosis?

(A) Breastfeeding jaundice
(B) Choledochal cyst
(C) Biliary atresia
(D) Neonatal hepatitis
(E) Breast milk jaundice

4. You are called to the delivery room to evaluate a newborn infant born at 37 weeks gestation who has an abdominal wall defect noted on delivery. Based on your initial physical examination, you diagnose an omphalocele. Which of the following statements is consistent with this clinical diagnosis?

(A) To rule out gastroschisis definitively, an abdominal computed tomographic scan is necessary.
(B) Compared with gastroschisis, omphalocele is more frequently associated with other congenital malformations.
(C) This abdominal wall defect is just lateral to the umbilicus.
(D) The incidence of bowel obstruction is higher in this infant than in one with gastroschisis.
(E) Omphaloceles may be associated with trisomy 21.

5. You are evaluating a 3-day-old infant with significant respiratory distress. He was delivered by emergency cesarean section at 42 weeks gestation because of fetal distress. You note that he has an oxygen saturation of 76% in room air that increases to 95% with administration of 100% oxygen. Which of the following statements most accurately supports your suspected diagnosis of persistent pulmonary hypertension of the newborn (PPHN)?

(A) This patient is likely to have an associated cyanotic congenital cardiac defect.
(B) PPHN occurs most frequently in premature infants, but may occur in post-term infants.
(C) PPHN usually resolves spontaneously.
(D) This infant is likely to have significant left-to-right shunting.
(E) Adequate oxygenation is the best preventive measurement and treatment.

6. A male infant was born at 32 weeks gestation via cesarean section because of bleeding from placenta previa. Soon after birth, he developed respiratory distress requiring supplemental oxygen and mechanical ventilation. Chest x-ray shows decreased lung volumes and a diffuse ground glass pattern with air bronchograms. Which of the following is the most likely cause of this condition?

(A) Persistent pulmonary hypertension of the newborn (PPHN)
(B) Deficient surfactant
(C) Fluid retention in the lungs
(D) Bronchopulmonary dysplasia
(E) Congenital heart disease

7. The parents of a term infant diagnosed with physiologic jaundice are very concerned that their child is at risk for brain damage. Which of the following statements regarding the infant's hyperbilirubinemia is most accurate?

(A) Breastfeeding, as compared with formula-feeding, is associated with higher peak serum bilirubin levels.
(B) Serum conjugated bilirubin concentration is the best predictor of bilirubin encephalopathy.
(C) Bilirubin encephalopathy does not occur in healthy term infants.
(D) Increased conjugated (direct) bilirubin levels cause neuronal damage, including choreoathetoid cerebral palsy, hearing loss, and opisthotonus.
(E) This infant's jaundice is expected to peak at 10–14 days of life.

8. A 2-day-old term male infant is being evaluated before discharge from the nursery. The parents are concerned about a skin rash on his face. As you perform the physical examination, you contemplate skin disorders that are benign as compared with those that may indicate underlying pathology. Which of the following skin findings is most likely to be associated with underlying pathology?

(A) Pustular melanosis
(B) Nevus simplex
(C) Milia
(D) Nevus flammeus
(E) Erythema toxicum neonatorum (ETN)

9. At a routine health maintenance visit, a 2-week-old infant appears jaundiced. Laboratory evaluation reveals a total bilirubin level of 12.6 mg/dL with a direct bilirubin level of 6.9 mg/dL. Which of the following is the most likely diagnosis?

(A) Breastfeeding jaundice
(B) Breast milk jaundice
(C) Crigler-Najjar syndrome
(D) ABO incompatibility
(E) Choledochal cyst

10. A female infant born at 30 weeks gestation develops abdominal distension, abdominal tenderness, and bloody stools on the third day of life. Which of the following statements regarding the most likely diagnosis is correct?

(A) The diagnosis is supported by a double-bubble sign on abdominal radiographs.
(B) The diagnosis is supported by pneumatosis intestinalis on abdominal radiographs.
(C) The diagnosis is supported by a soap-bubble appearance on abdominal radiographs.
(D) The infant will ultimately require pancreatic enzyme supplementation.
(E) The diagnosis has an increased association with Down syndrome.

Questions 11 and 12: The response options for statements 11 and 12 are the same. You will be required to select one answer for each statement in the set.

(A) 2
(B) 3
(C) 4
(D) 5
(E) 6
(F) 7
(G) 8

In each case, select the infant's 1-minute Apgar score.

11. At 1 minute of life, a newborn's respiratory rate is slow and irregular with a heart rate of 120 beats/min. There is some flexion of her upper and lower extremities; she grimaces when a catheter is placed into her nose; and she appears to be pink and well-perfused, except for some cyanosis of the distal extremities.

12. At 1 minute of life, a newborn's respiratory rate is slow and irregular with a heart rate of 80 beats/min. There is some flexion of his upper and lower extremities, he does not respond when a catheter is placed into his nose, and he is blue and pale.

Questions 13 and 14: The response options for statements 13 and 14 are the same. You will be required to select one answer for each statement in the set.

(A) Tetralogy of Fallot
(B) Pneumonia
(C) Respiratory distress syndrome (RDS)
(D) Meconium aspiration syndrome
(E) Truncus arteriosus

For each result of the 100% oxygen test, select the most likely diagnosis.

13. Almost no improvement in the PaO_2 (10 mm Hg)

14. A slight improvement in the PaO_2 (approximately 30 mm Hg)

Answers and Explanations

1. The answer is C [XII.A.3]. Esophageal atresia, if not detected at birth, is characterized by increased oral secretions as a result of the accumulation of saliva in the proximal esophageal pouch. Respiratory distress may occur if the infant aspirates this saliva. The presence of a distal tracheoesophageal fistula may also result in the passage of gastric contents to the trachea and lung, exacerbating the respiratory problem. Half of children with esophageal atresia have other congenital malformations, such as congenital heart disease. Both pneumonia and persistent pulmonary hypertension of the newborn also present with respiratory distress, but without increased oral secretions. Respiratory distress syndrome occurs less commonly in term infants, and increased oral secretions are not expected. Congenital diaphragmatic hernia usually presents with acute respiratory distress soon after birth in a newborn with a scaphoid abdomen. Bowel sounds can be heard on auscultation of the chest.

2. The answer is B [I.H.7 and I.I.1.b]. The most likely cause of an abdominal mass detected during the newborn period is of renal origin, with hydronephrosis being the most common cause. In female infants, an ovarian cyst, which is usually a benign tumor, is common, but not as common as hydronephrosis. Wilms' tumor and multicystic kidneys may present as abdominal masses but are also less common causes. Hydrometrocolpos, a retention of vaginal secretions, most commonly presents just after birth as a small cyst located between the labia, although during childhood, it may present as a lower midline abdominal mass.

3. The answer is A [X.C.1]. Breastfeeding jaundice is typically associated with indirect, or unconjugated, hyperbilirubinemia and is caused by suboptimal milk intake during the first week of life, which causes weight loss, poor hydration, and decreased stool output. The treatment of breastfeeding jaundice is hydration, which typically includes increasing the frequency of breastfeeding, along with observation and serial bilirubin assessments. Breast milk jaundice, which occurs later, after the first week of life, is thought to be associated with high levels of lipase and β-glucuronidase within breast milk. Choledochal cysts, biliary atresia, and neonatal hepatitis are more typical causes direct, or conjugated, hyperbilirubinemia.

4. The answer is B [XII.C]. Omphalocele is more frequently associated with congenital malformations, such as congenital heart defects, and with genetic conditions such as trisomy 13, and less commonly with trisomy 18, but not with trisomy 21. Omphalocele and gastroschisis are easily distinguished and diagnosed by inspection. An omphalocele occurs centrally through the umbilical ring, whereas gastroschisis is a lateral abdominal wall defect in which the abdominal contents herniate into the amniotic cavity. Because of this difference in clinical presentation, both omphalocele and gastroschisis are diagnosed clinically without the need for radiographic confirmation. In gastroschisis, exposure to the amniotic fluid may cause inflammation of the bowel with subsequent bowel damage and risk of bowel obstruction.

5. The answer is E [VII.B, VII.C, and VII.F]. One of the most common causes of persistent pulmonary hypertension of the newborn (PPHN) is perinatal asphyxia, resulting in increased pulmonary vascular resistance and significant right-to-left shunting through the foramen ovale or the ductus arteriosus. Oxygen is the most potent vasodilator of pulmonary vessels and, in most cases, increase of both alveolar and arterial partial pressures of O_2 produces a decrease in pulmonary vascular resistance and reversal of low blood flow to the lungs. By definition, PPHN excludes the presence of congenital heart disease. Left untreated, the hypoxemia caused by PPHN worsens the increased pulmonary vascular resistance, resulting in many cases in irreversible disease and death. In addition, PPHN occurs most commonly in near-term and full-term as well as in post-term infants.

6. The answer is B [VI.A–H]. Respiratory distress syndrome (RDS), which is most common in premature male infants, is caused by a lack or deficiency of surfactant, with alveolar atelectasis and hypoventilation. Chest x-ray findings usually include a diffuse ground glass pattern with air bronchograms. Pneumonia and sepsis should always be included in the differential diagnosis of

RDS because their clinical presentations may be quite similar. Persistent pulmonary hypertension of the newborn (PPHN) is more common in term infants than in premature infants and results most frequently from perinatal asphyxia and meconium aspiration syndrome (MAS). Fluid retention in the lungs may cause respiratory distress, but it is usually mild. The chest x-ray usually shows normal or increased lung volume with increased vascular markings. Bronchopulmonary dysplasia (BPD) is a chronic complication of RDS. Some causes of cyanotic congenital heart disease may cause hypoxemia and respiratory distress after birth; however, the chest x-ray does not show a ground glass appearance, nor air bronchograms.

7. The answer is A [X.A–G]. Newborn infants who breastfeed have higher peak serum bilirubin values. However, hyperbilirubinemia alone is not a reason to discontinue breastfeeding. Bilirubin encephalopathy is caused only by nonconjugated (indirect) bilirubin because of the ability of bilirubin to cross the blood-brain barrier. Encephalopathy caused by indirect hyperbilirubinemia does occur in healthy term newborns, and for this reason, high bilirubin levels in this group of infants should not be ignored. Benign physiologic indirect hyperbilirubinemia is expected to peak in term infants at 3–4 days of life and in preterm infants at 5–7 days of life.

8. The answer is D [I.B.11]. Nevus flammeus or "port wine stain" located over the V-1 branch of the trigeminal nerve may herald Sturge-Weber syndrome, with its associated, and potentially very significant, underlying intracranial vascular malformations and calcifications. Pustular melanosis is a benign rash, characterized by small, dry vesicles over a dark macular base, more frequently seen in African American infants. Nevus simplex is the most common vascular lesion of infancy and is also completely benign and often transient, appearing as a "salmon patch" or "stork bite" on the nape of the neck. Milia are benign very small cysts formed around the pilosebaceous follicles that appear as tiny whitish papules over the nose, cheeks, forehead, and chin. Erythema toxicum neonatorum (ETN) is a benign rash usually present in the first 72 hours of life and seen in approximately 50% of all infants. ETN is characterized by erythematous macules, papules, or pustules on the trunk and extremities.

9. The answer is E [Figures 4-2 and 4-3]. This infant's presentation with hyperbilirubinemia and a markedly elevated direct bilirubin level is consistent with a choledochal cyst, a disorder that causes obstruction of the biliary tree. Both breastfeeding and breast milk jaundice are characterized by indirect, not direct, hyperbilirubinemia. Crigler-Najjar syndrome, or hereditary deficiency of glucuronyl transferase, would also be expected to result in an indirect, or unconjugated, hyperbilirubinemia. ABO incompatibility would lead to hemolysis with predominantly an elevation of indirect bilirubin.

10. The answer is B [XII.E]. Necrotizing enterocolitis (NEC) is one of the most common surgical conditions in neonates, occurring most commonly in premature infants. Clinical features include abdominal distension, abdominal tenderness, residual gastric contents, bilious vomiting or bilious nasogastric aspirate, bloody stools, and, at times, abdominal wall erythema. Classic radiographic findings include abdominal distension, air-fluid levels, thickened bowel walls, and pneumatosis intestinalis (air within the bowel wall). In contrast, the double-bubble sign on abdominal radiograph is pathognomonic of duodenal atresia, which classically presents with nonbilious emesis and abdominal distension, but not with bloody stools. The presence of a soap-bubble appearance on abdominal radiographs is characteristic of meconium ileus, a presentation of cystic fibrosis during the neonatal period. Infants with meconium ileus would not be expected to pass bloody stools on the third day of life but may require pancreatic enzyme supplementation if they are ultimately diagnosed with fat malabsorption and cystic fibrosis. There is no known association between Down syndrome and NEC, although there is an association between Down syndrome and duodenal atresia.

11 and 12. The answers are E and B, respectively [Table 4.1]. The Apgar scoring system provides a simple, systematic, and objective assessment of intrapartum stress and neurologic depressions. The female newborn earns 2 points for a heart rate > 100 beats/min, 1 point for slow and irregular respirations, 1 point for having some flexion of the extremities, 1 point for reflex irritability or grimace when a catheter is placed in her nose, and 1 point for her peripheral cyanosis or acrocyanosis, for a total Apgar score of 6 points. The male newborn earns 1 point for a heart rate < 100 beats/min, 1 point for slow and irregular respirations, 1 point for having some flexion of the extremities, 0 points for the absence of reflex irritability when a catheter is placed into his nose, and 0 points for his cyanosis, for a total Apgar score of 3 points.

13 and 14. The answers are A and E, respectively [IV.D.2]. The 100% oxygen test helps distinguish whether cyanosis is caused by cardiac or respiratory disease. When administered 100% oxygen, infants with primary lung pathology, such as neonatal pneumonia, meconium aspiration syndrome, or respiratory distress syndrome, have a very significant increase in PaO_2 levels. In contrast, patients with cyanotic congenital heart disease would not be expected to have such a significant rise in their PaO_2 level. Patients with cyanotic congenital heart disease associated with reduced pulmonary blood flow, such as tetralogy of Fallot, would not be expected to respond with any increase of significance in PaO_2 level when given 100% oxygen. Those infants with cyanotic congenital heart disease associated with normal or increased pulmonary blood flow, such as truncus arteriosus, may have some increase in the PaO_2 level, but nowhere near as much of an increase as that seen in infants with primary pulmonary disease.

5

Genetic Disorders and Inborn Errors of Metabolism

Sharon L. Young, M.D.

I. Inheritance Patterns

A. Classic Mendelian patterns (Figure 5-1)

1. **Autosomal dominant** describes a disorder that is manifested if **only one abnormal allele** is present. If one parent is affected, the risk of having an affected child is 50%.

2. **Autosomal recessive** describes a disorder that is manifested if **two abnormal alleles** are present. If both parents are heterozygotes, neither parent is affected, and the risk of having an affected child is 25%.

3. **X-linked dominant** describes a disorder in which the allele is on the X chromosome. The disorder is manifested if **one abnormal allele** is present. X-linked dominant disorders are generally **more severe or lethal in males.** Affected females have a 50% risk of having an affected daughter.

4. **X-linked recessive** describes a disorder in which the allele is on the X chromosome and is only manifested if **no normal alleles** are present. Usually, **only males are affected** because the abnormal X chromosome is paired with a Y chromosome.

B. Nonclassic Patterns

1. **Unstable repeat sequences** occur when the number of specific nucleotide copies within a gene increases, resulting in increased disease severity (e.g., fragile X syndrome).

2. **Uniparental disomy** occurs when, instead of inheriting one gene or chromosome from each parent, both members of a chromosome or gene pair are inherited from the same parent.

3. **Translocations** occur when there is transfer of chromosomal material from one chromosome to another.

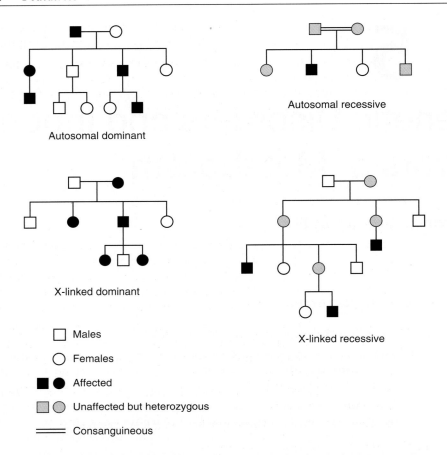

Figure 5-1. Pedigrees of different Mendelian inheritance patterns. (Modified with permission from Sakala EP. BRS Obstetrics and Gynecology. 2nd Ed. Philadelphia: Lippincott Williams & Wilkins, 2000:52.)

4. **Genomic imprinting** occurs when a gene defect is **expressed solely based on the sex of the parent** passing on the defective gene. For example, if a mother passes on an abnormal 11q region on chromosome 15, the offspring will have **Angelman syndrome,** but if a father passes on this same abnormal region, the offspring will have **Prader-Willi syndrome.** The mnemonic "Mom is an angel for Angelman syndrome, and P is for paternal and Prader-Willi syndrome" may be used to differentiate between the causes of the two syndromes.

C. **Abnormalities of Morphogenesis: malformation, deformation, disruption, syndrome**

1. **Malformation** occurs when an intrinsically abnormal process forms abnormal tissue (e.g., bladder extrophy results from the failure of infraumbilical mesenchyme to migrate and form the lower abdominal wall).

2. **Deformation** occurs when mechanical forces exerted on normal tissue result in abnormal tissues (e.g., constraint caused by an abnormally shaped uterus results in an abnormally shaped fetal skull).

3. **Disruption** occurs when normal tissue becomes abnormal after being

subjected to destructive forces (e.g., decreased blood flow to an organ causes tissue ischemia, eventually resulting in an atretic organ).

4. **Syndrome** occurs when a **collection of seemingly unrelated abnormal features occur in a familiar pattern** (e.g., because many of the clinical features of children with Down syndrome are similar, these children appear to be related to each other).

II. Fetal Evaluation and Prenatal Diagnosis

A. **Ultrasound** is used to assess gestational age and fetal growth and to evaluate for major fetal anomalies.

B. **Maternal serum markers**

1. **α-Fetoprotein (AFP)** is elevated with fetal neural tube defects, multiple gestation pregnancies, underestimated gestational age, ventral abdominal wall defects, fetal demise, or fetal conditions that cause edema or skin defects. Low AFP levels are associated with overestimated gestational age, trisomies 21 and 18, and intrauterine growth retardation.

2. **Triple marker** is used as a noninvasive method to assess the fetus for the possibility of trisomy syndromes. The three markers are **AFP, unconjugated estriol, and β subunit of human chorionic gonadotropin (β-HCG).**

   a. **Low AFP, low unconjugated estriol, and high β-HCG suggest Down syndrome.**

   b. Low values of all three markers suggest trisomy 18.

C. **Genetic evaluation of the fetus**

1. **Chorionic villus sampling (CVS)** collects villus tissue from the chorion of the trophoblast at **10–13 weeks** gestation. Karyotyping, DNA extraction, and enzyme analyses from CVS can be used to assess for genetic and metabolic diseases.

2. **Amniocentesis** collects amniotic fluid containing sloughed fetal cells at **16–18 weeks** gestation. This technique assesses for the same diseases as CVS.

3. **Percutaneous umbilical blood sampling** involves obtaining a sample of fetal blood to assess for hematologic abnormalities, genetic disorders, infections, and fetal acidosis. It can also be used to administer medications or blood transfusions to the fetus.

III. Common Genetic Disorders

A. **Common Syndromes**

1. **Marfan syndrome** is an **autosomal dominant** connective tissue disorder that affects primarily the **ocular, cardiovascular, and skeletal systems.** The gene defect has been mapped to a region on **chromosome 15** that codes for **fibrillin,** a protein that plays a major role in providing structure for connective tissues.

a. **Clinical features**

  (1) **Skeletal findings** include **tall stature with elongated extremities and long fingers** (i.e., arachnodactyly), joint laxity, chest wall deformities (e.g., pectus excavatum), and scoliosis or kyphosis. Marfan syndrome is suggested by a **decreased upper-to-lower segment ratio (U/L;** the lower segment is the distance from the symphysis pubis to the heel, and the upper segment is the height minus the lower segment).

  (2) **Ocular findings** include **upward lens subluxation** and retinal detachment.

  (3) **Cardiovascular findings** include **aortic root dilatation** (with or without aortic dissection), mitral valve prolapse, and aortic regurgitation.

b. **Diagnosis** is based on clinical findings; however, **homocystinuria** has many of the same clinical features. Therefore, screening tests to rule out homocystinuria are also generally performed (see section V.D).

c. **Complications** include endocarditis, retinal detachment, and **sudden death** as a result of aortic dissection.

  (1) **Hypertension** and chest trauma **increase dissection risk.** The overall risk is reduced with β-blocker medications and avoidance of contact sports.

  (2) **Endocarditis prophylaxis** and regular **ophthalmologic examinations** are warranted.

2. **Prader-Willi syndrome** is an example of **genomic imprinting** (see section I.B.4) and is caused by the absence of a region on the paternally derived **chromosome 15.**

a. **Clinical features**

  (1) **Craniofacial** findings include **almond-shaped eyes** and a down-turned, **fishlike mouth.**

  (2) **Growth** problems include **failure to thrive (FTT)** because of feeding difficulties in the **first year of life,** followed by **obesity** as a result of **hyperphagia later in childhood.** Patients also have **short stature** with small hands and feet.

  (3) **Neurologic features** include **hypotonia** (most pronounced during the newborn period), **mental retardation,** learning disabilities, and behavioral problems.

  (4) **Hypogonadism** manifests as a small penis, small testes, or cryptorchidism.

b. **Diagnosis,** based on fluorescent in situ hybridization (**FISH**) probes, detects the chromosomal deletion in almost all patients.

c. **Complications**

  (1) **In infancy,** hypotonia may lead to poor sucking, feeding problems, and developmental delay.

  (2) **In childhood,** obesity may lead to **obstructive sleep apnea.**

  (3) **In adulthood**, obesity may lead to **cardiac disease** and **type 2 diabetes mellitus.** Psychiatric illnesses may also be present.

3. **Angelman syndrome** is also known as the **"happy puppet"** syndrome because of its characteristic jerky, puppetlike gait and the happy demeanor with frequent laughter and smiling of affected individuals. Angelman syndrome is an example of **genomic imprinting** and is caused by a deletion of a region on the maternally derived **chromosome 15** (see section I.B.4).

   a. **Clinical features**

      (1) **Neurologic** findings include **jerky arm movements, ataxia,** and **paroxysms of inappropriate laughter. Mental retardation is severe** with significant speech delay.

      (2) **Craniofacial** findings include a small wide head, large mouth with widely spaced teeth, tongue protrusion, and prognathia. Most affected individuals have blond hair and pale blue deep-set eyes.

   b. **Diagnosis** is based on FISH probes to detect the chromosomal deletion on chromosome 15.

4. **Noonan syndrome** is often described as the male version of Turner syndrome, but females may also be affected. Cases are usually sporadic; however, an autosomal dominant pattern has been reported. A gene for the disorder has been mapped to **chromosome 12.**

   a. **Clinical features** (variable)

      (1) **Skeletal** findings include **short stature** and a **shield chest.**

      (2) **Craniofacial** findings include a **short webbed neck and low hairline,** hypertelorism (i.e., widely spaced eyes), epicanthal skin folds, downslanting palpebral fissures, and low-set ears.

      (3) **Cardiac defects** include **right-sided heart lesions,** most commonly **pulmonary valve stenosis.** (In contrast, patients with Turner syndrome have left-sided heart lesions.)

      (4) Mental retardation occurs in 25% of the patients.

   b. **Diagnosis** is based on clinical features.

5. **DiGeorge syndrome and velocardiofacial syndrome** are two distinct syndromes with a deletion at **chromosome 22q11.** Some experts support changing the name of both syndromes to **CATCH-22** (**C**—cardiac anomaly, **A**—abnormal facies, **T**—thymic hypoplasia, **C**—cleft palate, **H**—hypocalcemia, and a gene defect on chromosome **22**). Inheritance is both sporadic and autosomal dominant.

   a. **DiGeorge syndrome** is caused by a defect in the structures derived from the third and fourth pharyngeal pouches.

      (1) **Clinical features**

         (a) **Craniofacial** findings include short palpebral fissures, small chin, and ear anomalies.

         (b) **Cardiac** findings include aortic arch anomalies, ventricular septal defects, and tetralogy of Fallot.

         (c) **Thymus and parathyroid hypoplasia** cause **cell-mediated immunodeficiency** and **severe hypocalcemia.**

      (2) **Diagnosis** is based on FISH probes to detect the deletion on chromosome 22.

       (3) Complications include **infections** as a result of cell-mediated immunodeficiency and **seizures** caused by hypocalcemia (see Chapter 15, section X.E).

   b. Velocardiofacial syndrome

     (1) Clinical features

       (a) Craniofacial findings include cleft palate, wide prominent nose with a squared nasal root, short chin, and fish-shaped mouth.

       (b) Cardiac findings include ventricular septal defects and a right-sided aortic arch.

       (c) Neurologic findings include neonatal hypotonia, learning disabilities, and perseverative behaviors.

     (2) Diagnosis is based on FISH probes to detect the deletion on chromosome 22.

6. Ehlers-Danlos syndrome is characterized by production of **defective type V collagen** resulting in hyperextensible joints, fragile vessels, and loose skin. Inheritance is autosomal dominant.

   a. Clinical features

     (1) Musculoskeletal findings include **hyperextensible joints** with a tendency toward joint dislocation and scoliosis.

     (2) Dermatologic findings include soft, velvety textured, **loose, fragile skin.** Minor lacerations result in large wounds that heal poorly with broad, atrophic, **tissue paper-thin scars.**

     (3) Cardiovascular findings include mitral valve prolapse, aortic root dilatation, and fragile blood vessels that result in ease of bruising.

     (4) Gastrointestinal (GI) features include constipation, rectal prolapse, and hernias.

   b. Diagnosis is based on clinical findings.

   c. Complications include aortic dissection and GI bleeding as a result of blood vessel fragility.

7. Osteogenesis imperfecta (OI) results from mutations that cause production of **abnormal type I collagen**. OI is classified into four types based on clinical, radiographic, and genetic criteria. Type I is described below.

   a. Clinical features

     (1) Blue sclerae

     (2) Skeletal findings such as **fragile bones** resulting in frequent fractures, genu valgum (knock-knees), scoliosis or kyphosis, joint laxity, and osteoporosis or osteopenia.

     (3) Yellow or gray-blue teeth

     (4) Easy bruisability

   b. Diagnosis is based on clinical features and decreased type I collagen synthesis in fibroblasts.

   c. Complications include **early conductive hearing loss** and **skeletal deformities** as a result of fractures.

8. **VACTERL (VATER) association** is a group of malformations that occur sporadically.
   a. **Clinical features**
      (1) **V—vertebral defects**
      (2) **A—anal atresia**
      (3) **C—cardiac anomalies,** predominantly ventricular septal defects
      (4) **TE—tracheoesophageal fistula**
      (5) **R—renal** and genital defects
      (6) **L—limb defects,** including radial hypoplasia, syndactyly and polydactyly
   b. **Diagnosis** is based on clinical features.

9. **CHARGE association** is a group of malformations that occur sporadically.
   a. **Clinical features**
      (1) **C—colobomas** (absence or defect of ocular tissue), usually of the retina. Impaired vision is very common.
      (2) **H—heart defects,** most commonly tetralogy of Fallot
      (3) **A—atresia of the nasal choanae**
      (4) **R—retardation** of growth and cognition
      (5) **G—genital anomalies,** including genital hypoplasia
      (6) **E—ear anomalies,** including cup-shaped ears and hearing loss
   b. **Diagnosis** is based on clinical features.

10. **Williams syndrome** is most notable for the unique loquacious personality often described as a **"cocktail party" personality.** It is caused by a **deletion on chromosome 7** that includes the gene for elastin. Inheritance is autosomal dominant.
    a. **Clinical features**
       (1) **"Elfin facies"** with short palpebral fissures, flat nasal bridge, and round cheeks
       (2) **Mental retardation** and **loquacious personality**
       (3) **Supravalvular aortic stenosis**
       (4) **Idiopathic hypercalcemia** in infancy
       (5) **Connective tissue abnormalities,** including a hoarse voice and hernias
    b. **Diagnosis** is based on detection of the deletion with FISH probes.

11. **Cornelia de Lange (Brachmann-de Lange) syndrome** is most notable for a single eyebrow and very short stature without skeletal abnormalities. Inheritance is mostly sporadic, but autosomal dominant inheritance may occur.
    a. **Clinical features**
       (1) **Small for gestational age** and **FTT**
       (2) **Craniofacial** findings include **single eyebrow (synophrys),** long, curly eyelashes, **microcephaly,** thin, down-turned upper lip, and micrognathia.
       (3) **Infantile hypertonia**
       (4) **Mental retardation**

      (5) Small hands and feet

      (6) Cardiac defects

      (7) Behavioral findings include autistic features, lack of facial expression, and self-destructive tendencies.

    b. Diagnosis is based on clinical features.

12. Russell-Silver syndrome is known for the features of **short stature** and **skeletal asymmetry** with a **normal head circumference.** Inheritance is sporadic.

    a. Clinical features

      (1) Small for gestational age

      (2) Craniofacial findings include a **small triangular face,** prominent forehead, and down-turned mouth. Because of the small face, the head appears large, but the head circumference is normal.

      (3) Skeletal findings include **short stature** and **limb asymmetry.**

      (4) Café-au-lait spots on the skin

      (5) Excessive sweating

    b. Diagnosis is based on clinical features.

13. Pierre Robin syndrome

    a. Clinical features include **micrognathia, cleft lip and palate,** and a large protruding tongue. Feeding is often difficult because of the cleft palate.

    b. Diagnosis is based on clinical features.

    c. Complications include **recurrent otitis media** and **upper airway obstruction** that often requires tracheostomy.

14. Cri du chat syndrome is caused by a **partial deletion of the short arm of chromosome 5.** Most cases occur sporadically.

    a. Clinical features include slow growth, microcephaly, mental retardation, hypertelorism, downslanting palpebral fissures, and a characteristic **catlike cry.**

    b. Diagnosis is based on detection of the chromosomal deletion and the presence of clinical features.

B. Trisomy syndromes

   1. Down syndrome (trisomy 21) is the **most common trisomy syndrome** and involves **chromosome 21.** The risk of Down syndrome increases with maternal age because of the increased occurrence of nondisjunction within the ovum. Incidence is estimated to be 1:660 live births. **Table 5-1** describes the clinical features and complications of Down syndrome.

   2. Trisomy 18 is the **second most common** trisomy syndrome and is three times more common in **females.**

    a. Clinical features

      (1) Neurologic findings include **mental retardation** and **hypertonia** with **scissoring of the lower extremities.**

      (2) Delicate, small facial features

      (3) Musculoskeletal findings include **clenched hands** with **overlapping digits,** dorsiflexed big toes, and **rocker bottom feet.**

Table 5-1. Clinical Features and Complications Associated with Down Syndrome

Clinical Features	Complications

Craniofacial features
  Brachycephaly
  Epicanthal skin folds
  Upslanting palpebral fissures
  Brushfield spots (speckled irides)
  Protruding tongue
Hypotonia
Mental retardation
Musculoskeletal features
  Clinodactyly
  Single palmar creases
  Wide space between first and second toes
Gastrointestinal features
  Duodenal atresia
  Hirschsprung's disease and omphalocele
  Pyloric stenosis
Cardiac features (40%)
  Endocardial cushion defects (most
    common)
	Atlantoaxial cervical spine instability (20%)
	    Flexion-extension cervical spine radiographs
	      should be assessed by 3–5 years of age
	Leukemia (20 times more common than in
	    general population)
	Celiac disease
	    Total IgA and IgA anti-endomysium antibody
	      screen at 2 years of age
	Early Alzheimer's disease
	Obstructive sleep apnea
	Conductive hearing loss
	    Hearing screens needed every 1–2 years
	Hypothyroidism
	    Annual TSH screening
	Cataracts, glaucoma, and refractive errors
	    Annual ophthalmologic examinations

TSH = thyroid-stimulating hormone.

      b. Diagnosis is based on chromosomal analysis.

      c. Prognosis. Most affected individuals (95%) die within the first year of life.

    3. Trisomy 13 is associated with **midline defects,** particularly of the face and forebrain.

      a. Clinical features

        (1) Neurologic findings include **holoprosencephaly,** microcephaly, seizures, and **severe mental retardation.**

        (2) Ocular findings include **microphthalmia,** retinal dysplasia, colobomas, and, rarely, a single eye.

        (3) Cleft lip and palate

      b. Diagnosis is based on chromosomal analysis.

      c. Prognosis is poor, with death usually occurring within the first month of life.

  C. Sex Chromosome Syndromes

    1. Turner syndrome occurs when only one X chromosome is present. Incidence is 1:2,000 live births.

      a. Clinical features

        (1) Short stature

        (2) Webbed neck and low posterior hairline

        (3) Shield chest with broadly spaced nipples and scoliosis or kyphosis

        (4) Swelling of the dorsum of hands and feet (congenital lymphedema) may be present at birth.

        (5) Ovarian dysgenesis causes delayed puberty. **Turner syndrome should be considered in any female with pubertal delay.** Hormonal therapy is typically needed to stimulate puberty.

          (6) Cardiac defects usually include **left-sided** heart lesions, especially **coarctation of the aorta,** bicuspid aortic valve, and hypoplastic left heart.

          (7) Hypothyroidism may occur.

       b. Diagnosis is based on clinical features and chromosomal analysis.

    2. Fragile X syndrome is an X-linked disorder caused by a site on the X chromosome that contains a variable number of **CGG repeats.** Fragile X syndrome is an example of **anticipation.** As the disorder passes from generation to generation, there is an increase in the number of CGG repeats, corresponding to an increase in syndrome severity. Fragile X syndrome is **more severe in males,** but females may also have mental retardation. It occurs in 1:1,250 males and 1:2,500 females, making fragile X syndrome the **most common inherited cause of mental retardation.**

       a. Clinical features

          (1) Mild to severe mental retardation

          (2) Craniofacial findings include **large ears,** macrocephaly, thickened nasal bridge, and blue irides.

          (3) Large testes develop during puberty.

          (4) Behavioral findings include emotional instability, autistic features, and attention deficit/hyperactivity disorder.

       b. Diagnosis is based on chromosomal analysis.

    3. Klinefelter syndrome is the **most common cause of male hypogonadism and infertility.** Chromosomal analysis generally reveals an **XXY** genotype. Risk increases with advancing maternal age. Incidence is 1:500 live male births.

       a. Clinical features

          (1) Tall stature with long extremities

          (2) Hypogonadism, including small penis and testes, **delayed puberty** owing to lack of testosterone, and infertility.

          (3) Gynecomastia

          (4) Variable intelligence

          (5) Behavioral findings include antisocial behavior and excessive shyness or aggression. These findings may be noted before the appearance of the physical findings.

       b. Diagnosis is based on chromosomal analysis.

D. Skeletal dysplasias are a diverse group of inherited diseases characterized by **short stature caused by bone growth abnormalities.**

    1. Classification is based on the location of the bone abnormality or shortening.

       a. Rhizomelia refers to proximal long bone abnormalities (e.g., short humerus and femur).

       b. Mesomelia refers to medial long bone abnormalities (e.g., short ulna and tibia).

       c. Acromelia refers to distal abnormalities (e.g., small hands and feet).

       d. Spondylodysplasias involve abnormalities of the spine, with or without limb abnormalities.

2. **Achondroplasia** is the **most common skeletal dysplasia** and is characterized by **rhizomelia.** Although inheritance is **autosomal dominant,** most cases are **sporadic.** Achondroplasia is caused by a mutation in the fibroblast growth factor receptor 3 gene. Incidence increases with advancing paternal age.

   a. **Clinical features**

      (1) **Craniofacial findings** include **megalencephaly** (large brain), **foramen magnum stenosis,** frontal bossing, midface hypoplasia, and low nasal bridge.

      (2) **Skeletal findings**

         (a) **Lumbar kyphosis in infancy** evolving into **lumbar lordosis in later childhood** and adulthood

         (b) **Rhizomelic limb shortening,** bowed legs, and joint hyperextensibility

         (c) **Trident-shaped hands**

      (3) **Recurrent otitis media with conductive hearing loss**

   b. **Diagnosis** is based on clinical features and radiographs of the limbs demonstrating rhizomelic shortening.

   c. **Complications**

      (1) **Foramen magnum stenosis** may lead to **hydrocephalus** or **cord compression.** Head circumference must be monitored closely. Head sweating and dilated facial veins may be subtle signs of cord compression. **Sudden infant death** may occur as a result of cord compression.

      (2) **Obstructive sleep apnea** and respiratory compromise may occur from foramen magnum narrowing and upper airway obstruction.

      (3) **Orthopedic problems** such as severe bowed legs (genu varum) and back pain

E. **Environmental defects. Environmental factors** may cause congenital abnormalities and have an impact on the fetus.

   1. **Potter syndrome** is caused by **severe oligohydramnios,** which causes lung hypoplasia and fetal compression with limb abnormalities and facial features termed Potter facies. Severe oligohydramnios may occur as the result of a chronic amniotic fluid leak or intrauterine renal failure caused by bilateral renal agenesis, polycystic kidneys, or obstructive uropathy.

   2. **Amniotic band syndrome (amnion rupture sequence)** occurs as a result of rupture of the amniotic sac. Fluid leak leads to intrauterine constraint, and small strands from the amnion may wrap around the fetus, causing limb scarring and amputation.

F. **Syndromes caused by teratogens (Table 5-2)**

   1. **Fetal alcohol syndrome** is caused by alcohol, the **most common teratogen.** Fetal alcohol syndrome may occur if a woman chronically drinks alcohol or binges during her pregnancy. Features include small-for-gestational-age (SGA) at birth, FTT, microcephaly, a long smooth philtrum with a thin, smooth upper lip, mental retardation, attention deficit/hyperactivity disorder, and cardiac defects (ventricular septal defect is most common).

Table 5-2. Teratogens and Associated Anomalies

Drugs	Associated Anomalies
Alcohol	Microcephaly; short palpebral fissures; long, smooth philtrum; variable mental retardation
Cigarette smoking	Small-for-gestational age, polycythemia
Cocaine	Intrauterine growth retardation, microcephaly, genitourinary tract abnormalities
Diethylstilbestrol (DES)	Increased risk of cervical carcinoma, genitourinary anomalies
Isotretinoin	Central nervous system malformations, microtia, cardiac defects, thymic hypoplasia
Phenytoin	Wide anterior fontanelle, thick hair with a low hairline, small nails, cardiac defects
Propylthiouracil	Hypothyroidism, goiter
Thalidomide	Phocomelia (malformed extremities resulting in flipperlike appendages)
Valproic acid	Narrow head, high forehead, midface hypoplasia, spina bifida, cardiac defects, convex nails
Warfarin	Hypoplastic nose with a deep groove between the nasal alae and the nasal tip, stippling of the epiphyses, hypoplastic nails

2. **Fetal phenytoin syndrome** causes a spectrum of defects with mild to moderate mental retardation, cardiac defects, growth retardation, nail and digit abnormalities, and characteristic facial features. Pregnant women with seizure disorders face the dilemma of either exposing their unborn fetus to anticonvulsants (which may have teratogenic effects) or risk having a seizure (which may cause fetal injury).

G. **Defects of multifactorial inheritance**

1. **Cleft lip and palate.** A wide variety of syndromic and nonsyndromic diseases have cleft lip and palate as a feature, but the inheritance patterns are widely different.

2. **Neural tube defects (NTDs)** are the **most common congenital anomalies of the central nervous system.** Etiology is multifactorial and includes nutrition, genetic predisposition, drugs, and radiation exposure. Folic acid dosages of 400–800 μg/day may help prevent NTDs (see Chapter 12, section III.C).

3. **Congenital heart disease (CHD)** is a congenital defect with many causes, including syndromes, drugs, maternal disease, and genetic inheritance. Risk of CHD in the general population is approximately 1%, and **recurrence risk increases with each child affected.**

IV. **Inborn Errors of Metabolism (IEM) (Figure 5-2):** General Concepts. IEM are a heterogeneous group of diseases that can present in a variety of ways. Individually, each disease is rare, but collectively the overall incidence is 1:5,000 live births. Although most IEM are inherited in an autosomal recessive fashion, some are X-linked recessive, and many occur spontaneously.

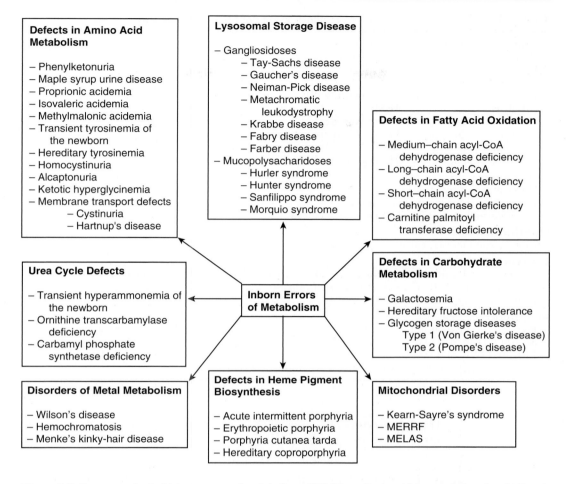

Defects in Amino Acid Metabolism

– Phenylketonuria
– Maple syrup urine disease
– Proprionic acidemia
– Isovaleric acidemia
– Methylmalonic acidemia
– Transient tyrosinemia of the newborn
– Hereditary tyrosinemia
– Homocystinuria
– Alcaptonuria
– Ketotic hyperglycinemia
– Membrane transport defects
   – Cystinuria
   – Hartnup's disease

Lysosomal Storage Disease

– Gangliosidoses
   – Tay-Sachs disease
   – Gaucher's disease
   – Neiman-Pick disease
   – Metachromatic leukodystrophy
   – Krabbe disease
   – Fabry disease
   – Farber disease
– Mucopolysacharidoses
   – Hurler syndrome
   – Hunter syndrome
   – Sanfilippo syndrome
   – Morquio syndrome

Defects in Fatty Acid Oxidation

– Medium–chain acyl-CoA dehydrogenase deficiency
– Long–chain acyl-CoA dehydrogenase deficiency
– Short–chain acyl-CoA dehydrogenase deficiency
– Carnitine palmitoyl transferase deficiency

Urea Cycle Defects

– Transient hyperammonemia of the newborn
– Ornithine transcarbamylase deficiency
– Carbamyl phosphate synthetase deficiency

Inborn Errors of Metabolism

Defects in Carbohydrate Metabolism

– Galactosemia
– Hereditary fructose intolerance
– Glycogen storage diseases
   Type 1 (Von Gierke's disease)
   Type 2 (Pompe's disease)

Disorders of Metal Metabolism

– Wilson's disease
– Hemochromatosis
– Menke's kinky-hair disease

Defects in Heme Pigment Biosynthesis

– Acute intermittent porphyria
– Erythropoietic porphyria
– Porphyria cutanea tarda
– Hereditary coproporphyria

Mitochondrial Disorders

– Kearn-Sayre's syndrome
– MERRF
– MELAS

Figure 5-2. Summary chart of inborn errors of metabolism. *MELAS = m*itochondrial *e*ncephalopathy, *l*actic acidosis, and *s*trokelike episodes; *MERRF = m*yoclonus *e*pilepsy and *r*agged-*r*ed *f*ibers.

A. Clinical features (Table 5-3)

  1. IEM should be suspected if a child:

    a. Is acutely ill and fails to respond to usual therapy

    b. Has unexplained seizures, developmental delay, progressive neurologic deterioration, persistent or recurrent vomiting, or FTT

    c. Has laboratory values inconsistent with the clinical presentation

  2. Onset of symptoms of an IEM often conjures an image of a critically ill neonate, but it is important to remember that each IEM may have subtypes that may present at an older age or in adulthood.

    a. Acute severe neonatal illness is the **classic presentation.** An apparently healthy newborn develops an acute severe illness within the first few hours to weeks of life.

    b. Recurrent intermittent episodes may present at **times of stress,** such as surgery, fasting, or illness.

    c. Chronic and progressive symptoms are typical of **mitochon-**

Table 5-3. Typical Clinical Features of Inborn Errors of Metabolism (IEM)

General symptoms:
 Lethargy or coma
 Poor feeding or failure to thrive
 Intractable hiccups
 Unusual odor (especially when acutely ill):

Odor:	IEM:
Mousey/musty	Phenylketonuria
Sweet maple syrup	Maple syrup urine disease
Sweaty feet	Isovaleric or glutaric acidemia
Rotten cabbage	Hereditary tyrosinemia

Neurologic:
 Hypertonia or hypotonia
 Unexplained developmental delay
 Unexplained and difficult-to-control seizures

Ophthalmologic:
 Cherry-red macula, cataracts, or corneal clouding

Gastrointestinal:
 Vomiting with metabolic acidosis should raise suspicion of an IEM because excessive
  vomiting normally causes metabolic alkalosis
 Hepatomegaly

Metabolic:
 Hypoglycemia with ketosis is suggestive of organic acidemias and carbohydrate disease
 Serum NH_3 > 200 mM is suggestive of urea cycle defects
 Elevated NH_3 and metabolic acidosis are suggestive of organic acidemias
 Urinary ketones in a newborn are always abnormal

NH_3 = ammonia.

drial disorders. Because of the slow progressive course, diagnosis is often delayed.

3. **Family history** suspicious for IEM includes:

   a. **Neonatal deaths** in siblings or affected males on the maternal side

   b. **Parental consanguinity**

   c. **Mental retardation** or neurologic disability

   d. **Unusual dietary preferences** in relatives

4. **Clinical pearl: Sepsis is much more common than metabolic disease.** However, it is important to keep in mind that the **presenting symptoms of IEM may be similar to those of sepsis,** and patients with IEM are vulnerable to sepsis.

B. **Initial laboratory evaluation** includes assessment for **metabolic acidosis** and **elevated serum ammonia** (Table 5-4). Further evaluation depends on whether metabolic acidosis or hyperammonemia are present.

C. **Management** includes stabilization and prevention of further catabolism.

   1. **Provide a source of energy. Intravenous glucose** is the most basic energy source.

   2. **Prevent exposure to the offending substance.** Initially, enteral feedings should be avoided and protein should be eliminated until a specific diagnosis is known. Lipids may be considered as a source of energy if a fatty acid oxidation defect is not suspected.

Table 5-4. Initial Evaluation for Inborn Errors of Metabolism

Test	Reason for Test
Initial studies	
Serum glucose	Rule out hypoglycemia
Serum Ca and Mg	Rule out hypocalcemia or hyper- or hypomagnesemia
CBC with differential	Assess for anemia, neutropenia, thrombocytopenia
Urinalysis	Assess for ketones
	Presence of ketones is especially suspicious in newborns because normally they do not produce ketones well
	In older children, absence of ketones with hypoglycemia is suspicious for fatty acid oxidation defect
Arterial blood gas and serum electrolytes	Assess for anion gap metabolic acidosis
Plasma NH_3	Rule out urea cycle defects (may also be elevated with hypoxia or severe dehydration)
Urine-reducing substance	If positive, dipstick for glucose; nonglucose-reducing substance is suggestive of galactosemia
If metabolic acidosis is present:	
Serum lactate and pyruvate	Rule out lactic acidemias or organic acidemias
Plasma amino acids	Rule out aminoacidemias or organic acidemias
If increased ammonia is present:	
Plasma amino acids	If elevated, then suspect aminoacidemias
Urine organic acids	If elevated orotic acid, suspect ornithine transcarbamylase deficiency

CBC = complete blood count; NH_3 = ammonia.

      3. **Correct acidosis or hyperammonemia.**

         a. **Sodium bicarbonate** corrects acidosis.

         b. **Sodium benzoate and sodium phenylacetate** increase ammonia excretion.

         c. **Oral Neosporin and lactulose** prevent bacterial production of ammonia in the colon.

         d. **Dialysis** may be necessary if other interventions fail to correct the electrolyte abnormalities.

V. Defects in Amino Acid Metabolism.

In general, individuals with these disorders may present with an unusual odor, vomiting with severe acidosis, lethargy, coma, and neutropenia. For characteristics of phenylketonuria (PKU), hereditary tyrosinemia, and maple syrup urine disease, see **Table 5-5.** Other examples of defects in amino acid metabolism are described in this section.

      A. **Homocystinuria.** This condition is caused by **cystathionine synthase deficiency.** Inheritance is **autosomal recessive.**

         1. **Clinical features** share some characteristics with Marfan syndrome (see section III.A.1).

           a. **Marfanoid body habitus without arachnodactyly**

           b. **Downward lens subluxation** (in Marfan syndrome, lens subluxation is upward)

Table 5-5. Characteristics of Selected Defects in Amino Acid Metabolism

	Phenylketonuria (PKU)	Maple Syrup Urine Disease	Tyrosinemia Type I
Inheritance	Autosomal recessive	Autosomal recessive	Autosomal recessive
Clinical features	Developmental delay Infantile hypotonia Mousy or musty odor Progressive mental retardation Eczema Decreased pigment (light eyes and hair) Mild PKU may present in early childhood with developmental delay, hyperactivity	Progressive vomiting and poor feeding Lethargy, hypotonia, and coma Developmental delay Maple syrup odor in urine Hypoglycemia and severe acidosis during episodes	Episodes of peripheral neuropathy Chronic liver disease Odor of rotten fish or cabbage odor Renal tubular dysfunction
Diagnosis	↑ Phenylalanine:tyrosine ratio in serum	↑ Serum and urine branched-chain amino acids	Succinylacetone in urine
Management	Phenylalanine-restricted diet	Dietary protein restriction	Dietary restriction of phenylalanine, tyrosine, NTBC Liver transplant
Prognosis	Near-normal intelligence if diet restriction begun < 1 month of age	Protein restriction within 2 weeks of life may avert neurologic damage	Death by 1 year of age if disease begins in infancy Increased risk of hepatocellular carcinoma and cirrhosis

NTBC = 2-2 nitro-4-trifluoromethylbenzoyl 1,3-cyclohexanedione.

    c. Hypercoagulable state increases the risk of stroke, myocardial infarction, and deep vein thrombosis.

    d. Cardiovascular abnormalities include mitral or aortic regurgitation. Aortic dilatation is absent (in contrast to Marfan syndrome).

    e. Scoliosis and large, stiff joints

    f. Developmental delay, mild mental retardation, and psychiatric illness

  2. Diagnosis is by finding **increased methionine** in urine and plasma, or by a positive urinary cyanide nitroprusside test.

  3. Management includes a **methionine-restricted diet, aspirin** to decrease risk of thromboembolism, and folic acid and vitamin B_6 supplementation.

B. Transient tyrosinemia of the newborn. This condition occurs in premature infants who receive high-protein diets.

  1. Clinical features begin during the first 2 weeks of life and may include poor feeding or lethargy. Patients may be asymptomatic.

  2. Diagnosis is based on **elevated serum tyrosine and phenylalanine levels.**

      3. **Management** includes decreasing protein intake during the acute episode. **Vitamin C** may help eliminate tyrosine.

      4. **Prognosis** is good. This **self-limited disease** should resolve within 1 month.

C. Membrane transport defects

      1. **Cystinuria** is an autosomal recessive disorder caused by a **defect in renal reabsorption of cystine, lysine, arginine, and ornithine** that leads to **renal stones.** Clinical features may include urinary tract infection, dysuria, abdominal or back pain, urgency, and urinary frequency.

      2. **Hartnup disease** is an autosomal recessive disorder caused by a defect in the transport of neutral amino acids. Most patients are asymptomatic but some may present with intermittent ataxia, photosensitive rash, mental retardation, and emotional lability.

D. Urea cycle defects. The urea cycle is responsible for the disposal of excess dietary nitrogen in the form of urea. Thus, defects in this cycle are manifested by **elevated ammonia (NH_3) > 200 μM.** Ammonia is toxic to the brain and the liver. Typical symptoms include poor feeding, hyperventilation, behavioral changes, seizures, ataxia, and coma.

      1. **Transient hyperammonemia of the newborn** is a **self-limited** disorder that may present in premature infants within the initial 24–48 hours of life. Symptoms are nonspecific and include respiratory distress, alkalosis, vomiting, and lethargy rapidly progressing to coma. Aggressive treatment of hyperammonemia is required to prevent neurologic sequelae (see section IV.D.3).

      2. **Ornithine transcarbamylase deficiency** is the **most common urea cycle defect.** Inheritance is **X-linked recessive,** and therefore males are more severely affected.

         a. **Clinical features** begin at the onset of protein ingestion and include vomiting and lethargy leading to coma. Some females with mild disease may present in childhood with cyclic vomiting and intermittent ataxia.

         b. **Diagnosis** is based on elevated urine orotic acid, decreased serum citrulline, and increased ornithine, as well as by liver biopsy.

         c. **Management** includes a low-protein diet and management of hyperammonemia. Liver transplant may be necessary.

         d. **Prognosis** depends on the neurologic sequelae of any hyperammonemic episode. Recurrent episodes with illness are common.

VI. Defects in Carbohydrate Metabolism

A. Galactosemia. This autosomal recessive disorder is caused by galactose-1-phosphate uridyltransferase deficiency. It should be **suspected in any newborn with hepatomegaly and hypoglycemia.**

      1. **Clinical features** begin after the newborn feeds a cow's milk-based formula or breastfeeds for the first time (both cow's milk and breast milk contain galactose).

    a. **Vomiting, diarrhea, and FTT**

    b. **Hepatic dysfunction** with **hepatomegaly**

    c. **Cataracts** with a characteristic **oil-droplet appearance**

    d. **Renal tubular acidosis**

2. **Diagnosis**

    a. **Nonglucose-reducing substance in urine** tested by a Clinitest. The usual urine dipstick or Clinistix only tests for glucose and is inadequate for the detection of galactose.

    b. Confirmation of enzyme deficiency in red blood cells

    c. Prenatal and newborn screening are available.

3. **Management** includes a **galactose-free diet,** such as soy or elemental formulas.

4. **Prognosis** is good with **normal intelligence if the disorder is treated early.** Mental retardation can be expected if diagnosis is delayed. Nearly **all** females suffer from ovarian failure. Death in early infancy, typically from ***Escherichia coli* sepsis,** is common if the diagnosis is not suspected and treated.

B. **Hereditary Fructose Intolerance.** This condition is caused by fructose-1-phosphate aldolase B deficiency and begins in infancy after the introduction of fruit or fruit juice to the infant's diet. Symptoms include severe hypoglycemia, vomiting, diarrhea, FTT, and seizures. Management includes avoidance of fructose, sucrose, and sorbitol.

C. **Glycogen storage diseases (GSDs)** are characterized by **organomegaly** and **metabolic acidosis.**

1. **Von Gierke's disease (GSD type 1)** is an autosomal recessive disorder caused by **glucose-6-phosphatase deficiency.** Presenting features may include persistent hypoglycemia, hepatomegaly, metabolic acidosis, hypertriglyceridemia, and enlarged kidneys. Management includes frequent feeding with a high-complex carbohydrate diet. Patients are at high risk for hepatocellular carcinoma.

2. **Pompe's disease (GSD Type 2),** caused by **α-glucosidase deficiency,** should be suspected in any infant with muscular weakness and cardiomegaly. It presents within the first 2 weeks of life with flaccid weakness, poor feeding, progressive cardiomegaly, hepatomegaly, and acidosis.

VII. **Fatty Acid Oxidation Defects.** These conditions present during an acute illness or fasting when fatty acids are normally used as an energy source. Patients with fatty acid oxidation defects are unable to utilize fatty acids and, as a result, develop **nonketotic hypoglycemia, hyperammonemia, myopathy, and cardiomyopathy. Medium-chain acyl-CoA dehydrogenase deficiency is the most common fatty acid oxidation disorder.** Diagnosis is based on tandem mass spectrometry detecting elevated plasma medium-chain fatty acids. Management includes frequent feedings with a high-carbohydrate, low-fat diet and carnitine supplementation during acute episodes.

VIII. Mitochondrial Disorders. One of these disorders should be suspected if a **common disease has an atypical presentation** or if a **disease involves three or more organ systems.** Examples include **Kearns-Sayre syndrome** (ophthalmoplegia, pigmentary degeneration of the retina, hearing loss, heart block, and neurologic degeneration) and **MELAS** (*m*itochondrial *e*ncephalopathy, *l*actic *a*cidosis, and *s*trokelike episodes). **Diagnosis is based on tissue biopsy revealing abnormal mitochondria.** Management is predominantly supportive and may include cofactor supplementation.

IX. Lysosomal Storage Diseases

A. Gangliosidoses

1. **Tay-Sachs disease** is an autosomal recessive disorder caused by **hexosaminidase A deficiency.** Incidence is higher in Ashkenazi Jews.
    a. **Clinical features**
       (1) **Infantile-onset Tay-Sachs disease** presents in early infancy with decreasing eye contact, hypotonia, mild motor weakness, and an increased startle as a result of **hyperacusis** (increased sensitivity to sound). Other findings include:
          (a) **Macrocephaly**
          (b) **Cherry-red macula**
          (c) Progressive blindness, seizures, and **severe developmental delay**
       (2) **Juvenile or adult-onset Tay-Sachs disease** begins after 2 years of age or in early adulthood. Clinical features include ataxia, dysarthria, and choreoathetosis. Cherry-red macula is absent.
    b. **Diagnosis** is based on decreased hexosaminidase A activity in leukocytes or fibroblasts.
    c. **Prognosis. Infantile Tay-Sachs disease is untreatable,** and death occurs by 4 years of age. Patients with the **juvenile or adult-onset** form have a poor prognosis with degeneration into a chronic debilitated state.

2. **Gaucher's disease,** caused by **glucocerebrosidase deficiency,** is the **most common gangliosidosis.** Inheritance is autosomal recessive. Typical features include hepatosplenomegaly, thrombocytopenia, a characteristic **Erlenmeyer flask-shape to the distal femur,** and early mortality by 4 years of age, if symptoms begin in infancy. Management includes enzyme replacement therapy.

3. **Niemann-Pick disease,** caused by **sphingomyelinase deficiency,** presents by 6 months of age with progressive neurodegeneration, ataxia, seizures, hepatosplenomegaly, and a cherry-red macula. Death occurs by 4 years of age.

4. **Metachromatic leukodystrophy** is a **neurodegenerative disorder** caused by **arylsulfatase A deficiency.** Presenting features are ataxia, seizures, and progressive mental retardation. Death occurs by 10–20 years of age.

B. **Mucopolysaccharidoses** are **lysosomal storage disorders** in which glucosaminoglycans accumulate in multiple organs. Common features include organomegaly, short stature, mental retardation, and specific skeletal abnormalities termed **dysostosis multiplex** (a constellation of bony abnormalities that include a thickened cranium, J-shaped sella turcica, malformed, ovoid or beaklike vertebrae, short and thickened clavicles, and oar-shaped ribs).

1. **Hurler syndrome,** caused by α-L-iduronidase deficiency, is the **most severe mucopolysaccharidosis.** Inheritance is autosomal recessive.

   a. **Clinical features** begin after 1 year of age with developmental delay, hepatosplenomegaly, and kyphosis. Other findings include **progressively coarsened facial features,** frontal bossing, prominent sagittal and metopic sutures, wide nasal bridge, thickening of the nasopharyngeal tissues, hydrocephalus, **corneal clouding,** and progressively stiff and contracted joints.

   b. **Diagnosis** is by finding dermatan and heparan sulfates in the urine and decreased α-L-iduronidase enzyme activity in leukocytes or fibroblasts.

   c. **Management** may include early bone marrow transplant to prevent neurodegeneration.

   d. **Prognosis** is poor, with death occurring by 10–15 years of age.

2. **Hunter syndrome** is unusual because it is inherited in an **X-linked recessive** fashion, and corneal clouding is absent.

   a. **Clinical features**

      (1) **Hepatosplenomegaly, hearing loss,** progressively stiff and contracted joints, small papules over shoulder, scapula, and lower back, and dysostosis multiplex

      (2) **Clinical pearl: The mnemonic "A hunter needs sharp eyes; therefore, no corneal clouding occurs"** may help distinguish between Hunter syndrome and Hurler syndrome.

   b. **Diagnosis** is the same as for Hurler syndrome (see IX.B.1.b).

   c. **Prognosis.** There is no treatment, and patients typically die by 20 years of age.

3. **Sanfilippo syndrome** is an autosomal recessive disorder that is characterized by rapid and severe mental and motor retardation.

4. **Morquio syndrome** differs from the other mucopolysaccharidoses in that **mental retardation is absent.** Severe scoliosis leading to cor pulmonale results in death by 40 years of age.

X. Defects in Heme Pigment Biosynthesis (Porphyrias). These defects cause an elevation of serum porphyrins that leads to skin photosensitivity and neurologic and abdominal symptoms. Acute intermittent porphyria is a classic example.

A. **Clinical features** are episodic and precipitated by drugs (e.g., alcohol, sulfa drugs, and oral contraceptives), hormonal surges (e.g., pregnancy or menses), or poor nutrition.

1. **Neurologic** findings include personality changes, emotional lability, paresthesias, and weakness (because these neurologic findings may not follow expected neural pathways, patients may be accused of malingering).

2. **GI** findings include **colicky abdominal pain,** vomiting, and constipation, often mimicking an acute abdomen.

3. **Autonomic instability** results in tachycardia, hypertension, sweating, and fever.

4. Dark burgundy-colored urine is present occasionally.

B. **Diagnosis** is based on **increased serum and urine porphobilinogen.**

C. **Management** includes intravenous glucose, correction of electrolyte abnormalities, and avoidance of fasting and precipitating drugs.

XI. Disorders of Metal Metabolism

A. **Wilson's disease** (hepatolenticular degeneration) is an autosomal recessive **defect in copper excretion** that causes copper deposition initially in the liver, followed by the brain, eyes, and heart.

1. **Clinical features** develop between 2 and 50 years of age.
   a. **Kayser-Fleischer rings** in the peripheral cornea (copper deposition in Descemet's membrane)
   b. **Neurologic** findings such as behavior changes, dystonia, dysarthria, tremors, ataxia, and seizures
   c. **Hepatic dysfunction**

2. **Diagnosis**
   a. **Decreased serum ceruloplasmin** is the **most commonly used screening test** for Wilson's disease.
   b. **Elevated serum and urine copper**
   c. Copper deposition in hepatocytes obtained by liver biopsy

3. **Management** includes **avoiding copper-containing food** (e.g., nuts, liver, shellfish, and chocolate), **chelation therapy** with oral penicillamine and zinc salts to prevent absorption, and, in some cases, liver transplant.

B. **Menkes kinky-hair disease** is an X-linked recessive disorder caused by **abnormal copper transport.** Affected patients have **low serum copper,** in contrast to those with Wilson's disease. Clinical features develop in the first few months of life and include myoclonic seizures, **pale kinky friable hair,** optic nerve atrophy, severe mental retardation, progressive neurologic degeneration, and early death. Diagnosis is based on **typical hair findings** and **low serum ceruloplasmin and copper.**

Review Test

1. A 1-week-old male infant is brought to the emergency department because of vomiting and diarrhea for 3 days. As his vital signs are being measured, he develops a generalized seizure. A stat serum glucose reveals profound hypoglycemia. On examination, you find that the edge of the liver reaches the pelvis. The infant is admitted to the neonatal intensive care unit, but later he dies of *Escherichia coli* sepsis. Which of the following is the most likely diagnosis?

(A) Gaucher's disease
(B) Galactosemia
(C) Hurler disease
(D) Transient hyperammonemia of the newborn
(E) Niemann-Pick disease

2. The parents of a 15-year-old boy consult you because they are concerned that their son has been acting strangely for the past 6 months. The boy has developed ataxia, tremors, and seizures. His father reports that his son seems to have developed a different personality. On examination, you note that the boy has brown rings at the edge of his corneas bilaterally. Which of the following is the best serum laboratory screen for the most likely diagnosis?

(A) Aluminum
(B) Lead
(C) Porphobilinogen
(D) Zinc
(E) Ceruloplasmin

3. A 6-year-old girl is brought to the clinic for a routine health maintenance visit. Her growth was normal until 2 years of age, when her height started to fall off of the growth curve, steadily decreasing to below the fifth percentile. On examination, she has a webbed neck with a normal range of motion, a shield chest with widely spaced nipples, and scoliosis. Past medical history is significant for repaired coarctation of the aorta at 3 years of age. Which of the following is the most likely diagnosis?

(A) Noonan syndrome
(B) Achondroplasia
(C) Turner syndrome
(D) Russell-Silver syndrome
(E) Marfan syndrome

4. The mother of a 6-year-old boy brings her son to the office for a second opinion regarding her child's developmental delay. Your nurse takes the initial history and reports that he was born at term by normal spontaneous vaginal delivery and seemed normal at birth but has not been meeting his developmental milestones. After assessing his vital signs, your nurse pulls you aside and states, "That mother has no control over her child! He is hyperactive, still in diapers, and he stinks!" You walk into the examination room and immediately notice a mousy, musty smell. Which of the following is the most likely diagnosis?

(A) Phenylketonuria
(B) Tyrosinemia type I
(C) Maple syrup urine disease
(D) Homocystinuria
(E) Cystinuria

5. During a health maintenance visit, the parents of a 9-month-old infant note that their infant is unable to sit alone or roll over and startles very easily to sound. On examination, you note a cherry-red macula and poor eye contact. Which of the following is correct regarding the likely diagnosis?

(A) No treatment is available, and death will occur early in childhood.
(B) Radiography of the lower extremity reveals an Erlenmeyer flask-shaped distal femur.
(C) Radiography of the extremities reveals dysostosis multiplex.
(D) Mild developmental delay is expected.
(E) Microcephaly should be apparent.

6. A 5-day-old male infant is brought to the emergency department in shock. The infant's diaper has a sickly sweet smell. Significant laboratory results include serum bicarbonate of 6 mmol/L, serum pH of 6.9, serum glucose of 19 mg/dL, and an elevated serum ammonia of 1,000 μmol/L. Maple syrup urine disease is in the differential diagnosis. Which of the following statements regarding the acute management of this patient is correct?

(A) Antibiotics are not indicated because the infant likely has an inborn error of metabolism.
(B) Oral glucose should be administered.
(C) Total parenteral nutrition with protein and lipids should be started.
(D) Sodium benzoate should be administered.
(E) Enteral feeds with a soy-based formula should be given to provide nutrition and to prevent intestinal villous atrophy.

7. A 14-year-old boy with mental retardation has been referred to you. The underlying cause of his mental retardation has never been identified. On physical examination, you note that he has large ears and large testes. Which of the following syndromes is associated with mental retardation and these physical findings?

(A) Klinefelter syndrome
(B) Down syndrome
(C) Prader-Willi syndrome
(D) Williams syndrome
(E) Fragile X syndrome

8. A 4-month-old male infant has been brought to your office for a routine health maintenance evaluation. You note that his height is below the third percentile, yet his head circumference is at the 75th percentile. Facial findings include a prominent forehead and hypoplasia of the midface region. He also has trident-shaped hands and bilateral short femurs and upper arms. Which of the following is a potential complication of this patient's likely disorder?

(A) Lumbar kyphosis in late childhood
(B) Atlantoaxial instability
(C) Spinal cord compression leading to sudden death during infancy
(D) Aortic dissection
(E) Delayed puberty

9. The mother of a 5-year-old boy is very concerned and shows you a note from his kindergarten teacher. The boy is very active, easily distracted, and unable to perform skills at the same level as others in his class, and the teacher expresses concern and wonders whether the boy could have a severe learning problem. On examination, you note that the boy's height and weight are at the 50th percentile, but his head appears very small. In addition, he has short palpebral fissures and a long, smooth philtrum with a thin upper lip. The remainder of the examination is normal. Which of the following is the most likely diagnosis?

(A) Angelman syndrome
(B) Down syndrome
(C) Fetal phenytoin syndrome
(D) Fetal alcohol syndrome
(E) Prader-Willi syndrome

10. A 12-year-old boy is brought to the office for a routine health maintenance visit by his parents. They report that he has struggled in school, requiring some special educational assistance since kindergarten, but has been otherwise healthy. Examination reveals that the boy is very tall (> 95th percentile) with long, thin arms with fingers of normal size. Mild scoliosis is evident. On auscultation, a murmur consistent with mitral regurgitation is audible. Based on the likely diagnosis, which of the following would you also expect to find on further evaluation?

(A) Increased upper-to-lower segment ratio
(B) Downward lens subluxation
(C) Aortic root dilatation
(D) Joint laxity
(E) Hypogonadism

11. You are called to the newborn nursery to evaluate a 1-day-old female infant with unusual physical findings. On examination, you note that the neonate's hands are clenched with overlapping digits and her lower extremities are extended and crossed. You also note the presence of rocker bottom feet and delicate, small facial features. Which of the following chromosomal abnormalities is the most likely cause of the patient's features?

(A) Trisomy 13
(B) Trisomy 18
(C) Trisomy 21
(D) Deletion on chromosome 7
(E) Absence of a region on paternally derived chromosome 15

The response options for statements 12–14 are the same. You will be required to select one answer for each statement in the set.

(A) Ehlers-Danlos syndrome
(B) Cri du chat syndrome
(C) Osteogenesis imperfecta
(D) Williams syndrome
(E) Angelman syndrome
(F) Hurler syndrome
(G) Hunter syndrome
(H) Tay-Sachs disease
(I) Gaucher's disease
(J) Homocystinuria

For each patient, select the most likely genetic condition.

12. Six-year-old boy with coarsened facial features, stiff joints, and a cloudy cornea

13. Four-year-old boy with microcephaly, hypertelorism, mental retardation, and a deletion on the short arm of chromosome 5

14. Fourteen-year-old girl with joint laxity, easily bruisable skin, and a defect in type V collagen

Answers and Explanations

1. The answer is B [VI.A]. Galactosemia should always be considered in the differential diagnosis of any newborn who develops hypoglycemia and has hepatomegaly. Infants with galactosemia develop vomiting and diarrhea after feeding with either breast milk or cow's milk-based formulas because both types of feedings contain galactose. Soy milk does not contain galactose, which means that an infant who is fed a soy formula will not be symptomatic; this delays the diagnosis. Infants with galactosemia are vulnerable to *Escherichia coli* sepsis, and if the condition is not diagnosed, they may die in early infancy. Children with Gaucher's disease present with neurodegeneration, splenomegaly, and bony changes (the most characteristic of which is an Erlenmeyer flask-shaped distal femur). After the first year of life, individuals with Hurler disease present with developmental delay, coarse facies, corneal clouding, and dysostosis multiplex. Individuals with transient hyperammonemia of the newborn may present with vomiting, and those with Niemann-Pick disease may present with hepatomegaly and seizures, but hypoglycemia and *E. coli* sepsis are not typical features of these diseases.

2. The answer is E [XI.A.2]. Wilson's disease should always be considered in a patient with personality changes, ataxia, and seizures. The patient's signs and symptoms are suggestive of Wilson's disease, which is caused by a defect in copper excretion leading to copper deposition in the brain, eyes, and liver. Kayser-Fleischer rings, which represent copper deposition in Descemet's membrane, are pathognomonic for Wilson's disease. The most commonly used screening test for Wilson's disease is a low serum ceruloplasmin, which is very suggestive of the disorder. None of the other answer choices are associated with the signs and symptoms present in this patient. Serum porphobilinogen is elevated in acute intermittent porphyria, which may present with weakness, abdominal pain, and autonomic instability. Neither aluminum, zinc, nor lead causes the signs and symptoms seen in this patient.

3. The answer is C [III.C.1]. Girls with Turner syndrome are usually diagnosed in childhood after an evaluation for short stature, or during adolescence after an evaluation for delayed puberty. Patients with Turner syndrome classically have a webbed neck with a low posterior hairline, a shield chest with widely spaced nipples, and transient swelling of the hands and feet during the newborn period. Noonan syndrome can occur in females and has similar physical findings, but affected patients usually have right-sided heart lesions (e.g., pulmonary stenosis). Patients with Turner syndrome have left-sided heart lesions (e.g., coarctation of the aorta). Patients with achondroplasia are short from birth with shortening of the proximal long bones (rhizomelic short stature), those with Silver-Russell syndrome have short stature with skeletal asymmetry, and those with Marfan syndrome are tall, not short.

4. The answer is A [Table 5-5]. Patients with mild phenylketonuria may present in childhood with developmental delay, hyperactivity, and a classic mousy or musty odor. Patients with tyrosinemia type I present with peripheral neuropathy and renal and liver disease, and may produce an odor of rotten fish or cabbage. Children with mild maple syrup urine disease may also present with developmental delay, but their urine has a sweet maple syrup odor. Neither homocystinuria nor cystinuria has a peculiar odor as a feature; however, patients with homocystinuria may have developmental delay as a result of strokes from their hypercoagulable state.

5. The answer is A [IX.A.1]. The infant has infantile Tay-Sachs disease, a devastating progressively neurodegenerative disease caused by hexosaminidase A deficiency. The onset of disease is in early infancy when the infant presents with a hyperactive startle and loses eye contact. Classic features include a cherry-red macula, enlarging head circumference, neurodegeneration with severe developmental delay, progressive blindness, and seizures. Death usually occurs by 4 years of age. An Erlenmeyer flask-shaped distal femur is a feature of Gaucher's disease and not Tay-Sachs disease. Dysostosis multiplex (bony abnormalities that include a thickened skull, malformed vertebrae, and abnormal ribs and clavicle) is found in patients with mucopolysaccharidoses (e.g., Hunter and Hurler syndromes).

6. The answer is D [IV.C]. In general, the acute management of an inborn error of metabolism involves supplying a source of energy that can be utilized, removing toxic metabolites, and preventing continued exposure to the offending substance. Because of this patient's hyperammonemia, sodium benzoate would be useful to facilitate ammonia excretion. Although the patient's condition is likely to be an inborn error of metabolism (maple syrup urine disease given the diaper odor consistent with the odor of maple syrup), sepsis is more common and can present in a similar fashion. Therefore, initial management should include intravenous antibiotics. Glucose is a basic energy source that can be used in any patient, regardless of the inborn error of metabolism, and should be administered intravenously, not orally, in a patient who is markedly hypoglycemic and in shock. Patients with maple syrup urine disease cannot metabolize branched-chain amino acids; therefore, offering parenteral nutrition with protein would continue the toxic exposure. In addition, until a diagnosis is made, initial management should include avoidance of any enteral feedings to limit continued exposure to the offending substance.

7. The answer is E [III.C.2]. The characteristic physical features of fragile X syndrome include large ears, macrocephaly, blue irides, and large testes. Klinefelter syndrome is characterized by tall stature, gynecomastia, and a small penis and testes; Down syndrome by characteristic facial features, endocardial cushion defects, duodenal atresia, mental retardation, single palmar creases, and a wide space between the first and second toes; Prader-Willi syndrome by infantile hypotonia, hypogonadism, short stature, and obesity and hyperphagia later in childhood; and Williams syndrome by a loquacious "cocktail party" personality, supravalvular aortic stenosis, and hypercalcemia. Testes are unaffected in Down syndrome and in Williams syndrome.

8. The answer is C [III.D.2.c]. This patient's physical features are consistent with achondroplasia, the most common skeletal dysplasia. Potential complications of this disorder include cord compression caused by foramen magnum stenosis that can lead to sudden death during infancy, obstructive sleep apnea, and orthopedic problems such as genu varum and back pain caused by lumbar lordosis during late childhood. Neither atlantoaxial instability (a complication of Down syndrome), aortic dissection (a complication of Marfan syndrome), nor delayed puberty is associated with achondroplasia.

9. The answer is D [III.F.1]. This patient's physical characteristics, along with learning problems and attention deficit/hyperactivity disorder, are consistent with fetal alcohol syndrome. Angelman syndrome is associated with severe mental retardation and a small head, although a puppetlike gait and inappropriate bouts of laughter are also characteristic. Down syndrome is also associated with mental retardation; however, the facial characteristics include upslanting palpebral fissures, epicanthal skin folds, and a protruding tongue. Fetal phenytoin syndrome is associated with mental retardation, nail and digit abnormalities, and cardiac defects. Prader-Willi syndrome is associated with hypogonadism, almond-shaped eyes, short stature, and hyperphagia with obesity during childhood.

10. The answer is B [V.A]. The clinical features of homocystinuria and Marfan syndrome overlap considerably; however, this patient most likely has homocystinuria based on the presence of a marfanoid body habitus with fingers of normal length (i.e., no arachnodactyly). In addition, patients with homocystinuria have downward lens subluxation (upward lens subluxation is found in Marfan syndrome); mitral or aortic regurgitation (aortic dilatation is absent but is present in Marfan syndrome); large, stiff joints (joint laxity is found in Marfan syndrome); and developmental delay and mild mental retardation (mental retardation is absent in Marfan syndrome). Patients with both disorders have a decreased upper-to-lower segment ratio. Hypogonadism is absent in both disorders.

11. The answer is B [III.B.2]. The findings of scissoring of the lower extremities, clenched hands with overlapping digits, rocker bottom feet, and delicate small facial features are consistent with the diagnosis of trisomy 18, the second most common trisomy syndrome after trisomy 21. Trisomy 21 is the cause of Down syndrome and is associated with hypotonia, prominent epicanthal folds, upslanting palpebral fissures, and single palmar creases. Trisomy 13 is associated with midline defects of the brain and forebrain. Features include microphthalmia, holoprosencephaly, and cleft lip and palate. Absence of a region on the paternally derived chromosome 15 is the cause of Prader-Willi syndrome, a disorder associated with neonatal hypotonia, hypogonadism, almond-shaped eyes, and short stature. A deletion on chromosome 7 causes Williams syndrome, characterized by elfin facies and a loquacious "cocktail party" personality.

12, 13, and 14. The answers are F [IX.B.1], **B** [III.A.14], **and A** [III.A.6], **respectively.** Hurler syndrome, a mucopolysaccharidosis in which glucosaminoglycans deposit in various tissues causing a progressive clinical picture, is characterized by corneal clouding, changes to the bone termed dysostosis multiplex, organomegaly, and progressively coarsened facies, including frontal bossing, widened nasal bridge, and thickening of the nasopharyngeal tissues.

Cri du chat syndrome, caused by a partial deletion on the short arm of chromosome 5, is characterized by slow growth, microcephaly, mental retardation, hypertelorism, and a classic catlike cry.

Ehlers-Danlos syndrome is caused by a defect in type V collagen that results in hyperextensible joints, fragile blood vessels that cause easily bruised skin, tissue paper-thin scars, and cardiovascular complications (e.g., mitral valve prolapse and aortic root dilatation that can lead to dissection).

6

Endocrinology

Ronald A. Nagel, M.D., and Lee Todd Miller, M.D.

I. Short Stature

A. **General Concepts**

1. **Definition.** Short stature is defined as **height that is two standard deviations (SDs) below the mean** (i.e., below the third percentile).

   a. **Normal variant short stature** describes a child whose height is below the third percentile but is growing with a normal growth velocity.

   b. **Pathologic short stature** describes a child whose height is below the third percentile (often more than 3 SDs below the mean) but is growing with a suboptimal growth velocity.

2. **Key point: It is critical to evaluate growth rate and not just absolute height** when evaluating short stature.

3. In the first 2 years of life, a normal downward shift in the height percentile may reflect genetic short stature.

4. **Key pearl:** Children who grow **2 inches per year (5 cm per year) between 3 years of age and puberty usually do not have an endocrinopathy or underlying pathologic disorder.**

5. All patients with short stature who are more than 3 SDs below the mean or who have a growth velocity less than 5 cm per year are considered to have a pathologic growth disorder until proven otherwise.

6. **Determining the targeted mid-parental height (MPH)** may be helpful in distinguishing a patient with normal variant short stature from pathologic short stature (**Figure 6-1**).

   a. Most children, when they have completed their growth, are within ±2 SDs, or 4 inches, of their MPH.

   b. A major discrepancy between a child's present growth percentile and the targeted MPH percentile suggests a pathologic state.

B. **History**

1. **Perinatal history.** Assess for prematurity or intrauterine growth retardation (IUGR). A history of hypoglycemia, prolonged jaundice, cryptorchidism, or microphallus suggests **hypopituitarism.**

$$\text{MALE MPH} = \frac{\text{Father's height} + (\text{Mother's height} + 5 \text{ inches})}{2}$$

$$\text{FEMALE MPH} = \frac{(\text{Father's height} - 5 \text{ inches}) + \text{Mother's height}}{2}$$

Figure 6-1. Determination of mid-parental height (MPH). Most patients, when they have completed their growth, will be within ±2 standard deviations, or 4 inches, of the MPH. For example, if a boy has a father who is 5 feet 9 inches in height and a mother who is 5 feet in height, then the MPH is 5 feet 7 inches ± 4 inches.

2. **Chronic diseases** such as renal failure, central nervous system (CNS) disease, severe asthma with frequent and prolonged steroid use, sickle cell anemia, and inflammatory bowel disease may manifest short stature.

3. **Chronic use of drugs,** such as steroids, or stimulants for attention deficit/hyperactivity disorder that result in significant appetite suppression and poor weight gain may lead to short stature.

4. **Family history, especially parental growth and pubertal histories, are important.** To evaluate for constitutional delay short stature and familial short stature (see section D.1), ask whether the family history is positive for "late growth spurts" or "late bloomers" in high school or college and the age of maternal menarche.

5. **Social history** is critical because children who live in neglected or hostile environments may exhibit short stature because of **psychosocial deprivation.**

6. **Review of systems** should include questions about cold intolerance, constipation (hypothyroidism), abdominal pain, diarrhea or bloody stools (inflammatory bowel disease), and headaches and vomiting (brain tumor).

7. **Dental history.** Delayed dental eruption may suggest a delayed bone age.

C. **Physical Examination**

1. **Accurate height and weight** should be plotted on a U.S. National Center for Health Statistics (NCHS) growth chart, along with previous growth points to assess the child's growth pattern.

2. **Measure the patient's upper-to-lower (U/L) body segment ratio.**

   a. **Lower segment** = pubic symphysis to the heel

   b. **Upper segment** = total height minus lower segment

   c. Normal ratios:

      (1) Birth = 1.7

      (2) 3 years of age = 1.3

      (3) > 7 years of age = 1.0

   d. **Abnormal U/L ratio** suggests **disproportionate short stature** (see section D.2.b).

3. Thorough physical examination should include a funduscopic examination, assessment of thyroid size, evaluation for stigmata of genetic syndromes (e.g., web neck, shield chest, and short fourth metacarpals are

suggestive of Turner syndrome; see Chapter 5, section III.C.1), scoliosis screening, and Tanner staging (see Chapter 3, section I).

D. Categorization of Short Stature (Figure 6-2).

    1. Normal variant short stature. The two most common categories of normal variant short stature (children whose height falls below the third percentile with **normal growth velocity**) are **familial** (or genetic) short stature and **constitutional growth delay** with delayed puberty.

        a. Familial (or genetic) short stature is defined as a height at least 2 SDs below the mean with a short MPH but with a **normal bone age, a normal onset of puberty,** and a minimum growth of 2 inches (or 5 cm) per year.

        b. Constitutional short stature is defined as a height at least 2 SDs below the mean with a history of delayed puberty in either or both parents, a **delayed bone age** and **late onset of puberty,** and a minimum growth of 2 inches (or 5 cm) per year.

    2. Pathologic short stature. Pathologic short stature (children whose heights fall more than 3 SDs below the mean with **abnormal growth velocity** (i.e., growth velocity less than 2 inches or 5 cm per year) may be categorized as **proportionate** or **disproportionate**.

        a. Proportionate short stature is defined as short stature with a normal U/L ratio (see section I.C.2.c). It is important to distinguish between prenatal onset and postnatal onset.

            (1) Causes of **prenatal onset proportionate** short stature include:

                (a) Environmental exposures (e.g., in utero exposure to tobacco and alcohol)

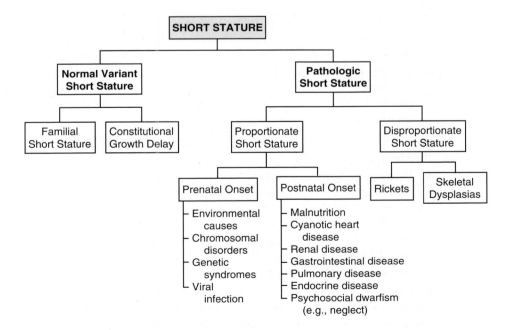

Figure 6-2. Differential diagnosis of short stature.

   (b) Chromosome disorders (e.g., Down syndrome, Turner syndrome)

   (c) Genetic syndromes (e.g., Russell-Silver syndrome, Prader-Willi syndrome; see Chapter 5, sections III.A.13 and III.A.2, respectively)

   (d) Viral infection early in pregnancy (e.g., cytomegalovirus, rubella)

(2) Causes of **postnatal onset proportionate** short stature

   (a) Malnutrition

   (b) Psychosocial causes (e.g., neglect, child abuse)

   (c) Organ system diseases, including gastrointestinal diseases (inflammatory bowel disease), cardiac diseases (cyanotic congenital heart disease), renal diseases (renal failure, renal tubular acidosis), chronic lung diseases (cystic fibrosis, asthma), and endocrinopathies (hypothyroidism, growth hormone deficiency, and cortisol excess; see also section I.F)

b. Disproportionate short stature is defined as short stature in patients are who very short-legged with an increased U/L ratio, suggesting rickets or a skeletal dysplasia.

   (1) Consider **rickets** for patients with frontal bossing, bowed legs, low serum phosphorus level, and high serum alkaline phosphatase (see section X.C).

   (2) Consider some form of **skeletal dysplasia** (e.g., achondroplasia) for patients who are short with short limbs (see Chapter 5, section III.D).

E. Evaluation of Pathologic Short Stature

1. Laboratory studies

   a. Complete blood count (CBC), erythrocyte sedimentation rate (ESR), thyroxine (T_4), serum electrolytes including calcium and phosphorus, and serum creatinine and bicarbonate levels should be obtained.

   b. Insulin growth factor **(IGF-1)** is an indirect test for growth hormone deficiency. Random growth hormone level should not be measured; most growth hormone is released during stage IV non-rapid eye movement sleep.

   c. Chromosome analysis in girls to evaluate for Turner syndrome

2. Radiographic studies

   a. Bone age determination (anterior-posterior [AP] film of the left hand and wrist to assess the characteristics of the epiphyses or growth plates) is very helpful to compare with chronologic age **(Table 6-1)**.

   b. AP and lateral skull radiographs are necessary to assess the pituitary gland (distortion of the sella turcica and suprasellar calcification suggest craniopharyngioma).

3. Key pearl: Patients with poor growth velocity with normal screening laboratory results but low IGF-1 and delayed bone age should have a workup for growth hormone deficiency.

Table 6-1. Using Bone Age in the Differential Diagnosis of Short Stature

Bone Age = Chronologic Age	Bone Age < Chronologic Age
Familial short stature	Constitutional short stature
Intrauterine growth retardation	Hypothyroidism
Turner syndrome	Hypercortisolism
Skeletal dysplasia	Growth hormone deficiency
	Chronic diseases

F. Endocrinopathies that Cause Short Stature

1. **Growth hormone (GH) deficiency** is uncommon.

   a. **Clinical features.** A history of prolonged neonatal jaundice, hypoglycemia, cherubic facies, central obesity, microphallus, cryptorchidism, and midline defects (e.g., cleft palate) may be present. The **growth curve** demonstrates poor growth velocity (less than 2 inches or 5 cm per year).

   b. **Causes** include brain tumors (**pearl: craniopharyngioma must be considered in any child older than 5 years of age who is not growing 2 inches per year**), prior CNS irradiation, CNS vascular malformations, autoimmune diseases, trauma, and congenital midline defects. (Consider GH deficiency in patients with a single central maxillary incisor or with cleft palate.)

   c. **Evaluation**

      (1) **Imaging studies.** Patients have a delayed bone age. All patients with GH deficiency must have an MRI of the head to rule out a CNS lesion.

      (2) **Laboratory studies.** Low IGF-1 levels, and a poor response on growth hormone stimulation testing (with L-dopa-Inderal, glucagon, or clonidine)

   d. **Management.** Treatment includes daily subcutaneous injections of recombinant growth hormone until a bone age determination shows that the patient has reached nearly maximal growth potential (by about 13–14 years of age in girls and 15–16 years of age in boys).

2. **Hypothyroidism.** The most common cause of hypothyroidism is Hashimoto's thyroiditis (see section VIII.B.2.b). Patients will present with increased TSH, low T_4, and positive antithyroid peroxidase antibodies.

3. **Hypercortisolism.** The most common cause of hypercortisolism is iatrogenic as a result of prolonged use of steroids (see section IV.E.1). Patients present with a history of poor growth and increasing weight gain, purpuric stretch marks and a dorsal neck fat pad on examination, and delayed bone age.

4. **Turner syndrome** (see also Chapter 5, section III.C.1). Female patients who are missing part or all of one of the X chromosomes may present with lack of puberty and poor growth velocity. Growth hormone treatment has been shown to improve the ultimate height of these patients.

II. Disorders of Puberty

A. Normal Puberty (see also Chapter 3, section I.A.2)

1. In the prepubescent state, sex steroids (testosterone and estradiol) are depressed by sensitive negative feedback at the level of the hypothalamus.

2. Puberty begins when there is a reduction in this hypothalamic inhibition, resulting in activation of the hypothalamic-pituitary-gonadal axis (HPGA).

3. The HPGA releases gonadotropin-releasing hormone (GnRH) from the hypothalamus, which binds to receptors in the pituitary gland and causes the release of follicle-stimulating hormone (FSH) and luteinizing hormone (LH).

4. **Female puberty.** Different stages of pubertal development are defined as follows. **It is important, however, to be aware that the age of onset and subsequent course of hormonal and physical changes during puberty are variable:**

   a. **Onset is between 7 and 13 years of age.**

   b. **Thelarche** is the onset of breast development as a result of the release of estrogen, and **adrenarche** is the onset of pubic or axillary hair development as a result of the release of adrenal androgens. **Breast buds** are usually the first sign of puberty, although in 15% of girls, pubic hair develops first.

   c. **Menarche** is the onset of the menstrual cycle. **Menstruation** begins at 9–15 years of age, with a mean onset of 12.5 years of age.

   d. **FSH** stimulates the ovaries to produce ovarian follicles, which in turn produce estrogen.

   e. **LH** is responsible for the positive feedback in the middle of the menstrual cycle resulting in the release of an egg.

   f. **Tanner staging.** See Chapter 3, section I.A.2.c.(2).

5. **Male puberty**

   a. **Onset is between 9 and 14 years of age.**

   b. **Testicular enlargement** is usually the first sign of puberty ($\geq$ 4 mL as measured with an orchidometer).

   c. Seventy-five percent of the testicular volume is the seminiferous tubules.

   d. **FSH** in boys stimulates the seminiferous tubules in the testes to produce sperm.

   e. **LH** in boys stimulates the testicular Leydig cells to produce androgens, which in turn are responsible for penile enlargement and the growth of axillary, facial, and pubic hair.

   f. **Tanner staging**. See Chapter 3, section I.A.2.c.(1).

6. African American children develop secondary sexual characteristics earlier than do most other children.

7. Moderate to severe obesity is associated with sexual precocity.

B. Precocious Puberty

1. **Definitions**

    a. Girls: presence of breast development or pubic hair before 7 years of age or menarche before 9 years of age

    b. Boys: presence of testicular changes, penile enlargement, or pubic or axillary hair before 9 years of age

2. Categories

    a. Premature thelarche

        (1) Definition. There is visible or palpable breast tissue only, with no other secondary sex characteristics. The growth pattern should be normal, and no pubic hair should be apparent.

        (2) Epidemiology. This very **common and benign** condition usually presents in the first 2 years of life.

        (3) Etiology. This condition is caused by a transient activation of the HPGA, resulting in transient ovarian follicular stimulation and a release of low levels of estrogen.

        (4) No workup is necessary and no treatment is indicated, unless there is pubic hair development or a rapid growth spurt.

    b. Premature adrenarche

        (1) Definition. Early onset of pubic or axillary hair occurs without the development of breast tissue or enlarged testes.

        (2) Epidemiology. This condition is more common in **girls** than in boys.

        (3) Classic presentation occurs after 5 years of age, with the onset of pubic hair growth, axillary hair growth, and apocrine odor. No breast tissue is noted, and there is no clitoromegaly. Growth is normal without advancement of bone age.

        (4) No treatment is indicated.

    c. Isosexual precocious puberty or central precocious puberty (CPP)

        (1) Definition. The early onset of gonadotropin-mediated (i.e., mediated by FSH and LH) puberty is a normal state, except that the hypothalamus has been activated earlier than usual.

        (2) Epidemiology. Girls have a higher incidence of isosexual precocious puberty than boys.

        (3) Clinical features

            (a) In girls, physical examination shows breast development, pubic hair, and rapid growth.

            (b) In boys, physical examination shows testicular enlargement, pubic hair, and rapid growth.

        (4) Etiology

            (a) In girls, most cases are **idiopathic.**

            (b) In boys, sexual precocity tends to be organic, and all cases need evaluation with an MRI of the head.

            (c) CNS abnormalities that may cause isosexual precocious puberty include hydrocephalus, CNS infections, cerebral palsy, benign hypothalamic hamartomas, malignant tumors such as astrocytomas and gliomas, and severe head trauma.

(d) Hypothyroidism may also present with isosexual precocious puberty, but in this case there is **poor growth and a delayed bone age** (unlike all other causes of sexual precocity).

(5) Evaluation

(a) FSH, LH, and **sex steroids** are elevated in the pubertal range.

(b) The **GnRH stimulation test** is an ideal test to demonstrate premature activation of the hypothalamus.

(i) By injecting synthetic GnRH into a patient, the LH response, and to a lesser degree the FSH response, can be used as an assessment of the activation of the HPGA. In response to synthetic GnRH, patients with CPP have a **dramatic increase in LH** secretion when compared with baseline levels.

(ii) On the other hand, prepubertal patients whose HPGA has not yet been activated, and patients with peripheral precocious puberty in which peripherally produced sex steroids suppress pituitary gonadotropin secretion, would be expected to have a **flat response** (i.e., no increase in LH secretion) on injection of synthetic GnRH.

(c) An MRI of the head should be performed in **all boys** and in very young girls with any neurologic symptoms (e.g., headaches or seizures) or with very rapid pubertal changes.

d. Peripheral precocious puberty (PPP) or heterosexual gonadotropin-independent puberty

(1) Definition. Precocious puberty that is independent of the HPGA (i.e., caused by the **peripheral production** of male or female sex steroids and not FSH- or LH-mediated). **The hallmark of PPP is a flat response on GnRH stimulation testing because the HPGA has not been activated.**

(2) Clinical features

(a) Boys present with either feminization (gynecomastia) or with premature onset of pubic hair. Note that there is usually **no testicular enlargement** because these patients do not have an increase in FSH, which would stimulate seminiferous tubule enlargement (see exceptions in section II.B.2.d.(3)(c)).

(b) Girls present with virilization or breast development.

(3) Etiology. Causes may differ in boys and girls, but in general include exposure to exogenous sex steroids (found in some skin lotions or foods), gonadal tumors, adrenal tumors, and nonclassic congenital adrenal hyperplasia (CAH; see section IV.C.4.a.(3)). **All of these causes are independent of the HPGA.**

(a) In boys, consider adrenal tumors, Leydig cell tumors (presenting with asymmetric testicular enlargement), nonclassic CAH, β-human chorionic gonadotropin (β-HCG)-producing tumors, McCune-Albright syndrome, and testotoxicosis.

(b) In girls, consider adrenal tumors, virilizing ovarian tumors (arrhenoblastomas), feminizing ovarian tumors (juvenile granulosa tumors), nonclassic CAH, and McCune-Albright syndrome.

(c) **Specific causes of PPP in males that result in testicular enlargement**

(i) **McCune-Albright syndrome** is characterized by bony changes (polyostotic fibrous dysplasia), skin findings (irregularly bordered hyperpigmented macules, or **"coast of Maine" café-au-lait spots**), and endocrinopathies (PPP or hyperthyroidism). Patients often have enlarged gonads but their secretion of sex steroids is independent of the HPGA.

(ii) **Testotoxicosis** is a rare disease in which the testes enlarge bilaterally independent of the HPGA.

(iii) **β-HCG–secreting tumors** are unique to boys. These tumors are found in the chest, pineal gland, gonad, or liver (hepatoblastoma). Because the β-HCG molecule crossreacts with LH, it too can bind to LH receptors and enlarge the testes slightly, stimulating Leydig cells and secreting androgens.

(4) **Evaluation.** A GnRH stimulation test may be warranted in addition to the following:

(a) **In boys,** check serum FSH, LH, testosterone, and β-HCG levels.

(b) **In girls,** check serum FSH, LH, and estradiol levels.

(c) Perform CNS imaging studies depending on the suspected etiology.

(5) **Management.** Treatment depends on the underlying cause.

C. **Delayed Puberty**

1. **Definitions**

a. **Boys:** No testicular enlargement by 14 years of age.

b. **Girls:** No breast tissue by 13 years of age, or no menarche by 14 years of age.

2. **Classification.** Two categories of disorders may result in delayed puberty.

a. **Hypogonadotropic hypogonadism.** Because of inactivity of the hypothalamus and pituitary gland, these patients have a low FSH, low LH, and, in turn, low testosterone and low estradiol, with a prepubertal (flat) GnRH stimulation test.

b. **Hypergonadotropic hypogonadism.** Because of end-organ dysfunction (i.e., gonadal failure), these patients have high FSH and high LH levels with low testosterone or low estradiol levels. There is no abnormality in the hypothalamus or pituitary gland.

3. **Etiology of hypogonadotropic hypogonadism**

a. **Constitutional delay of puberty** (i.e., immature hypothalamus or "late bloomers") is much more common in **boys** than in girls. Often there is a family history in one parent (i.e., mother had late menarche or father had his growth spurt late in high school or in college). Constitutional delay of puberty is frequently associated with constitutional delay of growth (see section I.D.1.b for a description of growth pattern).

b. **Chronic diseases** can cause pubertal delay (e.g., inflammatory bowel disease, anorexia nervosa, renal failure, and heart failure).

c. **Hypopituitarism** of any cause (e.g., brain tumors)

d. **Primary hypothyroidism**

e. **Prolactinoma**

f. **Genetic syndromes**

   (1) **Kallman syndrome.** Isolated gonadotropin deficiency associated with anosmia (inability to smell)

   (2) **Prader-Willi syndrome** (see Chapter 5, section III.A.2)

   (3) **Lawrence-Moon-Biedl syndrome.** Obesity, retinitis pigmentosa, hypogonadism, and polysyndactyly

4. **Etiology of hypergonadotropic hypogonadism**

   a. **Chromosomal disorders**

      (1) **In boys,** consider **Klinefelter syndrome (XXY;** see Chapter 5, section III.C.3).

      (2) **In girls,** consider **Turner syndrome** or gonadal dysgenesis (see Chapter 5, section III.C.1).

   b. **Autoimmune disorders** (e.g., hypogonadism in autoimmune oophoritis, which may also be associated with Hashimoto's thyroiditis or Addison's disease)

5. **Evaluation of delayed puberty.** A CBC, ESR, T_4, testosterone or estradiol, FSH, LH, prolactin level, and bone age are necessary.

III. Ambiguous Genitalia

A. **Normal Sexual Differentiation (Figure 6-3)**

1. **During the first 7 weeks of gestation,** the gonadal tissue remains undifferentiated. The final appearance of gonadal tissue is dependent on both genetic and hormonal influences.

2. **Male sexual differentiation** is an active process, whereas **female sexual differentiation** develops when genetic and hormonal influences are absent.

B. **Male sexual differentiation** is initiated by the *SRY* gene located on the short arm of the Y chromosome. By 9 weeks gestation, the *SRY* gene differentiates the gonads into fetal testes, which subsequently produce **testosterone** and **anti-müllerian hormone (AMH).**

1. **Internal ducts.** In the genetic XY male, testosterone made by fetal Leydig cells stimulates the development of the wolffian ducts (epididymis, vas deferens, and seminal vesicles), and anti-müllerian hormone made by fetal Sertoli cells inhibits the development of the müllerian structures (fallopian tubes, uterus, and upper one third of the vagina).

2. **External genitalia.** The conversion of testosterone to dihydrotestosterone (DHT) by 5α-reductase occurs in the skin of the external genitalia. DHT is responsible for penile enlargement, scrotal fusion, and the entire masculinization of the external genitalia. By 12 weeks this process is complete, except for penile growth, which continues to term.

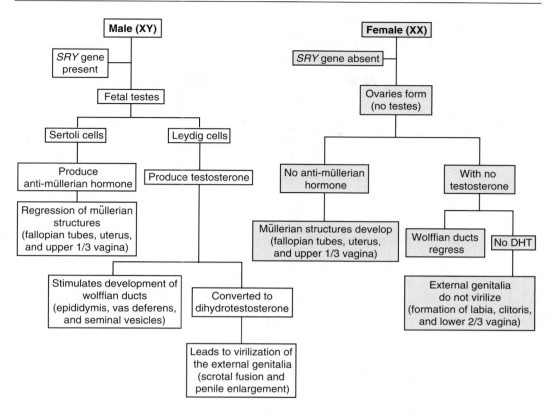

Figure 6-3. Normal sexual differentiation in utero. *DHT* = dihydrotestosterone.

C. Female sexual differentiation. In the absence of the *SRY* gene, the go-nads become ovaries.

    1. Internal ducts. Because there is no testicular tissue, there is no secre-tion of testosterone or of anti-müllerian hormone, resulting in the re-gression of the wolffian ducts and the development of the müllerian struc-tures, respectively.

    2. External genitalia. The external genitalia do not virilize because there is a lack of testosterone and of DHT. This results in the development of the labia, the clitoris, and the lower two thirds of the vagina.

D. Differential diagnosis of ambiguous genitalia in the undervirilized male (i.e., a **male pseudohermaphrodite,** who is usually a genetic 46,XY with ambiguous genitalia and one or both testes palpable; **Figure 6-4**)

    1. Inborn error in testosterone synthesis. Several inherited enzyme deficiencies result in low testosterone levels (i.e., any enzyme deficiency in the pathway of androgen synthesis in **Figure 6-5**).

    2. Gonadal intersex (i.e., conditions in which the internal structures are a combination of both male and female structures). These include two rare conditions:

        a. Mixed gonadal dysgenesis (MGD). These patients have a kary-otype with a 45,XO/46,XY mosaicism. Clinical presentation may be

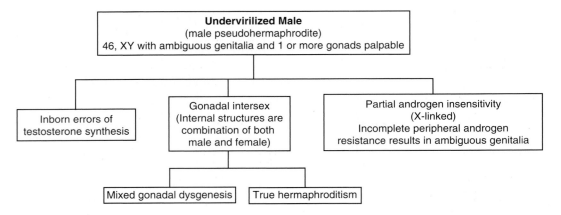

Figure 6-4. Differential diagnosis of ambiguous genitalia in an undervirilized male.

variable; however, most patients present with ambiguous genitalia and a testis and vas deferens on one side and a "streak gonad" on the contralateral side. Fallopian tubes may also be present bilaterally despite the presence of a testis.

   b. **True hermaphroditism.** These patients have ambiguous genitalia with both ovarian and testicular gonadal tissue. Usually the karyotype is 46,XX, but it can be 46,XY.

3. **Partial androgen insensitivity.** These patients have partial or incomplete peripheral androgen resistance resulting in defective androgen binding in the genital tissue (**Note:** Patients with **testicular feminiza-**

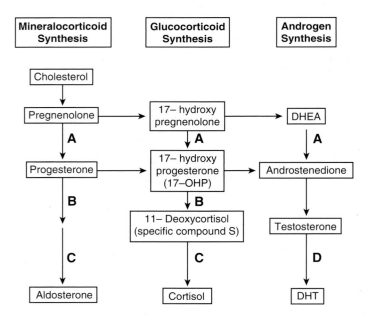

Figure 6-5. Steroid pathways in the adrenal cortex. *A* = 3β-hydroxysteroid dehydrogenase; *B* = 21-hydroxylase (21-OH); *C* = 11β-hydroxylase (11β-OH); *D* = 5α-reductase; *DHEA* = dehydroepiandrosterone; *DHT* = dihydrotestosterone.

tion syndrome have complete androgen insensitivity and present as normal phenotypic females [normal external genitalia] but with a 46,XY karyotype; see Chapter 3, Table 3-6).

E. **Differential diagnosis of ambiguous genitalia in the virilized female** (i.e., a **female pseudohermaphrodite,** who is a genetic XX with ambiguous genitalia and no gonads palpable; **Figure 6-6**).

1. **CAH caused by 21-hydroxylase deficiency is the most common cause of female pseudohermaphroditism** (see section IV.B). 11β-Hydroxylase (11β-OH) deficiency and 3β-hydroxysteroid dehydrogenase deficiency are other causes of CAH.

2. **Virilizing drug** used by mother during pregnancy

3. **Virilizing tumor** in mother during pregnancy

F. **Evaluation of the patient with ambiguous genitalia**

1. **Careful history.** Maternal history of drugs or virilization, family history of androgen insensitivity, CAH, or consanguinity

2. **Physical examination.** Presence or absence of gonads, labioscrotal swelling, bifid scrotum, labial fusion, urogenital sinus, or hypospadias. **(Pearl: Increased blood pressure suggests CAH with 11β-OH deficiency, and decreased blood pressure suggests adrenal insufficiency;** see sections IV.B.1.a and IV.C.3.b.)

3. **Chromosome studies**

4. **Radiographic studies** include pelvic ultrasound and genitogram to define the internal genitourinary anatomy.

5. **Laboratory studies**

   a. **Male pseudohermaphrodites.** DHT and testosterone levels are warranted. If serum testosterone is low, further evaluation for an inborn error in androgen synthesis is indicated.

   b. **Female pseudohermaphrodites.** Serum electrolytes, testosterone level, and further studies to look for evidence of CAH (17-OH progesterone, dehydroepiandrosterone [DHEA], and Compound S levels) are indicated (see Figure 6-5 and section IV.C.4).

6. **Management.** The focus is on gender assignment as soon as possible, with input from a pediatric urologist on surgical options. Hormonal therapy depends on etiology.

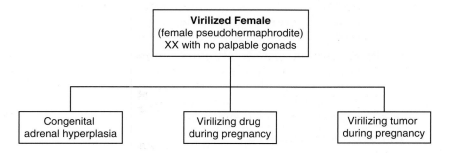

Figure 6-6. Differential diagnosis of ambiguous genitalia in a virilized female.

IV. Disorders of the Adrenal Gland

   A. **General Principles of Adrenal Function**

   1. The **adrenal gland** is composed of two parts, the **adrenal cortex,** which synthesizes a multitude of different steroid compounds, and the **adrenal medulla,** which produces catecholamines (i.e., epinephrine).

   2. **Three major pathways** in the adrenal cortex result in the production of **mineralocorticoids** (aldosterone), **glucocorticoids** (cortisol), and **androgens** (DHEA), as outlined in **Figure 6-5.**

   3. **Glucocorticoid and androgen synthesis** are regulated by a negative feedback loop by the hypothalamic-pituitary-adrenal axis via adrenocorticotropin hormone (ACTH). **Mineralocorticoid synthesis,** however, is controlled by the renin-angiotensin system and is **independent** of the pituitary gland and ACTH.

   4. Children may present with disorders of adrenal insufficiency and with disorders of glucocorticoid excess.

   B. **Classification of Adrenal Insufficiency**

   1. **Primary** or **secondary,** each with different clinical manifestations

      a. **Primary adrenal insufficiency**

         (1) This condition results from destruction of the adrenal cortex or from an enzyme deficiency **(i.e., a problem at the level of the adrenal gland).**

         (2) Patients present with signs and symptoms of both **cortisol deficiency** (anorexia, weakness, hyponatremia, hypotension, and increased pigmentation over recently healed scars) and **aldosterone deficiency** (failure to thrive, salt craving, hyponatremia, and **hyperkalemia**).

         (3) **Examples** include **Addison's disease, CAH,** and **adrenoleukodystrophy** (rare, X-linked recessive disorder with neurologic deterioration).

      b. **Secondary adrenal insufficiency**

         (1) This condition results from any process that interferes with the release of cortisol-releasing hormone (CRH) from the hypothalamus or ACTH from the pituitary **(i.e., a problem at the hypothalamic or pituitary level).**

         (2) In contrast to primary adrenal insufficiency, serum potassium may be normal in secondary adrenal insufficiency because there is **no aldosterone deficiency** given an intact renin-angiotensin system.

         (3) **Examples** include pituitary tumors, craniopharyngioma, and Langerhans cell histiocytosis. However, **the most common cause is iatrogenic;** this occurs when the hypothalamic-pituitary axis has been suppressed by exposure to long-term dosages of glucocorticoids (usually longer than 2 weeks).

   2. **Congenital** or **acquired**

      a. **Congenital adrenal insufficiency** includes CAH.

    b. Acquired adrenal insufficiency includes Addison's disease and patients taking chronic steroids resulting in adrenal suppression.

C. Congenital Adrenal Hyperplasia (CAH)

    1. This **autosomal recessive** congenital enzyme deficiency in the adrenal cortex is a classic example of primary adrenal insufficiency of childhood. CAH is also the **most common cause of ambiguous genitalia** when no gonads are palpable.

    2. The enzyme deficiency in patients with CAH may lead to underproduction of cortisol or aldosterone and a build-up of precursors that shunt into another pathway leading to **increased production of androgens** (see **Figure 6-5**).

    3. **Multiple enzyme deficiencies** may lead to CAH, and the clinical presentation varies depending on which enzyme is affected. The three main types include:

        a. 21-Hydroxylase deficiency (accounts for **90% of cases**). Three different subtypes of 21-hydroxylase deficiency affect the clinical presentation.

            (1) Classic salt-wasting CAH (i.e., both mineralocorticoid and glucocorticoid pathways are affected, resulting in both cortisol and aldosterone deficiency). Girls present with ambiguous genitalia, and at 1–2 weeks of life both boys and girls present with failure to thrive, vomiting, and electrolyte abnormalities.

            (2) Simple virilizing CAH (i.e., only the glucocorticoid pathway is affected, resulting only in cortisol deficiency). Because there is no aldosterone deficiency, there are usually no electrolyte abnormalities. Girls present with ambiguous genitalia at birth, and boys present later in life (1–4 years of age) with tall stature, advanced bone age, pubic hair, and penile enlargement.

            (3) Nonclassic CAH (i.e., late-onset with very mild cortisol deficiency and no mineralocorticoid involvement). These patients usually present at 4–5 years of age. Girls present with premature adrenarche, clitoromegaly, acne, rapid growth, hirsutism, and infertility. Boys present with premature adrenarche, rapid growth, and premature acne.

        b. 11β-Hydroxylase deficiency (accounts for 5% of cases). These patients present similarly to patients with the more common 21-hydroxylase deficiency, except that they are **hypertensive** and **hypokalemic.**

        c. 3β-Hydroxysteroid dehydrogenase deficiency (rare). These patients present with salt-wasting crises, glucocorticoid deficiency, and ambiguous genitalia as a result of an early block in all three adrenal cortex steroid pathways.

    4. **Diagnostic workup** varies with the type of CAH (see **Figure 6-5**):

        a. Patients with **21-hydroxylase deficiency** have increased **17-hydroxyprogesterone (17-OHP) levels.**

        b. Patients with **11β-hydroxylase deficiency** have increased levels of 11-deoxycortisol (also known as **specific compound S**).

    c. Patients with **3β-hydroxysteroid dehydrogenase deficiency** have increased levels of **DHEA** and **17-hydroxypregnenolone**.

  5. Management

    a. Cortisone is administered at a dose that sufficiently suppresses ACTH production so that androgen production decreases but is not excessive enough to interfere with proper growth.

    b. If patients are also aldosterone deficient, mineralocorticoid replacement (fluorocortisol) may be given at a dosage that normalizes the plasma renin activity (PRA).

    c. Frequent follow-up is essential, and growth velocity, physical examination, bone age, and laboratory tests (17-OHP, PRA) should be monitored carefully. Parents should be educated and warned about the importance of compliance with medicines and how febrile episodes, vomiting, and surgical operations may require additional steroid therapy to prevent adrenal shock.

D. Acquired Adrenal Insufficiency

  1. Etiology. Causes are multiple.

    a. Chronic supraphysiologic steroid use (usually greater than 2 weeks)

    b. Addison's disease is adrenal insufficiency resulting from **autoimmune destruction** of the adrenal cortex by lymphocytic infiltration. Antibodies to the adrenal gland may be detected, and there may be other associated endocrinopathies, including Hashimoto's thyroiditis and type 1 diabetes mellitus (**type I polyglandular syndrome**) or hypoparathyroidism and chronic mucocutaneous candidiasis (**type II polyglandular syndrome**).

    c. Less common causes of acquired adrenal insufficiency are acute adrenal hemorrhage in the neonate and septicemia (especially associated with meningococcemia, known as **Waterhouse-Friderichsen syndrome**).

  2. Evaluation

    a. A high index of suspicion is necessary because the symptoms may be very subtle and the conditions can be life-threatening.

    b. History of prior steroid use or autoimmune disorders should raise clinical suspicion.

    c. Random plasma cortisol levels are usually not helpful (although a cortisol level > 20 μg/dL in the presence of stress excludes adrenal insufficiency).

    d. ACTH stimulation test is the **test of choice** and measures adrenal cortisol reserve by comparing the baseline cortisol level with the cortisol level 1 hour after ACTH injection. Normally, the cortisol level doubles in response to ACTH stimulation. If there is a blunted response, it usually indicates primary adrenal insufficiency.

  3. Management

    a. Adrenal crisis is a medical emergency!

    b. Prompt treatment requires **intravenous fluids** with 5% dextrose in normal saline to correct hypotension and hyponatremia and to prevent hypoglycemia.

   c. Parenteral **steroids** are given until the patient is stabilized.

E. Glucocorticoid Excess

   1. Clinical features include poor growth with delayed bone age, central obesity, moon facies, nuchal fad pad, easy bruisability, purplish (hemorrhagic) striae, hypertension, and glucose intolerance.

   2. Major causes of hypercortisolism

      a. Iatrogenic. The **most common cause of glucocorticoid excess is iatrogenic,** as seen in patients who have been treated with chronic steroids for chronic diseases such as asthma, inflammatory bowel disease, and juvenile rheumatoid arthritis.

      b. Cushing syndrome. This is excessive glucocorticoid production caused by **benign or malignant adrenal tumors.** Note that most adrenal tumors are virilizing, but on occasion they may also feminize.

      c. Cushing disease. This is excessive glucocorticoid production caused by **excessive ACTH production** by a pituitary tumor, such as a microadenoma.

   3. Laboratory evaluation and diagnosis

      a. Elevated free cortisol in 24-hour urine collection.

      b. Absence of the expected cortisol suppression seen in an overnight **dexamethasone suppression test** (i.e., dexamethasone given in the evening normally suppresses the following morning's physiologic rise in cortisol)

   4. Key pearl: Cortisol excess states may be confused with **obesity.** Hypercortisolism presents with growth impairment and delayed bone age, but obese patients have normal to fast growth and an advanced bone age.

V. Diabetes Mellitus

A. Epidemiology

   1. Diabetes mellitus (DM) is the second most common chronic disease of childhood, affecting 1 of 500 children.

   2. Two times more common in **boys** than in girls

B. Types of Diabetes

   1. Type 1—insulin deficiency (insulin-dependent)

   2. Type 2—insulin resistant (non–insulin-dependent)

VI. Type 1 Diabetes Mellitus (Type 1 DM)

A. Etiology. Type 1 DM is likely multifactorial with genetic, environmental, and autoimmune factors.

   1. Genetic factors

    a. There are strong genetic influences, but inheritance has not been found to fit into classic Mendelian patterns (autosomal or X-linked).

    b. Approximately 95% of patients with type 1 DM have **HLA haplotype DR3 or DR4.**

    c. Monozygotic twins have a 50% concordance rate, whereas dizygotic twins have only a 30% concordance rate.

  2. Environmental triggers

    a. **Viral infections** have been implicated, including enteroviruses (coxsackie) and rubella.

    b. Whether the early introduction of cow's milk might trigger DM is controversial.

  3. Autoimmune factors. The autoimmune process begins with lymphocytic infiltration of the pancreas.

    a. **Islet cell antibodies (ICA)** are present in **85% of patients.**

    b. **ICA** may be detected in asymptomatic patients 10 years before the onset of clinical symptoms. **Other immunologic markers** may also be detected in patients long before the onset of clinical symptoms, including **antibodies against insulin** and **against glutamic acid decarboxylase (GAD).**

    c. Note that up to 10% of the general population may have ICA. Therefore, to develop type 1 DM, children must have a combination of ICA, environmental factors, and a genetic predisposition.

B. Clinical Features

  1. The **classic presentation** includes several weeks of **polyuria, polydipsia, nocturia,** and occasionally enuresis. As symptoms progress, weight loss, vomiting, and dehydration occur.

  2. Diabetic ketoacidosis (DKA) may be the initial presentation in **25% of patients** (see section VIII). The younger the patient, the shorter the course of symptoms before DKA occurs.

  3. Girls who have protracted cases of **monilial vulvovaginitis** may have early type 1 DM.

  4. Adolescents may present with type 1 DM during their pubertal growth spurt with hormones that are antagonistic to insulin action (specifically **growth hormone** and the **sex steroids**).

C. Diagnosis. Patients must have hyperglycemia documented by a random blood sugar above 200 mg/dL with polyuria, polydipsia, weight loss, or nocturia.

D. Management

  1. Insulin

    a. Types of insulin include **short-acting, intermediate-acting, long-acting,** and **very long-acting.**

    b. Administration in newly diagnosed patients may involve **combining the above types of insulin.**

    c. Insulin pumps are now being used in children to achieve better glucose control and to improve lifestyle.

  d. **Monitoring**
  (1) **Daily blood glucose** measurements using a glucose meter before all meals and at bedtime.
  (2) **Glycosylated hemoglobin level**, reflecting diabetic control for the past 2–3 months, should be checked every 3 months.
  (3) **Watch for hypoglycemia.** All patients should have parenteral **glucagon** available in case of seizure or coma secondary to low blood sugar.
  (4) **Watch for "honeymoon" period.** Within a few weeks after initial diagnosis, 75% of patients exhibit a temporary progressive reduction in their daily insulin requirements. This is because of a transient recovery of residual islet cell function, resulting in endogenous release of insulin in response to carbohydrate exposure. This honeymoon period may last anywhere from months to 1–2 years.
  (5) **Watch for Somogyi phenomenon.** This occurs when the evening dose of insulin is too high, causing hypoglycemia in the early morning hours, resulting in the release of counter-regulatory hormones (epinephrine and glucagon) to counteract this insulin-induced hypoglycemia. The patient then has high blood glucose and ketones in the morning. The **treatment** is to actually **lower** the bedtime insulin dose and not to raise it.
 2. **Diet.** Follow the **American Diabetic Association (ADA) diet.**
 3. **Education and close follow-up** every 3 months.

 E. **Long-Term Complications**
  1. **Microvascular complications** include diabetic retinopathy, nephropathy, and neuropathy.
  2. **Macrovascular complications are usually seen in adulthood** and include atherosclerotic disease, hypertension, heart disease, and stroke.
  3. **DKA** when ill or noncompliant

VII. Type 2 Diabetes Mellitus (Type 2 DM)

 A. **Epidemiology**
  1. **Occurs in 2–3% of all children with diabetes.**
  2. In the last decade there has been a 10-fold increase in the incidence of type 2 DM in children due to an increase in obesity.

 B. **Etiology**
  1. Very strong hereditary component (stronger for type 2 than for type 1)
  2. The cause is likely a combination of peripheral tissue resistance to insulin and progressive decline in insulin secretion, both of which result in a hyperglycemic state.

 C. **Clinical Features.** The clinical presentation is variable.
  1. Asymptomatic (50%) to mild DKA. **Serious DKA is uncommon** because type 2 DM is more of an insulin resistance than insulin deficiency.

2. **Obesity**

3. **Acanthosis nigricans** (velvety and hyperpigmented skin of the neck and axillary folds) is common.

D. **Management**

1. **Oral hypoglycemic agents** may be used if blood sugar levels are not very high.

2. **Insulin therapy** may be required for those patients who have high blood sugar or who fail oral agents.

VIII. Diabetic Ketoacidosis (DKA)

A. **Definition. Hyperglycemia usually greater than 300 mg/dL with ketonuria and a serum bicarbonate level <15 mmol/L or a serum pH < 7.30.**

B. **Pathophysiology**

1. **Insulin deficiency** creates a state of diminished glucose substrate at the cellular level, despite the high serum levels of glucose. The body's need for substrate to make energy therefore results in gluconeogenesis.

2. **Hyperglycemia** resulting from this insulin deficiency leads to an **osmotic diuresis** with polyuria and eventual dehydration.

3. **Counter-regulatory stress hormones** (i.e., glucagon, epinephrine, cortisol, and growth hormone) are released and contribute to fat breakdown (lipolysis).

   a. **Glucagon** stimulates conversion of free fatty acids into **ketone bodies** (acetone, acetoacetate, and β-hydroxybutyrate).

   b. The counter-regulatory stress hormones, in the face of insulin deficiency, lead to fat lipolysis and ketone formation and eventually DKA.

C. **Clinical Features**

1. Patients with **mild DKA** may present with vomiting, polyuria, polydipsia, and mild to moderate dehydration.

2. Patients with **severe DKA** may present with severe dehydration, severe abdominal pain that may mimic appendicitis, rapid and deep (Kussmaul) respirations, and coma.

3. It is the presence of ketones that gives the patient with DKA **"fruity breath." Ketones also contribute to coma in severe DKA.**

D. **Laboratory Findings**

1. **Anion gap metabolic acidosis**

2. **Hyperglycemia and glucosuria**

3. **Ketonemia and ketonuria**

4. **Hyperkalemia** caused by metabolic acidosis (potassium moves out of the cells in the face of acidosis) or normokalemia

E. Management

1. **Fluid and electrolyte therapy** and replacement of the depleted intravascular volume using isotonic saline should begin immediately.

2. A **gradual decline in osmolality** is critical to minimize the risks of cerebral edema, which is a very significant cause of morbidity and mortality in the treatment of DKA.

3. **Potassium repletion** (once urine output has been established) using potassium acetate and potassium phosphate is very important because all patients are potassium depleted, even with a normal serum potassium. Potassium acetate is helpful in managing the patient's metabolic acidosis. Potassium phosphate helps increase serum levels of 2,3-diphosphate glycerate (**2,3-DPG**), which in turn shifts the oxygen dissociation curve to the right and makes oxygen more readily available to the tissues.

4. **Regular insulin** (usually a continuous infusion of 0.1 U/kg per hour) with careful monitoring of serum glucose levels to ensure a gradual drop in the serum glucose levels

5. The **combination of intravenous fluids and insulin** should reverse the ketogenesis, stop the hepatic production of glucose, shut down the release of counter-regulatory hormones, and enhance peripheral glucose uptake.

F. Complications

1. **Cerebral edema**
   a. Usually occurs 6–12 hours into therapy and rarely after 24 hours
   b. Risk factors include patients younger than 5 years of age, initial drops in serum glucose levels faster than 100 mg/dL per hour, and fluid administration greater than 4 L/m^2 per 24 hours.
   c. Mortality rate may be as high as 70%.

2. Severe hypokalemia

3. Hypocalcemia, due to either excessive use of potassium phosphate or osmotic losses.

IX. Thyroid Disorders

A. Thyroid Physiology

1. **Hypothalamic-pituitary-thyroid axis** is regulated by a feedback loop between thyroxine (T$_4$), triiodothyronine (T$_3$), thyrotropin-releasing hormone (TRH), and thyroid-stimulating hormone (TSH).

2. **Both T$_4$ and T$_3$** circulate bound to **thyroid-binding proteins,** including thyroid-binding globulin (TBG) and thyroid-binding prealbumin (TBPA).

3. **The free (unbound) forms** of T$_4$ and of T$_3$ are the biologically active forms of each hormone.

B. Hypothyroidism

1. **Clinical presentation**

    a. Suboptimal growth velocity (less than 5 cm per year or 2 inches per year) with a **delayed bone age**

    b. Goiter sometimes may be found on gland palpation.

    c. Myxedema, or "puffy skin," dry skin, or, occasionally, orange-tinged skin

    d. Amenorrhea or oligomenorrhea in adolescent girls

2. Causes are extensive.

    a. Congenital hypothyroidism

        (1) Epidemiology. This condition is the **most common metabolic disorder.** It is evaluated on newborn screening and has an incidence of 1 in 4,000 births.

        (2) Etiology

            (a) Thyroid dysgenesis. This is the most common cause (90%) of congenital hypothyroidism. Two thirds of affected patients have an absent thyroid gland (thyroid aplasia) or thyroid hypoplasia. One third have an ectopic thyroid gland, which may be found anywhere between the base of the tongue (foramen cecum) to the mid-chest.

            (b) Thyroid dyshormonogenesis. This refers to multiple **inborn errors** of thyroid hormone synthesis, which account for about 10% of all cases of congenital hypothyroidism. These conditions are autosomal recessive and usually present with a goiter. **Pendred syndrome,** an organification defect, is the most common of these defects and is associated with **sensorineural hearing loss.**

            (c) Use of **propylthiouracil (PTU)** during pregnancy for maternal Graves' disease may result in transient hypothyroidism in the newborn because PTU crosses the placenta and may temporarily block fetal thyroid hormone synthesis.

            (d) Maternal autoimmune thyroid disease may also result in transient hypothyroidism, as maternal thyroid-blocking antibodies may cross the placenta and block TSH receptors on the newborn thyroid gland.

        (3) Clinical features. Most newborns are asymptomatic at birth and have an unremarkable physical examination (T_4 is not essential for fetal growth). However, thyroid hormone is essential for normal brain growth during the first 2 years of life, and with time, the following clinical features become more apparent if the patient goes untreated:

            (a) Classic historical features include a history of prolonged jaundice and poor feeding.

            (b) Classic symptoms include lethargy and constipation.

            (c) Classic physical examination findings include large anterior and posterior fontanelles, protruding tongue, umbilical hernia, myxedema, mottled skin, hypothermia, delayed neurodevelopment, and poor growth.

        (4) Management

            (a) Thyroid hormone replacement should begin immediately with L-thyroxine.

        (b) If treatment is delayed until after the signs and symptoms of hypothyroidism appear, most patients will have suffered permanent neurologic sequelae.

    b. Hashimoto's disease (chronic lymphocytic thyroiditis [CLT]). This autoimmune disorder is characterized by lymphocytic infiltration of the thyroid gland, resulting in varying degrees of follicular fibrosis and atrophy and follicular hyperplasia.

      (1) Epidemiology

        (a) Most common cause of acquired hypothyroidism with or without a goiter

        (b) More common in **girls**

      (2) Etiology. Thyroid autoantibodies develop because of a disturbance in immunoregulation, resulting in a state of thyroid cell cytotoxicity or stimulation. There is often a genetic predisposition.

      (3) Clinical features. Presentation is variable.

        (a) Asymptomatic

        (b) Goiter, which is classically firm and pebbly in nature

        (c) Short stature

        (d) Transient hyperthyroidism ("Hashitoxicosis") may occur in some patients.

      (4) Management. Thyroid hormone replacement with **L-thyroxine** to normalize the TSH level.

  3. Diagnosis of hypothyroidism

    a. Neonatal screening tests for congenital hypothyroidism (TSH is measured)

    b. Increased TSH, which is usually the first sign of thyroid failure

    c. Low T_4 level

    d. Antithyroid antibodies (especially **thyroid antiperoxidase antibodies**) as a marker for autoimmune thyroid disease

C. Hyperthyroidism

  1. Clinical features

    a. Eye examination may demonstrate lid lag and exophthalmos.

    b. Thyroid gland is enlarged and usually smooth in texture.

    c. Cardiac examination demonstrates tachycardia, and patients may complain of palpitations.

    d. Skin is warm and flushed. **(Pearl:** The presence of vitiligo or alopecia suggests the possible coexistence of other **autoimmune polyendocrinopathies,** including Addison's disease and diabetes mellitus.)

    e. CNS evaluation may be remarkable for nervousness and fine tremors with a history of fatigue and difficulty concentrating in school.

    f. Pubertal evaluation may be notable for delayed menarche and gynecomastia in boys.

  2. Graves' disease (diffuse toxic goiter). This **autoimmune disorder** is characterized by autonomous production of excessive thyroid hormone by the thyroid gland mediated by a TSH look-alike antibody.

a. **Epidemiology**. Graves' disease is the **most common cause of hyperthyroidism** in childhood. **Females** predominate (M:F = 1:3).

b. **Etiology**

(1) Strong genetic factors

(2) **Thyroid-stimulating immunoglobulin (TSI),** an IgG antibody, cross-reacts with TSH and binds to and stimulates the TSH receptors in the thyroid gland.

c. **Laboratory findings. Increased T_3 and T_4 levels** with **suppressed TSH level** in the presence of TSI.

d. **Management**

(1) **Antithyroid medications.** The two most commonly used antithyroid medications are **PTU** and **methimazole.** Although both medications inhibit thyroid hormone synthesis, PTU also impairs the peripheral conversion of T_4 to T_3. These medications are usually the first-line treatment.

(2) **Subtotal thyroidectomy** may be considered if antithyroid medication fails.

(3) **Radioactive iodine** is often used in adolescents if noncompliance with medication is an issue. Its use eventually results in permanent hypothyroidism.

X. Bone Mineral Disorders

A. **Physiology of calcium and vitamin D metabolism**

1. **Bone.** Both **vitamin D and parathormone (PTH)** release calcium and phosphorus from bone.

2. **Parathyroid gland**

a. **PTH** helps maintain a normal serum **calcium** level by releasing calcium from the bone and reabsorbing calcium from the kidneys.

b. **PTH** also releases **phosphorus** from the bone and excretes phosphorus from the kidneys.

3. **Kidney**

a. **PTH** is responsible for **calcium** and **bicarbonate reabsorption** and **phosphorus excretion.**

b. The enzyme **1α-hydroxylase vitamin D** made in the kidney converts 25-(OH) vitamin D (made by the liver) into the active vitamin D metabolite **1,25-(OH) vitamin D** (stimulated by PTH).

4. **Gastrointestinal (GI) tract.** The main source of calcium absorption is through the intestine, due to **1,25-(OH) vitamin D,** which is the **most potent form of vitamin D.**

B. **Hypocalcemia**

1. **Definitions**

a. **Hypocalcemia.** Serum calcium less than 8.0 mg/dL, or ionized calcium less than 2.5 mg/dL.

b. **Pseudohypocalcemia.** The factitious lowering of total calcium levels as a result of low serum albumin levels, as seen in nephrotic syndrome. Therefore, all low total calcium levels should have an ionized calcium level measured to verify true hypocalcemia.

2. **Clinical features**
    a. **Tetany** (neuromuscular hyperexcitability)
        (1) **Carpopedal spasm.** Hypocalcemia causes hyperexcitability of peripheral motor nerves, resulting in painful spasms of the muscles of the wrists and ankles.
        (2) **Laryngospasm.** Spasm of the laryngeal muscles
        (3) **Paresthesias**
    b. **Seizures.** Younger patients with hypocalcemia tend to present with seizures or coma, whereas older patients exhibit more signs of neuromuscular hyperexcitability.

3. **Etiology**
    a. **Early neonatal hypocalcemia (younger than 4 days of age)** is usually transient and may be associated with prematurity, IUGR, asphyxia, or infants of diabetic mothers. Hypomagnesemia may also result in hypocalcemia.
    b. **Late neonatal hypocalcemia (older than 4 days of age)**
        (1) **Hypoparathyroidism.** Patients have low calcium and elevated phosphorus levels, usually caused by asymptomatic maternal hyperparathyroidism, in which the mother's high serum calcium crosses the placenta and suppresses the fetus's PTH. After delivery this creates a temporary state of hypocalcemic hypoparathyroidism.
        (2) **DiGeorge syndrome** (see Chapter 5, section III.A.5)
        (3) **Hyperphosphatemia** leads to hypocalcemia by binding to calcium. It may result from **excessive phosphate intake** (found in some infant formulas) or from **uremia.**
    c. **Childhood hypocalcemia**
        (1) **Hypoparathyroidism (parathyroid failure).** This condition may be genetic (ring chromosome 16 or 18), autoimmune, or related to DiGeorge syndrome (see Chapter 5, section III.A.5) as above.
        (2) **Pseudohypoparathyroidism (parathyroid resistance).** This rare autosomal dominant disorder results in PTH resistance. Patients present with short stature, short metacarpals, developmental delay, and **elevated PTH levels.**
        (3) **Hypomagnesemia.** A **low magnesium** level, as seen in some renal and malabsorptive diseases, may cause hypocalcemia because it interferes with PTH release.
        (4) **Vitamin D deficiency** can cause hypocalcemia with low phosphorus levels (see section X.C).

4. **Laboratory evaluation**
    a. **Serum ionized calcium and phosphorus**
    b. **Serum magnesium**
    c. **Electrocardiogram** demonstrating a **prolonged QT interval** may be found with hypocalcemia.

    d. PTH level to distinguish between hypoparathyroidism (low PTH) and pseudohypoparathyroidism (increased PTH)

    e. Vitamin D level (in an older child) if both calcium and phosphorus levels are low

    f. Radiograph of wrists or knees to evaluate for **rickets** (see section X.C)

  5. Management

    a. Mild asymptomatic hypocalcemia does not require treatment.

    b. In newborns with serum calcium levels < 7.5 mg/dL (or ionized calcium < 2.5 mg/dL) or in older children with serum calcium levels < 8.0 mg/dL, calcium should be corrected to prevent CNS hyperexcitability.

    c. Calcium supplementation

      (1) Oral therapy is acceptable if there are no seizures or only moderate tetany.

      (2) Intravenous calcium gluconate should be given if patients are more symptomatic.

    d. 1,25 Vitamin D analog (calcitriol) should be given to patients with chronic hypoparathyroidism.

C. Rickets

  1. Definition. Rickets is a condition caused by vitamin D deficiency that results in deficient mineralization of growing bones with a normal bone matrix.

  2. Predisposing factors

    a. Exclusively breastfed infants with minimal sunshine exposure

    b. Fad diets

    c. Use of anticonvulsant medications (phenytoin, phenobarbital), which interfere with liver metabolism

    d. Renal or hepatic failure

  3. Etiology

    a. Vitamin D deficiency

    b. GI disorders associated with fat malabsorption resulting in vitamin D deficiency (e.g., cystic fibrosis, celiac disease)

    c. Nutritional causes (rare in the United States because of vitamin D supplementation)

    d. Defective vitamin D metabolism from renal and hepatic failure may cause a deficiency in the important enzymes that synthesize 1,25-(OH) vitamin D, resulting in renal osteodystrophy (see Chapter 11, section X.F). Anticonvulsants may also interfere with vitamin D metabolism through their effect on liver metabolism.

    e. Vitamin D–dependent rickets

      (1) This autosomal recessive condition is very rare.

      (2) Enzyme deficiency in the kidneys of 1α-hydroxylase vitamin D results in the lack of 1,25-(OH) vitamin D.

      (3) Patients present with increased PTH, low vitamin D levels, low calcium, low phosphorus, and increased alkaline phosphatase.

    f. **Vitamin D–resistant rickets (familial hypophosphatemia)**
      (1) **Most common form of rickets in the United States today**
      (2) **X-linked dominant** disorder
      (3) **Caused by a renal tubular phosphorus leak,** resulting in a low serum phosphorus level
      (4) Patients present with **rickets** in the face of normal calcium and low phosphorus.
      (5) Patients develop typical bowing of the legs, but never tetany.
      (6) **Treatment** includes **phosphate supplements** and 1,25 vitamin D analogs.
    g. **Oncogenous rickets** is a phosphate-deficient form of rickets caused by a bone or soft tissue tumor. It should be **considered in patients who present with bone pain or a myopathy.**

  4. **Clinical features**
    a. Rickets usually occurs during the **first 2 years of life** and in **adolescence,** when bone growth is most rapid.
    b. Rickets usually involves the **wrists, knees, and ribs** (where the growth velocity is the fastest), presenting with a knobby appearance.
    c. Weight-bearing bones become **bowed** once the patient begins ambulating.
    d. **Short stature**
    e. **"Rachitic rosary"** or prominent costochondral junctions
    f. **Craniotabes** or thinning of the outer skull create a "Ping-Pong ball sensation" on palpation.
    g. **Frontal bossing** and **delayed suture closure**

  5. **Radiographic findings. Wrist radiographs** show earliest changes of rickets with the distal end of the metaphysis appearing widened, frayed, and **cupped,** instead of showing a well-demarcated zone. There is also widening of the space between the epiphysis and the end of the metaphysis.

  6. **Laboratory findings.** A low serum phosphorus, low to normal serum calcium, elevated alkaline phosphatase, and elevated PTH levels are present.

  7. **Management.** Treatment depends on etiology.

XI. Diabetes Insipidus (DI)

A. Definition. Inability to maximally concentrate urine because of either low levels of antidiuretic hormone (ADH) or renal unresponsiveness to ADH.

B. Physiology. ADH is an octapeptide synthesized in the hypothalamic nuclei and transported via axons to the posterior pituitary. The action of ADH is to increase permeability of the renal collecting ducts to water, leading to increased water reabsorption. It is regulated by changes in volume, serum osmolality, and posture.

C. Classification
  1. **Central DI = ADH-deficient**

    2. Nephrogenic DI = ADH-resistant (kidney does not respond to ADH)

D. Etiology of Central DI

    1. Autoimmune. Antibodies target ADH-producing cells.

    2. Trauma and hypoxic ischemic brain injury

    3. Hypothalamic tumors (e.g., craniopharyngioma, glioma, germinoma)

    4. Langerhans cell histiocytosis. Twenty-five percent of patients develop DI.

    5. Granulomatous disease (e.g., sarcoidosis, tuberculosis)

    6. Vascular (e.g., aneurysms)

    7. Genetic (autosomal dominant inheritance)

E. Etiology of Nephrogenic DI. Inherited as an **X-linked recessive** disorder

F. Clinical Features. Children present with nocturia, enuresis, poor weight gain, polydipsia, and polyuria.

G. Evaluation and Diagnosis

    1. If thirst mechanisms are intact and child has access to water, then serum electrolytes will be normal. Otherwise, patients present with **hypernatremic dehydration** with an **inappropriately dilute urine in the face of increased serum sodium and increased serum osmolality.**

    2. An early morning urine specimen with a specific gravity > 1.018 rules out the diagnosis of DI.

    3. Water deprivation test in the hospital may be used to diagnose DI. A rising serum osmolality in the presence of persistent urine output and an inappropriately low urine osmolality is diagnostic. If, at the end of the test, the patient does not respond to administered ADH, then the patient has nephrogenic DI.

    4. In an **MRI of the head,** hyperintense signal normally found in the posterior pituitary is missing.

    5. A **bone scan** may be indicated to rule out Langerhans cell histiocytosis.

H. Management. The drug of choice for **central DI is DDAVP (synthetic ADH).**

XII. Hypoglycemia

A. General Principles

    1. Definition. Serum glucose less than 40 mg/dL, or whole blood glucose less than 45 mg/dL.

    2. It is important to recognize hypoglycemia early, especially in newborns and young infants, when the brain is dependent on glucose for proper neurodevelopment.

    3. The **symptoms of hypoglycemia** are age-dependent and vary in each patient.

    a. Newborns or infants may have varied symptoms that include lethargy, myoclonic jerks, cyanosis, apnea, or seizures.

    b. Older children may have symptoms similar to adults, including tachycardia, diaphoresis, tremors, headaches, or seizures.

B. Neonatal Hypoglycemia. This condition may be transient (most common) or persistent (less common).

  1. Transient neonatal hypoglycemia is usually detected by screening protocols established for high-risk infants.

    a. High-risk conditions associated with inadequate substrate include prematurity, a history of perinatal asphyxia or fetal distress, and small-for-gestational age (SGA) and large-for-gestational age (LGA) infants.

    b. High-risk conditions associated with inappropriate hyperinsulinism include SGA infants and infants of diabetic mothers.

  2. Persistent neonatal hypoglycemia is defined as hypoglycemia that persists for longer than 3 days. The differential diagnosis of persistent neonatal hypoglycemia includes:

    a. Hyperinsulinism, which may be caused by:

      (1) Islet cell hyperplasia (nesidioblastosis)

      (2) Beckwith-Wiedemann syndrome: Patients are LGA and present with visceromegaly, hemihypertrophy, macroglossia, umbilical hernias, and distinctive ear creases.

    b. Hereditary defects in carbohydrate metabolism (e.g., glycogen storage disease type I and galactosemia) or **amino acid metabolism** (e.g., maple syrup urine disease, methylmalonic acidemia and tyrosinemia; see Chapter 5, sections V and VI, and Table 5-5).

    c. Hormone deficiencies, including growth hormone deficiency and cortisol deficiency. **(Pearl: Congenital hypopituitarism should be suspected in the neonate who presents with hypoglycemia, microphallus, and midline defects such as a cleft palate.)**

C. Hypoglycemia in Infancy and Childhood. Hypoglycemia is relatively uncommon in older infants and children, but the differential diagnosis is extensive and includes the following:

  1. Ketotic hypoglycemia is the **most common cause of hypoglycemia in children 1–6 years of age.** This is defined as hypoglycemia occuring late in the morning in the presence of ketonuria and a low insulin level. This appears to be an inability to adapt to a fasting state. Typically these children are thin and become hypoglycemic after intercurrent infection.

  2. Ingestions must always be considered in the differential diagnosis of hypoglycemia in the older child, especially in adolescents.

    a. Alcohol metabolism in the liver can deplete essential cofactors needed for adequate gluconeogenesis, resulting in hypoglycemia (especially when the child is in the fasting state).

    b. Oral hypoglycemic agents

  3. Inborn errors of metabolism

  4. Hyperinsulinism, as described in section XII.B.2.a

Review Test

1. A 7-year-old boy is brought to the office for a routine health care maintenance visit. The nurse brings to your attention that he has grown only 1 inch during the past year. A review of his growth curve during the past 2 years shows that his height percentile has fallen from the 75th to the 40th percentile. His father is 66 inches tall, and his mother is 65 inches tall. He has recently had some early morning vomiting and headache. However, physical examination is unremarkable. A bone age study reveals a growth delay of just over 2.5 years. Complete blood count, erythrocyte sedimentation rate, and thyroid studies are all normal. The most likely cause of this patient's short stature is which of the following?

(A) Genetic short stature
(B) Constitutional growth delay
(C) Craniopharyngioma
(D) Skeletal dysplasia
(E) Cushing disease

2. You are called to the delivery room to evaluate a newborn infant with ambiguous genitalia. The mother had an amniocentesis showing a fetus with an XX genotype. Physical examination of the neonate indicates no palpable gonads, a small phallic structure, and labial fusion with a urogenital opening. Which of the following is the most likely diagnosis?

(A) Hermaphrodite
(B) Partial androgen insensitivity
(C) Congenital adrenal hyperplasia caused by 21-hydroxylase deficiency
(D) 5α-Reductase deficiency
(E) Hypopituitarism

3. An obese 12-year-old child is suspected of having the diagnosis of type 2 diabetes mellitus (DM). Which of the following statements regarding this suspected diagnosis is correct?

(A) This patient is likely to present with diabetic ketoacidosis during adolescence.
(B) Approximately 95% of patients with type 2 DM have HLA haplotypes DR3 or DR4.
(C) This patient is likely to have had islet cell antibodies before the onset of clinical symptoms.
(D) Type 2 DM has a very strong hereditary component (even stronger than in type 1 DM).
(E) In the last decade, there has been a decline in the incidence of type 2 DM, given greater public awareness of healthy eating habits.

4. A 13-year-old girl is brought to the office by her mother because of poor attention span and deteriorating grades. She is also fidgety and cannot sit still. Her mother is also concerned because her daughter has lost 5 pounds during the past 2 months. Physical examination shows a blood pressure of 130/75 mm Hg, a heart rate of 115 beats/min, and thyromegaly. You suspect Graves' disease. Which of the following statements regarding the suspected diagnosis is correct?

(A) Thyroid-stimulating immunoglobulins (TSI) are usually present and bind to thyrotropin (TSH) receptors.
(B) Girls with Graves' disease have an increased likelihood of developing precocious puberty.
(C) Subtotal thyroidotomy is the most appropriate initial management.
(D) This disease is more common in males.
(E) Radioactive iodine treatment is ineffective.

5. You have been following an 8-year-old child in your office for the past several years and have noted that during the past year, his height has remained below the third percentile. You are concerned about his short stature and decide to begin a workup. Your workup includes a bone age determination. The patient's bone age is discovered to be 3 years younger than his chronologic age. Which of the following diagnoses should be considered?

(A) Genetic short stature
(B) Skeletal dysplasias
(C) Intrauterine growth retardation
(D) Turner syndrome
(E) Growth hormone deficiency

6. You are called to the pediatric intensive care unit to evaluate a 4-year old girl with new onset type 1 diabetes mellitus who is in diabetic ketoacidosis (DKA). The nurse reports that she was alert and talking but *suddenly* has become obtunded and listless. Which of the following conditions is the likely cause of her change in mental status?

(A) Hyperglycemia
(B) Cerebral edema
(C) Hyperkalemia
(D) Hypercalcemia
(E) Stroke

The response options for statements 7–11 are the same. You will be required to select one answer for each statement in the set.

(A) Premature adrenarche
(B) Premature thelarche
(C) Central precocious puberty
(D) Peripheral precocious puberty
(E) Normal, no pubertal disorder

For each patient, select the most likely pubertal disorder.

7. A 13-month-old girl has a several month history of breast growth with Tanner stage 2 breast development on examination, but has no pubic hair. Her growth consistently follows the 75% growth curve.

8. A 7-year-old boy presents with pubic hair, acne, and rapid growth. His bone age evaluation reveals that his bones demonstrate advanced growth to the equivalent of a 10-year-old boy. Testicular examination shows prepubertal size testes.

9. A 5-year-old girl has a 1-year history of breast development and pubic hair. She is Tanner stage 3 on breast examination and Tanner stage 2 on pubic hair examination. Today she had her first menses. Bone age determination reveals her bone appearance is 5 years advanced, to that of a 10-year-old girl.

10. A 6-year-old girl has a strong apocrine odor, mild axillary hair, and Tanner stage 3 pubic hair. No clitoromegaly or breast development is seen. Bone age determination reveals her bone appearance is 2 years advanced, to that of an 8-year-old girl.

11. A 5-year-old girl is referred for vaginal bleeding. Physical examination shows breast development, multiple café-au-lait spots, and thyromegaly, and cystic bony changes are apparent on radiography of her legs.

The response options for statements 12–15 are the same. You will be required to select one answer for each statement in the set.

(A) Nesidioblastosis
(B) Hypopituitarism
(C) Beckwith-Wiedemann syndrome
(D) Glycogen storage disease
(E) Ketotic hypoglycemia

For each patient, select the most likely diagnosis.

12. A 4-year-old thin boy with a fever and vomiting went to sleep without dinner and has a hypoglycemic seizure at 8:00 AM.

13. A male newborn has a glucose of 15 mg/dL at 6 hours of age. Physical examination reveals a cleft palate, microphallus, and undescended testes.

14. A newborn who has had hypoglycemia for 1 week is nondysmorphic and requires a high rate of dextrose infusion to maintain blood sugar. The insulin level is inappropriately high.

15. A large-for-gestational age infant has hepatomegaly, macroglossia, moderate umbilical hernia, and hypoglycemia.

Answers and Explanations

1. The answer is C [I.F.1.b]. The decreased rate of growth in the face of early morning emesis should make one suspect a mass lesion within the central nervous system. The workup should begin with a skull radiograph followed by a cranial magnetic resonance imaging (MRI) scan. Both genetic short stature and constitutional growth delay are excluded from the diagnosis because patients with these conditions grow at a normal rate, at least 2 inches per year. Skeletal dysplasia may be ruled out because the delayed bone age is inconsistent with such a condition. Cushing disease may cause poor growth and bone age delay, but this rare disease is not associated with headaches and morning emesis.

2. The answer is C [III.D, III.E, and III.F]. Congenital adrenal hyperplasia (CAH) as a result of 21-hydroxylase deficiency is the most common form of female pseudohermaphrodism. The chromosomal analysis revealing XX chromosomes and the lack of gonads immediately exclude a male pseudohermaphrodite, such as that caused by partial androgen insensitivity, and inborn errors in testosterone synthesis, as in 5α-reductase deficiency. A true hermaphrodite is a possibility, but CAH is more common. Hypopituitarism in a newborn with an XX genotype would not present with ambiguous genitalia.

3. The answer is D [VII.A and VII.B]. Type 2 diabetes mellitus (DM) occurs in 2–3% of all children with diabetes mellitus, with a very significant increase in incidence during the last decade. There is a much stronger hereditary component in type 2 DM than in type 1 DM, and the etiology is likely a combination of peripheral tissue resistance to insulin and a progressive decline in insulin secretion. The clinical presentation of type 2 DM may be quite variable; however, the majority of patients do not present with diabetic ketoacidosis because type 2 DM reflects more of an insulin resistance than an insulin deficiency, and patients are not likely to present with insulin autoantibodies. Approximately 95% of patients with type 1 DM will have HLA haplotypes DR3 or DR4. Patients are often asymptomatic, with only glucosuria, and physical examination may be significant for obesity and acanthosis nigricans (velvety and hyperpigmented skin of the neck and axillary folds).

4. The answer is A [IX.C.2]. In patients with Graves' disease, thyroid-stimulating immunoglobulins are usually present because this is an autoimmune process and these antibodies are the cause of the thyrotoxic state. Girls with hyperthyroidism are more likely to have delayed menarche than to have precocious puberty. Both Graves' disease and Hashimoto's thyroiditis are examples of autoimmune disorders that are more common in females. First-line therapy is antithyroid medication. Surgery or radioactive iodine is effective and should be considered if medical treatment fails or is not tolerated. Radioactive iodine may also be considered for adolescents if noncompliance with medications is an issue.

5. The answer is E [I.E.2.a, I.F.1, and Table 6-1]. Bone age determination may be very helpful when compared with the patient's chronologic age in the evaluation of short stature. Because of slowed growth velocity, patients with growth hormone deficiency would be expected to have their bone age less than their chronologic age, as would patients with constitutional growth delay, hypothyroidism, and hypercortisolism. Patients with genetic short stature, skeletal dysplasias, intrauterine growth retardation, and Turner syndrome would all be expected to have their bone age approximately the same as their chronologic age.

6. The correct answer is B [VIII.F]. When treating diabetic ketoacidosis, especially in children younger than 5 years of age, the diagnosis of cerebral edema must be entertained if there is a sudden change in mental status. Risk factors for the development of cerebral edema include drops in serum glucose levels faster than 100 mg/dL per hour and excessive fluid administration. Changes in mental status can also result from hypoglycemia, hypocalcemia, and hypokalemia. If dextrose is not added to the insulin drip when the blood sugar drops below 250 mg/dL, the child may experience a sudden drop in glucose and exhibit lethargy, seizures, or coma. Hypocalcemia is caused by excessive phosphorus usage or osmotic losses and can cause a seizure or change in

179

mental status. Hypokalemia can result in an arrhythmia that, in turn, may result in hypotension and cardiac arrest. Stroke is a complication of long-standing poorly controlled DM.

7, 8, 9, 10, and 11. The answers are B, D, C, A, and D, respectively [II.B]. Most cases of sexual precocity are benign. Premature thelarche (question 7) is a transient state of isolated early breast development as is found in a girl younger than 7 years of age. Premature adrenarche is the early onset of pubic or axillary hair (question 10). Individuals with these conditions present with pubic hair and an apocrine odor but no breast development or very advanced bone age. Neither premature thelarche nor premature adrenarche are associated with activation of the hypothalamic-pituitary-gonadal axis.

Central precocious puberty (CPP) is puberty directed by the hypothalamus. A girl with CPP (question 9) presents with tall stature, advanced bone age, breast development, pubic hair, and sometimes menses. A boy with CPP is tall with pubic hair and enlarged testes.

Peripheral precocious puberty (PPP; questions 8 and 11) is sexual precocity that is not driven by the hypothalamus but rather originates from the ovaries, testes, or adrenal gland. In McCune-Albright syndrome (question 11), the girl shows breast development, café-au-lait spots, and fibrous dysplasia of the long bones. In another example of PPP (question 8), the boy's testes are prepubertal. If his androgens were driven by the hypothalamus, the testes would be enlarged.

12, 13, 14, and 15. The answers are E, B, A, and C, respectively [XII.B and XII.C]. Ketotic hypoglycemia is the most common cause of a low blood sugar in children. Patients are often thin, and symptoms develop after a prolonged fast. Congenital hypopituitarism should be considered in any newborn with a midline defect (e.g., cleft palate), hypoglycemia, and microphallus. Newborns with hypoglycemia persisting for longer than 4 days require further evaluation, and in these cases, hyperinsulinemia as a result of nesidioblastosis (beta cell hyperplasia) and Beckwith-Wiedemann syndrome should be considered. A newborn with nesidioblastosis will have no dysmorphic features but will have persistent low blood sugar owing to the high amounts of circulating insulin. Beckwith-Wiedemann syndrome is characterized at birth by large-for-gestational age, macroglossia, umbilical hernia, and hyperinsulinemic hypoglycemia.

7

Infectious Diseases

Deborah Lehman, M.D., Srinath Sanda, M.D.,
and Nirali P. Singh, M.D.

I. General Approach to the Child with Possible Infection

A. **Detailed history and physical examination is essential.**

1. **History** should include details about the present illness, significant past medical history, travel and animal contact, medications, unusual food ingestions (including raw meat and unpasteurized dairy products), and risk of infection with human immunodeficiency virus (HIV; e.g., intravenous drug use, remote history of blood transfusion, unprotected intercourse).

2. **Physical examination** should be comprehensive with special attention to general appearance, rashes, skin manifestations of endocarditis (see Chapter 8, section V.C), hepatosplenomegaly, evidence of joint effusion, and lymph node enlargement.

B. **Use of the laboratory.** Pathogens may be identified by direct or indirect laboratory methods.

1. **Direct methods**

a. **Cultures** for bacteria and viruses

b. **Microbiologic stains,** including **Gram stain, Ziehl-Neelsen stain** (acid-fast bacilli), **silver stain** (fungal elements), and **Wright stain** (stool white blood cells [WBCs])

c. **Fluorescent antibody-antigen staining** for herpes simplex virus (HSV) 1 and 2, varicella-zoster virus (VZV), and respiratory viruses, such as respiratory syncytial virus (RSV), adenovirus, influenza A and B, and parainfluenza

d. **Direct observation,** including **wet mount** for fungal elements and *Trichomonas vaginalis* and **dark-field microscopy** for *Treponema pallidum*

e. **Polymerase chain reaction (PCR)** is now available for identification and quantification of many pathogens.

2. **Indirect methods**
   a. **Intradermal skin testing** for *Mycobacterium tuberculosis* (TB) and *Coccidioides immitis*
   b. **Antibody testing** for viruses (Epstein-Barr virus, cytomegalovirus [CMV], VZV, and HIV), *Toxoplasma gondii, Bartonella henselae,* and *Mycoplasma pneumoniae.*

3. **Nonspecific** laboratory indications of infection typically include elevation of acute-phase reactants, such as C-reactive protein (CRP) and erythrocyte sedimentation rate (ESR).

II. Evaluation of the Child with Fever

A. **Fever** in children is defined as a **rectal temperature of 38°C (100.4°F) or higher.** Temperatures taken by axillary, oral, or tympanic methods may be less accurate.

B. Evaluation for serious bacterial infection (e.g., meningitis, pneumonia, sepsis, bone and joint infections, urinary tract infection, and enteritis) should occur in the following **high-risk groups:**

   1. **Young infants,** especially those younger than 28 days, because of immaturity of their immune system

   2. **Older infants** with **high fevers** (temperature > 39°C [102.2°F]) who appear ill

   3. Infants and children who are **immunodeficient,** have **sickle cell disease,** or have underlying chronic liver, renal, pulmonary, or cardiac disease

C. **Evaluation of fever in infants < 3 months**

   1. **Epidemiology. 3 to 10% of well-appearing,** and **17% of "toxic"-appearing,** febrile infants have serious bacterial infections. (Toxic appearance refers to a child appearing extremely ill with diminished interactivity or poor peripheral perfusion.)

   2. **Etiology**
      a. **Infections** may be acquired in several ways. Infections may be transplacental, acquired during passage through the birth canal, or transmitted postnatally in the nursery or at home.
      b. **Viruses are the most common organisms causing infection.**
      c. **Common bacterial organisms** causing infection in this age group are summarized in **Table 7-1.**

   3. **Clinical features** of infection in young infants are often **nonspecific** and include fever, diminished appetite, irritability, cough, rhinorrhea, vomiting, diarrhea, and apnea.

   4. **Diagnosis. Clinical and laboratory features may be used to identify infants at low risk for serious bacterial infection.**
      a. Infants who are well-appearing and previously healthy, who have had no recent antibiotic therapy, and who have no site of focal infection on examination are at low risk for serious bacterial infection. Infants who are ill-appearing or toxic and who have evidence of a fo-

Table 7-1. Typical Bacterial Pathogens and Empiric Antibiotics for Infants and Children with Suspected Sepsis or Meningitis

Age	Bacterial Pathogens	Empiric Intravenous Antibiotics
0–1 month	Group B streptococcus *Escherichia coli* *Listeria monocytogenes*	Ampicillin + gentamicin or cefotaxime
1–3 months	Group B streptococcus *Streptococcus pneumoniae* *Listeria monocytogenes*	Ampicillin + cefotaxime (+ vancomycin if bacterial meningitis suspected)
3 months–3 years	*Streptococcus pneumoniae* *Haemophilus influenzae type b* *Neisseria meningitidis*	Cefotaxime (+ vancomycin if bacterial meningitis suspected)
3 years–adult	*Streptococcus pneumoniae* *Neisseria meningitidis*	Cefotaxime (+ vancomycin if bacterial meningitis suspected)

cal infection on examination are at higher risk for serious bacterial infection.

b. **Laboratory evaluation** should include complete blood count (CBC), blood cultures, urinalysis, urine culture, chest radiograph if tachypnea or respiratory distress is present, and analysis of cerebrospinal fluid. Criteria that indicate an infant is at low risk for serious bacterial infection include:

(1) WBC > 5,000 and < 15,000 cells/mm^3

(2) Absolute band count < 1,500 cells/mm^3

(3) Normal urinalysis (< 10 WBCs per high-power field)

(4) If diarrhea is present, < 5 WBCs per high-power field on stool Wright stain

(5) Normal cerebrospinal fluid (CSF)

5. **Management**

a. **Hospitalization** is required for:

(1) **All infants ≤ 28 days of age**

(2) **Infants between 29 days and 3 months with any of the following:**

(a) **Toxic appearance on examination**

(b) Suspected **meningitis**

(c) **Pneumonia, pyelonephritis,** or **bone and soft tissue infections** unresponsive to oral antibiotics

(d) Patients in social circumstances in which there is **uncertain outpatient care and follow-up**

b. **Antibiotic management** is based on age, risk factors for infection, and etiology.

(1) Infants ≤ 28 days of age require intravenous antibiotics in the hospital until cultures of blood, urine, CSF, and stool, if diarrhea is present, are negative.

(2) Infants 29 days–3 months who satisfy low-risk clinical and laboratory criteria (see section II.C.4) and who have transportation

and good outpatient follow-up may be managed safely with empiric outpatient parenteral antibiotic therapy on a daily basis (i.e., intramuscular Ceftriaxone) while cultures are pending.

(3) Infants 29 days–3 months who do not meet low-risk clinical and laboratory criteria should be hospitalized for parenteral therapy while cultures are pending.

(4) Recommended parenteral antibiotic therapy for hospitalized infants is presented in **Table 7-1.**

D. Evaluation of fever in children 3–36 months

1. **Epidemiology.** Risk of serious bacterial infection is 3–10%, and the likelihood of bacteremia increases with increasing fever and peripheral WBC.

2. **Etiology** (see Table 7-1). *Streptococcus pneumoniae* is the **most common** organism. *Haemophilus influenzae* type b (**HIB**) is **less common** as a result of the introduction of HIB vaccine.

3. **Diagnostic evaluation** and **management** are based on the degree of the fever and whether the child appears toxic.

a. If the child is toxic-appearing, a complete evaluation for sepsis, intravenous antibiotics, and hospitalization are required.

b. If the child is nontoxic-appearing and the temperature is < 39°C (< 102.2°F), no laboratory tests are required and the child may be observed closely at home.

c. If the child is nontoxic-appearing and has a temperature > 39°C (> 102.2°F), the following studies are suggested:

(1) Urine culture for males < 6 months of age and females < 2 years of age

(2) Blood culture for all children or only for those whose WBC > 15,000 cells/mm^3

(3) Chest radiograph if respiratory distress, rales, or **tachypnea** is present

(4) Stool culture if there is blood and mucus in the stool or if there are ≥ 5 WBCs per high-power field on Wright stain

(5) Empiric antibiotics for all children or only for those whose WBC > 15,000 cells/mm^3. Reevaluation in 24–48 hours.

d. Recommended parenteral antibiotic therapy for hospitalized infants and children is presented in **Table 7-1.**

III. Fever of Unknown Origin (FUO)

A. **Definition.** Fever of unknown origin is a term used to describe a **fever lasting longer than 8 days to 3 weeks** (experts disagree about the length of time of fever necessary to diagnose fever as FUO) when **prior history, physical examination, and preliminary laboratory evaluation have all failed to lead to a diagnosis.**

B. **Etiology**

1. **Most children with FUO do not have a rare illness** but rather a common infection with an unusual presentation.

2. The **differential diagnosis** is extensive (**Table 7-2**).

3. **One fourth of cases of FUO resolve spontaneously** without a diagnosis having been made.

C. **Evaluation** should include the following:

1. **Comprehensive history,** focusing on a thorough **review of systems** (especially weight loss, rashes, fever, and stool patterns), **past medical and surgical history** (including prior blood transfusions), **travel history, animal exposure,** and **family and social history.**

2. **Detailed physical examination,** focusing on general appearance and growth curves, skin and mucous membrane findings, presence of lymphadenopathy and hepatosplenomegaly, and evaluation of joints and bones.

3. **Laboratory studies** are based on the history and physical examination and often include:

   a. **CBC with differential** to evaluate for infection or leukemia

   b. **ESR or CRP,** which are nonspecific indicators of tissue inflammation

   c. **Serum transaminases** to evaluate for hepatitis

   d. **Urinalysis and urine culture** to evaluate for infection

Table 7-2. Differential Diagnosis of Fever of Unknown Origin

Infectious disorders (most common cause of FUO)
  Occult infection (e.g., pyelonephritis, sinusitis, mastoiditis, otitis media)
  Viral syndromes (e.g., Epstein-Barr, cytomegalovirus, enterovirus, hepatitis B, HIV, parvovirus B19)
  Occult bacteremia (e.g., salmonellosis, tularemia, brucellosis, gonococcemia)
  Bacterial endocarditis
  Tuberculosis
  Occult abscess (e.g., liver, intra-abdominal, or perinephric)
  Musculoskeletal infections (e.g., diskitis, osteomyelitis, septic arthritis)
  Spirochete infections (e.g., Lyme disease, leptospirosis)
  Parasitic infections (e.g., malaria, toxoplasmosis)
  Cat scratch disease (*Bartonella henselae*)

Rheumatologic disorders (second most common cause of FUO)
  Systemic-onset juvenile rheumatoid arthritis (Still's disease)
  Kawasaki disease
  Systemic lupus erythematosus
  Acute rheumatic fever
  Polyarteritis nodosum

Malignancy (third most common cause of FUO)
  Lymphoma
  Leukemia

Periodic disorders characterized by spiking fevers at regular monthly intervals
  Familial Mediterranean fever: fever, peritonitis, pleuritis, and monoarthritis
  Periodic fever syndrome or periodic fever, aphthous stomatitis, pharyngitis, cervical adenitis syndrome (PFAPA)
  Cyclic neutropenia: neutropenia at time of fever occurring at regular 21-day intervals

Miscellaneous causes
  Inflammatory bowel disease
  Sarcoidosis
  Drug fever
  Factitious disorder

FUO = fever of unknown origin; *HIV* = human immunodeficiency virus.

e. **Blood cultures** to evaluate for bacteremia, including endocarditis

f. **Anti-streptolysin O titer** to evaluate for prior streptococcal infection, as seen in rheumatic fever

g. **Antinuclear antibody (ANA) and rheumatoid factor (RF)** to screen for rheumatic diseases

h. **Stool** for culture, ova and parasites, and *Clostridium difficile* toxin if diarrhea is present

i. **Tuberculosis skin test**

j. **HIV testing**

4. **Imaging options** may include chest radiography, echocardiography to evaluate for bacterial endocarditis, bone scanning to evaluate for osteomyelitis, gallium scanning to assess for sites of inflammation, and computed tomography (CT) and magnetic resonance imaging (MRI).

5. **Management.** Hospitalization is generally recommended for children with fever for greater than 2 weeks to facilitate evaluation and to document fever and coexisting symptoms. Specific management is based on the identified cause of the FUO.

IV. Meningitis

A. **Definition.** Meningitis is **inflammation of the meninges** and is classified as **bacterial** or **aseptic.**

B. **Bacterial Meningitis**

1. **Epidemiology**

a. Highest incidence of bacterial meningitis is during the **first month of life.**

b. Overall incidence during childhood has declined because of the introduction of the conjugate vaccine for HIB.

c. **Risk factors** for bacterial meningitis:

(1) **Young age**

(2) **Immunodeficiency** (e.g., asplenia, humoral-mediated immunodeficiency, and **terminal complement deficiency**)

(3) **Anatomic defects** (e.g., basilar skull fracture, ventriculoperitoneal shunt)

2. **Etiology.** Causes of infection are based on the age of the child (see Table 7-1).

3. **Clinical features**

a. Infants and young children often have minimal and **nonspecific signs and symptoms** (e.g., poor feeding, irritability, lethargy, respiratory distress). **Fever may be absent or minimal.** A bulging fontanelle may be present on physical examination.

b. Older children often present with **fever** and **signs suggestive of meningeal irritation.**

(1) **Alteration in level of consciousness,** with irritability, somnolence, or obtundation

      (2) Nuchal rigidity and positive **Kernig's and Brudzinski's signs** (these signs are less reliably present in infants and young children)

      (3) Seizures

      (4) Photophobia

      (5) Emesis

      (6) Headache

4. **Diagnosis. Index of suspicion for bacterial meningitis should be especially high in febrile, irritable infants.** Evaluation of all children with suspected bacterial meningitis should include:

    a. **Lumbar puncture,** which may demonstrate:

      (1) Pleocytosis with a predominance of **neutrophils.** The CSF WBC often exceeds 5,000 cells/mm^3.

      (2) Hypoglycorrhachia (low CSF glucose)—ratio of CSF to serum glucose < 0.40.

      (3) Increased protein

      (4) Positive Gram stain and culture

      (5) Bacterial antigens may be tested but have a low sensitivity and are not recommended on a routine basis.

      (6) Pretreatment with antibiotics may sterilize the CSF culture but should not alter the CSF cellular and biochemical profile above.

      (7) See **Table 7-3** for a comparison of the CSF profile in bacterial, viral, tuberculous, and fungal meningitis.

    b. **Blood culture** is positive in the majority of cases of bacterial meningitis.

    c. **CT scan with contrast** to evaluate for brain abscess is often recommended, especially for patients with focal neurologic findings.

5. **Management. Early, empiric treatment of bacterial meningitis is critical.**

    a. **Antibiotic therapy** varies based on age of child and the most likely pathogens:

      (1) Newborns (0–28 days): ampicillin plus aminoglycoside or third-generation cephalosporin. (Intravenous acyclovir for possible HSV infection should also be considered for ill neonates, especially those presenting with apnea, seizures, or cutaneous vesicles.)

      (2) Young infants (1–3 months): ampicillin plus third-generation cephalosporin. (Add vancomycin if bacterial meningitis is highly suspected, given the potential resistance pattern of pneumococcus.)

      (3) Older infants and children (> 3 months): third-generation cephalosporin. (Add vancomycin if bacterial meningitis is highly suspected, given the potential resistance pattern of pneumococcus.)

    b. **Corticosteroids** given before or with the first dose of antibiotics have been shown to be effective at reducing the incidence of hearing loss in HIB meningitis. Efficacy in other causes of bacterial meningitis has not been demonstrated.

    c. **Supportive care** includes attention to fluids with rehydration to normovolemic status, followed by administration of maintenance fluids with close attention to urine output, specific gravity, and serum

Table 7-3. Cerebrospinal Fluid Profiles in Meningitis

Pathogen	WBC Differential (cells/mm³)	Protein	Glucose	Gram Stain, Culture, and Other Definitive Tests
Acute bacterial	100–50,000 PMNs predominate	High	Low	Positive culture and Gram stain
Partially treated bacterial	1,000–10,000 Monos predominate	Normal to high	Low normal	Negative culture and usually negative Gram stain (+) CSF bacterial antigens
Viral	10–1,000 PMNs early, then monos + lymphs HSV encephalitis may show RBCs	Normal to high	Normal	Enterovirus may be recovered by culture Enterovirus and HSV may be identified by PCR
Tuberculosis	10–500 Lymphs predominate	Very high	Low to very low	AFB smear and culture rarely positive PCR may be positive
Fungal	25–500 Lymphs predominate	Normal to high	Low	Culture may be positive India ink (+) with *Cryptococcus*
Parameningeal focus (brain abscess)	10–200 Polys or monos predominate	High	Normal	Negative culture

AFB = acid-fast bacteria; *PMNs* = polymorphonuclear cells; *monos* = mononuclear cells; *lymphs* = lymphocytes; *CSF* = cerebrospinal fluid; *PCR* = polymerase chain reaction; *RBCs* = red blood cells; *HSV* = herpes simplex virus; *WBC* = white blood cell.

sodium to monitor for the development of the syndrome of inappropriate release of antidiuretic hormone (SIADH).

6. **Complications.** Complication rates are highest with meningitis caused by Gram-negative organisms, followed by *S. pneumoniae,* HIB, and, finally, *Neisseria meningitidis.* Mortality rates range from 5 to 50% depending on the infecting bacteria.

   a. **Hearing loss** is the **most common** complication occurring in up to 25% of patients.

   b. **Global brain injury** occurs in 5–10% of patients.

   c. Other complications include **SIADH, seizures, hydrocephalus, brain abscess, cranial nerve palsy, learning disability, and focal neurologic deficits.**

C. **Aseptic Meningitis**

   1. **Definition.** Aseptic meningitis is **inflammation of the meninges with a CSF lymphocytic pleocytosis** and, if caused by a virus, **normal CSF glucose and normal to minimally elevated CSF protein.**

2. **Etiology (Table 7-4).** Most causes of aseptic meningitis are viral.

3. **Clinical features** may be similar to those found in bacterial meningitis.

     a. Symptoms of viral meningitis may be mild with fever, headache, and emesis, or severe with altered level of consciousness and seizures.

     b. Symptoms in aseptic meningitis caused by *M. tuberculosis* (TB) may be nonspecific initially with lethargy or irritability, but during the second week of illness, symptoms progress rapidly with findings that include cranial nerve deficits, altered level of consciousness, coma, paraplegia, and eventual death if untreated.

4. **Diagnosis** (see **Table 7-3** for the CSF variables commonly seen in viral, fungal, tuberculous, and bacterial meningitis)

     a. **Viral meningitis**

         (1) Viral culture of CSF may be performed; however, the virus may not grow for 10–14 days.

         (2) PCR technology is available for the detection of Epstein-Barr virus (EBV), CMV, HSV, and enteroviruses.

         (3) Positive surface cultures for enterovirus from throat and rectum may be suggestive in cases of enteroviral meningitis.

     b. **TB meningitis.** CSF findings include lymphocytic pleocytosis, hypoglycorrhachia, and dramatically elevated protein. Brain imaging shows a characteristic **basilar enhancement.** Positive CSF acid-fast bacterial (AFB) stains (although rarely positive in TB meningitis), positive culture (may take as long as 6 weeks for growth), or positive PCR findings are diagnostic. Fifty percent of patients have a negative chest radiograph and tuberculin skin test at presentation.

Table 7-4. Causes of Aseptic Meningitis

Viral meningitis (most common cause of aseptic meningitis). If infection also involves the brain, it is termed a meningoencephalitis.

     Enteroviruses (most common cause of viral meningitis in the U.S.; most common in the summer and fall)

     Mumps

     Lymphocytic choriomeningitis

     Herpes viruses (herpes simplex virus, Epstein-Barr virus, cytomegalovirus, varicella zoster virus)

     Viruses that commonly cause encephalitis include arboviruses (St. Louis, Western equine, Eastern equine, West Nile virus), **influenza, and the herpes viruses**

Bacterial causes (some bacteria may cause an aseptic picture)
     Mycobacterium tuberculosis (most commonly seen in children younger than 5 years of age)
     Borrelia burgdorferi (Lyme disease)
     Treponema pallidum (syphilis)

Fungal causes
     Coccidioides immitis
     Cryptococcus neoformans
     Histoplasmosis capsulatum

Parasitic causes
     Taenia solium (etiologic agent of cysticercosis)
     Toxoplasma gondii (in immunocompromised patients)

---

    c. **Diagnostic studies that may identify other causes of aseptic meningitis** include CSF rapid plasma reagent (RPR) for syphilis, India ink for fungus (cryptococcus), cryptococcal antigen tests, and CSF and serum antibody testing for coccidioidomycosis, Lyme disease, and cysticercosis.

5. **Management**

    a. Most causes of viral meningitis are self-limited.

    b. TB meningitis is treated with four medications, including isoniazid, rifampin, pyrazinamide, and streptomycin. Corticosteroids are also commonly used.

6. **Prognosis** of aseptic meningitis is dependent on the causative agent and ranges from excellent in enteroviral meningitis to poor in TB meningitis (20% mortality in young children).

V. Upper Respiratory Infections

A. **General Concepts.** Upper respiratory infections (URIs) account for the majority of pediatric acute illness visits. Although generally benign illnesses, they may cause significant morbidity and parental anxiety.

B. **Simple Upper Respiratory Infection (common cold)**

1. **Etiology.** More than 100 viruses have been implicated and include **rhinovirus, parainfluenza virus, coronavirus, and respiratory syncytial virus.**

2. **Clinical features**

    a. Presenting symptoms include low-grade fever, rhinorrhea, cough, and sore throat. Symptoms resolve within 7–10 days.

    b. **Color of nasal discharge alone does not predict the presence of concurrent sinusitis** because purulent nasal discharge may occur early in the course of a URI.

    c. **Persistent symptoms** (> 10 days) **or fever should prompt the clinician to evaluate for bacterial superinfection** (e.g., sinusitis, acute otitis media).

3. **Diagnosis** is based on clinical features. The viral agent is rarely identified.

4. **Management.** The **most important step is to ensure adequate hydration, particularly in young children,** and to exclude more serious disorders such as sinusitis and acute otitis media. Over-the-counter medications (e.g., antihistamines, mucolytics, cough suppressant, decongestants) have minimal effectiveness and may cause side effects. **Antibiotics have no role in management.**

C. **Sinusitis**

1. **Development of the sinuses.** Ethmoid and maxillary sinuses form in the third to fourth month of gestation and are present at birth. The sphenoid sinuses develop between 3 and 5 years of age and frontal sinuses between 7 and 10 years of age.

2. **Categories of sinusitis.** Sinusitis is divided into **acute, subacute, and**

chronic forms on the basis of **duration of symptoms.** Clinical features, causes, and management of sinusitis are presented in **Figure 7-1.**

3. **Diagnosis** is based on clinical features. Note that physical examination (particularly sinus transillumination) is unreliable for diagnosis and that **imaging is not useful for the initial diagnosis or management of uncomplicated sinusitis.**

D. **Pharyngitis**

1. **Etiology**

   a. **Viral causes** include those viruses associated with simple URIs, as well as **coxsackievirus, EBV, and CMV.**

   b. **Bacterial causes** include *Streptococcus pyogenes* (group A β-hemolytic streptococcus [**GABHS**] or "**strep throat**"), *Arcanobacterium hemolyticum,* and *Corynebacterium diphtheriae* (diphtheria).

2. **Clinical features.** The **clinical features of viral pharyngitis and GABHS pharyngitis overlap,** resulting in difficulty differentiating between the two conditions solely on the basis of history and physical examination.

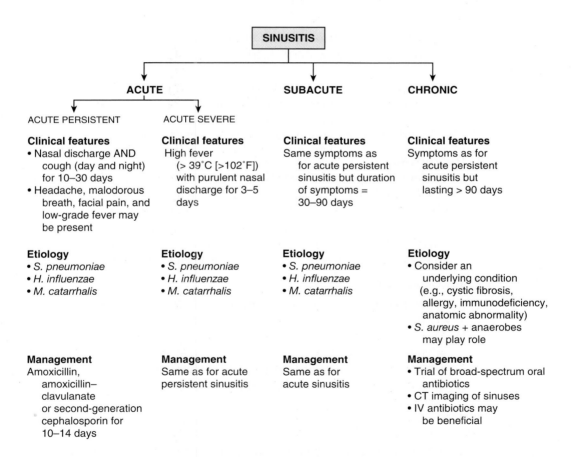

Figure 7-1. Diagnosis of sinusitis and clinical features, etiology, and management. *CT* = computed tomography; *IV* = intravenous.

   a. Viral pharyngitis may present with simple URI symptoms. **Tonsillar exudates may also be present.** Certain viral infections may have the following specific findings:

      (1) Children with **EBV pharyngitis** may present with enlarged posterior cervical lymph nodes, malaise, and hepatosplenomegaly.

      (2) Children with **coxsackievirus pharyngitis** may present with **painful vesicles or ulcers** on the posterior pharynx and soft palate (**herpangina**). Blisters may also be present on the palms and soles (**hand-foot-mouth disease**).

   b. Bacterial pharyngitis

      (1) GABHS pharyngitis (strep throat) is usually seen in school-age children (5–15 years of age) and in the winter and spring. Although it is difficult to distinguish GABHS pharyngitis from viral pharyngitis on the basis of signs and symptoms, GABHS infection has the following characteristics:

         (a) Lack of other URI symptoms (e.g., rhinorrhea, cough)

         (b) Exudates on the tonsils, petechiae on the soft palate, strawberry tongue, and enlarged tender anterior cervical lymph nodes

         (c) Fever

         (d) Scarlatiniform rash in some patients (see section IX.A.5)

         (e) Complications of GABHS infection are described in section IX.A.5.g.

      (2) Diphtheria is extremely rare in developed nations because of universal vaccination. Patients present with low-grade fever and a **gray, adherent tonsillar membrane.** Toxin-mediated cardiac and neurologic complications may also develop.

3. Diagnosis

   a. Patients with suspected GABHS pharyngitis should undergo culture (gold standard) or antigen testing ("rapid strep test") to confirm GABHS pharyngitis and to avoid overuse of antibiotics.

   b. Because 5% of the population carries GABHS in the pharynx (GABHS carriers), culture or rapid antigen testing should be limited to symptomatic patients who lack concomitant viral symptoms.

4. Management

   a. Management of viral pharyngitis is supportive and includes analgesics and maintenance of adequate hydration.

   b. Management of GABHS pharyngitis includes oral penicillin VK, a single dose of intramuscular benzathine penicillin, and for penicillin-allergic patients, oral erythromycin or macrolides.

   c. Management of severe EBV pharyngitis may sometimes include corticosteroids.

   d. Diphtheria is treated with oral erythromycin or parenteral penicillin, and a specific antitoxin that is available from the U.S. Centers for Disease Control and Prevention. Respiratory isolation is very important to prevent spread of infection.

E. Acute Otitis Media

1. **Definitions**
   a. **Acute otitis media (AOM)** is defined as an **acute infection of the middle ear space.**
   b. **Otitis media with effusion (OME)** is defined as fluid within the middle ear space without symptoms of infection.

2. **Etiology.** Bacterial pathogens include *S. pneumoniae*, **non-typeable** *H. influenzae,* and *Moraxella catarrhalis.* Viruses causing simple URIs also commonly cause AOM.

3. **Clinical features of AOM**
   a. AOM usually develops during or after a simple URI.
   b. Symptoms may include **fever, ear pain, and decreased hearing.** Symptoms are less reliably present in young children.
   c. If the tympanic membrane perforates, patients may report pus or fluid draining from the ear.

4. **Diagnosis**
   a. **Proper diagnosis of AOM depends on the identification of fluid within the middle ear space in the presence of symptoms of infection.**
      (1) **Pneumatic otoscopy** to identify abnormal movement of the tympanic membrane, and therefore fluid within the middle ear, is an essential component of the physical examination and is the **most reliable method of detecting middle ear fluid.**
      (2) **Erythema and loss of tympanic membrane landmarks are unreliable methods of identifying fluid within the middle ear space.**
   b. Although not routine, identification of the bacterial etiology may be made by tympanocentesis.
   c. A perforated tympanic membrane with purulent discharge within the external auditory canal is also consistent with the diagnosis of AOM.

5. **Management**
   a. Antibiotics are often prescribed for AOM; however, their use is controversial, especially in older children, because a majority of cases of AOM resolve spontaneously without complications.
   b. Initial antibiotic therapy, if used, is usually **amoxicillin.** If the patient attends a day care facility or has received antibiotics within the previous 1–2 months, then the likelihood of infection with penicillin-resistant *S. pneumoniae* increases. Initial therapy may then include high-dose amoxicillin, amoxicillin-clavulanic acid, or a cephalosporin. Macrolides may be used in penicillin-allergic patients.
   c. Antibiotics are not indicated for OME.

F. Otitis Externa

1. **Definition.** Otitis externa (OE) is defined as an **infection of the external auditory canal (EAC).**
2. **Pathogenesis.** Factors that interfere with the EAC protective mecha-

nisms (e.g., cerumen removal, trauma, maceration of skin from swimming, or excessive moisture or humidity) predispose to OE.

3. **Etiology.** Pathogens are most commonly *Pseudomonas aeruginosa, Staphylococcus aureus,* or *Candida albicans.* OE can also develop in a patient with a perforated tympanic membrane secondary to AOM.

4. **Clinical features.** Pain, itching, and drainage from the ear are usually present. Systemic symptoms are usually absent. A history consistent with AOM is helpful in determining whether there has been a tympanic membrane perforation.

5. **Diagnosis.** Findings on physical examination are the basis of diagnosis. **Erythema and edema of the EAC** may be present, sometimes with purulent or whitish material within the canal. There may also be tenderness on palpation or movement of the tragus. Visualization of the tympanic membrane is important to exclude perforation. In refractory cases, cultures of infected material may identify the etiologic agent.

6. **Management**
   a. The **key to successful management is to restore the EAC to its natural acidic environment.**
   b. For mild cases of OE (minimal pain and discharge), acetic acid solution may be sufficient to relieve the discomfort and to restore the natural environment of the EAC.
   c. For more severe cases, topical antibiotics (sometimes combined with a topical corticosteroid) are prescribed.
   d. Perforated AOM complicated by OE is treated with both oral and topical antibiotics.

VI. Middle and Lower Respiratory Infections, including pneumonia, bronchiolitis, epiglottitis, croup, and bacterial tracheitis, are described in Chapter 9, section III.

VII. Cervical Lymphadenitis

A. **Definition.** Cervical lymphadenitis is defined as an enlarged, inflamed, tender lymph node or nodes in the cervical area.

B. **Etiology and Differential Diagnosis**

1. **Localized bacterial infection**
   a. *S. aureus* is the **most common bacterial agent.**
   b. *S. pyogenes* is also common.
   c. **Mycobacterial infections,** including *M. tuberculosis* and atypical mycobacterium (*Mycobacterium avium* complex)
   d. *B. henselae,* which causes cat scratch disease (see section XVII.B)

2. **Reactive lymphadenitis** occurs in response to infections in the pharynx, teeth, and soft tissues of the head and neck.

3. **Viral infections,** such as EBV, CMV, and HIV, can also cause reactive lymphadenitis in the cervical area.

4. **Kawasaki disease** may present with unilateral cervical lymphadenitis. (An enlarged cervical lymph node is one of the diagnostic criteria of Kawasaki disease.)

5. *T. gondii* infection may cause a mononucleosis-like illness with cervical lymphadenopathy.

6. **Structural lesions in the neck** (e.g., branchial cleft cyst, cystic hygroma) can become secondarily infected and may present similarly to cervical lymphadenitis.

C. **Clinical Features**

1. The infected node is **mobile, tender, warm,** and enlarged, and the overlying skin is erythematous. Fluctuance may be present.

2. Nodes may be single, or multiple nodes may be clumped together in a mass.

3. Systemic symptoms (e.g., fever) may be present.

D. **Diagnosis** is based on clinical features.

1. Tests, such as placement of a tuberculin skin test, a CBC with differential, and antibody titers for *B. henselae* and *T. gondii,* may be indicated for infected nodes **unresponsive to therapy.**

2. **Antibody titers** for EBV, CMV, and HIV serology may be indicated if **lymphadenopathy is diffuse and persistent.**

3. **Imaging studies** may help define the anatomy of the cervical area and identify areas of suppuration or abscess that require surgical drainage. Imaging is essential if there is concern about airway compromise resulting from a deep infection.

E. **Management** includes empiric antibiotics directed toward the most common organisms (*S. aureus* and *S. pyogenes*). Initial treatment may include a first-generation cephalosporin or an anti-staphylococcal penicillin for 7–10 days. Intravenous antibiotics are indicated for the toxic-appearing child with adenitis or for the child who remains symptomatic despite appropriate oral therapy.

VIII. Parotitis

A. **Definition.** Parotitis is defined as inflammation of the parotid salivary glands.

B. **Etiology**

1. **Mumps and other viruses** (e.g., CMV, EBV, HIV, influenza) usually cause **bilateral involvement** of the parotid gland. **Before universal vaccination, mumps was the most common cause of parotitis.**

2. **Bacterial parotitis (acute suppurative parotitis)** is caused by *S. aureus*, *S. pyogenes,* and *M. tuberculosis* and usually results in **unilateral parotid involvement.** Bacterial parotitis is uncommon during childhood, although children with decreased salivary flow or stone formation are at increased risk.

C. **Clinical features** include swelling centered above the angle of the jaw and fever. Physical examination of the oropharynx may reveal pus that can be expressed from Stensen's duct.

D. Diagnosis is based on clinical features and may be confirmed by CT scan.

1. Culture of the drainage from Stensen's duct may reveal the microbiologic cause of bacterial parotitis.

2. Viral parotitis may be diagnosed by viral serology. Mumps virus may also be detected in the urine.

E. Management

1. Viral parotitis is treated with supportive care and analgesics.

2. Acute suppurative parotitis is treated with antibiotics directed against *S. aureus* and *S. pyogenes*. Rarely, surgical excision and drainage are required.

F. Complications

1. Mumps may also result in meningoencephalitis, orchitis and epididymitis, and pancreatitis.

2. Acute suppurative parotitis may result in formation of an abscess and osteomyelitis of the jaw.

IX. Skin and Soft Tissue Infections

A. Bacterial Infections

1. Impetigo

a. **Definition.** Impetigo is a superficial skin infection involving the upper dermis.

b. **Etiology.** *S. aureus* **is the most common agent, but GABHS (or** *S. pyogenes***)** may also cause infection.

c. *Clinical features. Honey-colored crusted* or bullous lesions are present, commonly on the face, especially around the nares. Fever is generally absent. **Infection is easily transmitted.**

d. **Diagnosis.** Visual inspection is the basis of diagnosis. Cultures are not required.

e. **Management.** Treatment may include topical mupirocin or oral antibiotics, such as dicloxacillin, cephalexin, or clindamycin.

f. **Complications.** Bacteremia, post-streptococcal glomerulonephritis (treatment of impetigo does not prevent this complication), and staphylococcal scalded skin syndrome (SSSS) are possible complications.

2. Erysipelas

a. **Definition.** Erysipelas is a skin infection that involves the dermal lymphatics.

b. **Etiology** is usually **GABHS.**

c. **Clinical features** include **tender, erythematous skin with a distinct border.** The face and scalp are common locations.

d. **Diagnosis** is by visual inspection.

e. **Management** includes systemic therapy with antibiotics targeted against GABHS.

    f. Complications include bacteremia, post-streptococcal glomerulonephritis, and necrotizing fasciitis.

3. Cellulitis

    a. Definition. Cellulitis is a skin infection that occurs within the dermis.

    b. Etiology. Causes include **GABHS** and ***S. aureus.*** Infection is usually caused by a break in the skin barrier allowing bacteria to gain entry beyond the protective layer of the epidermis.

    c. Clinical features. Cellulitis is characterized by erythema, warmth, and tenderness. The infected skin border is **indistinct.**

    d. Diagnosis is by visual inspection. Blood cultures are seldom positive. In more aggressive forms of cellulitis, biopsy and culture of the leading edge of infection may be useful to identify the pathogenic organism.

    e. Management includes oral or intravenous antibiotics directed against the typical causative agents, including first-generation cephalosporins or anti-staphylococcal penicillins.

4. Important variants of cellulitis

    a. Buccal cellulitis is a now uncommon form of cellulitis that occurs as a **unilateral bluish discoloration on the cheek of a young unimmunized child.** Patients are often febrile and may appear toxic. The causative agent is **HIB,** and blood cultures are often positive. Management includes intravenous antibiotics directed against *H. influenzae,* usually a second- or third-generation cephalosporin (e.g., cefuroxime or cefotaxime). Patients with buccal cellulitis caused by HIB have a high rate of concomitant bacteremia and meningitis; a lumbar puncture should be performed.

    b. Perianal cellulitis occurs as **well-demarcated erythema involving the skin around the anus.** Children may also present with constipation. The cause is usually GABHS. Diagnosis is by visual inspection or a positive rectal swab culture for GABHS. Management includes oral antibiotics (e.g., cephalexin, dicloxacillin).

    c. Necrotizing fasciitis is a **potentially fatal form of deep cellulitis. Patients** present with **pain and systemic symptoms out of proportion to physical findings.** Infection extends beyond the underlying fascia into the muscle. Examination may reveal crepitus and hemorrhagic bullae. The cause is polymicrobial and may involve GABHS and anaerobic bacteria. **Intravenous antibiotics and surgical debridement are essential components of therapy.**

    d. Staphylococcal scalded skin syndrome (SSSS) is caused by an *S. aureus* species that produces an exfoliative toxin. Presentation includes fever, **tender skin,** and bullae. Large sheets of skin slough several days after the illness begins, and the **Nikolsky sign is present** (extension of bullae when pressure is applied to the skin). Management includes good wound care and intravenous antibiotics directed against *S. aureus.*

5. Scarlet fever

    a. Definition. Scarlet fever is a toxin-mediated bacterial illness that results in a characteristic skin rash.

    b. Etiology. The cause of infection is strains of GABHS that produce an erythrogenic toxin.

    c. Epidemiology

        (1) Peak incidence is in the winter and spring.

        (2) Transmission is by large respiratory droplets or by infected nasal secretions.

    d. Clinical features

        (1) The exanthem may develop during any GABHS infection (e.g., impetigo, cellulitis, pharyngitis).

        (2) Before or during the exanthem, fever, chills, malaise, and often an exudative pharyngitis (see also section V.D) may occur.

        (3) The **exanthem is characterized by the following:**

            (a) Begins on the trunk and moves peripherally

            (b) Skin is **erythematous** with tiny skin-colored papules (scarlatiniform appearance) and has the texture of sandpaper (**sandpaper rash**). The rash blanches with pressure.

            (c) Petechiae are often localized within skin creases in a linear distribution ("**Pastia's lines**").

            (d) Desquamation of dry skin occurs as the infection resolves.

    e. Diagnosis. The basis of diagnosis is clinical features and a positive throat culture for *S. pyogenes* (gold standard) or positive rapid streptococcal tests that detect the GABHS antigen.

    f. Management

        (1) The **goal is to prevent development of rheumatic fever.**

        (2) Appropriate antibiotics include oral penicillin VK, intramuscular benzathine penicillin, or for penicillin-allergic patients, erythromycin or macrolides.

    g. Complications of GABHS infections

        (1) Post-streptococcal glomerulonephritis may occur several weeks after streptococcal pharyngitis. Patients present with hypertension and cola-colored urine. **Antibiotic therapy does not prevent this complication** (see Chapter 11, section IV.F.1).

        (2) Rheumatic fever (see Chapter 16, section VI)

        (3) Post-streptococcal arthritis is characterized by joint symptoms (without other features of rheumatic fever) that may last for weeks. **Antibiotic therapy does not prevent this complication.**

        (4) Pediatric autoimmune neuropsychiatric disorders associated with streptococcal infection (PANDAS) is a phenomenon in which patients develop the acute onset of **obsessive-compulsive symptoms** or a tic disorder after streptococcal infection. Antibiotic therapy prevents this complication.

6. Toxic shock syndrome (TSS)

    a. Definition. TSS is a **toxin-mediated** illness characterized by fever, shock, desquamating skin rash, and multiorgan dysfunction.

    b. Etiology and pathogenesis

        (1) *S. aureus* is the most common organism associated with TSS, although an increase in **GABHS**-associated TSS has been reported.

Table 7-5. Diagnostic Criteria for Toxic Shock Syndrome

Diagnostic criteria
(probable case = 5 of 6 criteria; confirmed case = 6 of 6 criteria)

1. **Fever > 38.5°C (> 101°F)**
2. Hypotension (SBP < 90 mm Hg or < fifth percentile for age)
3. Diffuse macular **erythroderma** (appears similar to sunburn)
4. **Desquamation** occurs 10–14 days after onset of illness
5. **Multisystem involvement,** including three or more of the following:
   a. Gastrointestinal—vomiting, diarrhea, and abdominal pain
   b. Myalgias or elevated creatine kinase levels
   c. Hyperemia of the mucous membranes (e.g., pharyngitis, vaginitis)
   d. Pyuria in the presence of negative urine cultures or elevated blood urea nitrogen and creatinine to twice normal limit
   e. Thrombocytopenia
   f. Central nervous system—altered level of consciousness, meningismus
6. **Negative cultures of blood, cerebrospinal fluid, and pharynx** (except for positive blood culture for *Staphylococcus aureus*)

Other clinical findings may include oral ulcers, acute respiratory distress syndrome, headache, edema, conjunctivitis, disseminated intravascular coagulation, elevated transaminases, hypocalcemia, and hypoalbuminemia.
SBP = systolic blood pressure.

In the early 1980s, the majority of TSS cases caused by *S. aureus* were in young women using **tampons.** However, only 50% of TSS cases are now related to tampon use.

    (2) Organisms produce toxins (exotoxins and toxic shock syndrome toxin) that result in the clinical features of TSS.

  c. Clinical features and diagnostic criteria (Table 7-5). Patients with TSS may present with a wide variety of signs and symptoms.

  d. Management. Treatment includes supportive measures to reverse shock, anti-staphylococcal antibiotics, and removal of the nidus of infection (tampon) if present. Intravenous immune globulin (IVIG) may have some benefit.

    7. Infection caused by animal and human bites (see Chapter 20, section IX.B–D)

B. Fungal infections of the skin (see Chapter 19, section V.A)

C. Viral infections of the skin (see Chapter 19, section V.C)

D. Ectoparasitic infections of the skin (see Chapter 19, section V.D)

X. Bone and Joint Infections (see Chapter 17, section III.B)

XI. Diarrhea

  A. Etiology. Diarrheal diseases and resulting dehydration are among the most common causes of childhood morbidity and mortality worldwide. Infection is one of the most common causes of acute diarrhea during childhood. Specific causes of diarrhea include:

1. **Viral causes** most commonly include **rotavirus and Norwalk virus.**
   a. **Rotavirus**
      (1) **Epidemiology. Rotavirus is the most common infectious agent causing gastroenteritis.** This RNA virus is usually seen in the **winter months** and is spread by the fecal-oral route.
      (2) **Clinical features.** Incubation period is 1–3 days. Patients may be asymptomatic, or may have **vomiting, diarrhea,** and **dehydration.** Diarrhea is usually self-limited and lasts 4–7 days. Symptoms of URI may sometimes be present.
      (3) **Diagnosis.** A positive stool enzyme-linked immunosorbent assay (ELISA) test is used to make the diagnosis. WBCs are absent from the stool.
      (4) **Management.** Treatment is **supportive** with particular attention to fluid management and early institution of feedings to prevent gut atrophy. Some children may develop transient lactose intolerance.
   b. **Norwalk virus**
      (1) **Epidemiology.** Norwalk virus is an RNA virus spread by the fecal-oral route and linked to **outbreaks of gastroenteritis in all age groups, particularly in closed populations** (e.g., day care centers, schools, cruise ships).
      (2) **Clinical features** are similar to those caused by rotavirus with **vomiting a prominent symptom.** Duration of illness is only 48–72 hours, a **shorter duration** as compared with the other viral causes.
      (3) **Diagnosis** is based on clinical features.
      (4) **Management** is supportive.
2. **Bacterial causes,** associated clinical features, and management (see **Table 7-6**)
3. **Parasitic causes** (see section XV)

B. **Evaluation** should include a detailed history, complete physical examination, and selective laboratory studies.
   1. **Specific historical features** include:
      a. Presence of fever, rash, abdominal pain, vomiting, and blood or mucus in the stool
      b. Recent antibiotic use (e.g., may result in *C. difficile* infection)
      c. **Day care attendance** or travel
      d. Unusual pets (e.g., lizards and turtles may transmit *Salmonella* species)
      e. Unusual foods or recent restaurant meal
   2. **Physical examination** should be detailed and focused, especially on assessment of hydration, particularly in young children.
   3. **Laboratory studies** may include CBC, serum electrolytes, and assessment of stool for gross or occult blood (i.e., stool guaiac), WBCs (i.e., Wright stain), ova and parasite evaluation (three separate ova and parasite stool specimens increase the yield) and culture. ELISA may be useful in the detection of rotavirus, *Giardia lamblia,* and *C. difficile* infection.

Table 7-6. Characteristics of Bacterial Causes of Infectious Diarrhea

Bacterium	Clinical Features	Diagnosis	Management
Enterotoxigenic *Escherichia coli* (ETEC)	**Major cause of traveler's diarrhea** Generally noninvasive with watery diarrhea	Stool WBCs **absent** Diagnosis is made clinically but can be confirmed on culture	Antibiotics (quinolones or sulfonamides in children) may shorten duration of symptoms Hydration is essential
Enteropathogenic *E. coli* (EPEC)	Noninvasive watery diarrhea seen in preschoolers	Stool WBCs **absent** Diagnosis made on stool culture	Oral sulfonamides or quinolones are indicated Hydration is essential
Enterohemorrhagic *E. coli* (EHEC)	**Strain 0157:H7 is responsible for hemolytic uremic syndrome (HUS)** via endotoxin release	Stool WBCs **present** Culture is diagnostic	**If HUS is present, antibiotic therapy is avoided** (HUS may worsen as a result of enhanced endotoxin release)
Shigella sonnei	**Bloody diarrhea predominates Children may develop seizures** secondary to neurotoxin release	Stool WBCs **present** Culture is diagnostic	Third-generation cephalosporins or fluoroquinolones are indicated
Salmonella species	May cause **bloody or nonbloody diarrhea** Spread by fecal-oral route, **poultry, milk, eggs, and exposure to lizards or turtles** Patients, especially those with sickle cell disease, may develop bacteremia or osteomyelitis	Stool WBCs may be **present or absent** Culture is usually diagnostic	Treatment is not indicated for uncomplicated gastroenteritis in immunocompetent hosts > 3 months of age because it increases carriage time Treatment for invasive disease includes a third-generation cephalosporin
Campylobacter jejuni	**Most common cause of bacterial bloody diarrhea in the U.S.** Disease is often self-limited and is spread by contaminated food (usually poultry)	Stool WBCs are usually present if blood is present Stool culture is diagnostic	Oral erythromycin is indicated but symptoms commonly resolve without antimicrobial intervention
Yersinia enterocolitica	May cause **mesenteric adenitis** along with gastroenteritis **that may mimic acute appendicitis**	Stool culture or mesenteric node culture grows the organism	Antibiotics may benefit patients; third-generation cephalosporins are commonly used
Clostridium difficile	A normal component of gut flora that may cause colitis if it overgrows the rest of the gut flora, as is seen **after antibiotic use**	Diagnosis is made by identifying toxin in the stool Endoscopy may demonstrate **pseudomem-branes**	Oral or intravenous metronidazole is effective Oral vancomycin is reserved for resistant cases

Table 7-6. Characteristics of Bacterial Causes of Infectious Diarrhea *(Continued)*

Bacterium	Clinical Features	Diagnosis	Management
Vibrio cholerae	Seen in developing countries Characterized by watery diarrhea with **massive water loss**	Diagnosis is based on history of massive watery diarrhea in a patient returning from or residing in an endemic area *V. cholerae* may be cultured from stool, but this is not routinely performed in the U.S. Serologic diagnosis is available from the Centers for Disease Control and Prevention	**Fluid replacement is critical** Antibiotics may shorten the duration but are generally not used

WBCs = white blood cells.

    a. The **classic electrolyte finding** is a **non–anion gap hyperchloremic metabolic acidosis** as a result of bicarbonate loss in the stool.

    b. In general, the presence of either gross or occult blood in stools predicts the presence of stool WBCs.

    c. The **utility of a culture when WBCs are absent in the stool is low.**

  C. Management principles

    1. Fluid management is the cornerstone of therapy.

    2. Antibiotics are indicated for only a few causes of diarrhea (**Table 7-6**).

XII. Urinary Tract Infections (see Chapter 11, section XIII)

XIII. Specific Viral Infections

  A. Human immunodeficiency virus (HIV) and acquired immunodeficiency syndrome (AIDS)

    1. Epidemiology. More than 10,000 children and adolescents in the United States are reported to be infected with HIV, although this is considered to be an underestimate. Worldwide, more than 1 million children have AIDS, and as many as 10 times this number are infected with HIV.

    2. Transmission

      a. Perinatal transmission currently accounts for > 95% of pediatric HIV cases.

        (1) In utero, intrapartum, or postpartum (through breastfeeding) **transmission** of HIV from an infected mother to her infant may occur. Transmission rates range from 5% in the United States, because of the common use of antiretroviral therapy during pregnancy, to 50% in the developing world.

    (2) Factors that **increase the risk of transmission:**

        (a) High maternal viral load (as measured by number of RNA copies)

        (b) Advanced maternal HIV disease

        (c) Primary maternal HIV infection

        (d) Concomitant maternal genital infections, including chorioamnionitis

        (e) Premature birth

        (f) Prolonged rupture of membranes

    (3) Factors that **decrease the risk of transmission:**

        (a) Undetectable maternal viral load

        (b) Cesarean section

        (c) Adherence to maternal antiretroviral therapy and infant postexposure prophylaxis

  b. Other modes of HIV transmission:

    (1) **Sexual contact,** an important mode of infection in adolescents

    (2) **Blood product** transmission, which is now rare because of mandatory blood product screening

    (3) **Sharing of intravenous and tattoo needles**

3. Clinical features

  a. Most infants with perinatally acquired HIV infection are **asymptomatic** for the first year of life.

  b. Early symptoms of HIV infection:

    (1) **Failure to thrive**

    (2) **Thrombocytopenia**

    (3) **Recurrent infections,** such as otitis media, pneumonia, and sinusitis

    (4) **Lymphadenopathy**

    (5) **Parotitis**

    (6) **Recurrent, difficult-to-treat thrush**

    (7) **Loss of developmental milestones**

    (8) **Severe varicella infection or zoster**

4. Diagnosis

  a. All infants born to HIV-infected mothers have transplacentally acquired maternal antibody that may persist for as long as 18–24 months.

  b. HIV-specific DNA PCR is performed at birth and monthly until 4 months of age to detect infants who are infected perinatally.

  c. Negative HIV-specific DNA PCR at 4 months is consistent with an infant who has not been infected. If the DNA PCR is negative for HIV, infants are followed until they lose their transplacentally acquired maternal antibody (by age 18–24 months).

5. Management

    a. Infants born to HIV-infected mothers should be tested for the presence of virus, as outlined above in section XIII.A.4, in addition to:

        (1) Zidovudine for 6 weeks for postexposure prophylaxis

        (2) Trimethoprim/sulfamethoxazole (TMP/SMX) for *Pneumocystis carinii* pneumonia (PCP) prophylaxis until HIV DNA PCR at age 4 months is negative

        (3) No breastfeeding

        (4) Urine CMV culture to detect coinfection with CMV (occurs in 5%)

    b. **HIV-infected children** should ideally be managed at an institution experienced in the care of children with HIV. Treatment includes administration of medications as well as nutrition and social work services and regular neurodevelopmental testing.

        (1) All HIV-infected infants and all symptomatic children should receive **antiretroviral agents** that may include nucleoside reverse transcriptase inhibitors (NRTIs), non–nucleoside reverse transcriptase inhibitors (NNRTIs), and protease inhibitors. **Combination therapy is the cornerstone of treatment to avoid selection of resistant viruses.** Close monitoring is essential because medications may cause bone marrow suppression, hepatitis, and pancreatitis.

        (2) **Prophylaxis for opportunistic infections is important.** The decision to begin prophylaxis is based on the patient's age and CD4 count.

        (3) **Immunizations** and usual **well child care are critical.** HIV-infected children should receive all routine childhood vaccines except the live varicella vaccine. The measles, mumps, and rubella (MMR) vaccine, although a live viral vaccine, is currently recommended for all but the most severely immunocompromised HIV-infected children. Annual influenza vaccine, pneumococcal vaccine, and annual tuberculin skin testing are all recommended.

        (4) Regular monitoring of T-cell subsets and HIV RNA PCR to assess viral load

        (5) Annual ophthalmologic examination to assess for CMV retinitis in HIV-infected children who are CMV antibody positive

6. Complications of HIV infection

    a. Opportunistic infections

        (1) PCP

            (a) Epidemiology

                (i) Most common opportunistic infection in HIV-infected children

                (ii) Risk of infection correlates with CD4 cell number and percentage.

            (b) Clinical features. Fever, hypoxia, and interstitial pulmonary infiltrates are present.

            (c) Management. Prophylaxis against PCP infection is with oral **TMP/SMX.** Treatment of PCP infection may include TMP/SMX, pentamidine, or atovaquone.

    (2) *M. avium* **complex (MAC).** MAC is characterized by fever, weight loss, night sweats, abdominal pain, bone marrow suppression, and elevated liver transaminases. Risk is highest when the CD4 count falls to less than 50 cells/mm^3.

    (3) Fungal infections. Candidal infections (e.g., thrush, esophagitis), cryptococcal infections (e.g., meningitis, pneumonia), histoplasmosis, coccidioidomycosis, and aspergillosis may occur.

    (4) Viral infections. CMV (e.g., retinitis, esophagitis, colitis), HSV, and varicella zoster virus (VZV) may occur.

    (5) Parasitic infections. Toxoplasmosis and infections caused by *Cryptosporidium* and *Isospora belli* may occur.

  b. Lymphoma, especially B cell, caused by EBV.

7. Prognosis. The expanded testing of pregnant women for HIV, coupled with aggressive prenatal antiretroviral therapy, has dramatically reduced the perinatal HIV transmission rate in the United States. Morbidity and mortality of HIV-infected children have also declined, correlating with the licensure of new antiretroviral agents, especially protease inhibitors.

B. Infectious Mononucleosis

  1. Etiology and epidemiology

    a. EBV, a member of the herpes virus family, is the **major etiologic agent.** EBV is commonly acquired during adolescence, although infection also often occurs in young children. EBV is **transmitted primarily by saliva** and seems to infect the B lymphocyte.

    b. Other agents, including **toxoplasmosis, CMV, and HIV,** may cause a similar clinical syndrome.

  2. Clinical features

    a. Young children may be asymptomatic.

    b. Older children develop **typical signs and symptoms.**

      (1) Fever, which may last up to 2 weeks

      (2) Malaise and fatigue

      (3) Pharyngitis (typically exudative, resembling **GABHS pharyngitis**)

      (4) Posterior cervical lymphadenopathy (lymphadenopathy may also be diffuse)

      (5) Hepatosplenomegaly. Spleen is enlarged in 80%.

      (6) A minority of patients may also develop a **macular or scarlatiniform rash.**

      (7) Symptoms resolve in weeks to months.

  3. Diagnosis

    a. CBC may demonstrate **atypical lymphocytes.** Other laboratory abnormalities include neutropenia, thrombocytopenia, and elevated transaminases.

    b. Monospot is a first-line test in diagnosing EBV infectious mononucleosis. A monospot measures the presence of heterophile antibody, the ability to agglutinate sheep red blood cells (RBCs). It has an overall sensitivity of 85% but is **less sensitive in children under 4 years of age** because these antibodies do not reliably form in younger children. CMV causes the majority of monospot-negative cases of infectious mononucleosis in older children.

    c. EBV antibody titers are the preferred method of diagnosing EBV infection in children younger than 4 years of age.

        (1) To diagnose EBV, antibodies to **viral capsid antigen (VCA), early antigen (EA), and Epstein-Barr nuclear antigen (EBNA)** are tested.

        (2) Acute infection is diagnosed by finding **elevated levels of IgM–VCA** and absent antibodies to EBNA. Antibodies to EBNA are detected 2–3 months after acute infection.

    d. PCR testing may also be used for diagnosis.

  4. Management. Therapy for most cases of EBV infection is supportive. Corticosteroids are sometimes used for severe pharyngitis.

  5. Complications

    a. Neurologic complications, including cranial nerve palsies and encephalitis

    b. Severe pharyngitis, which may cause **upper airway obstruction**

    c. Amoxicillin-associated rash. Patients with EBV infection who are misdiagnosed with GABHS pharyngitis and prescribed amoxicillin often develop a **diffuse pruritic maculopapular rash** 1 week after starting the antibiotic. This is not an allergic reaction but is idiosyncratic.

    d. Splenic rupture. Children with infectious mononucleosis with splenomegaly should be restricted from contact sports until the spleen has returned to normal size.

    e. Malignancy. EBV has been isolated from nasopharyngeal carcinoma and Burkitt's lymphoma. EBV may also result in lymphoproliferative disease, a lymphomalike illness, in immunosuppressed patients.

C. Measles

  1. Etiology. Measles is also known as rubeola and 10-day measles and is caused by an RNA virus of the **Paramyxoviridae family.**

  2. Epidemiology

    a. Owing to routine measles vaccination, the incidence of measles has declined in the United States during the past 40 years, with fewer than 100 cases per year now reported.

    b. Measles is **highly infectious** and spreads easily among susceptible individuals in households and schools.

  3. Clinical features. Manifestations develop after an **8- to 12-day incubation period.** Clinical features include a classic clinical prodrome, followed by a transient enanthem (rash on mucous membranes) and a characteristic exanthem (rash on the skin).

    a. The **three C's (cough, conjunctivitis, and coryza)** is a mnemonic to help remember the **classic prodrome.** Other early symptoms include photophobia and low-grade fever.

    b. The **enanthem** is characterized by **Koplik spots,** small gray papules on an erythematous base located on the buccal mucosa. **Koplik spots are pathognomonic of measles and are present before the generalized exanthem.** They are transient and may be absent by the onset of other clinical features.

    c. The **exanthem** is characterized as an erythematous maculopapular eruption that **begins around the neck and ears and spreads down the chest and upper extremities during the subsequent 24 hours.** The exanthem covers the lower extremities by the second day, becomes confluent by the third day, and lasts for 4–7 days.

    d. Fever, usually > 101°F (> 38.3°C) accompanies the onset of symptoms.

4. Complications

    a. Bacterial pneumonia is the most common complication and the most common cause of mortality.

    b. Otitis media is also common.

    c. Laryngotracheitis

    d. Encephalomyelitis (i.e., inflammation of both the brain and spinal cord)

    e. Subacute sclerosing panencephalitis is a rare **late** complication.

5. Diagnosis. The basis of diagnosis is clinical features and confirmation of measles infection by serologic testing.

6. Management

    a. Supportive care is most important.

    b. Vitamin A has been shown to improve outcome.

    c. Immunoglobulin can be used for postexposure prophylaxis in high-risk individuals (e.g., children with HIV and other immunodeficiency states) who are exposed to measles.

D. Rubella

1. Etiology. Rubella, which is also known as German measles or 3-day measles, is caused by an RNA virus in the **togavirus family.**

2. Epidemiology. Like measles, the incidence of rubella has declined during the past 40 years as a result of routine immunization during childhood. Rubella is also **highly infectious.**

3. Clinical features. Unlike measles, rubella is mild and often **asymptomatic.** Incubation period is 14–21 days.

    a. The **prodrome** includes mild upper respiratory symptoms and low-grade fever.

    b. Painful lymphadenopathy, especially of the suboccipital, posterior auricular, and cervical nodes

    c. The **exanthem** follows the adenopathy and is characteristically **nonpruritic, maculopapular, and confluent.** It begins on the face, spreads to the trunk and extremities, and lasts 3–4 days.

    d. The **fever is usually mild** ($< 101°F$ or $< 38.3°C$) and accompanies the other clinical symptoms.

  4. Complications

    a. **Meningoencephalitis**

    b. **Polyarteritis** is seen primarily in teenage girls and young women and may last several weeks.

    c. **Congenital rubella syndrome (CRS)** is the **most serious complication of an otherwise relatively benign disease.**

      (1) **CRS occurs after primary maternal infection during the first trimester. Fetal anomalies occur in 30–50% of infected fetuses.**

      (2) **Presenting clinical features** include thrombocytopenia, hepatosplenomegaly, jaundice, and purpura ("**blueberry muffin baby**").

      (3) **Structural abnormalities** include **congenital cataracts** and **patent ductus arteriosus.** Other findings include **sensorineural hearing loss** and meningoencephalitis.

      (4) **Late complications** may include mental retardation, hypertension, type 1 diabetes mellitus, and autoimmune thyroid disease.

  5. Diagnosis is by viral culture and by serology.

  6. Management is supportive.

 E. Hepatitis (see Chapter 10, section XI.E)

 F. Varicella (see Chapter 19, section V.C.6)

XIV. Specific Fungal Infections

 A. Aspergillosis. *Aspergillus* species are ubiquitous molds that cause **both invasive disease and noninvasive allergic disease.**

  1. Invasive disease occurs in severely immunocompromised patients, such as recipients of bone marrow or solid organ transplant. Management includes high-dose systemic antifungal therapy with amphotericin B and often surgery to resect the aspergilloma, a tumorlike mass formed by the fungus. Prognosis is poor.

  2. Allergic bronchopulmonary aspergillosis is characterized by **wheezing, eosinophilia, and pulmonary infiltrates.** It occurs most commonly in patients with chronic lung disease (e.g., cystic fibrosis). Patients have elevated aspergillus-specific immunoglobulin E levels, and management includes corticosteroids and, in some cases, antifungal therapy.

 B. Candidiasis

  1. Epidemiology and etiology. *Candida* species, especially *C. albicans*, are present on the skin and throughout the gastrointestinal tract.

    a. In immunocompetent individuals, overgrowth of yeast may occur normally or under the influence of systemic antibiotics, causing mild superficial infection.

      b. In immunocompromised individuals, overgrowth of yeast may occur readily, causing severe invasive infection.

   2. Clinical features and management

      a. Overgrowth of *Candida* on the skin or mucous membranes may lead to diaper dermatitis, **oral thrush,** or vulvovaginal candidiasis. Treatment includes topical antifungal therapy.

      b. Invasive candidal infections in immunocompromised patients may include fungemia, meningitis (see Table 7-3 for CSF profile), osteomyelitis, and endophthalmitis. Treatment includes systemic antifungal therapy.

C. Coccidioidomycosis

   1. Etiology. *C. immitis* is a fungus found in the soil in the southwestern United States and Mexico.

   2. Clinical features

      a. Infection occurs when *Coccidioides* is inhaled into the lungs.

      b. Most infections are **asymptomatic** or cause a **mild pneumonia.**

      c. African Americans, Filipinos, pregnant women, neonates, and immunocompromised individuals are at highest risk for **disseminated disease,** which may include severe pneumonia, meningitis, and osteomyelitis.

   3. Management. Mild pulmonary disease in immunocompetent patients generally does not require treatment. Disseminated disease and illness in immunocompromised hosts are treated with systemic antifungal therapy.

D. Cryptococcal infection

   1. Etiology. *Cryptococcus neoformans* is a yeast found in the soil.

   2. Clinical features

      a. Infection is acquired when *Cryptococcus* is inhaled into the lungs.

      b. Most infections are asymptomatic.

      c. Spread to the central nervous system (CNS) occurs primarily in immunocompromised patients. Cryptococcal meningitis is one of the AIDS-defining illnesses.

      d. Disseminated infection, including infection of the bones, joints, and skin, may also occur in immunocompromised hosts but is rare in children.

   3. Management. Treatment of disseminated and CNS cryptococcal infection includes systemic antifungal therapy.

XV. Specific Parasitic Infections

A. Amebiasis

   1. Etiology. Infection is by the protozoan ***Entamoeba histolytica.*** Infection is acquired by **ingestion of the cyst in contaminated food or water.** Symptoms begin 1–4 weeks later as the trophozoite form emerges from the cyst and invades the colonic mucosa.

   2. Epidemiology. Amebiasis is present worldwide with the highest incidence in developing nations.

3. **Clinical features**
   a. **Most patients are asymptomatic.**
   b. **Symptomatic intestinal disease** ranges from **mild colitis to severe dysentery.** Young children, pregnant women, and immunocompromised patients have more severe disease.
      (1) **Symptoms** include **cramping abdominal pain, tenesmus, and diarrhea** that may contain blood or mucus. Weight loss, fever, tender hepatomegaly, chest pain, right shoulder pain, respiratory distress, and jaundice may also occur.
      (2) **Abdominal complications** include intestinal perforation, hemorrhage, strictures, and a local inflammatory mass or **ameboma.**
   c. **Extraintestinal amebiasis** manifests as an **abscess,** most commonly in the liver, although it may form in the brain, lung, or other organs.

4. **Diagnosis.** Identification of the trophozoites or cysts in the stool is diagnostic. Colonoscopy with biopsy or **serum antibody assays** may also be helpful. Ultrasound or CT scan can identify an abscess in the liver or other organs.

5. **Management.** Treatment is based on the site of involvement and includes elimination of both the invading organism and those within the intestinal lumen. **Metronidazole** is the **mainstay of therapy** and is recommended along with a luminal amebicide, such as iodoquinol.

B. **Giardiasis**

1. **Etiology.** Infection is by the protozoan *G. lamblia.* Infection occurs by fecal-oral contamination when the cyst is accidentally ingested.

2. **Epidemiology.** Giardiasis occurs worldwide. Travelers to Russia and individuals who **drink contaminated mountain water in the western United States are at higher risk.** Giardiasis may occur as endemic disease or as large waterborne or **day care center** outbreaks. It may also be transmitted by person-to-person spread or from animals, such as dogs and cats.

3. **Clinical features.** Signs and symptoms are variable and range from asymptomatic disease to explosive diarrhea. Symptoms occur 1–2 weeks after ingestion of the cyst and may persist for 2–6 weeks.
   a. Infection **localizes within the small bowel,** causing **diarrhea** that is typically described as **voluminous, watery, and foul-smelling.**
   b. Abdominal pain, cramping, **bloating, flatulence, weight loss,** and low-grade fever may also occur.

4. **Diagnosis. Direct examination** of stool for **cysts and trophozoites** or by **stool ELISA tests** are used to make the diagnosis. Small bowel biopsy is sometimes indicated in difficult-to-diagnose cases.

5. **Management.** Treatment includes **metronidazole** or furazolidone.

C. **Malaria**

1. **Etiology.** Malaria is an obligate intracellular bloodborne parasitic infection caused by four species of ***Plasmodium**: P. falciparum* (responsible for the most severe disease), *P. vivax, P. malariae,* and *P. ovale.*

2. **Epidemiology**

    a. **Malaria is the most important parasitic cause of morbidity and mortality in the world,** responsible for 2–3 million deaths each year, mostly in young children.

    b. Malaria is endemic in tropical and subtropical regions of the world. The **risk of malaria** is high for travelers to these endemic areas.

    c. **Transmission** of *Plasmodium* occurs via the bite of the infected female ***Anopheles* mosquito,** a night-biting mosquito.

3. **Clinical features**

    a. **Initial findings** include vague flulike symptoms that typically include headache, malaise, anorexia, and fever.

    b. **Cyclical fevers** follow the flulike prodrome and occur every 48–72 hours; they **correlate with RBC rupture and subsequent parasitemia.** Chills, vomiting, headache, and abdominal pain may also occur.

    c. **Other features** include **hemolytic anemia,** splenomegaly, jaundice, and hypoglycemia. Cerebral malaria, renal failure, shock, and respiratory failure all may occur.

4. **Diagnosis.** Identification of the parasite on **thin and thick Giemsa-stained peripheral blood smears** is diagnostic. The thick smear is for malarial screening, and the thin smear is for malarial identification and staging (determination of the level of parasitemia) of the particular *Plasmodium* species.

5. **Management.** Choice of antimalarial therapy is based on resistance patterns, species type, and severity of illness. Medications include chloroquine, quinine, quinidine gluconate, mefloquine, and doxycycline.

6. **Prevention**

    a. **Avoidance of mosquito bites is the mainstay of prevention.** DEET (*N,N*-diethyl-*m*-toluamide)-containing repellants, insecticide-impregnated bed nets, and protective clothing are essential.

    b. **Chemoprophylaxis,** which may include oral chloroquine, mefloquine, doxycycline, or atovaquone and proguanil hydrochloride (dependent on the area visited and its *Plasmodium* species and resistance patterns).

    c. **Control of the *Anopheles* mosquito** is important for individuals living in endemic areas.

D. **Toxoplasmosis**

1. **Etiology.** Infection is by the intracellular parasite ***T. gondii.***

2. **Epidemiology. Transmission** occurs through **direct contact with cat feces** (the cat is the definitive host for the parasite), ingestion of undercooked meat, fruits, or vegetables contaminated with cysts, transplacental passage, exposure to contaminated blood products, or organ transplantation.

3. **Clinical features**

    a. **Most patients are asymptomatic.**

    b. **Symptoms,** if present, include a **mononucleosis-like illness** consisting of malaise, fever, sore throat, myalgias, and lymphadenopathy. Rash and hepatosplenomegaly may be present. Symptoms are self-limited and generally benign.

    c. **Reactivation of disease may occur** if patients become **immuno-suppressed.** In this situation, the symptoms are often more severe and may include encephalitis, focal brain lesions, pneumonitis, or, rarely, disseminated disease. Toxoplasmosis is an important opportunistic infection in HIV-infected patients, and patients **commonly present with focal seizures.**

    d. **Ocular toxoplasmosis** may occur. *T. gondii* **is the most common cause of infectious chorioretinitis.**

    e. **Congenital toxoplasmosis** is characterized by the **triad of hydrocephalus, intracranial calcifications, and chorioretinitis.**

  4. Diagnosis. Serologic testing, PCR, or identification of the organism in cultures of amniotic fluid, CSF, or blood are used for diagnosis.

  5. Management. Most infections do not require specific therapy. Treatment is indicated for infants with congenital toxoplasmosis, pregnant women with acute toxoplasmosis, and immunocompromised individuals with reactivation resulting in toxoplasma encephalitis. Treatment includes sulfadiazine and pyrimethamine.

  6. Prevention. Pregnant women and immunocompromised individuals are at highest risk. Therefore, they should avoid cat feces and undercooked meats and should clean all fruits and vegetables before consumption. Gloves should be used when gardening or preparing meat.

XVI. Specific Helminth Infections

  A. General Concepts (characteristics of specific infections are noted in Table 7-7)

    1. Groups at highest risk include immigrants, travelers, and homeless individuals.

    2. Common clinical features

      a. **Most infections are asymptomatic.**

      b. **Abdominal symptoms** include pain, anorexia, nausea, rectal prolapse, and obstruction.

    3. Diagnosis is usually made by **three separate stool examinations for ova and parasites.** To detect **pinworms,** a **cellulose tape test** may be performed; the tape is placed sticky side down on the perianal region before sleep and is removed immediately on awakening and examined for eggs.

  B. Cysticercosis

    1. Epidemiology

      a. **Worldwide distribution** with high incidence in **Mexico** and Central America

      b. In endemic areas, **20–50% of cases of epilepsy are caused by cysticercosis.**

Table 7-7. Characteristics of Specific Helminth Infections

Infection	Epidemiology	Clinical Features	Management
Enterobius vermicularis (pinworm)	**Most common helminthic infection in the U.S.** Fecal-oral transmission of eggs Preschool and school-age children	**Anal or, less commonly, vulvar pruritus** Insomnia, anorexia, enuresis, nighttime teeth-grinding	Single dose of mebendazole, albendazole, or pyrantel pamoate Treat all close contacts
Ascaris lumbricoides (roundworms)	Largest and most common intestinal roundworm Fecal-oral transmission of eggs	Löffler syndrome— transient pneumonitis as larvae migrate through lungs causing fever, cough, wheezing, and eosinophilia Small bowel obstruction	Mebendazole, albendazole, or pyrantel pamoate Screen all close contacts
Trichuris trichiura (whipworm)	Worldwide distribution Often seen in association with *Ascaris* infection	Most are asymptomatic Abdominal pain, tenesmus, bloody diarrhea, rectal prolapse	Mebendazole, albendazole, or pyrantel pamoate Screen all close contacts
Necator americanus and *Ancylostoma duodenale* (hookworm)	Rural, tropical, and subtropical areas where soil is contaminated with human feces Percutaneous infection through a bare foot; larvae migrate to lungs and are coughed up and then swallowed	**Rash and pruritus at site of penetration** **Iron-deficiency anemia** with fatigue, pallor, and failure to thrive	Mebendazole, albendazole, or pyrantel pamoate Screen close contacts Iron supplementation
Strongyloides stercoralis	Tropics, subtropics, and southern and southwestern U.S. Life cycle same as hookworm	**Transient pruritic papules** at site of penetration **Pneumonitis** **Gastrointestinal symptoms** **Eosinophilia**	Ivermectin, thiabendazole, or albendazole
Cutaneous larva migrans	Intradermal migration of dog or cat hookworms Contact with feces-contaminated soil	**Migrating, pruritic, serpiginous, erythematous tracks on skin** Self-limited, lasting weeks to months	Resolves without treatment in most cases Ivermectin, thiabendazole, or albendazole for severe disease
Toxocara canis or *cati* (**toxocariasis** or **visceral larva migrans— VLM**)	Most common in children 1–4 years who have pica Ingestion of eggs in contaminated soil or dog fur Larvae released from eggs and migrate through tissues	**Generalized VLM:** fever, eosinophilia, leukocytosis, hepatomegaly; may have malaise, anemia, cough, myocarditis **Ocular larva migrans:** retinal granulomas or endophthalmitis	Albendazole or mebendazole Steroids may also be used for ocular involvement

2. **Etiology.** Infection occurs via the **fecal-oral route** when the eggs of *Taenia solium*, the pork tapeworm, are accidentally ingested.

3. **Clinical features**
   a. No symptoms are present until the tapeworm **encysts in muscle, subcutaneous tissue, or brain.**
   b. **Subcutaneous nodules** may be palpated or seen as calcifications on radiography.
   c. **Neurocysticercosis**
      (1) The **fourth ventricle** is the **most common site of involvement,** although brain parenchyma, meninges, spine, or eyes may be affected.
      (2) **Signs and symptoms** include **seizures (presenting symptom in 70% of cases),** hydrocephalus, and stroke.

4. **Diagnosis**
   a. **Ova and parasite stool evaluation** detects the *Taenia* eggs in only 25% of cases.
   b. Serology is available in some laboratories.
   c. **Head CT or MRI scans** may show a solitary parenchymal cyst or single or multiple calcifications. Calcified lesions represent areas of old, nonviable parasitic infection.

5. **Management.** Antiparasitic medications are reserved for individuals infected with the adult tapeworm. Those with neurocysticercosis with brain imaging that shows only calcified lesions require only anticonvulsant therapy.

XVII. Miscellaneous Infections

A. **Rickettsial Infections**

1. **Lyme disease** (see Chapter 16, section VII)

2. **Rocky mountain spotted fever (RMSF)**
   a. **Etiology.** RMSF is caused by *Rickettsia rickettsii,* a Gram-negative intracellular coccobacillus that is transmitted by the bite of a tick.
   b. **Epidemiology**
      (1) RMSF is endemic across the United States but occurs primarily in the **southeastern regions of the United States.**
      (2) Incidence is highest in school-age children, and infection usually occurs in the spring and summer.
      (3) Fewer than 50% of patients recall a tick bite.
   c. **Clinical features.** Symptoms and signs range from mild to life-threatening and may include:
      (1) **Fever**
      (2) **Petechial rash** that **begins on the extremities** (ankles and feet) and moves in a caudal and centripetal direction (i.e., wrists and hands and then to trunk and head)
      (3) **Myalgias**

        (4) Hepatosplenomegaly and jaundice

        (5) CNS symptoms, such as **headache,** coma, and seizures

        (6) Hypotension

    d. Laboratory findings. Thrombocytopenia, elevated transaminases, and **hyponatremia** may occur. CSF findings may show an aseptic meningitis picture (see Table 7-3).

    e. Diagnosis. The diagnosis is made clinically but should be confirmed with serologic tests for *Rickettsia.*

    f. Management. Treatment includes oral or intravenous doxycycline and supportive care. Antibiotics are usually started empirically on the basis of clinical presentation before the results of diagnostic testing, given the possibility of significant morbidity and mortality in untreated infection.

    g. Prevention. Methods include tick avoidance and prompt tick removal. Prophylactic antibiotics after tick bites are not indicated.

  3. Ehrlichiosis (human monocytic ehrlichiosis and human granulocytic ehrlichiosis)

    a. Etiology. Ehrlichiosis is caused by ***Ehrlichia chaffeensis,*** which is transmitted by the bites of several tick species.

    b. Epidemiology. Most cases occur in the spring and summer in the same regions as RMSF.

    c. Clinical features. Ehrlichiosis is often referred to as **"spotless RMSF"** because it has many of the same symptoms as RMSF but usually no rash. Symptoms include fever, headache, myalgias, and lymphadenopathy.

    d. Laboratory findings. These are similar to those seen in RMSF (see section XVII.A.2.d).

    e. Diagnosis. The diagnosis is confirmed by serology and PCR technology in some laboratories.

    f. Management. Treatment includes doxycycline and supportive care.

B. Cat Scratch Disease

  1. Etiology. Cat scratch disease is caused by the Gram-negative bacteria ***Bartonella henselae.***

  2. Clinical features

    a. Regional lymphadenopathy (especially in the axillary, cervical, or inguinal region), distal to and **after a cat or kitten scratch,** is the **most common presentation.**

    b. The initial scratch results in a papule along the line of the scratch, followed by lymphadenopathy 1–2 weeks later.

    c. The involved lymph node is commonly erythematous, warm, and tender. Suppuration occurs in approximately 10%.

    d. Fever may occur in one third of patients.

    e. Less common findings include **Parinaud oculoglandular syndrome** (conjunctivitis and preauricular lymphadenitis), encephalitis, osteomyelitis, hepatitis, pneumonia, and hepatic or splenic lesions.

  3. Diagnosis. Serology that demonstrates elevated serum IgM antibody to *B. henselae* is diagnostic.

4. **Management.** Treatment usually consists of **supportive care.** Antibiotics are generally reserved for patients with systemic disease or immunodeficiency. Antibiotics used include oral azithromycin, TMP/SMX, and ciprofloxacin. Surgery is not indicated and may result in persistent fistulous tracks.

C. **Tuberculosis (TB)**

1. **Etiology.** The cause of TB is *Mycobacterium tuberculosis.*

2. **Categories**

   a. **Exposure** is the term used to describe an individual who has been in **recent contact** with an individual with **contagious pulmonary TB.** Physical examination, tuberculin skin test, and chest radiograph are all normal.

   b. **Latent tuberculosis infection (LTBI)** is the term used to describe an asymptomatic individual with a positive tuberculin skin test, normal physical examination, and a chest radiograph that either is negative or shows only pulmonary granulomas or calcifications with or without regional lymph nodes.

   c. **Tuberculosis disease** is the term used to describe an individual with **signs and symptoms of TB** with or without positive findings on chest radiograph (see section XVII.C.5). Disease may be pulmonary or extrapulmonary.

3. **Epidemiology**

   a. TB is most common among urban, low-income, and minority groups, although it may be seen in children of any socioeconomic status.

   b. Those at **highest risk** include **immigrants** from highly endemic regions of the world, health care personnel, **homeless** individuals, residents of institutions or **correctional facilities,** and individuals with **immunodeficiency conditions** (e.g., HIV, chronic disease, immunosuppressive medications).

   c. **Transmission** of TB occurs by inhalation of small airborne droplets from an individual with contagious pulmonary TB. **Children younger than 12 years of age are generally not contagious** because their cough is minimal and their pulmonary lesions are usually small.

4. **Clinical features**

   a. **In LTBI, most children with a positive tuberculin skin test are asymptomatic and do not progress to TB disease. Infants younger than 12 months of age are at greatest risk of developing disease.**

   b. **Symptoms of TB disease** include **fever, chills, weight loss, cough, and night sweats.**

   c. **Extrapulmonary TB disease** may include:

      (1) **Cervical lymphadenitis (scrofula), the most common form of extrapulmonary TB disease in children**

      (2) **Meningitis** (for CSF findings, see Table 7-3)

      (3) Abdominal involvement (ileitis)

      (4) Skin and joint involvement

    (5) Skeletal disease, which may involve the vertebrae (**Pott's disease**)

    (6) Disseminated or miliary disease

5. Radiographic features of TB disease

    a. Hilar or mediastinal lymphadenopathy

    b. Ghon complex—small parenchymal infiltrate with enlarged hilar lymph nodes

    c. Lobar involvement, pleural effusion, or cavitary disease, which typically affects the upper lung segments.

6. Diagnosis. Diagnosis and categorization of TB infection is based on an individual's risk factor for infection, tuberculin skin test findings, chest radiographic findings, and culture.

    a. Tuberculin skin test or Mantoux skin test contains 5 tuberculin units of purified protein derivative **(PPD).**

        (1) It is administered intradermally and read 48–72 hours later by health care personnel trained in interpretation.

        (2) The tuberculin skin test becomes positive **2–12 weeks after exposure.**

        (3) A positive tuberculin skin test is identified by measuring the area of **induration** (not erythema) and is interpreted on the basis of clinical and individual risk factors:

            (a) ≥ 5 mm is considered positive in children who have had close contact with an individual with TB disease, who have clinical or chest radiographic findings consistent with TB disease, or who are immunocompromised.

            (b) ≥ 10 mm is considered positive if children are younger than 4 years of age, have a chronic medical condition, or live in an area endemic for TB.

            (c) ≥ 15 mm is considered positive in children older than 4 years of age who do not have other risk factors.

    b. Definitive diagnosis involves the following:

        (1) Positive culture for *M. tuberculosis* from early morning **gastric aspirates** obtained by a nasogastric tube (gastric aspirate samples are preferred for diagnosis in children because children are generally unable to cough up sputum for culture but instead swallow the sputum into the stomach), pleural fluid, CSF, or other body fluids.

        (2) Positive staining of fluid for acid-fast bacilli (AFB)

        (3) Positive histology (caseating granulomas) from a biopsy specimen

7. Management. Treatment is based on the TB category.

    a. Patients with **LTBI** are treated with **isoniazid** (INH) for 9 months. Older adolescents, pregnant adolescents, and adults are also given daily pyridoxine (vitamin B_6) to prevent neurologic complications of INH therapy.

    b. Patients with TB disease are treated on the basis of the location of TB disease and the susceptibility pattern of the organism. Treatment generally includes 2 months of INH, rifampin, and pyrazinamide, followed by 4 months of INH and rifampin.

Review Test

1. A 13-day-old male infant presents with a fever (temperature to 100.6°F [38.1°C]), mild irritability, and diminished appetite. His parents report no change in the number of wet diapers. Which of the following statements regarding this patient's management or prognosis is correct?

(A) Careful observation at home is appropriate because of the relatively low fever and normal urine output.
(B) The risk of bacteremia in this patient is approximately 25%.
(C) Intramuscular ceftriaxone and close home monitoring are appropriate after evaluation with a complete blood count, blood culture, urinalysis, and urine culture.
(D) Irrespective of the results of initial laboratory testing, management should include intravenous antibiotics and hospitalization.
(E) Bacteria likely to cause fever in this patient include *Streptococcus pneumoniae* and *Haemophilus influenzae* type b.

2. A 7-month-old female infant presents with a fever (temperature to 103.5°F [39.7°C]) for the past 2 days. She was previously healthy. Her parents report no symptoms other than the fever. On examination, she is well hydrated and appears nontoxic, and no focus of infection is identified. Which of the following is the next appropriate management step?

(A) Complete blood count (CBC) and blood culture; if the white blood count (WBC) is normal, home observation is indicated.
(B) Urine culture, urinalysis, CBC, and blood culture; if the WBC is $\geq$ 15,000 cells/mm^3, empiric intramuscular ceftriaxone should be administered.
(C) No laboratory studies are indicated because the patient appears nontoxic.
(D) Hospitalization and empiric intravenous cefotaxime
(E) CBC, blood culture, urinalysis, urine culture, lumbar puncture, and chest radiograph; intramuscular ceftriaxone should be given because of the high risk of bacteremia.

3. A 2-year-old girl presents with fever. On examination, she has exudative pharyngitis, enlarged posterior cervical lymph nodes, and splenomegaly. Which of the following statements regarding her evaluation and management is correct?

(A) Amoxicillin should be prescribed after throat culture for suspected "strep throat."
(B) Monospot testing is highly sensitive and is the best test to make a diagnosis in this case.
(C) Human immunodeficiency virus is the most likely cause of this infection.
(D) Amoxicillin may result in a pruritic rash in this patient.
(E) Supportive care will lead to rapid improvement and resumption of full activity.

4. A 6-year-old girl is sent home from summer camp with a fever of 101.3°F (38.5°C), stiff neck, photophobia, and headache. Lumbar puncture in the emergency department reveals the following results: white blood count 380 cells/mm^3, with 65% polymorphonuclear cells and 35% lymphocytes; normal protein and glucose; and negative Gram stain. Which of the following pathogens is the most likely cause of her meningitis?

(A) *Neisseria meningitidis*
(B) *Streptococcus pneumoniae*
(C) Enterovirus
(D) *Borrelia burgdorferi*
(E) *Mycobacterium tuberculosis*

5. A previously healthy 18-month-old girl is admitted to the hospital with fever (temperature to 102.8°F [39.3°C]), vomiting, and lethargy. She was well until 2 days ago, when she was diagnosed with a viral upper respiratory infection. Lumbar puncture to evaluate the cerebrospinal fluid shows the following results: white blood cells 3,050 cells/mm³, with 98% polymorphonuclear cells; very low glucose; and elevated protein. Gram stain shows Gram-positive diplococci. Initial management should include which of the following?

(A) Vancomycin and third-generation cephalosporin
(B) Third-generation cephalosporin alone
(C) Ampicillin and third-generation cephalosporin
(D) Third-generation cephalosporin and acyclovir
(E) Third-generation cephalosporin and corticosteroids

6. A 25-year-old woman is pregnant with her first child. The woman has human immunodeficiency virus (HIV) infection that was diagnosed 2 years before this pregnancy. Which of the following has been shown to increase her risk of transmitting HIV to her infant?

(A) Treatment with highly active antiretroviral therapy during pregnancy and before delivery
(B) Exclusive bottle formula feeding
(C) Prolonged rupture of membranes
(D) Birth by cesarean section
(E) Orally administered zidovudine given to the infant after birth

7. An 8-year-old girl presents with sore throat, fever, and a rough sandpaper-like rash over her trunk and extremities. A throat culture is positive for group A β-hemolytic streptococcus. Treatment of her infection with antibiotics will prevent which of the following complications?

(A) Reactive arthritis
(B) Rheumatic fever
(C) Post-streptococcal glomerulonephritis
(D) Guillain-Barré syndrome

8. A 1-year-old girl presents with weight loss and a 2-week history of large, bulky, nonbloody, foul-smelling stools. She has been attending day care and recently received amoxicillin for an ear infection. Which of the following is the most likely cause of her diarrhea?

(A) *Entamoeba histolytica*
(B) Enterotoxigenic *Escherichia coli*
(C) *Clostridium difficile*
(D) *Giardia lamblia*
(E) Norwalk virus

9. A 19-year-old boy, a college sophomore, presents with high fever, headache, cough, conjunctivitis, and a diffuse macular rash over his trunk and face. He is unsure of his immunization status. You suspect measles infection. Which of the following is correct regarding this diagnosis?

(A) Vitamin A may improve his outcome.
(B) Koplik spots would likely be present on examination of his mouth.
(C) Mortality is most commonly caused by measles encephalitis.
(D) Diagnosis is based on culture and direct fluorescent antigen testing.
(E) Corticosteroids will decrease symptoms and improve outcome.

The response options for statements 10–14 are the same. You will be required to select one answer for each statement in the set.

(A) Malaria *Plasmodium* species
(B) *Toxoplasma gondii*
(C) *Giardia lamblia*
(D) *Entamoeba histolytica*
(E) *Coccidioides immitis*
(F) *Cryptococcus neoformans*
(G) *Aspergillus fumigatus*
(H) *Candida albicans*

For each clinical description, select the most likely cause.

10. At birth, a term infant is noted to have hydrocephalus and intracranial calcifications on computed tomography of the head. Eye examination reveals bilateral chorioretinitis.

11. A 5-year-old boy is admitted with a fever of unknown origin. An abdominal computed tomographic scan reveals a large hepatic abscess.

12. A 12-year-old girl with cystic fibrosis has an exacerbation of her disease and presents with wheezing, pulmonary infiltrates, and eosinophilia.

13. A 16-year-old boy is admitted to the hospital for a workup of cyclical fevers after a trip to India. His illness began with flulike symptoms.

14. An 18-month-old girl and three of her day care classmates present with 2 weeks of watery diarrhea and some weight loss.

15. A 2-year-old boy has a positive tuberculin skin test that measures 12 mm. It was placed during a routine well child care visit. He is well, without fever, chills, cough, weight loss, or night sweats. No known tuberculosis contacts are identified. Which of the following statements regarding this patient's management is correct?

(A) A chest radiograph should be ordered because the tuberculin skin test is positive.
(B) He should be placed into respiratory isolation immediately because he is likely to spread tuberculosis to others.
(C) Isoniazid is not indicated because this tuberculin skin test is negative.
(D) Triple-drug therapy for tuberculosis should be started immediately.
(E) Gastric aspirates should be ordered.

The response options for statements 16–20 are the same. You will be required to select one answer for each statement in the set.

(A) *Salmonella* species
(B) *Shigella sonnei*
(C) *Yersinia enterocolitica*
(D) *Clostridium difficile*
(E) *Campylobacter jejuni*
(F) *Vibrio cholerae*
(G) Enterotoxigenic *Escherichia coli*
(H) *E. coli* 0157:H7
(I) Enteropathogenic *E. coli*

Match the clinical description with the likely causative organism.

16. While visiting Monterey, Mexico, a 16-year-old boy develops watery, nonbloody diarrhea, without fever.

17. A 3-year-old boy presents with an acute onset of high fevers, bloody diarrhea, and a generalized tonic-clonic seizure. The stool Wright stain reveals sheets of white blood cells.

18. An 8-year-old girl presents with a 1-week history of diarrhea and low-grade fever. The family reports that they have recently acquired a pet turtle.

19. A 10-year-old boy is admitted to the hospital and taken directly to the operating room for suspected acute appendicitis. Surgeons discover a normal appendix but enlarged mesenteric lymph nodes.

20. A group of travelers to Bangladesh suddenly develop massive, watery, nonbloody diarrhea that results in severe dehydration and electrolyte imbalance.

The response options for statements 21–24 are the same. You will be required to select one answer for each statement in the set.

(A) Buccal cellulitis
(B) Impetigo
(C) Necrotizing fasciitis
(D) Erysipelas
(E) Staphylococcal scalded skin syndrome
(F) Toxic shock syndrome

Match the clinical description with the likely diagnosis.

21. A 9-month-old girl with mild facial eczema has fever and a facial skin rash. The skin lesion is weepy with a honey-colored crust.

22. An unvaccinated 4-month-old boy has a facial skin rash and a positive blood culture for *Haemophilus influenzae* type b.

23. An infant boy has fever, an erythematous skin rash, and a positive Nikolsky sign.

24. A 7-year-old girl develops fever and a rapidly expanding tender skin rash with a well-demarcated border.

Answers and Explanations

1. The answer is D [II.C.5 and Table 7-1]. Fever in an infant younger than 28 days of age must be taken very seriously because the neonate's immune system is immature. As a result, the current appropriate management for any neonate with fever (temperature >100.4°F [>38°C]) includes a complete workup for serious bacterial infection that includes evaluation of blood, urine, and cerebrospinal fluid for evidence of bacterial infection; administration of empiric intravenous antibiotics; and hospitalization. The risk of serious bacterial infection in a nontoxic infant younger than 3 months of age is approximately 3–10%. Usual bacteria resulting in infection in this age group include group B streptococcus, *Escherichia coli,* and *Listeria monocytogenes*.

2. The answer is B [II.D.3 and Table 7-1]. Because of the patient's elevated fever, evaluation for bacteremia and urinary tract infection, including urine culture, urinalysis, complete blood count, and blood culture, is indicated. After these laboratory studies, intramuscular ceftriaxone may be given either empirically or only if the white blood count is ≥ 15,000 cells/mm^3. Hospitalization is generally not required unless the patient is toxic in appearance, dehydrated, or has poor ability to return to the physician for follow-up. Neither evaluation of spinal fluid nor a chest radiograph is indicated in this nontoxic patient without respiratory signs or symptoms. Neither intravenous antibiotics nor hospitalization is indicated because the infant is nontoxic and well hydrated.

3. The answer is D [XIII.B]. This patient's clinical presentation with fever, lymphadenopathy, pharyngitis, and splenomegaly is most consistent with infectious mononucleosis. If a child with infectious mononucleosis is mistakenly given amoxicillin, a diffuse pruritic rash may develop. Monospot testing is highly sensitive in older children, but heterophile antibodies do not reliably form in children younger than 4 years of age. Antibody titers are therefore the preferred diagnostic test in such young children. The most common cause of infectious mononucleosis is Epstein-Barr virus. Although supportive care for infectious mononucleosis is appropriate, symptoms of infection may last weeks, and contact sports restriction is advised because of the risk of splenic rupture. Splenomegaly is not consistent with the diagnosis of streptococcal pharyngitis.

4. The answer is C [IV.C.3 and Tables 7-3, 7-4]. This cerebrospinal fluid (CSF) evaluation is most consistent with aseptic meningitis, specifically viral meningitis. Enteroviruses are the most common cause of viral meningitis and most often occur during the summer and fall. Early in viral meningitis, the white blood count (WBC) in the CSF may demonstrate a polymorphonuclear cell predominance that shifts to a lymphocyte predominance within 24–48 hours. The normal protein and glucose and negative Gram stain are also consistent with viral meningitis. Meningitis caused by *Neisseria meningitidis* or *Streptococcus pneumoniae* would be reflected by a higher CSF WBC, lower glucose, and higher protein. Although patients with Lyme meningitis, which is caused by *Borrelia burgdorferi,* may present with an aseptic CSF profile, the onset is not as acute as in this patient. Patients with *Mycobacterium tuberculosis* present with a low to very low glucose and elevated protein level in the CSF.

5. The answer is A [IV.B.5]. Empiric therapy of presumed bacterial meningitis should include a third-generation cephalosporin and the addition of vancomycin until sensitivities are available, because of the high level of pneumococcal antibiotic resistance in many communities. Ampicillin is not indicated; this child is out of the age range at which *Listeria* infection occurs. Acyclovir is not indicated; the cerebrospinal fluid profile is most consistent with bacterial meningitis. Corticosteroids are effective in reducing the incidence of hearing loss in *Haemophilus influenzae* type b meningitis but have not been shown to be effective for other bacterial pathogens.

6. The answer is C [XIII.A.2]. Factors that increase the risk of HIV transmission from mother to infant include high maternal viral load (measured by RNA copy number) at delivery, concomitant chorioamnionitis or other genital tract infections, primary or advanced maternal HIV infection, premature birth, and prolonged rupture of membranes. Transmission may also occur through breast milk. Transmission is decreased through the use of maternal antiretroviral therapy, newborn prophylaxis with antiretroviral agents (e.g., zidovudine), birth by cesarean section, and low maternal viral load.

7. The answer is B [IX.A.5.f]. This patient's clinical presentation of a sandpaper-like rash associated with pharyngitis and fever is consistent with scarlet fever, caused by erythrogenic toxin-producing strains of group A β–hemolytic streptococcus (GABHS). Although there are multiple complications of GABHS infection, including rheumatic fever, glomerulonephritis, reactive arthritis, and pediatric autoimmune neuropsychiatric disorders associated with streptococcal infection (PANDAS), only PANDAS and rheumatic fever will be prevented by treatment with antibiotics.

8. The answer is D [Tables 7-6, 7-7, XV.B.3]. Infection with the protozoan *Giardia lamblia* is associated with bulky, foul-smelling stools, weight loss, and day care attendance. *Entamoeba histolytica* and *Clostridium difficile* generally cause bloody diarrhea. *Escherichia coli* infection generally results in short-term watery diarrhea. Day care attendance is also associated with Norwalk virus; however, symptoms of Norwalk virus infection generally last only 48–72 hours.

9. The answer is A [XIII.C.3, XIII.C.4, XIII.C.5]. This patient's presentation is most consistent with measles infection. Management includes supportive care, and vitamin A therapy may also be beneficial. Koplik spots are transient, and by the time the rash is present, Koplik spots are no longer appreciated. Bacterial pneumonia is the most common complication of measles infection and is the most common cause of mortality. Diagnosis is based on confirmation by serologic testing in the presence of typical clinical features. Corticosteroids do not play a role in the therapy of measles.

10–14. The answers are B, D, G, A, and C, respectively [XV.D.3, XV.A.3, XIV.A.2, XV.C.3, and XV.B.3]. The triad of intracranial calcification, hydrocephalus, and chorioretinitis is consistent with congenital toxoplasmosis, which is caused by *Toxoplasma gondii*. *Entamoeba histolytica* may result in asymptomatic infection or colitis. The most common extraintestinal complication is a liver abscess. *Aspergillus* infection may result in invasive disease or in noninvasive allergic disease characterized by wheezing, eosinophilia, and pulmonary infiltrates. Malaria classically presents with a flulike illness followed by the development of high fevers that cycle in 48- to 72-hour paroxysms. *Giardia lamblia* typically presents with bulky, large-volume, watery stools that eventually lead to weight loss.

15. The answer is A [XVII.C]. A tuberculin skin test is considered positive depending on a patient's specific risk factor(s) for acquisition of tuberculosis. A tuberculin skin test ≥ 10 mm is considered positive if the patient is younger than 4 years of age or if the patient resides or has lived in an area endemic for tuberculosis. Therefore, given that the tuberculin skin test is positive, a chest radiograph to evaluate for pulmonary tuberculosis is indicated. Children younger than 12 years of age with tuberculosis are unlikely to be contagious because of minimal cough and pulmonary involvement. Medications for tuberculosis disease (e.g., triple-drug regimen) are indicated if the patient has signs and symptoms of tuberculosis. Gastric aspirates are indicated only if the chest radiograph reveals pulmonary disease.

16–20. The answers are G, B, A, C, and F, respectively [Table 7-6]. Enterotoxigenic *Escherichia coli* is the major cause of traveler's diarrhea and results in nonbloody watery stools. Bloody stools may result from infection with *Salmonella, Shigella, Yersinia, Campylobacter,* enterohemorrhagic *E. coli,* and *Clostridium difficile. Shigella* may be associated with seizures caused by the release of a neurotoxin. *Salmonella* may be acquired by ingestion of contaminated poultry or by exposure to turtles and lizards that carry the organism. *Yersinia* may result in mesenteric adenitis that causes pain mimicking acute appendicitis. Infection with *Vibrio cholerae* generally occurs in developing countries and causes massive fluid loss from the gut.

21–24. The answers are B, A, E, and D, respectively [IX.A]. Buccal cellulitis is characterized by a bluish color to the cheeks of a young child; this condition is typically caused by infection with *Haemophilus influenzae* type b, which is identified on blood culture. Impetigo typically presents with honey-crusted lesions on the face; it is caused by infection with *Staphylococcus aureus* and group A β-hemolytic streptococcus. Staphylococcal scalded skin syndrome is manifested by Nikolsky sign, or the extension of bullae with lateral pressure applied to the skin. Fever, tender skin, and widespread bullae are present. Erysipelas is characterized by tender, erythematous skin, but the border is well demarcated.

8

Cardiology

David Ferry, M.D., and David Chun, M.D.

I. Congestive Heart Failure (CHF)

A. **Definition.** CHF is a clinical syndrome defined as **inadequate oxygen delivery** by the myocardium to meet the metabolic demands of the body.

B. **Pathophysiology.** Signs and symptoms of CHF often result from compensatory mechanisms that lead to increased demand on an already compromised myocardium.

1. **Hypoperfusion of end organs** stimulates the heart to maximize contractility and heart rate in an attempt to increase cardiac output.

2. **Hypoperfusion** also signals the kidneys to **retain salt and water** through the renin-angiotensin system in an attempt to increase blood volume.

3. **Catecholamines** released by the sympathetic nervous system also increase heart rate and myocardial contractility.

C. **Etiology.** CHF may result from congenital heart disease, acquired heart disease, and a variety of miscellaneous disorders.

1. **Congenital heart disease (CHD)** may result in CHF.
   a. **Increased pulmonary blood flow** may cause CHF. Examples of congenital lesions that cause increased pulmonary blood flow include a large ventricular septal defect (VSD), a large patent ductus arteriosus (PDA), transposition of the great arteries (TGA), truncus arteriosus, and total anomalous pulmonary venous connection (TAPVC).
   b. **Obstructive lesions** may also cause CHF. Examples include severe aortic, pulmonary, and mitral valve stenosis, coarctation of the aorta, interrupted aortic arch, and hypoplastic left heart syndrome.
   c. **Other causes** include arteriovenous malformations and mitral or tricuspid regurgitation, which overload portions of the heart.

2. **Acquired heart disease** may also lead to CHF.
   a. **Viral myocarditis is a common cause of CHF** in older children and adolescents.
   b. Other cardiac infections (e.g., endocarditis, pericarditis), metabolic

diseases (e.g., hyperthyroidism), medications (e.g., doxorubicin, a chemotherapeutic agent), cardiomyopathies, and ischemic diseases

   c. Dysrhythmias, including tachycardia and bradycardia

  3. **Miscellaneous** causes of CHF include:

   a. **Severe anemia,** which may cause **high-output CHF**

   b. Rapid infusion of intravenous fluids, especially in premature infants

   c. Obstructive processes of the airway, such as enlarged tonsils or adenoids, laryngomalacia, and cystic fibrosis, which may cause CHF as a result of chronic hypoxemia that results in right-sided heart failure

D. Clinical Features

  1. **Tachypnea, cough, wheezing, and rales** on examination and **pulmonary edema** on chest radiograph (CXR) are evidence of pulmonary congestion.

  2. **Tachycardia, sweating, pale or ashen skin color, diminished urine output, and enlarged cardiac silhouette** on CXR are evidence of impaired myocardial performance.

  3. **Hepatomegaly and peripheral edema** are evidence of systemic venous congestion.

  4. Other signs and symptoms include **failure to thrive, poor feeding (common symptom in newborns), and exercise intolerance (common symptom in older children and adolescents).**

  5. **Cyanosis and shock** are **late manifestations.**

E. Management

  1. **Goals of medical management** are to improve myocardial function and relieve pulmonary and systemic congestion.

   a. **Cardiac glycosides** (e.g., digoxin) increase the efficiency of myocardial contractions and relieve tachycardia.

   b. **Loop diuretics** (e.g., furosemide, ethacrynic acid) reduce intravascular volume by maximizing sodium loss, which in turn leads to diminished ventricular dilation and improved function.

   c. **Inotropic medications** administered intravenously (e.g., dobutamine, dopamine) may be used to treat severe CHF.

   d. Other medications, such as amrinone and milrinone (phosphodiesterase inhibitors) improve contractility and reduce afterload.

  2. **Interventional catheterization** procedures may address some of the underlying causes of CHF (e.g., **balloon valvuloplasty** for critical aortic and pulmonary valve stenosis).

  3. **Surgical repair** is often the definitive treatment of CHF secondary to CHD.

II. Innocent Cardiac Murmurs

  A. Definition. Innocent murmurs result from turbulent blood flow, are **not caused by structural heart disease,** and have no hemodynamic significance.

B. **Epidemiology.** Approximately **50%** of children have an innocent heart murmur at some point during childhood.

C. **Clinical Features.** The most common innocent heart murmurs are presented in **Table 8-1.**

III. Acyanotic Congenital Heart Disease

A. Normal cardiac anatomy is depicted in Figure 8-1.

B. **Clinical and Diagnostic Features.** Physical examination, CXR, and electrocardiographic (ECG) findings of acyanotic CHD are presented in **Table 8-2. Echocardiography confirms the specific anatomic lesions.**

C. **Atrial Septal Defect (ASD)** (Figure 8-2)

1. **Classification**

   a. **Ostium primum.** This type of ASD is a defect in the lower portion of the atrial septum. A cleft, or division, in the anterior mitral valve leaflet may also be present and may cause mitral regurgitation. Ostium primum ASD is a common congenital heart lesion in **Down syndrome.**

   b. **Ostium secundum.** This type of ASD is a defect in the middle portion of the atrial septum. Ostium secundum is the **most common type** of ASD.

   c. **Sinus venosus.** This type of ASD is a defect high in the septum near the junction of the right atrium and superior vena cava (SVC). In sinus venosus, the right pulmonary veins usually drain anomalously into the right atrium or SVC instead of into the left atrium.

2. **Pathophysiology.** Blood flows across the septal defect **from the left atrium to the right atrium** (i.e., **left-to-right shunt**). The direction of the blood flow is determined by the compliance of the right and left ven-

Table 8-1. Clinical Features of Innocent Heart Murmurs

Murmur	Age	Location	Characteristics
Still's murmur	Ages 2–7 years	Mid-left sternal border	Grade 1–3, systolic Vibratory, twanging, or buzzing Loudest supine Louder with exercise
Pulmonic systolic murmur (systolic ejection murmur)	Any age	Upper left sternal border	Grade 1–2, peaks early in systole Blowing, high-pitched Loudest supine Louder with exercise
Venous hum	Any age, but especially school age	Neck and below the clavicles	Continuous murmur Heard only sitting or standing Disappears if supine; changes with compression of the jugular vein or with neck flexion or extension

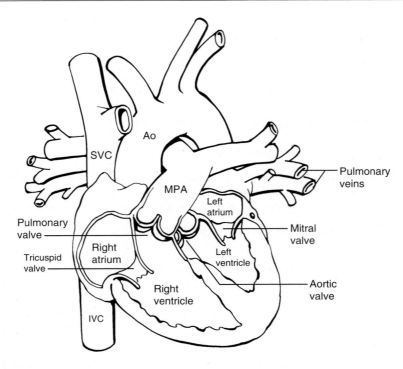

Figure 8-1. Anatomy of the normal heart. *Ao* = aorta; *MPA* = main pulmonary artery; *SVC* = superior vena cava; *IVC* = inferior vena cava.

tricles (compliance is determined by systemic and pulmonary vascular resistances). **Blood therefore flows from areas of higher resistance to areas of lower resistance.** Increased blood flow across the ASD leads to an increase in size of the right atrium and right ventricle, and to increased pulmonary blood flow.

3. **Clinical features**

   a. **Symptoms are minimal,** if any, except in patients with an ostium primum defect who develop mitral regurgitation that results in CHF.

   b. **Physical examination** findings include:

      (1) **Increased right ventricular impulse** as a result of right ventricular overload

      (2) **Systolic ejection murmur** (from excessive pulmonary blood flow) best heard at the **mid and upper left sternal borders.** A mid-diastolic filling rumble representing excessive blood flow through the tricuspid valve may also be heard.

      (3) **Fixed-split second heart sound.** Because of the excessive pulmonary blood flow, the normal physiologic variation in timing of aortic and pulmonic valve closure with respiration is absent.

4. **Management.** Treatment is **closure by open heart surgery** to prevent right-sided heart failure, pulmonary hypertension, atrial dysrhythmias, and paradoxic embolism. Some centers close ASDs using interventional catheterization procedures.

Table 8-2. Key Differentiating Clinical Features of Acyanotic Congenital Heart Disease

Heart Lesion	Physical Examination Findings	ECG	Chest X-Ray
Atrial septal defect	Systolic ejection murmur mid-left sternal border and ULSB Fixed split S$_2$ Diastolic rumble LLSB	RAD, RVH, and RAE	Right atrial and ventricular enlargement Increased PVM
Ventricular septal defect	High-pitched **holosystolic** murmur at LLSB, with or without a thrill Diastolic rumble at apex if pulmonary blood flow is high	If small: normal, or mild LVH If moderate: LVH RVH if pulmonary hypertension present	If small, normal If moderate or large, cardiomegaly and increased PVM If elevated PVR, decreased PVM
Patent ductus arteriosus	Continuous murmur at ULSB; machinery-like Brisk pulses	LVH RVH if pulmonary hypertension present	Cardiomegaly with increased PVM
Coarctation of the aorta (older child)	Elevated BP in right arm Reduced BP in legs Dampened and delayed femoral pulse Bruit left upper back	Normal or LVH	Normal heart size Rib-notching (evidence of collateral flow)
Aortic stenosis	Ejection click Systolic ejection murmur at base with radiation to URSB, apex, suprasternal notch, and carotids Thrill at URSB and suprasternal notch	Normal or LVH	Normal or mild cardiomegaly Prominent ascending aorta (poststenotic dilatation)
Pulmonary stenosis	Ejection click Systolic ejection murmur at ULSB	RVH	Normal Prominent main pulmonary artery

ECG = electrocardiogram; *ULSB* = upper left sternal border; *LLSB* = lower left sternal border; *URSB* = upper right sternal border; *S$_2$* = second heart sound; *LVH* = left ventricular hypertrophy; *RVH* = right ventricular hypertrophy; *BP* = blood pressure; *RAD* = right axis deviation; *PVM* = pulmonary vascular markings; *PVR* = pulmonary vascular resistance.

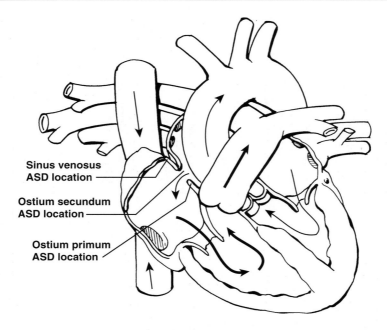

Figure 8-2. Location of atrial septal defects (ASD). Arrows designate the direction of blood flow. Thick arrows designate increased blood flow. The right atrium and the right ventricle are enlarged. The location of the sinus venosus ASD is the posterior-superior aspect of the atrial septum.

D. Ventricular Septal Defect (VSD)

1. **Classification.** VSDs are classified by location as **inlet, trabecular (muscular), membranous,** and **outlet (supracristal)** (Figure 8-3).

2. **Pathophysiology.** After birth, as pulmonary vascular pressure decreases, blood flows across the VSD from the left ventricle to the right ventricle owing to the lower resistance within the pulmonary circulation compared with the resistance within the systemic circulation. However, with time, the pulmonary vessels hypertrophy in response to this increased pulmonary flow. This hypertrophy may lead to increased pulmonary vascular resistance (pulmonary hypertension).

3. **Clinical features and course** vary greatly depending on the magnitude of the left-to-right shunt across the VSD. **The amount of blood flow directed from one side of the heart to the other side (i.e., the shunt) is determined by both the size of the VSD and the degree of pulmonary vascular resistance (PVR).** For example, the larger the VSD and the lower the PVR, the greater the blood flow across the VSD and into the pulmonary vessels. The greater the pulmonary blood flow, the more symptomatic the patient. Typical clinical presentations include:

    a. **Small VSDs** have little to no shunt across the VSD and **may close spontaneously.** On examination, a thrill at the lower left sternal border and a grade 4 high-pitched **holosystolic** murmur may be present, indicative of a very restrictive defect with a high flow velocity across the VSD. Key pearl: **As the size of the VSD decreases, the intensity of the murmur increases.**

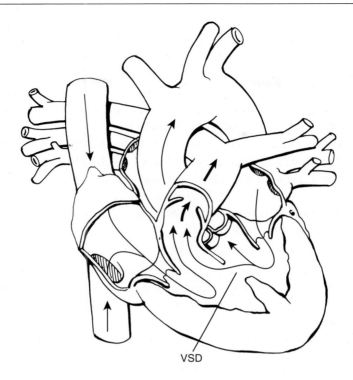

Figure 8-3. Trabecular (muscular) ventricular septal defect (VSD). Arrows designate the direction of blood flow. Thick arrows designate increased blood flow.

    b. Moderate VSDs may have a large shunt across the VSD that may result in signs and symptoms of CHF. A holosystolic murmur is usually present, and its intensity depends on the size of the shunt. If excessive blood flows across the VSD (2:1 pulmonary-to-systemic flow; twice as much blood flows to the lungs as to the systemic circulation), then a diastolic murmur of mitral turbulence (mitral filling rumble representing the excess blood from the lungs now passing through the mitral valve) may be heard at the apex.

    c. Large VSDs often cause signs and symptoms of CHF. They have less turbulence across the VSD, so the systolic murmur is shorter and lower in pitch. A mitral filling rumble may be heard at the apex.

    d. PVR may eventually become elevated in moderate or large VSDs in response to chronically high pulmonary flow. When this occurs, clinical features change.

        (1) When PVR becomes elevated, the right ventricular impulse is noticeably increased and the second heart sound may be single and loud. The mitral filling rumble disappears because of diminished pulmonary blood flow as a result of decreased left-to-right shunting. Symptoms of CHF also diminish as PVR increases because of the decrease in pulmonary blood flow.

        (2) If PVR remains elevated, pulmonary hypertension becomes irreversible, even if the VSD is surgically closed. In the extreme situation in which PVR exceeds systemic vascular resistance (SVR), shunting changes from left-to-right to right-to-left (a condition termed **Eisenmenger syndrome**).

4. **Management**

    a. **Medical management** of CHF is indicated in a symptomatic child. Large shunts are also associated with a high incidence of pulmonary infections from excessive blood flow.

    b. **Surgical closure** is indicated in the following circumstances:

        (1) **Heart failure refractory to medical management**

        (2) **Large VSDs with pulmonary hypertension** are usually surgically closed at 3–6 months of age.

        (3) **Small to moderate VSDs** are usually surgically closed between 2 and 6 years of age.

E. Patent Ductus Arteriosus (PDA)

1. **Definition.** In the fetus, the ductus arteriosus connects the pulmonary artery to the aorta. After birth, as the PaO_2 rises, the ductus normally fibroses. If it remains open, it is termed a PDA. Incidence of PDA is especially high in preterm infants.

2. **Pathophysiology.** In a PDA, blood flows through the ductus from the aorta to the pulmonary artery (left-to-right shunt), leading to increased pulmonary blood flow (Figure 8-4).

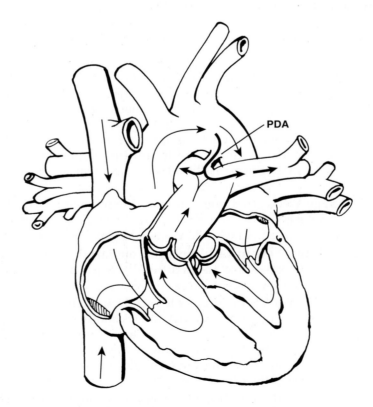

Figure 8-4. Patent ductus arteriosus (PDA). Arrows designate the direction of blood flow. Thick arrows designate increased blood flow.

3. **Clinical features.** Signs and symptoms depend on the size of the PDA and on the relationship between SVR and PVR.

   a. **Small PDAs** usually produce **no symptoms,** but **moderate or large PDAs** generally result in signs and symptoms of **CHF** due to increased pulmonary blood flow.

   b. **Physical examination findings**

      (1) The classic murmur is a **"machinery-like" continuous murmur** at the **upper left sternal border.**

      (2) **If the left-to-right shunt is large,** there may also be a **diastolic rumble** of blood flow across the mitral valve at the apex, a **widened pulse pressure** (> 30 mm Hg) and **brisk pulses.**

   c. **Risk of pulmonary hypertension** caused by excessive pulmonary blood flow is significant in children older than several years of age.

4. **Management**

   a. **Indomethacin** is used in premature infants to close a PDA medically.

   b. **PDAs** may also be closed surgically by coil embolization, video-assisted thoracoscopic surgery, and ligation in a thoracotomy.

F. **Coarctation of the Aorta**

   1. **Definition.** Coarctation of the aorta is narrowing of the aortic arch, just below the origin of the left subclavian artery and typically at, or just proximal to, the ductus arteriosus. It may be a discrete narrowing (hourglass) or a long-segment obstruction.

   2. **Pathophysiology.** The narrowed segment obstructs or diminishes flow from the proximal to the distal aorta (Figure 8-5).

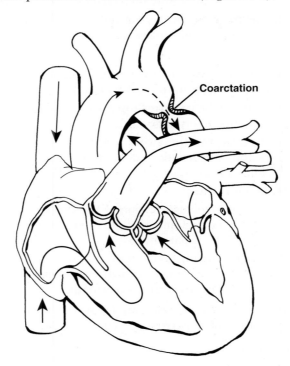

Figure 8-5. Coarctation of the aorta. Arrows designate the direction of blood flow.

3. **Clinical features.** Signs and symptoms depend on the severity of the obstruction and on the presence of any other associated cardiac abnormalities.

a. **Neonates or infants with severe coarctation** may **depend on a right-to-left shunt through the PDA** for perfusion of the lower thoracic and descending aorta. Such infants may be **minimally symptomatic initially,** but **symptoms of CHF develop** and progress as the **PDA closes.**

   (1) Blood pressure may be elevated in the upper extremities and low in the lower extremities before the onset of CHF.

   (2) Once the infant or neonate develops CHF, pulses in all four extremities are poor, any murmur is absent, and hypotension may develop.

b. **Older children or adolescents** may have no symptoms and may have only hypertension or a heart murmur. **Hypertension** is typically noted in the **right arm,** and **blood pressure is reduced in the lower extremities.**

   (1) **Femoral pulse,** which normally precedes the radial pulse, is **dampened and delayed** until after the radial pulse (**radiofemoral delay**).

   (2) **Blood pressure and pulse findings** may be less prominent if collateral vessels (intercostal arteries) develop that allow the ascending aortic pressure and flow to circumvent the coarctation.

   (3) **Bicuspid aortic valve** or aortic stenosis is present in 50% of patients. If either of these conditions is present, a systolic murmur of aortic stenosis may be heard (see section III.G.3).

   (4) **Bruit of turbulence** through the coarctation may be audible at the left upper back near the scapula.

4. **Management**

a. **Initial management** in the **symptomatic neonate** is directed at improving circulation to the lower body.

   (1) **Intravenous prostaglandin E** (PGE) is given urgently to open the ductus arteriosus.

   (2) **Inotropic medications** are given to overcome myocardial depression, and low-dose dopamine is used to maximize renal perfusion and function.

b. **Corrective repair**

   (1) **Surgery** involves excision of the narrowed segment followed by end-to-end anastomosis. Late recurrence of narrowing may occur in up to 50% of patients.

   (2) **Balloon angioplasty** may be successful in coarctations that have not undergone surgical correction and is the **therapy of choice** for **recurrent coarctation.**

5. **Prognosis** is excellent, but long-term concerns include recurrence of coarctation and upper extremity hypertension with exercise.

G. **Aortic Stenosis**

1. **Definition.** Aortic stenosis is narrowing of the aortic valve. Pathologi-

cally, aortic stenosis appears as commissural fusion of the three normal leaflets leading to a bicuspid or unicuspid valve.

2. **Pathophysiology.** Aortic stenosis results in reduced left ventricular output. At the myocardial level, aortic stenosis results in an imbalance between myocardial oxygen demand (which is higher than usual owing to the increased ventricular work as a result of outflow obstruction) and supply. This may lead to myocardial ischemia. In the neonate, severe aortic stenosis may be associated with hypoplasia of the left ventricle as a result of impaired fetal left ventricular development.

3. **Clinical features.** Signs and symptoms depend on the severity of the stenosis and age. **Physical examination** findings are presented in Table 8-2.

   a. **Neonates with severe stenosis ("critical aortic stenosis")** appear normal at birth but develop signs and symptoms of CHF at 12–24 hours of age. Once the PDA closes, all systemic flow must be ejected through the aortic valve. However, in critical aortic stenosis (like coarctation of the aorta), this is not possible and adequate perfusion to the body cannot be maintained.

   b. **Older children** generally have **no symptoms** until the stenosis becomes severe. Once severe, symptoms include **exercise intolerance, chest pain, syncope,** and even **sudden death.**

4. **Management. Indications for intervention** include CHF, symptoms such as chest pain or syncope, and documentation of high resting pressure gradient across the aortic valve (> 50–70 mm Hg).

   a. **Balloon valvuloplasty** is often the initial management approach for aortic stenosis without insufficiency.

   b. **Surgery** is often required for aortic stenosis with insufficiency and **5–10 years after palliative valvuloplasty** because of recurrent stenosis or progressive insufficiency. The aortic valve is replaced with either the patient's own pulmonary valve (**Ross procedure**) or with a prosthetic valve.

H. Pulmonary Stenosis

1. **Definition.** Pulmonary stenosis is narrowing of the pulmonary valve. Pathologically, fusion of the valve commissures is typically seen.

2. **Pathophysiology.** Pulmonary stenosis results in increased right ventricular pressure and reduced right ventricular output.

3. **Clinical features. Physical examination** findings are presented in Table 8-2.

   a. **Severe** pulmonary stenosis **in the neonate** may be manifested by cyanosis as a result of **right-to-left shunting** at the atrial level through a patent foramen ovale.

   b. For most children, outflow obstruction is **mild to moderate** and **symptoms are absent.**

4. **Management.** Treatment is **balloon valvuloplasty** for symptomatic infants with critical pulmonary stenosis and for older children with significant gradients across the pulmonary valve (> 35–40 mm Hg) or high right ventricular pressures.

IV. Cyanotic Congenital Heart Disease

A. General Concepts

1. **Cyanosis** may be peripheral, central, or both. **Peripheral cyanosis** is usually caused by vasomotor instability or vasoconstriction as a result of cold temperature. **Central cyanosis,** especially apparent in the tongue and inner mucous membranes, may be attributable to both cardiac and noncardiac causes:

   a. **Noncardiac causes of central cyanosis** include pulmonary disease, sepsis, hypoglycemia, polycythemia, and neuromuscular diseases that impair chest wall movement.

   b. The **most common cardiac causes of central cyanosis** may be remembered using the **mnemonic "5 Ts":** *t*etralogy of Fallot, *t*ransposition of the great arteries, *t*ricuspid atresia, *t*runcus arteriosus, and *t*otal anomalous pulmonary venous connection.

2. **Evaluation**

   a. Thorough physical examination is essential.

   b. Other studies initially include pulse oximetry (in room air), complete blood count (CBC), arterial blood gas (ABG), ECG, and CXR. The degree of pulmonary blood flow seen on CXR may be useful in diagnosis (**Table 8-3**).

   c. The **100% oxygen challenge test** suggests cyanotic CHD when the PaO2 fails to rise despite administration of 100% oxygen.

   d. **Echocardiogram** provides a definitive diagnosis.

3. **Diagnosis.** The distinguishing features of the five types of cyanotic CHD are presented in **Table 8-4.**

B. Tetralogy of Fallot is the most common cause of central cyanosis presenting beyond the newborn period.

1. **Definition.** Tetralogy of Fallot has four anatomic components:

   a. **VSD**

   b. **Overriding aorta** (aorta overlies a portion of the ventricular septum)

   c. **Pulmonary stenosis**

   d. **Right ventricular hypertrophy**

2. **Pathophysiology.** As a result of right ventricular outflow tract obstruction (RVOT; pulmonary stenosis), blood flows right to left across the VSD

Table 8-3. Cyanotic Congenital Heart Disease Lesions and Pulmonary Blood Flow on Chest Radiograph

Increased Pulmonary Flow	Decreased Pulmonary Flow
Transposition of the great arteries	Tetralogy of Fallot
Total anomalous pulmonary venous connection	Pulmonary atresia
Truncus arteriosus	Tricuspid atresia
Single ventricle	

Table 8-4. Key Differentiating Features of Cyanotic Congenital Heart Disease

Heart Lesion	Physical Examination Findings	ECG	Chest X-Ray
Tetralogy of Fallot	Systolic ejection murmur of pulmonary stenosis (Table 8-2)	RVH	Upturned cardiac apex (**"boot shaped"**) Decreased PVM Right aortic arch (commonly)
Transposition of the great arteries	No murmur Single S_2	Normal or RVH	Small heart with narrow mediastinum (**"egg-on-a-string"** appearance) Increased PVM
Tricuspid atresia	No murmur and single S_2 if no VSD If VSD is present, systolic murmur of VSD (Table 8-2)	LAD, RAE, and LVH	Small heart Decreased PVM
Truncus arteriosus	Single S_2 Systolic ejection murmur along left sternal border Diastolic murmur at apex	CVH	Enlarged heart Increased PVM Right aortic arch (commonly)
Total anomalous pulmonary venous connection	Pulmonary ejection murmur along left sternal border	RVH and RAE	Enlarged heart in older, unrepaired children with supracardiac drainage ("snowman appearance") Increased PVM If obstruction is present, small heart and pulmonary edema

RVH = right ventricular hypertrophy; *LAD* = left axis deviation; *RAE* = right atrial enlargement; *CVH* = combined ventricular hypertrophy; *PVM* = pulmonary vascular markings; *LVH* = left ventricular hypertrophy; *VSD* = ventricular septal defect; S_2 = second heart sound.

and into the overriding aorta (Figure 8-6). As a result of diminished pulmonary blood flow, cyanosis results.

3. **Clinical features.** Signs and symptoms depend on the severity of the RVOT obstruction.

  a. **Physical examination** findings include an **increased right ventricular impulse** because of right ventricular hypertrophy (RVH), a **systolic ejection murmur representing pulmonary stenosis** (see Table 8-2), and **cyanosis.**

  b. **Cyanosis** depends on the interplay between the resistance to flow out of the RVOT and the SVR. **It is important to remember that blood always flows from higher resistance to lower resistance.**

   (1) **Actions** that **decrease SVR** (e.g., exercise, vasodilation, volume depletion) or **increase resistance through the RVOT** (e.g., crying, tachycardia) **increase right-to-left shunting** from the right ventricle through the VSD and to the aorta, resulting in cyanosis.

   (2) **Actions** that **increase SVR** or **reduce resistance through the RVOT** (e.g., volume infusion, systemic hypertension, Valsalva maneuver, bradycardia) **reduce the right-to-left shunt** through the VSD and therefore increase systemic arterial saturation.

   (3) Neonates with severe pulmonary stenosis or atresia present with **cyanosis** immediately after birth **once the PDA closes;** such patients are dependent on the PDA for blood flow to the lungs.

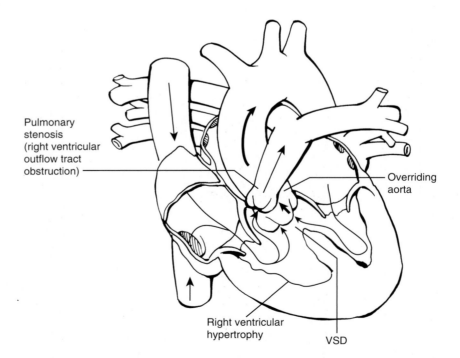

Pulmonary stenosis (right ventricular outflow tract obstruction)

Overriding aorta

Right ventricular hypertrophy

VSD

Figure 8-6. Tetralogy of Fallot. Arrows designate direction of blood flow. Thick arrows designate increased blood flow. *VSD* = ventricular septal defect.

   c. Tetralogy of Fallot (hypercyanotic or "tet") spells are characterized by **sudden cyanosis** and **decreased murmur intensity.**

     (1) The **trigger** may be any maneuver that decreases arterial oxygen
saturation.

     (2) With desaturation, the child typically becomes irritable and cries,
which increases resistance through the RVOT, worsening the
cyanosis by increasing the right-to-left shunt, resulting in a cycle
of increasing cyanosis.

     (3) **Alterations in consciousness and hyperpnea** may occur as a
result of severe hypoxia and acidosis.

     (4) **To compensate,** a child with tetralogy of Fallot learns to **squat.**
This position (knee-chest position in an infant) increases venous
return to the heart and increases SVR, thereby decreasing the
right-to-left shunt.

  4. Management (Table 8-5 describes management of "tet" spell)

   a. Definitive management is complete surgical repair at 4–8
months of age.

   b. Some infants with poor anatomy (small pulmonary arteries) or with
recurrent tetralogy of Fallot spells may initially undergo a palliative
procedure to improve systemic saturation and encourage pulmonary
growth. The procedure involves either a modified **Blalock-Taussig
shunt** (Gore-Tex graft interposed between the subclavian and ipsilateral pulmonary artery) or balloon pulmonary valvuloplasty.

C. Transposition of the Great Arteries (TGA)

  1. Definition. TGA occurs when the aorta arises from the right ventricle
and the main pulmonary artery from the left ventricle.

  2. Pathophysiology (Figure 8-7)

   a. Pulmonary and systemic circulations are **in parallel,** rather than in
series.

   b. Adequate saturation can only be achieved by **shunting blood
from one circulation to the other** through a patent foramen ovale
(PFO), ASD, VSD, or PDA.

  3. Clinical features

   a. Cyanosis is present **at, or shortly after, birth.** Cyanosis is more intense if the PFO is small. Cyanosis is less intense if the PFO is large,
or if there are additional sites of mixing, such as an ASD or VSD.

Table 8-5. Acute Management of a Tetralogy of Fallot ("Tet" or Hypercyanotic) Spell

Placement in knee-chest position (mimics squatting position)
Intravenous fluid bolus
Oxygen
Sedation (morphine) to decrease agitation, which will then slow heart rate
β-Adrenergic blocker (e.g., propranolol) to slow heart rate, reduce contractility in right
   ventricular outflow tract, and augment pulmonary blood flow
Intravenous sodium bicarbonate to correct any acidosis from prolonged hypoxia
Correction of significant anemia with transfusion
Rarely, general anesthesia and surgery

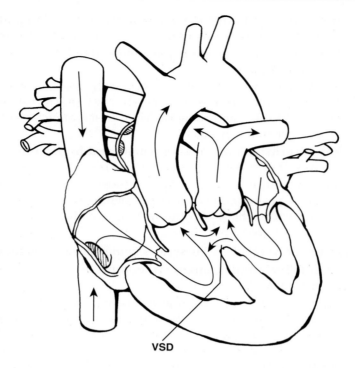

VSD

Figure 8-7. Transposition of the great arteries. A ventricular septal defect (VSD) is present. Arrows designate the direction of blood flow.

       b. Physical examination findings include an infant who appears healthy but who has **central cyanosis,** a quiet precordium, and on auscultation, a **single S_2** (because the aortic valve is anterior and the pulmonary valve is posterior in TGA, the closure of the pulmonary valve is difficult to hear) and **no murmur.**

    4. Management

       a. Neonates may require **initial management** with **PGE** to improve oxygen saturation by keeping the ductus patent, or **emergent balloon atrial septostomy** (Rashkind procedure), an often life-saving procedure that increases the size of an ASD or PFO.

       b. Definitive repair is the **arterial switch operation,** in which the great arteries are incised above their respective valves and implanted in the opposite root. The coronary arteries are attached to the original aorta, so the coronaries must also be incised and reimplanted.

D. Tricuspid Atresia

    1. Definition. Tricuspid atresia is defined anatomically as a plate of tissue located in the floor of the right atrium in the location of the tricuspid valve. An **ASD or PFO is always present.**

    2. Pathophysiology. Whether or not a VSD is also present determines the direction of blood flow, the presence of other anatomic features, and the degree of cyanosis.

a. If no VSD is present and the **ventricular septum is intact, pulmonary atresia is also present.** For blood to flow to the lungs in this situation, a PDA must be present. As the PDA constricts after birth, visible cyanosis develops.

b. If a **VSD is present,** blood flow from the left ventricle through the VSD and into the pulmonary artery (left-to-right shunt) may be adequate, facilitating acceptable systemic oxygen saturations (Figure 8-8).

3. **Clinical features. Signs** also depend on anatomy.

   a. Patients with an **intact ventricular septum and pulmonary atresia** have **no murmur** and a **single S_2.**

   b. Patients with a **VSD** have a VSD murmur (see Table 8-2).

   c. **ECG** shows right atrial enlargement, **left axis deviation (LAD), and left ventricular hypertrophy (LVH). Tricuspid atresia is the only cause of cyanosis in the newborn period that results in LAD and LVH.**

4. **Management.** Treatment includes staged surgery with eventual **Fontan** procedure at 3–6 years of age.

   a. In the **Fontan procedure,** flow from the inferior vena cava is directed into the pulmonary arteries, usually by means of an extracardiac conduit or intra-atrial baffle or tunnel.

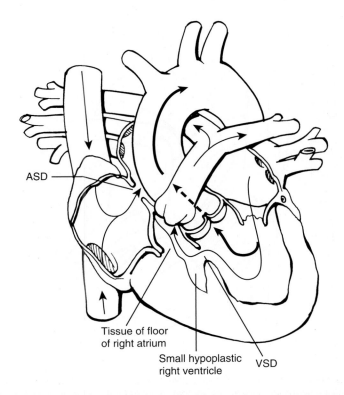

Figure 8-8. Tricuspid atresia with atrial septal defect (ASD) and ventricular septal defect (VSD). Arrows designate direction of blood flow. Thick arrows designate increased blood flow.

      b. Before the Fontan, a bidirectional **Glenn shunt** (superior vena cava is anastomosed to the right pulmonary artery) is usually placed.

      c. The **net result of these procedures is systemic venous return directed to the pulmonary artery.**

E. Truncus Arteriosus

  1. Definition. Truncus arteriosus occurs when the aorta and pulmonary artery originate from a common artery, the **truncus.** The pulmonary arteries usually originate from the proximal truncus, and the truncal valve may be regurgitant or stenotic. A VSD is almost always present.

  2. Pathophysiology. Because the aorta and pulmonary arteries are connected and the pulmonary arteries are well-formed, excessive blood flows to the lungs and CHF commonly develops. Mixing of desaturated and saturated blood occurs within the truncus, and patients are commonly only mildly desaturated and sometimes cyanotic (Figure 8-9).

  3. Clinical features

    a. Signs and symptoms of CHF are common.

    b. Physical examination findings

      (1) Systolic ejection murmur at the base from increased flow across the truncal valve and a **single S$_2$** caused by the presence of only one atrioventricular valve

      (2) Diastolic murmur of flow across the mitral valve at the apex as

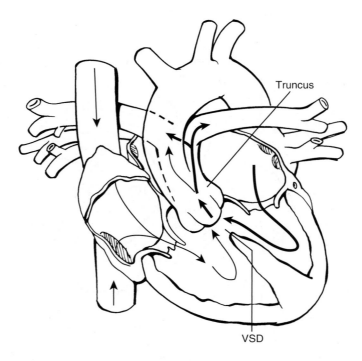

Figure 8-9. Truncus arteriosus with ventricular septal defect (VSD). Arrows designate the direction of blood flow. Thick arrows designate increased blood flow. The dashed line represents the other border of the pulmonary artery at the back of the truncus.

a result of excessive pulmonary blood flow that returns to the left atrium

(3) **High-pitched systolic murmur** at the base indicates insufficiency of the truncal valve.

4. **Management.** Treatment includes medications for CHF and surgical repair early in infancy to close the VSD and to place a homograft between the right ventricle and pulmonary artery.

F. **Total Anomalous Pulmonary Venous Connection (TAPVC)**

1. **Definition.** TAPVC occurs when the pulmonary veins drain into the systemic venous side rather than into the left atrium. Sites of TAPVC include supracardiac (into the right superior vena cava or innominate vein), cardiac (into the right atrium or coronary sinus), and infracardiac (into the portal system).

2. **Pathophysiology. Systemic and pulmonary venous blood enters the right atrium and mixes together.** As a result, this mixture of systemic and pulmonary venous blood is present in all four cardiac chambers (blood also passes across a PFO or ASD into the left heart), pulmonary arteries, and aorta, resulting in desaturated systemic blood and cyanosis visible on examination. Obstruction of pulmonary venous return can occur if the PFO or ASD is small, by compression of the returning vein(s) by an adjacent structure, or by obstruction in the liver once the ductus venosus closes.

3. **Clinical features**
   a. **Cyanosis** is present, and if severe, may indicate obstruction of pulmonary venous return.
   b. **Pulmonary flow murmur** at the mid-left sternal border is caused by increased pulmonary blood flow.

4. **Management.** Treatment is surgical repair shortly after diagnosis; the pulmonary veins are anastomosed to the back of the left atrium, and the PFO or ASD is closed.

V. Acquired Heart Disease

A. **Kawasaki disease** is the **most common cause of acquired heart disease in children in the United States** and is discussed in Chapter 16, section II.

B. **Acute rheumatic fever** is the **most common cause of acquired heart disease worldwide** and is discussed in Chapter 16, section VI.

C. **Infective endocarditis**

1. **Definition.** Infective endocarditis is a microbial infection of the endocardium, or internal surface, of the heart.

2. **Epidemiology**
   a. **Eighty percent of cases** occur in children who have **structural abnormalities of the heart.** Endocarditis may also occur in

anatomically normal hearts, especially in the hearts of neonates and infants.

    b. **Fifty percent of cases** occur soon **after cardiac surgery.**

3. **Etiology**

    a. **Gram-positive cocci,** including α-**hemolytic streptococcus** *(Streptococcus viridans) and* **Staphylococcus** species, are the most common bacterial agents.

    b. **Gram-negative** organisms are **rare causes of endocarditis.**

    c. **Fungal** endocarditis is extremely rare but may occur in a chronically ill child.

4. **Pathophysiology**

    a. **Bacteria are introduced into the blood** spontaneously or during an invasive procedure. Bacteria then infect injured cardiac endothelium.

    b. **Fibrin and platelets adhere** to the site of injury, creating a growth or **vegetation.** The **vegetation** may induce valve incompetency.

    c. **Distal manifestations** of disease may occur, including embolic phenomena and immunologic sequelae (e.g., nephropathy).

5. **Clinical features (Table 8-6)**

6. **Diagnosis.** History and physical examination, in addition to several other studies, are the basis of diagnosis.

    a. **Blood culture** is the **single most important laboratory test.** Three aerobic and anaerobic blood cultures should be drawn to maximize the likelihood of identifying the infecting organism. Because bacteremia is continuous in endocarditis, blood cultures may be drawn even if the patient is afebrile.

    b. The **erythrocyte sedimentation rate (ESR)** is usually **elevated,** unless polycythemia is present. (Patients with cyanotic CHD may have polycythemia.)

Table 8-6. Clinical Features of Bacterial Endocarditis

Symptoms
Fever (most common symptom)
Nonspecific complaints, such as malaise, arthralgia, headache, weight loss, night sweats, and anorexia

Signs
New or changing murmur
Splenomegaly
Microscopic or gross hematuria (as a result of embolism or endocarditis-associated glomerulonephritis)
Splinter hemorrhages (linear hemorrhages beneath the nails)
Retinal hemorrhages
Osler's nodes (small, raised pink, red, or blue swollen tender lesions on the palms, soles, or pads of the toes or fingers)
Janeway lesions (small, erythematous hemorrhagic lesions on the palms or soles)
Roth's spots (round or oval white spots seen in the retina)

    c. **Other acute-phase reactants** (e.g., **rheumatoid factor**) are found in **50% of patients.**

    d. **Transthoracic echocardiography** detects most vegetations. However, a normal transthoracic echocardiogram does not exclude endocarditis. **Transesophageal echocardiography** is **more sensitive** than transthoracic echocardiography at identifying vegetations.

7. Management

    a. **Intravenous antimicrobial therapy** is directed against the identified organism. Treatment for 4–6 weeks is required.

    b. Because endocarditis is rarely a medical emergency, therapy may be safely withheld until an adequate number of blood cultures are obtained.

8. Antibiotic prophylaxis for endocarditis is recommended before invasive procedures in certain patients. Such procedures include dental work likely to produce bleeding, surgery (including tonsillectomy), and invasive gastrointestinal (GI) or urologic procedures. This applies to:

    a. **All patients with structural heart disease, except secundum ASD**

    b. **All postoperative** cardiac surgery patients for up to 6 months after surgical repair

    c. **All postoperative** cardiac surgery patients for an indefinite period if any hemodynamic residua of the initial lesion remain

D. Pericarditis

1. Definition. Pericarditis is inflammation of the pericardial space.

2. Etiology. Causes most commonly include **infection, collagen vascular disease** (e.g., systemic lupus erythematosus [SLE]), **uremia,** and **inflammatory response after cardiac surgery (postpericardiotomy syndrome).**

    a. **Viral infection** is the **most common** cause of pericarditis in children. Viruses include coxsackievirus, echovirus, adenovirus, influenza, parainfluenza, and Epstein-Barr virus (EBV).

    b. **Purulent pericarditis** is usually caused by **bacterial infection,** either primary or disseminated from pneumonia or meningitis.

        (1) *Staphylococcus aureus* and *Streptococcus pneumoniae are the most common agents.*

        (2) Patients with purulent pericarditis have a **high incidence of constrictive pericarditis** owing to the intense inflammatory response.

    c. **Postpericardiotomy syndrome** may occur in as many as one third of patients whose pericardium has been opened during surgery. The cause is unknown but is thought to be an autoimmune response to a concomitant viral infection.

3. Pathophysiology. Inflammation of parietal and visceral pericardial layers leads to exudation or transudation of fluid and impairment of venous return and cardiac filling. **Cardiac tamponade,** or critically impaired left ventricular output, may occur.

4. Clinical features

    a. Symptoms include fever, dyspnea, malaise, and **chest pain most intense while supine and relieved when sitting upright.**

    b. Physical examination findings include a **pericardial friction rub, distant heart sounds** if the effusion is large, **pulsus paradoxus** (> 10 mm Hg reduction in systolic blood pressure on deep inspiration), and **hepatomegaly.**

5. Diagnosis

    a. Pericarditis should be considered in any child with dyspnea and fever, and in any patient who recently underwent cardiac surgery and has hemodynamic instability or nonspecific complaints of dyspnea or malaise.

    b. Pericardiocentesis, in which a needle is inserted into the pericardial sac and fluid is withdrawn, is both diagnostic and therapeutic. Fluid should be sent for cell and serologic analysis and for culture.

    c. ESR, although not specific for pericarditis, is **elevated.**

    d. Imaging studies

        (1) ECG may show ST-segment changes or low-voltage QRS complexes in patients with large pericardial effusions.

        (2) CXR shows an enlarged heart shadow in patients with large effusions.

        (3) Echocardiogram demonstrates the extent and quality of the pericardial effusion.

6. Management

    a. Appropriate antibiotics should be given if bacterial pericarditis is suspected.

    b. Anti-inflammatory agents, such as aspirin or steroids, are indicated for viral pericarditis or postpericardiotomy syndrome.

    c. Drainage of pericardial effusion by placement of a pericardial catheter or surgical window may be indicated.

E. Myocarditis

1. Definition. Myocarditis is inflammation of the myocardium, characterized by cellular infiltrate and myocardial cell death.

2. Epidemiology. Myocarditis is one of several **common causes of sudden death** in young athletes. Overall incidence is unknown, but evidence of myocarditis is apparent in 20% of children who die suddenly.

3. Etiology

    a. Viruses, such as enteroviruses, especially coxsackievirus

    b. Bacteria, such as *Corynebacterium diphtheriae, Streptococcus pyogenes, Staphylococcus aureus,* and *Mycobacterium tuberculosis*

    c. Fungi, such as *Candida* and *Cryptococcus*

    d. Protozoa, such as *Trypanosoma cruzi* (Chagas' disease)

    e. Autoimmune diseases, such as SLE, rheumatic fever, and sarcoidosis

    f. Kawasaki disease

4. **Pathophysiology.** Myocarditis may involve infectious infiltration that damages myocardial cells, or activated lymphocytes that are misdirected to attack the myocardium.

5. **Clinical features**
   a. **Myocarditis frequently follows a viral or flulike illness.**
   b. **Symptoms** include dyspnea and malaise.
   c. **Physical examination** shows **resting tachycardia, muffled heart sounds,** gallop heart rhythm, hepatomegaly, tachypnea, and pulmonary rales.

6. **Diagnosis**
   a. **Laboratory studies. Findings** include **elevated ESR, creatinine kinase (CK) MB fraction,** and **C-reactive protein (CRP)** in most, but not in all, cases. The etiologic organism may be identified by viral serology or polymerase chain reaction (PCR) of **endomyocardial biopsy** specimens.
   b. **Accessory tests**
      (1) **ECG** may show T-wave and ST-segment changes. Atrial or ventricular dysrhythmias may be present.
      (2) **Echocardiogram** shows an anatomically normal heart with **global ventricular dysfunction.** Pericardial effusion and valvular insufficiency may be present.

7. **Management.** Treatment is largely supportive, with use of inotropic agents, diuretics, and afterload-reducing drugs as needed. Intravenous immune globulin may be helpful in some cases. **Cardiac transplantation** is an option for patients with CHF refractory to medical management.

8. **Prognosis.** Outlook is variable. Mortality is 10–20% and is especially high in young infants and in those with ventricular dysrhythmias.

F. **Cardiomyopathy**

1. **Definition.** Cardiomyopathy is defined as an abnormality of cardiac muscle manifested by systolic or diastolic dysfunction. There are three types of cardiomyopathy.

2. **Dilated cardiomyopathy**
   a. **Definition.** This primary myocardial disorder (i.e., not attributable to valvular, coronary artery, pericardial, or CHD) is characterized by ventricular dilation and reduced cardiac function.
   b. **Etiology.** Dilated cardiomyopathy is frequently **idiopathic,** but many causes have been identified.
      (1) **Viral myocarditis** (see section IV.E)
      (2) **Mitochondrial abnormalities**
      (3) **Carnitine deficiency**
      (4) **Nutritional deficiency,** such as selenium and thiamine deficiency

      (5) Hypocalcemia

      (6) Chronic tachydysrhythmias

      (7) Anomalous origin of left coronary artery from the pulmonary artery (ALCAPA), which results in myocardial ischemia and infarction

      (8) Medications (e.g., doxorubicin)

  c. Clinical features. Signs and symptoms of CHF may be present.

  d. Diagnosis. Evaluation should include **viral serologies** and **serum carnitine level.** In addition:

      (1) ECG shows sinus tachycardia, low cardiac voltage, and ST-segment and T-wave changes. With ALCAPA, evidence of infarction is typically noted.

      (2) Echocardiogram shows a dilated left ventricle with poor ventricular function.

  e. Management

      (1) Medical management of CHF

      (2) Treatment of underlying metabolic or nutritional problem

      (3) Surgical repair of ALCAPA (implantation of left coronary artery into aortic sinus)

      (4) Cardiac transplantation if CHF is unresponsive to medical management

3. Hypertrophic cardiomyopathy

  a. Definition. Hypertrophic cardiomyopathy is LVH in the absence of any systemic or cardiac disease known to cause the hypertrophy. The **most typical anatomic finding is asymmetric septal hypertrophy** (also termed *idiopathic hypertrophic subaortic stenosis*).

  b. Etiology. Inheritance is **autosomal dominant** in 60% of cases. Infants of mothers with diabetes mellitus may have transient septal hypertrophy.

  c. Pathophysiology

      (1) Poor left ventricular filling

      (2) Dynamic left ventricular outflow tract (LVOT) obstruction is present and caused by the anterior mitral leaflet being swept into the subaortic region during systole.

      (3) Mismatch between myocardial oxygen demand and supply (owing to hypertrophy) may result in myocardial ischemia.

  d. Clinical features. Hypertrophic cardiomyopathy is **the most common cause of sudden death** in athletes.

      (1) Symptoms may be absent until syncope or sudden death occurs, or may include **chest pain and exercise intolerance.**

      (2) Physical examination shows a classic **harsh, systolic ejection murmur at the apex** that is accentuated with physiologic maneuvers that reduce left ventricular (LV) volume, such as **Valsalva or standing** (by reducing LV volume, these maneuvers worsen the outflow obstruction, increasing the intensity of the murmur).

  e. Diagnosis

(1) **ECG** shows LVH, ST-segment and T-wave changes, LAD, and abnormally deep and wide Q waves in the inferior and lateral leads.

(2) **Echocardiogram** shows the hypertrophy.

f. **Management.** Treatment is generally reserved for patients with symptoms.

(1) β-Adrenergic blockers or **calcium-channel blockers** reduce the LVOT obstruction and improve diastolic compliance.

(2) **Surgical myomectomy** has been recommended for patients with severe obstruction refractory to medical management.

(3) **Antiarrhythmic medications** may be needed (ventricular dysrhythmias are common).

(4) **Dual-chamber pacing** has been shown to reduce septal hypertrophy and LVOT obstruction in some studies.

(5) Participation in competitive athletic sports should be prohibited.

4. **Restrictive cardiomyopathy**

a. **Definition.** Restrictive cardiomyopathy is defined as excessively rigid ventricular walls that impair normal diastolic filling.

b. **Etiology**

(1) **Amyloidosis**

(2) **Inherited infiltrative disorders** (e.g., Fabry disease, Gaucher disease, hemosiderosis, hemochromatosis)

c. **Clinical features**

(1) **Symptoms** include **exercise intolerance** (because of limitation of cardiac output), **weakness,** and **dyspnea.**

(2) **Physical examination** shows edema, hepatomegaly, and ascites. These **findings** are caused by **elevated central venous pressure (CVP).**

d. **Management.** Treatment is related to reducing CVP with diuretics and improving diastolic compliance with β-blockers and calcium-channel blockers.

VI. Dysrhythmias.

The most common dysrhythmias of childhood include supraventricular tachycardia, heart block, and long QT syndrome.

A. **Supraventricular Tachycardia (SVT)**

1. **Definition.** SVT is an abnormally accelerated heart rhythm that originates proximal to the bifurcation of the bundle of His. **SVT is the most common dysrhythmia in childhood.** It is necessary to distinguish SVT from sinus tachycardia, as detailed in **Table 8-7.**

2. **Pathophysiology.** Two types of SVT occur.

a. **Atrioventricular re-entrant tachycardia (AVRT).** Retrograde conduction through an accessory pathway leads to SVT.

b. **Atrioventricular node re-entrant tachycardia (AVNRT).** The conduction abnormality occurs in different pathways within the atrioventricular node itself.

c. When anterograde conduction occurs through a bypass tract between

Table 8-7. Features Differentiating Sinus Tachycardia from Supraventricular Tachycardia

Feature	Sinus Tachycardia	Supraventricular Tachycardia
Rate (beats/min)	< 230 in newborns < 210 in children	Frequently > 250
Heart rate variation	Present	Absent
P waves on ECG	Normal (axis is 0–90°)	Absent or abnormal axis
Predisposing factors	Fever, infection, anemia	None
Response to intervention (e.g., adenosine)	Gradual	Rapid

ECG = electrocardiogram.

the atria and ventricles, **Wolff-Parkinson-White (WPW) syndrome** is present. WPW is associated with **sudden cardiac death.**

3. **Clinical features.** Symptoms include **palpitations, chest pain,** dyspnea, and, sometimes, **altered level of consciousness.** Prolonged SVT may lead to signs and symptoms of **CHF,** especially in the neonate.

4. **Diagnosis.** WPW may be identified on ECG by the presence of a **delta wave** (i.e., slurred upslope of the QRS complex with a short PR interval).

5. **Management**

   a. **Vagal maneuvers**, such as Valsalva, placement of an **ice pack to the face,** unilateral carotid massage, placing the child upside down, and orbital pressure in older children may all convert SVT into a sinus rhythm.

   b. **Intravenous adenosine** is the primary medication used for acute conversion to a sinus rhythm. Other medications used acutely include propranolol, digoxin, procainamide, and amiodarone.

   c. **Synchronized cardioversion** may be used in patients who are hemodynamically unstable.

   d. **Chronic medical management** typically includes digoxin or propanolol, although the use of digoxin in the presence of WPW is controversial.

   e. **Radiofrequency catheter ablation** may be used to destroy the accessory pathway in chronic SVT.

B. **Heart Block or Atrioventricular (AV) Block**

   1. **Definition and classification**

      a. **Definition. Heart block** is delayed or interrupted conduction of sinus or atrial impulses to the ventricles.

      b. **Classification.** Heart block is classified on the basis of ECG findings (e.g., first-, second-, or third-degree) and by the ratio of atrial to ventricular impulses (e.g., 1:1, 3:1, 3:2, and so on).

         (1) **First-degree** AV block is prolongation of the PR interval.

         (2) **Second-degree** AV block

            (a) **Type I,** also known as **Wenckebach,** is progressive prolongation of the PR interval leading to failed AV conduction.

            (b) **Type II** is abrupt failure of AV conduction without progressive prolongation of the PR interval.

(3) **Third-degree** AV block is **complete block,** with no conduction of atrial impulses to the ventricles.

2. **Etiology**

   a. **Congenital third-degree AV block** is associated with children born to mothers with **SLE.**

   b. **Postsurgical AV block** may occur as a result of cardiac surgery, especially after closure of a VSD that lies close to the conduction system.

   c. **Bacterial endocarditis** may be associated with AV block.

3. **Clinical features.** Fatigue, syncope, and, rarely, sudden death may occur.

4. **Management.** Treatment of symptomatic AV block is cardiac pacing (pacemaker).

C. **Long QT Syndrome**

1. **Definition.** Long QT syndrome is prolongation of the QT interval. Prolongation increases the risk of lethal ventricular arrhythmias known as **torsades de pointes.**

2. **Etiology**

   a. In **50%** of cases, inheritance is either **autosomal recessive (Jervell-Lange-Nielsen syndrome, associated with congenital deafness) or autosomal dominant (Romano-Ward syndrome, not associated with deafness).**

   b. Some cases may result from use of **drugs,** which may directly, or in combination, prolong the QT interval (e.g., phenothiazines, tricyclic antidepressants, erythromycin, terfenadine).

   c. The remainder of cases are **idiopathic.**

3. **Clinical features.** Presenting signs and symptoms include **syncope (most common),** seizure, palpitation, or **sudden cardiac arrest.** Exercise and increased emotion are often inciting factors.

4. **Diagnosis.** Diagnosis is made on the basis of **ECG** showing a long QT interval with a corrected QT interval (**QTc**) greater than 0.44 seconds (up to 0.49 seconds may be normal in the first 6 months of life). The QTc interval is calculated by taking the measurement of the QT interval divided by the square root of the previous RR interval.

5. **Management.** Treatment of symptomatic patients includes a β-blocker to reduce symptoms, although the QT interval usually remains prolonged. Treatment of asymptomatic individuals is controversial. Other therapeutic modalities include cardiac pacing, left stellate ganglionectomy, and an automatic implantable cardiac defibrillator (AICD).

VII. **Chest Pain.** Chest pain is a common presenting complaint in children and adolescents. However, this symptom is rarely of cardiac origin. Figure 8-10 schematically presents the differential diagnosis of chest pain.

A. **Cardiac Chest Pain**

1. **Pericarditis** is the most common cause (see section V.D).

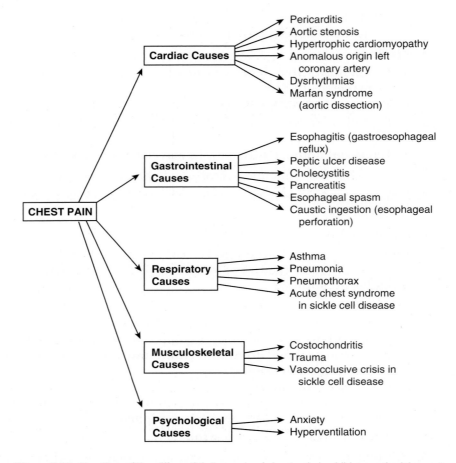

Figure 8-10. Algorithm of the differential diagnosis of chest pain in children and adolescents.

2. Chest pain or chest pressure that occurs with exercise or is associated with syncope, shortness of breath, or abnormal heart rhythm should be further investigated by a cardiologist. Appropriate testing (e.g., continuous ECG monitoring, echocardiography, exercise stress test) is necessary.

B. **Noncardiac Chest Pain.** Causes include asthma, esophagitis, and costochondritis (tenderness in one or more costochondral joints).

Review Test

1. You are called to the newborn nursery to evaluate a 2-hour-old newborn who has suddenly become cyanotic. The oxygen saturation breathing room air is 69%, and the patient is tachycardic and tachypneic. Oxygen is administered without improvement in the patient's oxygen saturation. On examination you hear a loud S_2 and no murmur. A chest radiograph shows increased pulmonary vascular markings, a narrow mediastinum, and a small heart. Which of the following would be the next step in management?

(A) Start digoxin.
(B) Refer the patient to surgery for placement of a Blalock-Taussig shunt.
(C) Refer the patient to surgery for repair of the ventricular septal defect.
(D) Proceed with pulmonary balloon valvuloplasty.
(E) Begin infusion of prostaglandin E (PGE).

2. A 20-month-old boy with tetralogy of Fallot is admitted for evaluation of cyanosis that is increasing in frequency. As you conclude your history and physical examination, you witness an episode of cyanosis when the patient's brother makes him cry. As the crying increases, the patient becomes more and more cyanotic. On examination, his cardiac murmur is now much softer than before he began crying. What is the next most appropriate step in management?

(A) Intubate and begin mechanical ventilation.
(B) Administer intravenous dopamine.
(C) Place the patient in a knee-chest position.
(D) Administer subcutaneous epinephrine.
(E) Call for a cardiology consult.

3. A 10-year-old girl is seen for a routine health maintenance evaluation. Five years ago, she underwent surgical repair of coarctation of the aorta. On examination, the blood pressure in her right arm is 173/81 mm Hg, and her oxygen saturation is 97% in room air. Auscultation reveals a systolic ejection murmur audible throughout the precordium. The patient is otherwise asymptomatic. Which of the following would be the most appropriate next step in management?

(A) Check the blood pressure in all extremities.
(B) Refer the patient to a cardiac surgeon promptly.
(C) Obtain an echocardiogram to rule out a bicuspid aortic valve.
(D) Recheck the oxygen saturation in 100% oxygen.
(E) Have the patient return in 6 months for re-evaluation.

4. A 7-year-old boy presents with a 3-day history of fever (temperature to 103.5°F [39.7°C]), shortness of breath, and weakness. He also complains of chest pain, which is most intense when he lies down and improved when he sits upright. His past medical history is significant for closure of a ventricular septal defect 2 weeks ago. Which of the following findings is consistent with the most likely diagnosis?

(A) Splinter hemorrhages
(B) Pulsus paradoxus
(C) Heart rate of 260 with absent P waves
(D) Prolongation of his QT interval
(E) Tenderness at two of his costochondral joints

5. A 1-month-old female infant is seen in your office for a routine health maintenance evaluation. On examination you hear a grade IV holosystolic murmur at the left sternal border. Femoral pulses and oxygen saturation in room air are normal. The infant is otherwise well and growing normally. Which of the following statements regarding this patient's condition is correct?

(A) Without intervention, congestive heart failure will develop.
(B) Eisenmenger syndrome will eventually occur.
(C) Surgical closure of the patent ductus arteriosus is indicated.
(D) The murmur may disappear without intervention.
(E) Balloon valvuloplasty is indicated.

6. You are called to the nursery to evaluate a male newborn with cyanosis. On auscultation, you hear a single S_2 but no murmur. Pulse oximetry shows an oxygen saturation of 72% in room air. An electrocardiogram reveals left axis deviation and left ventricular hypertrophy. What is his likely diagnosis?

(A) Tetralogy of Fallot
(B) Transposition of the great arteries
(C) Truncus arteriosus
(D) Total anomalous pulmonary venous connection
(E) Tricuspid atresia with intact ventricular septum

7. A 4-year-old boy is in the office for a routine health maintenance evaluation. His examination is normal except for multiple deep dental cavities. You plan on referring him for dental evaluation and possible dental extraction. His mother reminds you that he has a "heart condition." Which of the following cardiac conditions requires antibiotic prophylaxis against endocarditis?

(A) Ventricular septal defect repaired 8 months ago
(B) History of uncomplicated Kawasaki disease
(C) Wolff-Parkinson-White syndrome
(D) Patent ductus arteriosus
(E) Ostium secundum atrial septal defect

8. You see a 7-week-old male infant with cough and poor feeding. Examination reveals a respiratory rate of 72 breaths/min and a heart rate of 170 beats/min. His weight is 7 pounds 6 ounces, just 2 ounces more than his birth weight. You hear diffuse rales throughout the lung fields and a systolic murmur on auscultation. The liver is 4 cm below the right costal margin. Which of the following conditions is the most likely cause of his signs and symptoms?

(A) Large ventricular septal defect
(B) Ostium secundum atrial septal defect
(C) Small patent ductus arteriosus
(D) Critical or severe aortic stenosis
(E) Mild-to-moderate pulmonary stenosis

9. A thin 5-year-old boy presents for a routine health maintenance evaluation. He feels well and is growing normally. On examination, you hear a continuous murmur below the right mid-clavicle. The murmur is loudest while the patient is sitting and disappears while he is supine. The femoral pulses are normal. Which of the following conditions is the most likely diagnosis?

(A) Aortic stenosis with insufficiency
(B) Venous hum
(C) Patent ductus arteriosus
(D) Still's murmur
(E) Pulmonic systolic murmur

10. A 15-year-old boy complaints of chest pain that occurs during basketball practice. He is otherwise healthy and has no prior history of cardiac problems. Examination is normal except for a harsh systolic ejection murmur at the apex that worsens with standing and the Valsalva maneuver. An electrocardiogram demonstrates left ventricular hypertrophy and left axis deviation. Which of the following is the most appropriate initial management at this time regarding the likely diagnosis?

(A) Start propranolol to reduce left ventricular outflow tract obstruction.
(B) Admit for urgent aortic balloon valvuloplasty.
(C) Reassure the patient that the murmur is innocent and allow complete athletic participation.
(D) Admit for surgical myomectomy for septal hypertrophy.
(E) Begin albuterol, as the patient's chest pain is likely caused by asthma.

The response options for statements 11–13 are the same. You will be required to select one answer for each statement in the set.

(A) Sinus tachycardia
(B) Supraventricular tachycardia
(C) Third-degree atrioventricular (AV) heart block
(D) Wolff-Parkinson-White syndrome
(E) Second-degree AV heart block, Wenckebach type
(F) Prolonged QT syndrome
(G) First-degree AV heart block

For each patient, select the most likely associated heart rhythm abnormality.

11. A female newborn is born to a mother with systemic lupus erythematosus.

12. A 10-year-old girl has congenital deafness.

13. A 5-year-old boy has an electrocardiogram that demonstrates a slurred upslope of the QRS complex.

The response options for statements 14–17 are the same. You will be required to select one answer for each statement in the set.

(A) Tetralogy of Fallot
(B) Truncus arteriosus
(C) Transposition of the great arteries
(D) Total anomalous pulmonary venous connection with supracardiac drainage
(E) Tricuspid atresia with ventricular septal defect

For each clinical description, select the cyanotic congenital heart disease lesion.

14. A male newborn has cyanosis and no heart murmur on auscultation.

15. When a 4-year-old boy with cyanosis squats, his cyanosis improves.

16. A male newborn with cyanosis has an electrocardiogram that demonstrates left ventricular hypertrophy.

17. An 8-year-old boy has a chest radiograph that shows cardiomegaly with a "snowman" appearance.

Answers and Explanations

1. The answer is E [IV.C.4]. This patient's clinical presentation and physical examination are most consistent with transposition of the great arteries (TGA). Because the pulmonary and systemic circulations are in parallel, rather than in series, blood must be shunted from one circulation to the other for survival, either by a patent ductus arteriosus or a patent foramen ovale. Intravenous prostaglandin E (PGE) helps keep the ductus patent, which improves oxygen saturation. This patient's presentation is not consistent with a ventricular septal defect. Neither digoxin, pulmonary balloon valvuloplasty, nor a Blalock-Taussig shunt is indicated in the management of a patient with TGA.

2. The answer is C [IV.B.3.c and Table 8-5]. Tetralogy of Fallot (hypercyanotic or "tet") spells are defined as paroxysmal episodes of hyperpnea, irritability, and prolonged crying that result in increasing cyanosis and decreasing intensity of the heart murmur. This condition is often triggered by crying. Initial management is to increase systemic vascular resistance by placing the patient in a knee-chest position. Other therapeutic modalities include the administration of morphine sulfate, sodium bicarbonate, and intravenous fluids, and the use of oxygen. Mechanical ventilation in combination with general anesthesia may be effective but would only be used once other management options fail to reverse the cyanosis. Dopamine and epinephrine are contraindicated because they may worsen the spell. A cardiology consultation may be useful, but the acuity of the patient's clinical presentation requires immediate intervention.

3. The answer is A [III.F.3.b]. Restenosis is a known complication from repair of coarctation of the aorta, and these clinical features are consistent with restenosis. Patients with coarctation of the aorta classically present with hypertension in the right arm and reduced blood pressures in the lower extremities. Therefore, the most appropriate initial step in this patient would be to obtain blood pressures in all four extremities. Balloon angioplasty is the treatment of choice for restenosis, rather than surgical repair, after the patient undergoes a complete evaluation. Confirmation of a bicuspid aortic valve is important because it may accompany coarctation in up to half of patients; however, it is not the most appropriate initial step in this patient's management. The oxygen saturation is normal in room air, and therefore does not require reassessment in 100% oxygen. Given the significantly elevated blood pressure, it is not appropriate to wait 6 months for reevaluation.

4. The answer is B [V.D.2.c, V.D.4]. This patient's clinical presentation is most consistent with pericarditis. The likely cause of his pericarditis is postpericardiotomy syndrome, given the closure of his ventricular septal defect (11 days) before the onset of his symptoms. Postpericardiotomy syndrome is believed to be an autoimmune response to a concomitant viral infection and is associated with opening of the pericardium during cardiac surgery. Pulsus paradoxus, or a greater than 10 mm Hg drop in systolic blood pressure on deep inspiration, is found in patients with pericarditis. Splinter hemorrhages are noted in patients with endocarditis, which is also associated with fever. Supraventricular tachycardia, which would present as a rapid heart rate with absent P waves on electrocardiogram, may cause chest pain, but the pain would not change with position and fever would be absent. Prolonged QT syndrome is most often associated with syncope and sudden cardiac arrest. Costochondritis is a common cause of chest pain, but fever is not associated with this disorder.

5. The answer is D [III.D.3]. This patient's murmur is consistent with a small ventricular septal defect (VSD). With a small VSD, a patient is likely to remain asymptomatic with normal growth and development. Typically, the smaller the VSD, the louder the murmur. Small muscular or membranous VSDs may close on their own without intervention. Small VSDs do not generally result in congestive heart failure or in Eisenmenger syndrome. A patent ductus arteriosus would more commonly present with a machinery-like continuous murmur at the upper left sternal border. Balloon valvuloplasty is not indicated for a VSD.

6. The answer is E [IV.D.3 and Table 8-4]. Tricuspid atresia is the only cause of cyanosis in the newborn period that manifests with left axis deviation and left ventricular hypertrophy on electrocardiogram (ECG). Patients with tricuspid atresia without a ventricular septal defect have a single S_2 as a result of the usual coexistence of pulmonary atresia and do not have a murmur. Patients with tetralogy of Fallot present with a systolic murmur of pulmonary stenosis and right ventricular hypertrophy (RVH) on ECG. Patients with transposition of the great arteries also have no murmur and a single S_2 but RVH on ECG. Similarly, RVH is present in total anomalous pulmonary venous connection, along with a systolic murmur. Truncus arteriosus manifests as combined ventricular hypertrophy with both a systolic and diastolic murmur.

7. The answer is D [V.C.8]. Before any invasive procedure that may result in bacteremia, such as a gastrointestinal, urologic, or dental procedure, prophylaxis against bacterial endocarditis is required for any patient with structural heart disease (e.g., patent ductus arteriosus) or for any patient who had structural heart disease repaired within the past 6 months. The major exception to this would be patients with ostium secundum atrial septal defects in whom the risk of endocarditis is very low. Patients with uncomplicated Kawasaki disease and cardiac dysrhythmias, including Wolff-Parkinson-White syndrome, do not require antibiotic prophylaxis.

8. The answer is A [I.C.1.a]. This patient's signs and symptoms are consistent with congestive heart failure (CHF). Forms of congenital heart disease that increase pulmonary blood flow, obstruct outflow, or overload portions of the heart through valvular regurgitation are among the many causes of CHF. Of the choices listed, only a large ventricular septal defect, which has a large left-to-right shunt with increased pulmonary blood blow, would cause CHF in a child of this age. Atrial septal defects, small patent ductus arteriosus defects, and mild-to-moderate pulmonary stenosis do not typically cause CHF. Critical or severe aortic stenosis may cause CHF, but this usually occurs within 24 hours of birth.

9. The answer is B [Table 8-1]. This murmur is most consistent with a venous hum, an innocent heart murmur. Aortic stenosis with insufficiency presents with systolic ejection and decrescendo diastolic murmurs. The murmur of a patent ductus arteriosus (PDA) is generally continuous and machinery-like and does not vary with position. Patients with PDAs generally also have brisk pulses. Both a Still's murmur and a pulmonic systolic murmur are innocent systolic murmurs. A Still's murmur is usually a grade I–III systolic murmur best heard at the mid-left sternal border. A pulmonic systolic murmur is a grade I–II high-pitched systolic murmur best heard at the upper left sternal border. Both the Still's murmur and the pulmonic systolic murmur are loudest supine.

10. The answer is A [V.F.3]. This patient's presentation, including the heart murmur and electrocardiogram findings, is consistent with hypertrophic cardiomyopathy. Initial management typically includes medications, such as β-adrenergic blockers or calcium-channel blockers, to reduce the left ventricular outflow tract obstruction and improve ventricular compliance. Aortic balloon valvuloplasty is a treatment for aortic stenosis. In aortic stenosis, the murmur would not be expected to increase with Valsalva maneuver or standing. Patients with hypertrophic cardiomyopathy are at risk for sudden death and should be restricted from athletic participation. Myomectomy is recommended for severe obstruction refractory to medical management. Albuterol is a $β_2$-agonist and is contraindicated in hypertrophic cardiomyopathy.

11–13. The answers are C, F, and D, respectively [VI.A–VI.C]. Congenital third-degree atrioventricular block is a complete heart block, with no conduction of atrial impulses to the ventricles. It is associated with infants born to mothers with systemic lupus erythematosus. Long QT interval is a lengthening of the QT interval, which increases the risk of lethal ventricular arrhythmias. There are two inherited forms of the disorder, one associated with congenital deafness (autosomal recessive; Jervell-Lange-Nielsen syndrome) and one not associated with congenital deafness (autosomal dominant; Romano-Ward syndrome). Wolff-Parkinson-White syndrome is a form of supraventricular tachycardia that is identified by the presence of a delta wave (slurred upslope of the QRS complex) on electrocardiogram.

14–17. The answers are C, A, E, and D, respectively [IV.B–IV.D, IV.F, and Table 8-4]. Transposition of the great arteries presents with no murmur and a single S_2 on auscultation. Squatting, or knee-chest positioning, increases systemic vascular resistance, which decreases the right-to-left shunt through a ventricular septal defect in tetralogy of Fallot. It is usually the first maneuver attempted to resolve a "tet" or hypercyanotic spell. Tricuspid atresia is the only cyanotic congenital heart disease lesion that manifests left ventricular hypertrophy on electrocardiogram in the newborn period. The classic chest radiograph in older children with unrepaired total anomalous pulmonary venous connection and with supracardiac drainage is cardiomegaly with a "snowman" appearance.

9

Pulmonology

Lauren J. Witcoff, M.D.

I. Anatomy and Physiology of the Respiratory System

A. Development

1. By 16 weeks gestation, the **bronchial tree** has developed. By 26–28 weeks gestation, sufficient air sacs and pulmonary vasculature have developed so that the fetus is able to survive.

2. **Ninety percent of alveolar development** occurs **after birth,** and alveoli increase in number until 8 years of age.

B. Anatomy

1. The **right lung contains three lobes,** and the **left lung contains two lobes,** including the lingula.

2. **Infants are at higher risk for respiratory insufficiency** than older children and adults because infants have anatomically smaller air passages, less compliant (stiffer) lungs with a more compliant chest wall, and less efficient pulmonary mechanics.

3. **Congenital malformations** of the respiratory tract may be associated with other congenital anomalies, especially of the cardiovascular system.

C. Physiology

1. **Pulmonary vascular resistance** decreases after birth when the fetal pulmonary and systemic circulations separate and the lungs ventilate for the first time.

2. The **primary function** of the lungs is gas exchange.

3. **Lung problems** may be classified as obstructive or restrictive.

   a. **Obstructive defects** are secondary to decreased airflow through narrowed airways. Examples include asthma, bronchiolitis, and foreign body aspiration.

   b. **Restrictive defects** are secondary to pulmonary processes that decrease lung volume (the amount of air filling the alveoli). Examples include pulmonary edema, scoliosis, pulmonary fibrosis, and respiratory muscle weakness.

II. Clinical Assessment of Pulmonary Disease

A. **History** is most important in determining the diagnosis of pulmonary disorders.

1. The **antenatal, prenatal, and neonatal histories** are very important because complications of pregnancy, fetal or postnatal tobacco exposure, prematurity, and airway instrumentation can cause pulmonary problems.

2. **Past medical history** should include previous respiratory problems, including frequent respiratory tract infections, cough, wheeze, stridor, snoring, and exercise intolerance.

3. **Review of systems** should include documentation of atopy (asthma), failure to thrive or steatorrhea (cystic fibrosis), choking (aspiration), or recurrent infections (immunodeficiencies).

4. **Family history** should include assessment for genetic diseases (e.g., cystic fibrosis, asthma).

5. **Environmental history** is extremely important because fumes, strong odors, tobacco smoke, allergens, animals, and day care attendance may cause or exacerbate pulmonary disease.

B. **Physical examination** should emphasize the chest and respiratory system.

1. In the **general assessment,** assess for **evidence of increased work of breathing,** such as tachypnea, nasal flaring, expiratory grunting, and chest wall retractions.

2. Evaluate **ears, nose, and throat** for signs of obstruction, atopy, or infection.

3. **Perform a chest examination.**

   a. **Inspiratory stridor** suggests extrathoracic obstruction, such as in croup and **laryngomalacia** (softening and weakness of laryngeal cartilage that collapses into the airway, especially when in the supine position).

   b. **Expiratory wheezing** suggests intrathoracic obstruction, as in asthma and bronchiolitis.

   c. **Crackles or rales** suggest parenchymal disease, such as in pneumonia and pulmonary edema.

4. **Assess for related findings in other organs**, such as heart murmurs, increased second heart sound (elevated pulmonary pressure), eczema, and digital clubbing.

C. **Accessory tests to evaluate pulmonary function**

1. **Imaging studies** such as chest x-ray (CXR), computed tomography (CT) scan, magnetic resonance imaging (MRI), and nuclear studies (e.g., ventilation-perfusion scans).

2. **Arterial blood gas** (ABG) is the gold standard to measure oxygenation (PO_2) and ventilation (PCO_2).

3. **Pulse oximetry** noninvasively measures oxygen saturation (SaO_2).

4. **Pulmonary function testing** (PFT) helps determine the type and

severity of pulmonary dysfunction. PFTs measure airflow as a function of time (**spirometry**) and **lung volumes.**

D. **Laryngoscopy and bronchoscopy** are performed in some conditions to visualize the upper or lower airways or to obtain bronchoalveolar lavage specimens for laboratory analysis. Common indications include **persistent pneumonia, cough, stridor, or wheezing.**

III. Infectious Disorders of the Respiratory Tract

A. **Epiglottitis**

1. **Definition.** Epiglottitis is **acute inflammation and edema** of the epiglottis, arytenoids, and aryepiglottic folds.

2. **Epidemiology.** The disorder is **most common** in children **2–7 years of age,** with equal incidence in males and females.

3. **Etiology**
   a. **Infection** with ***Haemophilus influenzae* type b (HIB)** was the most common cause before HIB immunization. Epiglottitis is now rare because of the success of the HIB immunization program.
   b. **Group A β-hemolytic streptococcus,** *Streptococcus pneumoniae,* and *Staphylococcus* species may also cause epiglottitis.

4. **Clinical features**
   a. **Abrupt onset** of **rapidly progressive** upper airway obstruction without prodrome. The following signs and symptoms may occur:
      (1) **High fever and toxic appearance**
      (2) **Muffled speech** and quiet stridor
      (3) **Dysphagia with drooling**
      (4) **Sitting forward in tripod** position with neck hyperextension
   b. **Complete airway obstruction** with respiratory arrest **may occur suddenly.**
   c. **Laboratory studies** demonstrate leukocytosis with left shift. **Ninety percent of patients have a positive blood culture,** if the epiglottitis is secondary to HIB.
   d. **Epiglottis** appears like a **"thumbprint" on a lateral radiograph of the neck.**

5. **Differential diagnosis.** Croup, bacterial tracheitis, and retropharyngeal abscess are diagnoses to also consider. Table 9-1 compares the clinical features that differentiate supraglottic disorders (e.g., epiglottitis) from subglottic disorders (e.g., viral croup).

6. **Diagnosis.** Epiglottitis should be suspected on the basis of clinical features. Visualization of a **cherry red** swollen epiglottis is made when the airway is established.

7. **Management**
   a. **Epiglottitis is a medical emergency.**
   b. **Controlled nasotracheal intubation** should be performed by **experienced personnel.**

Table 9-1. Differentiating Features of Supraglottic and Subglottic Disorders*

Feature	Supraglottic Disorders	Subglottic Disorders
Stridor	Quiet	Loud
Cough	None	Barky
Voice	Muffled	Hoarse
Dysphagia/drooling	Present	Absent
Fever	High	Low to moderate (croup)
		High (tracheitis)
Toxicity	Present	Absent, unless tracheitis is present
Posture	Neck extended, tripod position	Normal

*Supraglottic disorders include epiglottitis and retropharyngeal abscess. Subglottic disorders include bacterial tracheitis and viral croup.

    c. **Before intubation, minimize stimulation** while offering humidified oxygen. **Avoid causing distress** or examining the throat with a tongue depressor as this may cause respiratory arrest.

    d. **Antibiotic therapy** typically includes a second- or third-generation intravenous cephalosporin. If epiglottitis is secondary to HIB, **rifampin** prophylaxis is indicated for unimmunized household contacts younger than 4 years of age.

B. Laryngotracheobronchitis (Croup)

    1. **Definition.** Croup is **inflammation and edema** of the **subglottic** larynx, trachea, and bronchi.

    2. **Epidemiology.** There are **two forms of croup.**

        a. **Viral croup** is the **most common cause of stridor.** It typically occurs in children 3 months of age to 3 years of age in the late fall and winter. The male to female ratio is 2:1.

        b. **Spasmodic croup** occurs year round in preschool age children.

    3. **Etiology**

        a. **Viral croup**

            (1) **Parainfluenza** viruses are the most common cause.

            (2) **Other organisms** include respiratory syncytial virus (RSV), rhinovirus, adenovirus, influenza A and B, and *Mycoplasma pneumoniae.*

        b. **Spasmodic croup** is likely secondary to a **hypersensitivity reaction.**

    4. **Clinical features**

        a. **Viral croup**

            (1) **Begins with** upper respiratory infection prodrome for 2–3 days, followed by stridor and cough.

            (2) **Symptoms include inspiratory stridor,** fever, **barky cough,** and hoarse voice, which typically last 3–7 days. Respiratory distress may occur.

            (3) **Stridor** and cough **worsen at night and with agitation.**

            (4) **Wheezing** may occur.

            (5) **Anterior-posterior radiograph of the neck** demonstrates the "steeple sign" of subglottic narrowing.

    b. Spasmodic croup

       (1) Characteristic acute onset of stridor usually occurs at night.

       (2) Spasmodic croup typically recurs and resolves without treatment.

5. Diagnosis. Croup should be suspected on the basis of clinical features.

6. Management

    a. Supportive care involves using **cool mist** and fluids. Improvement is also noted when patients are exposed to cool night air.

    b. Children with stridor at rest benefit from **systemic corticosteroids,** such as intramuscular dexamethasone, nebulized budesonide, or oral corticosteroids, which reduce airway edema.

    c. Children with respiratory distress benefit from **racemic epinephrine aerosols,** which vasoconstrict subglottic tissues.

    d. β_2-Agonists (e.g., albuterol) are useful when wheezing is appreciated on examination.

    e. Hospitalization is indicated for children in respiratory distress.

C. Bacterial tracheitis is an uncommon, but reemerging, cause of stridor.

1. Definition. Bacterial tracheitis is **acute inflammation** of the trachea.

2. Etiology. Causes include *Staphylococcus aureus* (60%), *Streptococcus,* and nontypeable *Haemophilus influenzae.*

3. Clinical features

    a. Abrupt onset

    b. Toxicity, high fever, and mucous and pus in the trachea

4. Management. Appropriate antistaphylococcal antibiotics and airway support are indicated.

D. Bronchiolitis

1. Definition. Bronchiolitis is **inflammation of the bronchioles.** The term is most commonly used to refer to a **viral infection** that causes **inflammatory bronchiolar obstruction.**

2. Epidemiology

    a. Bronchiolitis is the **most common lower respiratory tract** infection in the first 2 years of life.

    b. This disorder **predominantly affects children younger than 2 years of age.**

    c. The male to female ratio is 2:1.

    d. Epidemics occur from November to April.

    e. Risk of infection is increased with day care attendance, multiple siblings, exposure to tobacco smoke, and lack of breastfeeding.

    f. More significant disease occurs in patients with **chronic lung disease,** congenital heart disease, history of prematurity, immunodeficiency diseases, and in infants younger than 3 months.

3. Etiology

    a. RSV is most common.

    b. Less common causes include parainfluenza, adenovirus, rhinovirus, influenza, and *Mycoplasma pneumoniae.*

4. **Clinical features**
   a. **Onset is gradual,** with upper respiratory symptoms, such as rhinorrhea, nasal congestion, fever, and cough occurring initially.
   b. **Progression** of respiratory symptoms takes place.
      (1) **Tachypnea, fine rales, wheezing,** and evidence of respiratory distress
      (2) The **spleen and liver** may appear enlarged as a result of lung hyperinflation.
   c. **Hypoxemia** may occur.
   d. **Apnea may occur,** especially in young infants and in children with a history of apnea of prematurity.
   e. **CXR** reveals **hyperinflation** with air trapping, **patchy infiltrates,** and **atelectasis.**
   f. **Improvement is noted within 2 weeks. More than 50% have recurrent wheezing.**
   g. **Complications** may include **apnea,** respiratory insufficiency, respiratory failure, and death. Bacterial superinfection occurs rarely.

5. **Diagnosis** is made on the basis of clinical features and may be confirmed with viral antigen or antibody testing.

6. **Management**
   a. Treatment is **primarily supportive** with nasal bulb suctioning, hydration, and oxygen as needed.
   b. **Careful handwashing** to prevent spread of infection is necessary.
   c. **Nebulized bronchodilators** are controversial and may only be effective in up to **50%** of patients.
   d. **Steroids** are controversial and may be most effective in patients with a prior history of wheezing.
   e. **Nebulized racemic epinephrine** may be effective in reducing airway constriction.
   f. **Aerosolized ribavirin**, a nucleoside analog with in vitro activity against RSV, may be considered for very ill infants. Evidence of definitive benefit is lacking.
   g. **Hospitalization** is indicated for respiratory distress, hypoxemia, apnea, dehydration, or underlying cardiopulmonary disease.
   h. **RSV monoclonal antibody** (palivizumab [Synagis]) may be given prophylactically by monthly intramuscular injection during RSV season to prevent severe disease in infants with a history of prematurity, chronic lung disease, or cyanotic or hemodynamically significant congenital heart disease.

E. **Pneumonia**

1. **Definition.** Pneumonia involves **infection and inflammation of lung parenchyma.**

2. **Epidemiology.** Pneumonia is associated with poverty, multiple siblings, exposure to tobacco smoke, and prematurity, as well as urban residence.

3. **Etiology.** Causes may be classified based on the child's age (**Table 9-2**).

Table 9-2. Age and Its Relationship to Pneumonia Etiology

Age	Typical Causes
0–3 months	Congenital infections, such as syphilis, toxoplasmosis, CMV, rubella, herpes simplex virus, and tuberculosis Intrapartum acquired infections, such as group B streptococcus (most common infection), Gram-negative rods, and *Listeria monocytogenes* Postpartum infections, such as RSV and other respiratory viruses Afebrile pneumonitis caused by *Chlamydia trachomatis, Ureaplasma urealyticum, Mycoplasma hominis,* CMV, and PCP
3 months–5 years	Viruses, such as adenovirus, influenza A and B, parainfluenza, and RSV (note that RSV pneumonia is generally uncommon beyond 2–3 years of age) Bacteria, most commonly *Streptococcus pneumoniae,* but may also include *Staphylococcus aureus* and HIB
Age 6 and older	*Mycoplasma pneumoniae* and *Chlamydia pneumoniae* increasingly common Viruses, such as adenovirus, influenza A and B, and parainfluenza Bacteria, most commonly *S. pneumoniae*

CMV = cytomegalovirus; *RSV* = respiratory syncytial virus; *HIB = Haemophilus influenzae* type b; *PCP = Pneumocystis carinii* pneumonia.

   a. **Viruses are the most common cause of pneumonia in all age groups.**

   b. **Recurrent or persistent pulmonary infiltrates** may have many causes (**Table 9-3**).

4. **Clinical features, diagnosis, and management** vary depending on etiologic agent.

   a. **Viral pneumonia**

      (1) **Symptoms** often begin with upper respiratory complaints, such as nasal congestion and rhinorrhea. Fever, cough, and dyspnea typically follow.

      (2) **Physical examination** may demonstrate tachypnea, wheezing, rales, or respiratory distress.

      (3) **Diagnosis** is suggested by **interstitial infiltrates** on CXR and a **white blood cell (WBC) count** < **20,000 cells/mm³** with a lymphocyte predominance.

      (4) **Management** is supportive.

   b. **Bacterial pneumonia**

      (1) **Symptoms** have more rapid onset and greater severity. Fever, cough, and dyspnea typically occur without preceding upper respiratory symptoms.

      (2) **Physical examination** may demonstrate rales, tachypnea, decreased breath sounds, and evidence of respiratory distress.

      (3) **Diagnosis** is suggested by a **WBC count** > **20,000 cells/mm³** with a neutrophil predominance, and **lobar consolidation** on CXR.

      (4) **Management** includes appropriate antibiotics and supportive care.

   c. ***Chlamydia trachomatis*** is a common cause of **afebrile** pneumonia at **1–3 months** of age.

Table 9-3. Causes of Recurrent or Persistent Pulmonary Infiltrates

Single Lobe	Multiple Lobes

Intraluminal obstruction
  Foreign body
  Tumor
  Mucus plug
Extraluminal obstruction
  Enlarged lymph node from infection
    or malignancy
Structural abnormalities
  Bronchial stenosis
  Bronchiectasis
  Right middle lobe syndrome
  Congenital lung abnormalities, such
    as cysts or sequestration
	Aspiration
	  Impaired gag or swallow
	  Esophageal obstruction or dysmotility
	  GERD
	Mucociliary clearance dysfunction
	  Cystic fibrosis
	  Ciliary dyskinesia (e.g., immotile cilia
	    syndrome)
	Bronchopulmonary dysplasia (chronic
	  lung disease)
	Miscellaneous
	  Congenital heart disease
	  α_1-Antitrypsin deficiency
	  Sickle cell disease
	  Hypersensitivity pneumonitis
	  Pulmonary hemosiderosis
	Asthma
	Immunodeficiency diseases

GERD = gastroesophageal reflux disease.

      (1) Symptoms include a **staccato-type** cough, dyspnea, and absence of fever. A history of conjunctivitis after birth may be identified in 50% of patients.

      (2) Physical examination may demonstrate tachypnea and wheezing.

      (3) Diagnosis is suggested by **eosinophilia** and CXR with **interstitial infiltrates. Definitive diagnosis** is by positive culture or direct fluorescent antibody (DFA) staining of cells from conjunctiva or nasopharynx.

      (4) Management includes oral **erythromycin or azithromycin.**

    d. *Mycoplasma pneumoniae* is one of the most common causes of pneumonia in older children and adolescents.

      (1) Symptoms include low-grade fever, chills, nonproductive cough, headache, pharyngitis, and malaise. The cough may last 3–4 weeks.

      (2) Lung examination may demonstrate widespread rales. Examination findings are often worse than expected by history.

      (3) Diagnosis

        (a) Positive cold agglutinins are suggestive but **not specific.**

        (b) CXR findings vary but may show bilateral diffuse infiltrates.

        (c) Definitive diagnosis is by elevation of serum IgM titers for *Mycoplasma.*

      (4) Management includes oral **erythromycin** or azithromycin.

  F. Pertussis. Pertussis is an acute respiratory infection also known as **"whooping cough."**

    1. Etiology. *Bordetella pertussis* is the major pathogen responsible for infection. *B. parapertussis* causes illness that appears clinically very similar to pertussis.

2. **Epidemiology**
   a. Routine immunization beginning at 2 months of age has been effective in reducing the overall incidence of pertussis infection (see Chapter 1, section III.C.2).
   b. **Infants younger than 6 months of age** are most at risk for **severe disease.**
   c. **Adolescents and adults** whose immunity has waned are the **major source** for pertussis infection of unimmunized or underimmunized children.
   d. Infection is **highly contagious.**

3. **Clinical features**
   a. Incubation period is typically 7–10 days.
   b. Pertussis is characterized by **3 stages.**
      (1) **Catarrhal stage** (lasts **1–2 weeks**) is characterized by upper respiratory symptoms such as rhinorrhea, nasal congestion, conjunctival redness, and low-grade fever.
      (2) **Paroxysmal stage** (lasts **2–4 weeks**) is characterized by fits of forceful coughing ("paroxysms") that are the hallmark of pertussis. A **whoop** is an inspiratory gasp heard at the very end of a coughing fit (the whoop is heard rarely in young infants). The coughing fits are exhausting, and post-tussive vomiting is common. Young infants may have **cyanosis, apnea, and choking** during the paroxysms of cough. Between the fits, children appear well and are afebrile.
      (3) **Convalescent phase** (lasts **weeks to months**) is a recovery stage in which paroxysmal cough continues but becomes less frequent and less severe over time.

4. **Diagnosis**
   a. Diagnosis is suspected based on clinical features.
   b. White blood cell count is elevated with a **lymphocytosis.**
   c. Diagnosis is confirmed by identification of the organism on **culture** (gold standard) of nasopharyngeal secretions plated on Regan-Lowe or Bordet-Gengou media, or by positive **direct fluorescent antibody tests** of nasopharyngeal secretions.

5. **Management**
   a. **Hospitalization** of young infants often occurs during the paroxysmal phase because of choking, apnea, or cyanosis. Supportive care and oxygen (if needed) are important therapies.
   b. **Antibiotics** are given to all patients to **prevent the spread of infection** (azithromycin or erythromycin is used). Antibiotics do not alter the patient's clinical course unless they are administered during the catarrhal phase or very early in the paroxysmal phase.
   c. **Respiratory isolation** is needed until antibiotics have been given for at least 5 days.

IV. Noninfectious Disorders of the Respiratory Tract

A. **Asthma (Reactive Airway Disease)**

1. **Definition**

   a. Asthma is a **chronic inflammatory** disorder of the airways that causes recurrent episodes of wheezing, cough, dyspnea, and chest tightness.

   b. **Symptoms** are typically associated with widespread, variable **airflow obstruction that is at least partially reversible,** either spontaneously or with therapy.

   c. **Inflammation** causes **airway hyperresponsiveness** to many stimuli.

2. **Epidemiology.** Asthma is the **most common chronic pediatric disease.**

   a. **Fifty percent** of children have symptoms by 1 year of age and ninety percent by 5 years of age.

   b. **Thirty to fifty percent** have **remission** by puberty.

3. **Etiology**

   a. **Predisposing factors** include atopy, family history of asthma, and exposure to tobacco smoke. Infection, diet, and pollution increase susceptibility in predisposed patients.

   b. **Trigger factors** of exacerbations include respiratory infections, exercise, cold air, emotions, allergens, gastroesophageal reflux, and exposure to pollutants.

   c. Asthma may accompany other acute or chronic lung diseases, such as cystic fibrosis.

4. **Pathophysiology.** Mechanisms include **smooth muscle bronchoconstriction, airway mucosal edema, increased secretions with mucous plugging, eventual airway wall remodeling, and production of inflammatory mediators (e.g., IgE).**

5. **Clinical features**

   a. **Typical features during an exacerbation** include tachypnea, dyspnea, nasal flaring, retractions, and multiphonic wheezing with a prolonged expiratory phase.

   b. Some patients have **only chronic or recurrent cough.**

   c. **CXR** often reveals **hyperinflation, peribronchial thickening, and patchy atelectasis.**

   d. **PFTs** reveal increased lung volumes and **decreased expiratory flow rates.**

6. **Diagnosis**

   a. **The basis of diagnosis is** clinical features and, usually, a therapeutic response to a bronchodilator trial.

   b. **"All that wheezes is not asthma."**

      (1) Differential diagnosis of acute wheezing (Figure 9-1)

      (2) Differential diagnosis of recurrent or chronic wheezing (Figure 9-2)

7. **Management.** Treatment depends on the severity of illness and trigger factors. Self-management with a normal lifestyle is the primary goal.

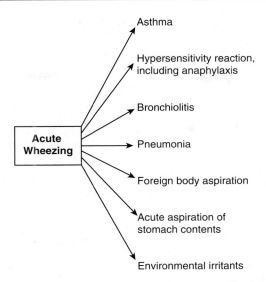

Figure 9-1. Differential diagnosis of acute wheezing.

a. **Prevention** of initial disease development and of secondary exacerbations is critical to effective management.

b. **Effective** control of asthma

   (1) **Assessment and monitoring** of asthma symptoms involve home assessments of peak expiratory flow rates (**peak flows**) and a symptom diary. Parents and patients should be instructed concerning using peak flow measurements to guide changes in medication or to know when to seek acute medical care.

   (2) **Control of trigger factors** includes avoidance of causal allergens, dust mites, molds, animal dander, cockroaches, pollens, smoke, pollution, and irritants.

   (3) **Patient and family education**

   (4) **Pharmacologic therapy** is added in a stepwise fashion based on disease severity (**Table 9-4**).

   (a) **Sympathomimetics**

   (i) **β_2-Adrenergic agonists** may be given by inhaler or by nebulization.

   (ii) **Short-acting bronchodilators** (e.g., albuterol) are first-line therapies for exacerbations. They can also be used for prevention of exercise-induced symptoms.

   (iii) **Long-acting** preparations may be used for chronic control.

   (iv) **If the asthma is persistent (i.e., more severe than intermittent), it is more effectively controlled by the addition of anti-inflammatory medications.**

   (b) **Cromolyn sodium and nedocromil sodium**

   (i) **Anti-inflammatory** prophylaxis is induced by inhibition of activation and release of inflammatory mediators.

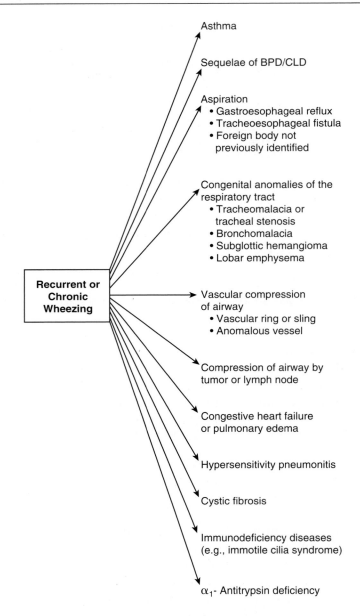

Figure 9-2. Differential diagnosis of recurrent or chronic wheezing. *BPD/CLD* = bronchopulmonary dysplasia/chronic lung disease.

    (ii) These drugs have **no effect on acute symptoms** but may help prevent exacerbations.

  (c) Corticosteroids

    (i) These drugs are the **most effective anti-inflammatory** agents.

    (ii) Systemic steroids are given for 5–10 days for moderate to severe exacerbations.

Table 9-4. Categories of Asthma Severity and Their Management

Category	Clinical Characteristics	Management
Intermittent	Daytime symptoms ≤ 2×/week Nighttime symptoms ≤ 2×/month	No daily medication Short-acting inhaled β_2-agonist for symptom relief Anti-inflammatory agents not needed
Mild persistent	Daytime symptoms > 2×/week, but < 1×/day Nighttime symptoms > 2×/month FEV_1 ≥ 80% predicted (normal)	Short-acting inhaled β_2-agonist for symptom relief Low-dose inhaled corticosteroid (preferred) or cromolyn sodium or leukotriene modifier
Moderate persistent	Daily symptoms Nighttime symptoms > 1×/week FEV_1 60–80% predicted Daily use of inhaled short-acting β_2-agonist	Short-acting inhaled β_2-agonist for symptom relief Medium-dose inhaled corticosteroid OR Low-dose inhaled corticosteroid and long-acting inhaled β_2-agonist
Severe persistent	Continuous symptoms Frequent nighttime symptoms Limited physical activity FEV_1 ≤ 60% predicted	Short-acting inhaled β_2-agonist for symptom relief High-dose inhaled corticosteroid and long-acting β_2-agonist Long-term systemic corticosteroids, if needed

FEV_1 = forced expiratory velocity in 1 second.
Adapted from the National Heart, Lung, and Blood Institute, National Asthma Education and Prevention Program Expert Panel Report: Guidelines for the Diagnosis and Management of Asthma—Update On Selected Topics 2002.

> (iii) **Inhaled steroids** are very effective in **preventing** exacerbations.
>
> **(d) Anticholinergic agents** (e.g., atropine or ipratropium bromide [Atrovent])
>
> > (i) These agents are used as second-line bronchodilators.
> >
> > (ii) These agents **decrease airway vagal tone** and block reflex bronchoconstriction, and they may be useful in severe exacerbations.
>
> **(e) Leukotriene modifiers** (montelukast, zafirlukast) are oral anti-inflammatory agents for long-term control of mild, persistent asthma.
>
> **(f) Methylxanthines (theophylline)** play a controversial role in asthma management. They are bronchodilators with possible anti-inflammatory effects but have a narrow toxic–therapeutic ratio, and their use has therefore decreased.

B. Cystic Fibrosis (CF)

> **1. Definition.** CF is a **multisystem disorder** that results in altered content of **exocrine gland secretions.**

2. **Epidemiology**
   a. CF affects **1 in 2,500 Caucasians,** with equal incidence in males and females.
   b. **Five percent of Caucasians are carriers.**
   c. **Median age of survival** is 31 years.

3. **Etiology.** CF is an **autosomal recessive** disease resulting from a genetic mutation on **chromosome 7.**

4. **Pathophysiology**
   a. The **genetic defect** produces an **abnormal ion-channel regulator (CFTR) protein** that causes sodium and chloride transport dysfunction in epithelial cells.
   b. **Abnormal mucus** produced in airways helps create **airway obstruction, inflammation, and infection.**

5. **Clinical features. Classic hallmarks of CF** include **chronic progressive pulmonary insufficiency, pancreatic insufficiency,** and **high sweat electrolytes.** Clinical expression is variable. **See Table 9-5** for the multisystem signs and symptoms of CF.
   a. **Meconium ileus at birth** is present in 20% of patients.
   b. **Recurrent** or **chronic respiratory symptoms, steatorrhea, and failure to thrive** (FTT) are typical **presenting features.**
   c. **Respiratory signs and symptoms** include chronic productive cough, dyspnea, lung hyperinflation, lung crackles, wheezing, digital clubbing, and progressive hypoxemia.
      (1) **PFTs** show **decreased respiratory flow rates** (consistent with obstruction) and eventually **decreased lung volumes** (consistent with restriction).
      (2) **Pneumonia** develops as lungs become colonized, first with *Staphylococcus aureus,* and later with *Pseudomonas aeruginosa.*

Table 9-5. Clinical Features of Cystic Fibrosis (CF)

Organ System	Specific Feature
Chronic sinopulmonary disease	Persistent colonization or infection with CF pathogens, such as *Staphylococcus aureus, Pseudomonas aeruginosa,* or *Burkholderia cepacia* Chronic cough, wheeze, sputum production Mucus plugging Nasal polyps and chronic sinusitis Chest radiograph abnormalities including bronchiectasis, atelectasis, pulmonary infiltrates, and hyperinflation
Gastrointestinal abnormalities	Meconium ileus and distal intestinal obstruction syndrome Rectal prolapse Pancreatic insufficiency and recurrent pancreatitis Chronic hepatic disease
Nutritional abnormalities	Failure to thrive, hypoproteinemia, and edema Fat-soluble vitamin deficiencies (A, D, E, K)
Metabolic abnormalities	Salt depletion, classic electrolytes: hyponatremic, hypochloremic, hypokalemic metabolic alkalosis
Other	Digital clubbing and obstructive azoospermia

      (3) Common pulmonary complications include hemoptysis, pneumothorax, asthma, chronic sinusitis, and **nasal polyps. Recurrent pneumonia,** bronchiectasis, pulmonary fibrosis, cor pulmonale, and respiratory failure eventually occur.

    d. Pancreatic insufficiency occurs in **90%** of patients, with malabsorption predisposing to malnutrition and **FTT.**

  6. Diagnosis requires:

    a. One or more phenotypic features **or** positive family history **or** increased immunoreactive trypsinogen on newborn screen.

    b. Laboratory evidence of abnormal CFTR, including sweat chloride > 60 mmol/L **or** two CF mutations **or** a characteristic ion transport abnormality across the nasal epithelium.

  7. Management. Treatment requires a team approach and includes:

    a. Antibiotics for pulmonary exacerbations

    b. Pulmonary toilet with chest percussion and antimucous therapy

    c. Bronchodilators for wheezing

    d. Good nutrition, pancreatic enzyme replacement, and **fat-soluble vitamins** (vitamins A, D, E, and K)

    e. Oxygen as needed for hypoxemia

    f. Anti-inflammatory and immunosuppressive therapy

    g. Lung transplantation and, ultimately, future gene therapy

    h. Psychological support for patients and families

C. Chronic Lung Disease (CLD; also termed bronchopulmonary dysplasia [BPD]; see also Chapter 4, section VI.G.2.a).

  1. Definition. CLD is oxygen dependency beyond 28 days of life.

  2. Epidemiology. CLD **most commonly** occurs in children born prematurely who suffered from **respiratory distress syndrome** (hyaline membrane disease or surfactant deficiency syndrome).

  3. Etiology and pathophysiology. CLD follows acute lung injury and results in a continuum of altered lung repair and function.

    a. Causes of **acute lung injury** may include barotrauma from mechanical ventilation, meconium aspiration syndrome, or infection.

    b. Secondary lung injury caused by oxidants and proteases typically follows the acute injury.

    c. Healing of lung tissue is typically abnormal and is characterized by altered airway and parenchymal remodeling with resultant lung tissue fibrosis, chronic airflow limitations, and diminished lung compliance. This results in both obstructive and restrictive lung disease.

  4. Clinical features vary and range from transient oxygen dependency to prolonged need for ventilatory support.

    a. Diminished oxygenation (PaO_2) and **hypercarbia** ($PaCO_2$) are often found on ABG testing.

    b. Intermittent episodes of tachypnea, wheezing, sputum production, and respiratory distress typically occur.

    c. Frequent respiratory tract infections, airway hyperreactivity, and pulmonary hypertension may result.

    d. **CXR** typically demonstrates hyperinflation, atelectasis, and linear or cystic radiodensities.

    e. **Nonpulmonary manifestations** may include increased caloric needs and delayed growth and development.

5. **Management**

    a. Administer **supplemental oxygen** or ventilatory support as needed.

    b. **Optimize pulmonary function** with bronchodilators, diuretics, anti-inflammatory agents, and fluid restriction.

    c. **Optimize caloric intake** and growth.

    d. **Prevent complicating infections** through appropriate immunization practices and early antibiotic treatment.

    e. Focus on **early identification of complications,** such as subglottic stenosis, gastroesophageal reflux disease, and tracheobronchomalacia.

6. **Prognosis.** Pulmonary symptoms and disease often diminish with time and growth. Some patients have increased risk of sudden death, continued airway hyperreactivity, hyperinflation, and increased risk of respiratory infections.

D. **Foreign Body Aspiration**

1. **Epidemiology.** Children **3 months–5 years** of age are at greatest risk for small object aspiration.

2. **Etiology. Typical aspirated objects** include seeds, popcorn, hot dogs, candy, grapes, and small toy parts.

3. **Clinical features depend on location and biologic reactivity** of material aspirated.

    a. **History** may elicit **choking episode** in 50–80% of cases.

    b. **Laryngotracheal foreign bodies** (extrathoracic) result in cough, hoarseness, and **inspiratory stridor.**

    c. **Bronchial foreign bodies** (intrathoracic; right bronchus slightly more common than left)

        (1) **Asymmetric findings on auscultation**

        (2) **Complete** obstruction with atelectasis, **partial ball-valve** obstruction with unilateral emphysema, **or no obstruction** that initially can be asymptomatic

        (3) **Localized wheezing, persistent pneumonia,** chronic cough, or hemoptysis

    d. **Esophageal foreign bodies may compress the trachea, producing respiratory symptoms.**

4. **Diagnosis** is challenging. **Have a high index of suspicion!**

    a. **A radiopaque** object is evident on CXR in **only 15% of cases.**

    b. **Consider inspiratory and expiratory films, bilateral decubitus films** in young children who cannot inspire and expire on command, or fluoroscopy to identify air trapping distal to a foreign body.

5. **Management**

    a. **Basic life support** is the initial management for a severe choking episode.

    b. Natural cough, if present, is the most effective expulsive mechanism.

    c. Foreign bodies that **remain in the airway** must be removed by **bronchoscopy.**

E. Apnea, apparent life-threatening event (ALTE), and sudden infant death syndrome (SIDS)

  1. Definitions

    a. Apnea of infancy is the unexplained **cessation of breathing for ≥ 20 seconds,** or a shorter respiratory pause associated with bradycardia, cyanosis, pallor, or hypotonia in a full-term infant.

      (1) Respiratory pause may be **central** (no respiratory effort), **obstructive** (efforts at respiration are made, but are unsuccessful usually because of upper airway obstruction), or both.

      (2) Short central apnea for ≤ **15 seconds is normal** at all ages.

    b. Apnea of prematurity is the unexplained cessation of breathing for ≥ 20 seconds in a premature infant (see also Chapter 4, section IX).

    c. Periodic breathing is a breathing pattern with three or more respiratory pauses lasting at least 3 seconds each, with less than 20 seconds of normal respiration in between.

    d. ALTE is a frightening event characterized by some combination of apnea, color change, change in muscle tone, choking, or gagging, in which recovery occurs only after stimulation or resuscitation.

    e. SIDS is the sudden death of a child younger than 1 year of age that is unexplained after a thorough investigation, including a complete autopsy, an examination of the death scene, and a review of the clinical history.

  2. Epidemiology

    a. SIDS reaches its **peak incidence at 2–4 months** of age, and 95% of cases occur before 6 months of age.

    b. Risk factors for SIDS

      (1) Prone sleeping position

      (2) Soft bedding, overbundling, and **overheating**

      (3) Prematurity

      (4) Being the **twin** of a sibling who died of SIDS

      (5) Low birth weight or growth retardation

      (6) Recent illness

      (7) Lack of breastfeeding

      (8) Maternal smoking, drug abuse, or infection

  3. Etiology

    a. Apnea of prematurity is usually caused by **immature central respiratory center control.**

    b. Obstructive apnea may be secondary to **craniofacial anomalies, adenotonsillar hypertrophy, obesity, or hypotonia.**

    c. The **cause of SIDS is unknown.**

    d. No definite cause and effect relationship has been proven among apnea, ALTE, and SIDS.

4. Differential diagnosis of ALTE
   a. **Seizure disorder**
   b. **Gastroesophageal reflux disease (GERD)**
   c. **Upper airway obstruction**
   d. **Intracranial mass lesion**
   e. **Sepsis or other infections,** including RSV, pertussis, and meningitis
   f. **Metabolic abnormalities, including electrolyte imbalance** and **hypoglycemia**
   g. **Inborn errors of metabolism**
   h. **Arrhythmia,** including **long QT syndrome**
   i. **Abnormal central control** of breathing
   j. **Munchausen by proxy**
   k. **Nonaccidental trauma** (shaken baby syndrome)

5. Evaluation
   a. **Detailed history and physical examination** is necessary.
   b. **Further testing** is based on clinical impression from the history and physical and may include:
      (1) **Hospital observation** and monitoring
      (2) **Blood work,** including complete blood count, ABG, electrolytes, and evaluation for infection
      (3) **CXR, electrocardiogram, and electroencephalogram**
      (4) **Multichannel recording (sleep study),** which simultaneously evaluates oxygen saturation, airflow, chest wall movement, and cardiac rhythm
      (5) **Barium esophagram or pH probe study** to evaluate for **GERD.**
      (6) **Imaging** studies of the head and neck
      (7) **Workup** for **metabolic disease**

6. Management
   a. **Teach caregivers cardiopulmonary resuscitation techniques.**
   b. The **efficacy of home monitoring** in reducing infant morbidity and mortality is **not well established.** Recommended indications for home cardiorespiratory monitoring include:
      (1) **History of ALTE**
      (2) **Documentation** of clinically significant **apnea** on sleep study
      (3) **Apnea of prematurity**
      (4) **Documented central hypoventilation**
      (5) **Consider monitors** for siblings of SIDS victims, infants of substance-abusing mothers, and oxygen-dependent infants.

7. Prevention of SIDS
   a. **Sleep on back**
   b. **Firm bedding**
   c. **Avoid overheating**
   d. **Smoke-free environment**
   e. **Early prenatal care and regular well child care**
   f. **Breastfeed**

Review Test

1. A 2-year-old toddler presents with a 3-day history of increasing inspiratory stridor, cough, and increased work of breathing. On examination, you confirm the inspiratory stridor and also note intercostal retractions and tachypnea with a respiratory rate of 44 breaths/min. Which of the following is correct regarding the cause and management of the probable diagnosis?

(A) Parainfluenza virus is the most likely cause.
(B) Foreign body aspiration is unlikely because of the absence of a history of choking.
(C) Albuterol nebulization should be administered.
(D) A "thumbprint sign" will be found on a lateral radiograph of the neck.
(E) Antibiotics against *Staphylococcus aureus* are indicated.

2. A 5-month-old female infant in a day care facility develops a low-grade fever to 100.8°F (38.2°C), rhinorrhea, and cough. A few days later, she is brought to the emergency department with tachypnea, chest retractions, diffuse expiratory wheezing, and fine inspiratory crackles bilaterally. Which of the following is correct regarding her likely diagnosis?

(A) Chest radiography will demonstrate decreased lung volumes with bilateral lobar consolidation.
(B) *Chlamydia trachomatis* should be considered as a possible etiologic agent.
(C) Supportive care is the most important management.
(D) Intravenous erythromycin should be started.
(E) Ribavirin should be administered.

3. A previously healthy 13-year-old boy presents with a 2-week history of nonproductive cough and low-grade fever. On examination, you note a normal respiratory rate and no evidence of respiratory distress, but are surprised to also hear inspiratory rales at the bilateral lung bases. Which of the following is the most likely cause of pneumonia in this adolescent?

(A) *Pneumocystis carinii*
(B) *Staphylococcus aureus*
(C) Group B streptococcus
(D) *Haemophilus influenzae* type b
(E) *Chlamydia pneumoniae*

4. A 7-month-old male infant presents with failure to thrive, and he has had two previous episodes of pneumonia. Past medical history is also significant for meconium ileus during the neonatal period. Which of the following is correct regarding his likely diagnosis?

(A) Electrolytes demonstrate hypernatremic, hyperchloremic metabolic alkalosis.
(B) His lungs are likely colonized with *Staphylococcus aureus*.
(C) Pulmonary function studies show increased lung volume consistent with restrictive lung disease.
(D) There is a 50% chance that a subsequent sibling will have the same illness.
(E) Pathophysiology involves abnormal calcium transport.

5. A 5-year-old girl presents with failure to thrive. Workup reveals a sweat chloride level of 90 mmol/L, which is consistent with cystic fibrosis. Which of the following is true regarding this patient's management?

(A) True malabsorption is uncommon and if it occurs, the malabsorption responds well to good nutrition.
(B) Antibiotic therapy should be avoided to prevent development of resistant organisms.
(C) Bronchodilators are ineffective in this condition.
(D) Replacement of vitamin K is necessary.
(E) Chest physical therapy provides little added benefit.

6. A male infant born at 29 weeks gestation was diagnosed with surfactant deficiency syndrome. He required 3 months of mechanical ventilatory support and oxygen therapy. Now he is ready for discharge from the neonatal intensive care unit and will go home on 0.25 L/min of oxygen. Which of the following is likely to be correct regarding his lung function?

(A) He will probably develop obstructive lung disease.

(B) Because of the difficulties breathing and swallowing in young premature infants, his caloric intake should be minimized.

(C) His lung function will continue to deteriorate with time and further growth.

(D) His chest radiograph will be normal because he has clinically improved.

(E) His lung disease should not affect his development.

7. A 3-month-old female infant required mouth-to-mouth resuscitation by her mother when she became blue and limp after feeding. In the emergency department, the physical examination is completely normal. Which of the following is correct regarding her presentation?

(A) A home apnea monitor should be ordered and will prevent sudden infant death syndrome in this high-risk infant.

(B) Her presentation likely represents periodic breathing, and reassurance should be given.

(C) Sweat chloride test should be performed to rule out cystic fibrosis.

(D) Even though no seizure activity was witnessed, an electroencephalogram should be considered as part of the evaluation.

(E) Given a normal examination in the emergency department, the patient may be discharged home with close follow-up.

8. A 3-year-old boy presents with acute onset of fever to 103.5°F (39.7°C), diminished appetite, and drooling. He has been previously well, and inspection of his immunization records reveals that all are up-to-date for his age. On examination, you note that he appears very ill and prefers to sit leaning forward on his hands with his neck hyperextended. His voice is muffled. Which of the following is correct regarding his likely diagnosis?

(A) This patient likely has bacterial tracheitis and should be started on antistaphylococcal antibiotics.

(B) Racemic epinephrine should be immediately administered.

(C) Anesthesiology should be consulted and should visualize his airway and intubate him in a controlled environment (e.g., operating room).

(D) An anterior-posterior radiograph of the neck will show a "steeple sign."

(E) The throat should be examined with a tongue depressor to rule out retropharyngeal abscess.

9. A 6-week-old female infant presents with increased work of breathing and a staccato-type cough for 3 days. On physical examination you note a temperature of 98.8°F (37.1°C), a respiratory rate of 60 breaths/min, and bilateral conjunctival erythema. The lungs are clear except for mild wheezing at the bilateral lung bases. Which of the following is correct regarding her likely diagnosis?

(A) Pneumonia is unlikely given the absence of fever, and therefore a noninfectious cause of the patient's symptoms should be sought.

(B) Eosinophilia will be found on complete blood count.

(C) Blood culture will be positive in 25% of cases.

(D) Corticosteroids are indicated and will improve the patient's clinical course.

(E) Ribavirin should be considered.

10. A 9-year-old girl with asthma is brought to the office for the first time. On average, she uses her albuterol inhaler three times per week, but for the past 10 days, she has been wheezing both day and night and is using the inhaler three to four times per day. On examination, you note diffuse wheezing and moderate subcostal retractions. Which of the following is the next step in management?

(A) Order a chest radiograph to assess for pneumonia.
(B) Refer her to an allergist for allergen immunotherapy.
(C) Start an oral leukotriene modifier.
(D) Start a low-dose inhaled corticosteroid.
(E) Start a 5-day course of systemic corticosteroids.

The response options for statements 11 and 12 are the same. You will be required to select one answer for each statement in the set.

(A) Short-acting inhaled β_2-agonist for symptom relief plus medium-dose inhaled corticosteroid
(B) Short-acting inhaled β_2-agonist for symptom relief
(C) Short-acting inhaled β_2-agonist for symptom relief plus long-acting β_2-agonist and high-dose inhaled corticosteroid
(D) Short-acting inhaled β_2-agonist for symptom relief plus low-dose inhaled corticosteroid

(E) Inhaled cromolyn sodium for symptom relief

For each description of a patient with asthma, select the most appropriate pharmacologic therapy.

11. A 12-year-old girl with daily wheezing and nighttime symptoms two times per week.

12. A 10-year-old boy with wheezing every other month associated with cold symptoms.

Answers and Explanations

1. The answer is A [III.B]. Croup is the most common cause of acute stridor and cough in toddlers, and parainfluenza virus causes the majority of these infections. Foreign body aspiration may cause stridor or cough and should be considered as a cause because in as many as 50% of foreign body aspirations, choking is not witnessed. Albuterol plays no role in management of croup unless associated asthma or wheezing is present. An anterior-posterior radiograph of the neck will show a "steeple sign" characteristic of subglottic narrowing; however, a "thumbprint sign" is associated with epiglottitis. Antibiotics are not indicated for croup.

2. The answer is C [III.D.3–6]. This patient's clinical features are consistent with bronchiolitis, a lower respiratory tract infection. Supportive care is the most effective management, although inhaled albuterol and racemic epinephrine may have some benefit for some patients. Respiratory syncytial virus (RSV) is the most common cause of bronchiolitis. Chest radiography usually demonstrates hyperinflation and atelectasis. *Chlamydia trachomatis* pneumonia generally occurs in a young infant, 1–3 months of age, and would be very unlikely in a 5-month-old infant. Erythromycin is not effective for bronchiolitis. Evidence for benefit of ribavirin in the treatment of bronchiolitis is lacking, and ribavirin should only be considered for severely ill infants.

3. The answer is E [Table 9-2 and III.E.3]. The most common cause of pneumonia in older children and adolescents is infection with *Mycoplasma pneumoniae* and *Chlamydia pneumoniae*. Pneumonia in immunocompromised patients may be caused by *Pneumocystis carinii*. Although pneumonia as a result of *Staphylococcus aureus* may occur in adolescents, it is less common than *Mycoplasma* and *Chlamydia* infection. Group B streptococcus is an organism unique to the neonatal period. *Haemophilus influenzae* type b (HIB) typically causes pneumonia in infants and toddlers, although the incidence has declined markedly as a result of effective vaccination against HIB.

4. The answer is B [IV.B.3–5, IV.B.7, Table 9-5]. The likely diagnosis is cystic fibrosis (CF). Lung disease eventually develops in all individuals with CF; the lungs are initially colonized with *Staphylococcus aureus* and subsequently with *Pseudomonas aeruginosa*. Twenty percent of neonates with CF present with meconium ileus, an impaction of inspissated meconium that causes congenital intestinal obstruction. Classic electrolytes reveal a hyponatremic, hypochloremic, hypokalemic metabolic alkalosis. Pulmonary function studies demonstrate decreased respiratory flow rates consistent with obstructive lung disease early in the disease process. Later, restrictive lung disease patterns are present. The autosomal recessive inheritance of CF means that each subsequent sibling has a 25% chance of having the disease. Pathophysiology involves an altered ion-channel regulator (CFTR) protein, resulting in abnormal sodium and chloride transport in epithelial cells.

5. The answer is D [IV.B.7]. Pancreatic insufficiency and malabsorption are very common and require pancreatic enzyme replacement and the administration of fat-soluble vitamins (vitamins A, D, E, and K). Nutritional support is very important as patients commonly have failure to thrive with difficulty gaining weight, and high-calorie diets are therefore prescribed. Broad-spectrum antibiotics should be used for treatment of pulmonary exacerbations. Other effective modalities in CF are bronchodilators for wheezing and aggressive pulmonary toilet, including chest physical therapy.

6. The answer is A [IV.C]. Prematurity and barotrauma from prolonged mechanical ventilation are significant risk factors for the development of bronchopulmonary dysplasia or chronic lung disease. Lung injury typically causes a combination of obstructive (from dysplastic and narrowed airways) and restrictive (from lung tissue fibrosis) lung disease. To meet their metabolic demands and facilitate growth, patients require very high caloric intakes. Pulmonary disease improves with time and lung growth, although chest radiographs may remain abnormal for years. Development is often delayed in children with chronic lung disease.

7. The answer is D [IV.E]. This patient had an apparent life-threatening event (ALTE). The evaluation of an ALTE should include attempts to identify an underlying cause, and workup may include an electroencephalogram to rule out a seizure disorder, an electrocardiogram to rule out a dysrhythmia such as long QT syndrome, electrolytes, a barium esophagogram or pH probe study to rule out gastroesophageal reflux disease, and a sleep study. An ALTE is not a presentation of cystic fibrosis (CF), and therefore a sweat chloride test is not indicated. Patients with CF generally present with failure to thrive, repeated pulmonary infections, or evidence of pancreatic insufficiency. After an ALTE, many experts recommend observation and monitoring of the infant in the hospital and, sometimes, discharge home on an apnea monitor. However, the effectiveness of an apnea monitor in preventing sudden infant death syndrome has not been established. The patient's presentation is not consistent with periodic breathing, which is defined as a breathing pattern with three or more respiratory pauses lasting 3 seconds each, with less than 20 seconds of normal respirations in between.

8. The answer is C [III.A.7]. This patient's presentation with fever, toxic appearance, muffled speech, tripod positioning when seated, drooling, and neck hyperextension all point to epiglottitis as a possible diagnosis. Epiglottitis is now a very uncommon infection as a result of the successful immunization of children against *Haemophilus influenzae* type b (HIB); however, epiglottitis may still occur secondary to infection with streptococcal and staphylococcal species. Management includes avoidance of excessive stimulation, including examination of the pharynx with a tongue depressor, because this may induce respiratory distress. Evaluation of the airway and intubation by experienced personnel in a controlled setting is necessary. Racemic epinephrine is not effective in epiglottitis. A "steeple sign" on a radiograph of the neck is consistent with the diagnosis of croup, not epiglottitis (which demonstrates a "thumbprint sign" on lateral radiograph of the neck). Bacterial tracheitis presents with fever and stridor (rather than a muffled voice), and drooling and neck hyperextension are unlikely to be present.

9. The answer is B [III.E.3, III.E.4.c, Table 9-2]. This patient's clinical features point to a likely diagnosis of pneumonia secondary to infection with *Chlamydia trachomatis,* which is a common cause of pneumonia in patients 1–3 months of age. Patients are afebrile, have a characteristic staccato-type cough, and may have a history of conjunctivitis (in 50% of cases). Diagnosis is suggested by the presence of elevated eosinophils on complete blood count. Blood cultures are not positive in this infection. Management includes oral erythromycin or azithromycin. Neither corticosteroids nor ribavirin are effective treatments for *C. trachomatis* pneumonia.

10. The answer is E [IV.A.7, Table 9-4]. This patient presents with a moderate exacerbation of her chronic asthma and therefore would benefit from a 5- to 10-day course of systemic corticosteroids. Both inhaled corticosteroids and leukotriene inhibitors are effective management options for the prevention and long-term management of asthma, and these agents should be considered for this patient after the systemic corticosteroids. Allergen immunotherapy may also be beneficial but would not be the initial step in management. Pneumonia is unlikely, and therefore a chest radiograph is not indicated.

11 and 12. The answers are A and B, respectively [Table 9-4 and IV.A.7]. Asthma is graded on a severity scale on the basis of the frequency of asthma symptoms during the day and night and also on pulmonary function testing. The 12-year-old girl's asthma would be characterized as moderate persistent asthma because of the presence of daily symptoms and nighttime wheezing more often than once per week. The best treatment for moderate persistent asthma is medium-dose inhaled corticosteroids added to as needed inhaled β_2-agonists. The 10-year-old boy's asthma would be characterized as intermittent asthma because his asthma symptoms occur twice weekly or less, and nighttime symptoms twice monthly or less. The best treatment for intermittent asthma is short-acting inhaled β_2-agonist medication.

10

Gastroenterology

Tiffany Merrill Becker, M.D., Frederick D. Watanabe, M.D., and Lloyd J. Brown, M.D.

I. Nutrition

A. General Concepts

1. **Essential nutrients** cannot be synthesized by the body and must be derived from the diet. These include certain vitamins, minerals, amino acids, fatty acids, and a carbohydrate source.

2. **Nonessential nutrients** can be synthesized from other compounds or may be derived from the diet.

3. **Macronutrients** supply energy and essential nutrients needed for growth, development, disease prevention, and activity.

    a. **Carbohydrates** make up approximately 50% of a typical diet and are converted by the body to glucose and other monosaccharides.

    b. **Proteins** are converted to peptides and amino acids. Of the 20 amino acids, nine are essential. As compared with adults, infants require more protein in their diet (2.2 g/kg during infancy decreasing to 0.8 g/kg during adulthood).

    c. **Fats** are broken down into fatty acids and glycerol. **Essential fatty acids** play an **important role in infant brain development.** Less than 30% of all calories should come from fats.

    d. **Minerals,** including sodium, chloride, potassium, calcium, phosphorus, and magnesium, are also required daily.

4. **Micronutrients**

    a. **Water-soluble vitamins** include vitamin C and the B-complex vitamins (thiamine, riboflavin, niacin, pyridoxine, folic acid, cobalamin, biotin, and pantothenic acid).

    b. **Fat-soluble vitamins** include vitamins A, D, E, and K.

    c. **Essential trace minerals,** such as iron, iodine, fluorine, zinc, chromium, selenium, and copper, play important roles in metabolism and as enzyme cofactors.

    d. **Certain clinical features are associated with vitamin and mineral deficiencies (Table 10-1).**

Table 10-1. Clinical Features of Selected Vitamin and Mineral Deficiencies

Nutrient	Signs and Symptoms
Vitamin A	Night blindness, xerophthalmia (dry conjunctiva and cornea)
Vitamin D	Rickets/osteomalacia, dental caries, hypocalcemia, hypophosphatemia
Vitamin E	Anemia/hemolysis, neurologic deficits, altered prostaglandin synthesis
Vitamin K	Coagulopathy/prolonged prothrombin time, abnormal bone matrix synthesis
Vitamin B_1 (thiamine)	**Beriberi** (cardiac failure, peripheral neuropathy, hoarseness or aphonia, Wernicke's encephalopathy)
Vitamin B_6 (pyridoxine)	Dermatitis, cheilosis, glossitis, microcytic anemia, peripheral neuritis
Vitamin B_{12} (cobalamin)	Megaloblastic anemia, demyelination, methylmalonic acidemia
Vitamin C	**Scurvy** (hematologic abnormalities, edema, spongy swelling of gums, poor wound healing, impaired collagen synthesis)
Folic acid	Megaloblastic anemia, neutropenia, impaired growth, diarrhea
Niacin	**Pellagra** (diarrhea, dermatitis, dementia), glossitis, stomatitis
Zinc	Skin lesions, poor wound healing, immune dysfunction, diarrhea, growth failure

B. Malnutrition

1. **Marasmus** is the **most common energy depletion state** and is characterized by near starvation from **protein and nonprotein deficiencies.** The patient is typically **very thin from loss of muscle and body fat.**

2. **Kwashiorkor** is **less common** and is seen in the parts of the world in which starches are the main dietary staple. This **protein-deficient** state is characterized by **generalized edema, abdominal distension, changes in skin pigmentation, and thin, sparse hair.**

3. Most patients suffering from malnutrition have a combination of energy and protein depletion. The term **protein-energy malnutrition** is used to describe this state.

II. Malabsorption

A. General Concepts

1. **Definition.** Malabsorption is the **inadequate absorption of nutrients** and is **most often characterized by diarrhea, abdominal distension, and impaired growth.**

2. **Normal physiology**

   a. **Digestion** is an intraluminal event requiring digestive enzymes and bile acids for micelle formation.

   b. **Absorption** requires an adequate intestinal mucosal surface and villous brush border with intact transport mechanisms.

3. **Pathophysiology and etiology**

a. **Carbohydrates**
   (1) **Undigested sugars are osmotically active** and draw water into the intestinal lumen, causing increased stool volume, increased peristaltic activity, and decreased transit time. This results in diminished digestion and absorption of nutrients.
      (a) Unabsorbed sugars are fermented by colonic bacteria, which produce hydrogen gas, carbon dioxide, and acids.
      (b) The resulting stool is watery and **acidic** and contains unabsorbed sugars detected as **reducing substances** by a **positive Clinitest** reaction. A stool pH below 5.6 suggests carbohydrate malabsorption.
   (2) **Causes** of carbohydrate malabsorption include **isolated congenital enzyme deficiency** (e.g., lactase deficiency) or **mucosal atrophy,** which can cause a loss of enzymes or a disruption of transport mechanisms.

b. **Proteins**
   (1) Dietary proteins are broken down into amino acids or oligopeptides by pepsinogen and pancreatic proteases in the proximal small intestine.
   (2) **Causes** of protein malabsorption
      (a) **Congenital enterokinase deficiency** is a rare cause of massive protein and nitrogen loss in the stool. **Hypoproteinemia** with resultant **edema and growth impairment** develops.
      (b) **Protein-losing enteropathies** result in hypoproteinemia as a result of transudation of protein from inflamed intestinal mucosa.
      (c) **Inflammatory disorders** of the intestinal mucosa, such as Crohn's disease (see section IX) and colitis, may also result in protein loss.
   (3) **Fecal α_1-antitrypsin levels** may be used to document enteric protein losses.

c. **Lipids**
   (1) Fats are insoluble in water and must be incorporated into bile salt micelles to be absorbed. Pancreatic lipase is a necessary enzyme that hydrolyzes triglycerides for emulsification.
   (2) **Decreased lipase activity** results in **steatorrhea** (fat in stool) and **decreased absorption of fat-soluble vitamins (vitamins A, D, E, and K).**
   (3) **Causes** of fat malabsorption
      (a) **Exocrine pancreatic insufficiency** (e.g., cystic fibrosis, Schwachman-Diamond syndrome, chronic pancreatitis)
      (b) Intestinal mucosal atrophy, bile acid deficiency, and abetalipoproteinemia

4. **Evaluation**
   a. **Stool studies** for fat, carbohydrates, pH, reducing substances, and α_1-antitrypsin should be performed.

b. A **compete blood count (CBC)** may be suggestive.

   (1) A macrocytic blood smear suggests folic acid or vitamin B_{12} deficiency.

   (2) Acanthocytosis of erythrocytes is seen in abetalipoproteinemia.

   (3) Neutropenia may suggest Schwachman-Diamond syndrome, an autosomal recessive disorder characterized by pancreatic exocrine insufficiency, failure to thrive (FTT), short stature, neutropenia, and sometimes pancytopenia.

c. **Low serum albumin** may be seen in protein-losing enteropathies.

d. **Infection with *Giardia lamblia*** can cause chronic malabsorption and can be diagnosed by stool studies (see Chapter 7, section XV.B.4).

e. **Small bowel biopsy** is used to diagnose celiac disease (see section II.C), abetalipoproteinemia, and some infectious disorders and enzyme deficiencies.

B. **Protein Intolerance**

1. **Definition.** Protein intolerance is characterized by diarrhea, vomiting, and colicky abdominal pain that occur after exposure to dietary protein.

2. **Epidemiology.** Protein intolerance occurs in up to 8% of children. **Cow's milk protein** causes the majority of these reactions. Other causes include soy and egg proteins.

3. **Clinical features**

   a. **Enteropathy,** which is characterized by progressive onset of diarrhea, vomiting, irritability, and abdominal pain. Chronic blood loss in the stool may lead to anemia, and significant stool protein loss may cause edema and FTT.

   b. **Enterocolitis,** which typically presents acutely with diarrhea, rectal bleeding, mucus in the stool, abdominal distension, and irritability. As with enteropathy, hypoproteinemia, edema, and FTT may develop.

4. **Diagnosis** is made by resolution of acute symptoms within a few days after complete withdrawal of the suspected antigen. Chronic symptoms usually resolve within 1–2 weeks.

5. **Management** includes withdrawal and avoidance of suspected dietary protein. Most protein intolerance is transitory and resolves by 1–2 years of age.

C. **Celiac Disease (Gluten-Sensitive Enteropathy)**

1. **Definition.** This autoimmune disorder of the proximal small intestine is characterized by **intolerance to gluten,** which results in mucosal damage.

2. **Epidemiology**

   a. Celiac disease is most common in regions where wheat is a staple in the diet (e.g., North America, Europe, Australia). In the United States, the incidence is as high as 1 in 250 individuals.

   b. Celiac disease generally presents between **6 months and 2 years of age** when gluten, found in **wheat, rye, barley,** and **oats** (if the oats are harvested in fields that also contain wheat), is introduced into the diet. The disease may sometimes present in adulthood.

  c. Individuals who are susceptible to celiac disease may have a **genetic predisposition.**

3. **Clinical features**
   a. The **primary symptoms** are **diarrhea, vomiting, bloating, anorexia, and sometimes FTT.** Diarrhea may not be present in all patients.
   b. Irritability is common in infants.
   c. Abdominal pain and large, foul-smelling stools are also common.

4. **Evaluation**
   a. **Small bowel biopsy** is the **gold standard** for diagnosis and demonstrates short, flat villi, deep crypts, and vacuolated epithelium with lymphocytes.
   b. A **clinical response** with weight gain and resolution of symptoms **when gluten is removed from the diet** also helps confirm the diagnosis.
   c. **Serum IgA-endomysial** and **serum tissue transglutaminase antibody testing** are extremely sensitive and specific screens for celiac disease, except in individuals with IgA deficiency. Serum antigliadin IgG antibody testing is useful for patients who are IgA deficient.

5. **Management**
   a. A strict **gluten-free diet for life** is necessary and results in complete reversal of intestinal damage. Vitamin and iron supplements may be required.
   b. Corticosteroids are used for severe diarrhea.
   c. Dietary changes in children often yield a rapid response, but noncompliance in adolescents is common and may lead to **growth failure** and **delayed sexual maturity.**

D. **Short Bowel Syndrome**

1. **Definition.** Patients with a shortened small intestine may have malabsorption resulting in malnutrition and compromised bowel function.

2. **Etiology**
   a. **Congenital lesions of the gut,** such as gastroschisis, volvulus, or intestinal atresia, may require surgical resection of the small intestine resulting in an inadequate absorptive surface area.
   b. Infants who have undergone intestinal surgery for necrotizing enterocolitis may have short bowel syndrome.
   c. Crohn's disease, tumors, and radiation enteritis may also lead to short bowel syndrome.

3. **Pathophysiology**
   a. The absorptive capacity of the bowel depends on the length and location of the resected segment and on the condition of the residual gut.
   b. After gut resection, **carbohydrate and fat malabsorption** with **steatorrhea** are common.
   c. Dehydration, hyponatremia, and hypokalemia may all occur if resorptive capacity is limited.
   d. **Distal** small bowel resection (i.e., ileum) limits **vitamin B_{12}** and **bile acid absorption.**

4. **Clinical features** include diarrhea, malabsorption, and FTT.

5. **Management**
   a. Short bowel syndrome was formerly a fatal disorder. The development of **total parenteral nutrition (TPN)** now allows patients to maintain adequate nutrition and significantly improves survival.
   b. **Early enteral feedings** are important to ensure adaptive growth of the remaining small bowel, proper hepatic function, and proper oral motor development.
   c. With proper management, patients may be able to wean off parenteral nutrition and survive. Adaptation of the intestine depends on the length and quality of the residual small bowel and on the presence of an intact ileocecal valve.
   d. **Small bowel transplantation** has been performed but is reserved for patients with coexisting life-threatening TPN-associated liver disease. Liver transplantation may also be required.

6. **Complications** include **TPN cholestasis** with resultant gallstones and cholestatic liver disease, **intestinal bacterial overgrowth, nutritional deficiencies, poor bone mineralization** and **renal stones** from hyperoxaluria, and **secretory diarrhea** as a result of the osmotic load on the remaining intestine.

III. Gastroesophageal Reflux

A. **Definitions**
   1. **Gastroesophageal reflux (GER)** is the **normal physiologic state** in which stomach contents move retrograde into the esophagus.
   2. **Gastroesophageal reflux disease (GERD)** is a **pathologic state** associated with **gastrointestinal (GI) or pulmonary symptoms and sequelae.** Ten percent of infants with GER have GERD.

B. **Normal physiology.** Normal periodic peristaltic waves of contraction of the esophagus transport ingested food into the stomach. The **lower esophageal sphincter (LES)** is a contracted circular muscle at the distal end of the esophagus that relaxes in a coordinated fashion with the peristaltic wave to allow esophageal contents to enter the stomach.

C. **Pathophysiology**
   1. **Inappropriate transient lower esophageal sphincter relaxation (TLESR) is the predominant cause of GERD during childhood.** Inappropriate TLESR allows excessive gastric refluxate to enter the esophagus and even the oropharynx. With time, prolonged contact of esophageal mucosa with gastric contents results in inflammation.
   2. **Gastric emptying delay** may also play a role in GERD by increasing the quantity of gastric refluxate and by increasing gastric distension, which induces more TLESR.

D. **Clinical features of physiologic reflux (GER)**
   1. Infants are termed "**happy spitters**" because they are without other re-

flux-associated symptoms. Up to 60% of all infants have episodes of spitting up or vomiting not related to overfeeding or gastrointestinal disease.

2. **Emesis is benign,** but often dramatic and traumatic for parents.

3. Efforts at parental education and reassurance are vital. Avoidance of aimless formula changes, inappropriate early weaning, medications, homeopathic remedies, or costly seats, straps, and slings is the goal.

4. Emesis generally resolves by 6–12 months of age.

E. **Clinical features of pathologic reflux (GERD)**

1. **Infants** may present with the following:

   a. **Emesis** is the **most common presentation.**

   b. Emesis may not always be present, or it may be so severe that it results in suboptimal calorie retention and **FTT.**

   c. **Sandifer syndrome** is a characteristic torticollis with arching of the back caused by painful esophagitis.

   d. **Feeding refusal** with irritability or **constant hunger** may indicate esophagitis. The irritated esophagus may be painful, negatively reinforcing feeding, or the child may desire the buffering action of milk to reduce acid irritation.

2. **Older children** usually present with the following:

   a. Symptoms of esophagitis, including **midepigastric pain** ("heartburn") that is temporarily relieved with food or antacids and is exacerbated by fatty foods, caffeine, and the supine position.

   b. Associated symptoms include nausea (especially on awakening), hoarseness, halitosis, and wheezing.

3. **Sequelae of GERD**

   a. **Upper and lower airway disease** may be induced or worsened by GERD. Acidic refluxate induces **bronchopulmonary constriction** and can also lead to frank aspiration or microaspiration. Common signs and symptoms include chronic laryngitis, hoarseness, wheezing, vocal cord nodules, and subglottic stenosis.

   b. **Gastrointestinal sequelae** include FTT, esophageal strictures, and **Barrett's esophagus** (conversion of the normal stratified squamous epithelium of the esophagus into columnar epithelium; this condition may be associated with esophageal adenocarcinoma).

4. Infants who remain symptomatic past 1 year of age and older children are unlikely to have spontaneous resolution of GERD and usually require long-term medical management or surgery.

F. **Diagnosis. Diagnostic evaluation** focuses on ensuring normal anatomy and confirming any abnormalities.

1. **Barium upper gastrointestinal (UGI) study** examines the **anatomy** of the esophagus, stomach, and duodenum. The UGI is a **poor test for diagnosis of GERD,** even if the refluxate is seen rising up to the oropharynx. Because TLESR is induced during administration of barium through a nasogastric tube, the sensitivity for GERD is high (85–90%) but the specificity is low (50%). Only frank aspiration of barium can be interpreted as GERD.

2. **Scintigraphy** uses a radioactive marker (e.g., technetium 99m) mixed into age-appropriate foods to measure the rate of gastric emptying. When slow-decay markers are used, radioactive tracer detected in the lungs confirms aspiration.

3. **pH probe measurement** is the **gold standard** for diagnosis.
   a. The pH of the esophagus is continuously monitored for at least 18 hours.
   b. Diagnosis of GERD is based on the number of acidification episodes, the total duration of esophageal acidification, and the time required for the pH to normalize in the presence of symptoms.
   c. **To interpret the pH probe correctly, results should be correlated with the clinical presentation.**

4. **Endoscopy with biopsy** to detect inflammation may be indicated when the diagnosis is uncertain.

5. **Bronchoscopy with alveolar lavage** is performed when aspiration is strongly suspected.

G. **Management. Treatment** includes attempts at reducing entry of stomach contents into the esophagus and relieving symptoms.

1. **Conservative management**
   a. **Positioning** in an **upright or sitting position** or raising the head of the bed after feedings or when asleep
   b. **Dietary** recommendations include frequent small meals and **thickening of feeds** using infant cereal or a commercial thickener, which attempts to hinder GERD by making the stomach contents more viscous. **Acid inhibition** with antacids, histamine H_2-blockers, and proton pump inhibitors is effective in reducing the irritation caused by the refluxate.

2. **Motility agents** increase the LES tone or increase gastric emptying. The most commonly used agent is **metoclopramide,** although side effects occur in up to one third of patients (e.g., drowsiness, restlessness, dystonic reactions).

3. **Surgery** may be required for patients who fail medical and conservative management.
   a. The **Nissen fundoplication** wraps the fundus of the stomach around the distal 3.5 cm of esophagus, resulting in reduction of TLESR in as many as 90% of children.
   b. Gastric antroplasty may be performed to improve gastric emptying.
   c. In infants, placement of a **gastrostomy tube** often accompanies a Nissen fundoplication. Reduction in stomach volume by the Nissen procedure requires a period of adaptation and expansion of the stomach best assisted with tube feedings.

IV. Intestinal Anatomic Obstructions That Result in Vomiting

A. **Hypertrophic Pyloric Stenosis**
1. **Definition.** Thickening of the circular pylorus muscle results in gastric outlet obstruction with projectile vomiting.

2. **Epidemiology**
   a. Incidence is 1 in 250 live births.
   b. **Caucasians and first-born male children are affected more commonly.** The male-to-female ratio is 4:1.

3. **Etiology**
   a. The **etiology is unknown.** Abnormal muscle innervation, breast-feeding, early administration of oral erythromycin, and decreased production of nitric oxide synthase have all been implicated.
   b. Associated conditions include duodenal atresia, tracheoesophageal fistula, trisomy 18, and Cornelia de Lange syndrome.

4. **Clinical features**
   a. Vomiting of **nonbilious,** milky fluid starts during the second or third week of life.
   b. Vomiting becomes more forceful, is often described as **projectile,** and typically occurs immediately after feeding.
   c. Affected infants may be **irritable but hungry.**
   d. Jaundice occurs in 5% of patients, and it is associated with low levels of glucuronyl transferase enzyme.
   e. Dehydration from vomiting may occur.

5. **Evaluation**
   a. **Physical examination**
      (1) The hypertrophied pylorus muscle may be palpable just above and to the right of the umbilicus. It is often referred to as the **"olive."**
      (2) Abdominal peristaltic waves may be visible after feeding.
   b. Prolonged vomiting of gastric contents classically results in **hypochloremic, hypokalemic, metabolic alkalosis.**
   c. **Diagnostic studies**
      (1) **Ultrasound** is able to measure the pylorus muscle length and thickness and is the **diagnostic method of choice.**
      (2) **UGI** may demonstrate an elongated, narrow pyloric channel **("string sign").**

6. **Management**
   a. **Electrolyte abnormalities and dehydration** should be corrected before surgery.
   b. Surgical correction is with a **partial pyloromyotomy,** in which the circular pylorus muscle fibers are transected.

B. **Malrotation and Midgut Volvulus**
   1. **Definition.** Malrotation is an anatomic abnormality of intestinal rotation that allows the midgut to twist around the superior mesenteric vessels (i.e., volvulus). This may obstruct and infarct the bowel.
   2. **Epidemiology**
      a. Incidence of malrotation is 1 in 500 live births, with a 2:1 **male predominance.**
      b. Malrotation is common in patients with heterotaxy and may be associated with small bowel atresia, Hirschsprung's disease, and intussusception.

3. **Pathogenesis.** The intestines normally return to the abdomen through the umbilical cord during the 10th week of gestation and undergo counterclockwise rotation about the axis of the superior mesenteric artery. The intestines are then fixed to the abdominal wall. Malrotation occurs when normal bowel rotation is interrupted.

   a. Lack of fixation of the small bowel results in peritoneal bands (**Ladd's bands**) that can compress the duodenum, causing mechanical obstruction.

   b. The narrow pedicle, which suspends the small bowel and the base of the superior mesenteric vessels, can easily twist, leading to ischemia and midgut volvulus.

4. **Clinical features**

   a. **Bilious vomiting** and **sudden onset of abdominal pain in an otherwise healthy infant** are the classic presentation. Older children may have intermittent, crampy abdominal pain and vomiting.

   b. Anorexia, distension, and blood-tinged stools are common.

   c. Physical examination may be initially normal with peritonitis occurring later. Shock and cardiovascular collapse may occur as bowel ischemia progresses.

5. **Evaluation**

   a. **Abdominal radiographs** may show gastric or proximal intestinal distension and obstruction, often with little or no distal bowel gas.

   b. **Upper intestinal contrast imaging** is the **diagnostic tool of choice** and shows abnormal position of the ligament of Treitz to the right of midline, partial or complete duodenal obstruction, and the jejunum to the right of midline.

   c. **Lower intestinal contrast studies** may reveal the cecum in the left abdomen or right upper quadrant.

6. **Management**

   a. Volvulus is a **surgical emergency** requiring immediate exploration, untwisting of the gut, resection of any nonviable segments of intestine, and fixation of the gut to prevent recurrence.

   b. **Fluid resuscitation,** nasogastric suctioning, and broad-spectrum parenteral antibiotics should be administered.

   c. TPN may be required if a large segment of bowel is resected.

C. **Atresias**

1. **Duodenal atresia and stenosis**

   a. **Definition.** Duodenal atresia is a congenital obstruction of the duodenum caused by failure of the lumen to recanalize at 8–10 weeks gestation.

   b. **Epidemiology**

      (1) Intestinal atresia is the **most common cause of obstruction** in the neonatal period.

      (2) Incidence is approximately 1 in 10,000 live births, with a **male predominance.**

      (3) One fourth of cases occur in patients with **Down syndrome.**

c. **Clinical features**

(1) Diagnosis may be suspected if prenatal ultrasound demonstrates gastric dilation with **polyhydramnios.**

(2) At birth, physical examination of patients with duodenal atresia may reveal a **scaphoid abdomen with epigastric distension.** Infants have feeding intolerance and vomiting.

(3) Duodenal stenosis may present with emesis, weight loss, and FTT.

(4) Other congenital defects (e.g., malrotation, esophageal atresia, congenital heart disease, renal anomalies) may also be present.

d. **Evaluation**

(1) **Abdominal radiography** shows air in the stomach and proximal duodenum, creating a **"double bubble"** sign.

(2) **Intestinal contrast studies** are very effective at diagnosing atresia and stenosis.

e. **Management**

(1) Nasogastric decompression, hydration, and correction of electrolyte abnormalities (typically hypochloremic metabolic alkalosis) are necessary.

(2) Atresia is surgically corrected by duodenoduodenostomy.

(3) Exploration for malrotation and other luminal obstructions is also performed at the time of surgical correction.

2. **Jejunoileal atresia**

a. **Definition.** This congenital obstruction of the jejunum or ileum is caused by a mesenteric vascular accident during fetal life.

b. **Epidemiology.** The incidence is approximately 1 in 3,000 live births. It is not usually associated with other anomalies.

c. **Clinical features.** Bilious emesis and abdominal distension occur within the first few days of life.

d. **Evaluation.** Abdominal **radiographs** reveal air-fluid levels, and **contrast studies** reveal the atresia.

e. **Management.** Patients should receive nasogastric suctioning and fluid resuscitation before surgical resection and anastomosis of the atretic segment of small bowel.

D. **Intussusception**

1. **Definition.** Intussusception is the telescoping or invagination of a more **proximal portion of intestine into a more distal portion.**

2. **Epidemiology.** The incidence is 1.5–4 in 1,000 live births, with a slight **male predominance.** Peak incidence occurs at **5–9 months of age.** It is the most common cause of bowel obstruction after the neonatal period in infants less than 2 years of age.

3. **Pathogenesis and etiology**

a. Intussusception may occur at a variety of sites within the intestine, but **ileocolic intussusception is the most common location.**

b. Etiology is generally unknown, but a **lead point** such as Meckel's diverticulum, polyp, intestinal duplication, Peyer's patch, or lymphoma may act to draw the proximal intestine inward. However, a lead point is identified in only 5% of cases and is **more common in older children.**

   c. Intussusception causes bowel wall edema and hemorrhage and may lead to bowel ischemia and infarction.

4. Clinical features

   a. Previously healthy infants or children may present with **sudden on-set of crampy or colicky abdominal pain.** The pain often occurs in intervals followed by periods of calm. Infants may cry and draw their legs toward the chest.

   b. Vomiting and lethargy are common.

   c. Stools may be normal or have a bloody, **"currant jelly"** appearance because of intestinal ischemia and mucosal sloughing.

   d. Occasionally, a **sausage-shaped mass** may be palpated in the abdominal right upper quadrant, representing the intussusception.

5. Evaluation

   a. Initial management should include fluid resuscitation.

   b. Radiographs are of limited usefulness but may reveal dilated loops of bowel, or pneumoperitoneum if perforation has occurred.

   c. Abdominal ultrasound may be a useful diagnostic tool, but **air or contrast enema** (barium or Gastrografin) **remains the gold standard,** both to establish the diagnosis and to reduce the intussusception. (Contrast enema may show the classic **"coil spring" sign** representing the intussusception.)

6. Management

   a. **Contrast enemas** with air or hydrostatic pressure successfully reduce the intussusception in 80–90% of cases.

   b. If the contrast enema fails to reduce the intussusception, or if the child has signs of peritonitis or pneumoperitoneum, **operative reduction** is indicated.

   c. The **risk of recurrence** is 5% after contrast reduction and 1% after surgical repair.

E. Hirschsprung's disease. This disorder may also cause vomiting and is described in Chapter 4, section XII.D.4.

V. Acute Abdominal Pain

A. General Concepts

   1. Definition. The term **acute abdomen** describes the sudden onset of abdominal pain that requires urgent evaluation, diagnosis, and treatment. Although most acute abdominal pain is self-limited, the pain may result from a serious medical or surgical cause and may require prompt surgical evaluation.

   2. Etiology (Figure 10-1)

   3. Evaluation

   a. **Complete history,** specifically including assessment for recent trauma, prior abdominal pain or surgery, infections, and medications. **Review of systems** should focus on associated symptoms of fever,

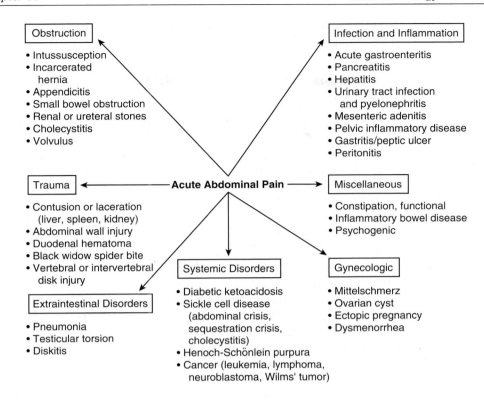

Figure 10-1. Etiology of acute abdominal pain during childhood.

vomiting, diarrhea, constipation, anorexia, dysuria, or worsening pain with eating. The timing of symptoms may provide key diagnostic information.

  b. Physical examination should include evaluations of the abdomen, chest, back, head and neck, and genitourinary system.

   (1) General assessment. Restlessness may indicate colicky pain. Abdominal rigidity is seen with a peritoneal process. Constant pain suggests strangulation of the gut or torsion.

   (2) Abdominal examination

   (a) Intestinal obstruction may present with high-pitched bowel sounds, abdominal distension, tenderness, and, at times, visible peristalsis.

   (b) Peritonitis presents with diminished or absent bowel sounds, abdominal wall rigidity, involuntary guarding, and often rebound tenderness.

  c. Accessory tests

   (1) Imaging studies may include abdominal radiography to identify obstruction, mass, or free air; ultrasound for evaluation of viscera and fluid; and CT scan (often with oral, intravenous, and/or rectal contrast) to visualize abdominal anatomy and pathology.

   (2) Laboratory evaluation should include a CBC, urinalysis, and metabolic panel. Hepatic function tests, amylase and lipase, and testing for pregnancy and sexually transmitted diseases should be performed, if indicated.

B. Specific Causes of Abdominal Pain

1. Appendicitis

a. **Definition.** Appendicitis is obstruction and inflammation of the appendix.

b. **Epidemiology.** Appendectomy is the **most common pediatric emergency operation.** Peak incidence is **10–12 years of age.**

c. **Pathophysiology.** The lumen of the appendix is obstructed by either a fecalith or by lymphoid tissue causing appendiceal distension and ischemia. This distension produces visceral pain referred to the T-10 dermatome or periumbilical region and the release of inflammatory mediators. Without surgical intervention, this process usually leads to perforation within 36 to 48 hours.

d. **Clinical features**

(1) **Symptoms** usually **begin with periumbilical pain,** followed by vomiting. Within hours, the pain usually localizes to the **right lower quadrant.** Fever and anorexia are usually present.

(2) **Physical examination** classically demonstrates tenderness to palpation at **McBurney's point** (an area two thirds of the way from the umbilicus to the anterior superior iliac spine). Voluntary guarding may progress to involuntary guarding and rebound tenderness as peritoneal irritation increases.

(3) **Laboratory findings** include leukocytosis with a polymorphonuclear predominance.

e. **Diagnosis** may be difficult in children, which contributes to a high rate of perforation (20–50%). Although **abdominal ultrasound or CT** often aids in diagnosis, the patient may undergo an appendectomy without having a definitive diagnosis in an attempt to prevent perforation.

f. **Management** consists of fluid resuscitation, preoperative antibiotics, and an appendectomy, often by laparoscopy. Perforated appendicitis requires drainage of purulent material, irrigation of the peritoneal cavity, and parenteral antibiotics.

2. Acute pancreatitis

a. **Definition.** Pancreatitis is an acute inflammatory process of the pancreas that may involve peripancreatic tissues and other organ systems.

b. **Epidemiology.** Pancreatitis is **uncommon** in children.

c. **Pathophysiology.** An initial insult, such as ductal obstruction or viral infection, causes premature activation of pancreatic proenzymes and autodigestion of pancreatic cells. Inflammatory mediators and cytokines damage the pancreas and cause interstitial edema and necrosis. Necrosis of blood vessels may lead to parenchymal hemorrhage.

d. **Etiology. Causes** include blunt **trauma (most common), infections** (e.g., mumps, enterovirus, Epstein-Barr virus [EBV], HIV, hepatitis A and B), drugs and toxins, congenital anomalies, and obstruction. Less commonly, acute pancreatitis may be the result of a systemic illness, such as systemic lupus erythematosus or cystic fibrosis. **Idiopathic pancreatitis accounts for up to 25% of cases in children and is the second most common cause of pancreatitis during childhood.**

e. **Clinical features**

(1) Abdominal pain occurs in the **periumbilical or epigastric area** and may radiate to the back.

(2) Fever, anorexia, nausea, and vomiting are common.

(3) Physical examination reveals epigastric tenderness, abdominal distension, and decreased bowel sounds. **Gray-Turner sign** (bluish discoloration of the flanks) or **Cullen sign** (bluish discoloration of the periumbilical area) may be present in severe cases and is caused by blood tracking along fascial planes.

(4) Hypotension, tachycardia, hypoxia, and capillary leak may be seen in severe, acute hemorrhagic pancreatitis.

f. **Evaluation**

(1) **Serum amylase** levels rise within hours of pain onset and remain elevated for 4–5 days. **Serum lipase** level elevation is **more specific** for acute pancreatitis and remains elevated longer than serum amylase levels.

(2) **Other laboratory abnormalities** may include leukocytosis, hyperglycemia, hypocalcemia, elevated transaminases, and coagulopathy.

(3) **Abdominal ultrasound** is the most common method used for diagnosing and monitoring acute pancreatitis. **Abdominal CT** is useful in diagnosing complications, such as **pseudocyst,** abscess, or necrosis.

g. **Management**

(1) **Supportive care** includes bed rest, hydration, electrolyte correction, analgesia, and nasogastric suctioning. Oral feedings usually are restricted to minimize pancreatic stimulation.

(2) **TPN** is essential to prevent protein catabolism because some patients may not be able to tolerate oral feedings for weeks.

(3) **Antibiotics** are indicated for severe, acute necrotizing pancreatitis.

(4) **Surgery** to remove necrotic tissue within and around the pancreas may be indicated. However, surgical intervention for early, acute pancreatitis is controversial.

h. **Complications.** Conditions include respiratory insufficiency and acute respiratory distress syndrome (ARDS), renal failure, shock, and gastrointestinal bleeding. A **pseudocyst** (collection of fluid rich in pancreatic enzymes that arises from pancreatic tissue) may develop. A small pseudocyst resolves on its own; however, a large, persistent pseudocyst may require surgical drainage.

3. **Cholecystitis**

a. **Definition.** Inflammation of the gallbladder with transmural edema that may be associated with gallstones, or less commonly, without stones (termed **acute acalculous cholecystitis**).

    b. Epidemiology. In contrast to adults, acute cholecystitis is uncommon in healthy children. However, it may occur in children with predisposing conditions such as **sickle cell disease,** cystic fibrosis, or prolonged TPN therapy.

    c. Pathophysiology and etiology

       (1) Obstruction of the cystic duct causes increased intraluminal pressure and distension, increased secretion of enzymes and prostaglandins, and progressive inflammation. Infection, necrosis, and perforation may all occur.

       (2) Acute acalculous cholecystitis is usually caused by infection (e.g., *Salmonella, Shigella, Escherichia coli*) but may also be seen after abdominal trauma, burns, or vasculitis.

    d. Clinical features

       (1) Abdominal pain is initially diffuse but eventually worsens and localizes to the **right upper quadrant.**

       (2) Fever, anorexia, and vomiting are common.

       (3) Jaundice may be a late finding.

       (4) Physical examination may reveal **Murphy's sign** (i.e., palpation of the right upper quadrant during inspiration elicits intense pain and causes the patient to stop inspiratory effort). Guarding and peritoneal signs may also be present.

    e. Evaluation

       (1) Diagnosis is confirmed by **abdominal ultrasound,** which can detect stones and a thickened gallbladder wall.

       (2) Cholescintigraphy may be useful.

       (3) Laboratory findings may include mild elevations of bilirubin and serum transaminases.

    f. Management. Treatment includes fluid resuscitation, parenteral antibiotics, and analgesia. If the disease progresses or if peritonitis develops, **cholecystectomy** is indicated. This procedure is often performed laparoscopically and may be done electively after the acute episode resolves.

VI. Chronic Abdominal Pain

  A. Definitions. Chronic abdominal pain (CAP) is defined as **abdominal pain that occurs each month for at least 3 consecutive months.**

    1. Organic (caused by a disease process or disorder; one third of cases)

    2. Nonorganic (functional; two thirds of cases). Functional CAP occurs more commonly in **females.**

  B. Epidemiology. CAP occurs in 20–40% of children and adolescents.

  C. Etiology

    1. Organic CAP (Table 10-2)

    2. Nonorganic CAP. Note: It is important to understand that the **patient senses real pain, even in the absence of an underlying organic cause.**

Table 10-2. Organic Causes of Chronic Abdominal Pain

Constipation
Peptic ulcer disease
Carbohydrate intolerance (e.g., lactose, fructose, sorbitol)
Inflammatory bowel disease
Pancreatitis
Parasitic infection (e.g., *Giardia lamblia* infection)
Genitourinary disorders (e.g., pyelonephritis, hydronephrosis)
Congenital structural abnormalities of the gastrointestinal tract (e.g., malrotation, intestinal duplication, hernia)

   a. Classification is based on clinical features.
     (1) Epigastric pain, associated with belching, bloating, nausea, vomiting, and early satiety, is the childhood equivalent of **nonulcer dyspepsia** in adults.
     (2) Periumbilical pain represents **classic functional abdominal pain (FAP)**. FAP is most likely in a child **older than 5 years of age.**
       (a) The **pain may be varied in character,** including paroxysmal, dull, sharp, or cramping.
       (b) The **pain confers secondary gain, does not interfere with pleasurable activities or sleep,** and has no consistent temporal correlation to activity, meals, or bowel patterns.
     (3) Infraumbilical pain, associated with abdominal cramping, bloating, and alterations in stool, is the childhood equivalent of **irritable bowel syndrome** in adults.
   b. Etiology. Although the cause in unknown, the following are risk factors that predispose to the development of nonorganic CAP:
     (1) Psychosocial risk factors include **personality** (e.g., timid, nervous, anxious, overachiever), **birth order** (e.g., first-born and last-born), **life stressors,** including change in daily routine (e.g., nanny, change in school), family stressors (e.g., divorce, separation, parental fighting), and methods of discipline that are either too extreme or submissive.
     (2) Risk factors relating to family history include alcoholism, antisocial or conduct disorders, attention deficit hyperactivity disorder, and family members with functional pain syndromes (e.g., headaches, CAP, musculoskeletal pain).
     (3) Risk factors relating to past medical history
       (a) Maternal: pregnancy problems, intrapartum problems (e.g., labor difficulties, cesarean section)
       (b) Child: neonatal problems (e.g., colic), childhood problems (e.g., enuresis, nightmares)
     (4) Some children also have **minor GI disturbances** in motility or in their sympathetic or parasympathetic nervous systems that make them susceptible to risk factors for nonorganic CAP.
D. Evaluation. A detailed history focusing on symptoms and risk factors for nonorganic CAP, and a comprehensive physical examination with special attention to the abdominal and genitourinary systems are necessary to ex-

clude organic disease. **The healthier the child appears, the more likely the pain is functional.**

1. **Laboratory evaluation** should be tempered and based on examination or clinical symptoms.

   a. **Screening laboratories** include CBC, electrolytes, liver function panel, stool for occult blood, stool for parasite screening, and erythrocyte sedimentation rate (ESR) or C-reactive protein.

   b. Screening for *Helicobacter pylori* should be reserved for children with symptoms of dyspepsia because the asymptomatic carriage rate of *H. pylori* is high during childhood.

   c. **Lactose breath hydrogen testing** to rule out lactose intolerance is a reasonable option because lactose intolerance may be present in as many as 10% of otherwise asymptomatic children.

2. **Radiographic studies** are not routinely indicated unless warranted by the history or physical examination.

E. **Management**

1. **Organic CAP** is treated on the basis of the specific diagnosis.

2. **FAP**

   a. **Goals of therapy** include normalization of the child's activities, education of parents as to the nature of the disorder, and development of methods to empower the child and family to control the discomfort.

   b. **Family and individual counseling** are usually necessary.

   c. **Symptomatic medications,** such as antispasmodics, sedatives, or analgesics, are ineffective.

F. **Prognosis.** Long-term prognosis of FAP is poor. Only 50% of patients have complete symptom resolution during childhood, and at least 25% of patients have abdominal pain as adults. Poor prognostic factors include male gender, age of onset < 6 years, duration of symptoms > 6 months, maximum parental education less than high school, lower socioeconomic status, a history of abdominal operations, and having unresolved family issues.

VII. Constipation and Encopresis

A. **Definitions**

1. **Constipation** is defined as a **reduction in defecation** that causes adverse symptoms that may include difficult defecation, painful defecation, abdominal discomfort, and stool retention. Stools are often dry and hard.

2. **Encopresis** is defined as the **developmentally inappropriate release of stool,** unrelated to an organic etiology. **Encopresis is almost always associated with severe constipation:** liquid stool leaks around a hard, retained stool mass and is involuntarily released through the distended anorectal canal.

B. **Epidemiology**

1. Constipation is **very common** during childhood.

   2. Age of onset usually occurs during infancy for organic causes of constipation, and after toilet training for functional constipation.

   3. Encopresis is seen predominantly in **males.**

C. Normal stool patterns. Normal defecation frequency varies with age with
   an adult pattern developed by 4 years of age.

   1. Frequency averages 4×/day during the first week of life, 2×/day by 1 year
   of age, and 1×/day by 4 years of age.

   2. Adult defecation ranges from 3×/day to 3×/week.

   3. Breastfed infants defecate more frequently during the first months
   of life; however, this decreases rapidly so that there is no difference in
   stool pattern between breastfed and formula-fed infants by 4 months of
   age.

D. Etiology. Constipation may be **functional** or **organic.**

   1. Functional fecal retention (FFR) is the **most common form of constipation during childhood** and results from inappropriate constriction of the external anal sphincter.

   a. Pathophysiology and etiology

   (1) Infants and toddlers may inappropriately retain stool as a **result
   of traumatic events** (e.g., hard stool, painful diarrhea, diaper
   rash, physical abuse) leading to a self-fulfilling cycle of increased
   fecal mass, fecal hardness, and painful defecation.

   (2) Although **behavioral** in pathophysiology, some FFR patients
   also have subclinical disturbances in the defecation process predisposing them to constipation.

   b. Clinical features. FFR becomes a behavioral pattern of stool with-
   holding that may lead to large amounts of retained feces with secondary anorectal distension, encopresis, fecal halitosis, abdominal
   distension and pain, anorexia, urinary tract problems (from pelvic
   displacement), and psychosocial problems.

   2. Organic causes represent **fewer than 5%** of cases of childhood constipation and are **usually present early in infancy.**

   a. Hirschsprung's disease is the **most common cause of organic
   constipation** in an otherwise healthy child (see Chapter 4, section
   XII.D.4 for details).

   b. Table 10-3 lists other organic causes of constipation.

E. Evaluation. It is necessary to focus on determining whether organic constipation or FFR exists. While FFR is the most likely cause, a thorough history and physical examination (including a complete neurologic examination) must be conducted to identify the presence of an organic etiology.

   1. Delayed meconium passage (> 48 hours after birth), onset of constipation during infancy, history of pelvic surgery, encopresis before 3 years of
   age, and inability to toilet train all suggest an **organic cause.**

   2. Development of constipation after toilet training, identification of a **sen-
   tinel event** (e.g., diarrhea, change in psychosocial environment, inappropriate toilet training methods, abuse) with continued normal growth
   and development all suggest **FFR.**

Table 10-3. Organic Causes of Constipation

Hirschsprung's disease
Neuroenteric dysfunction secondary to ischemia, trauma, spinal cord abnormality
Medications (e.g., narcotics, sedatives)
Low-fiber feeding regimens
Anatomic abnormalities (e.g., stricture, adhesion, anteriorly displaced anus)
Systemic disease (e.g., **dehydration,** celiac disease, **hypothyroidism, cystic fibrosis,** diabetes mellitus)
Infant botulism
Lead toxicity
Anorexia nervosa

        3. **Diagnostic studies** are only necessary when organic disease is suspected, or if the patient with FFR is failing management. Radiographic studies may include a barium enema, rectal biopsy to rule out Hirschsprung's disease, and manometry studies.

    F. **Management.** Treatment is based on the suspected cause.

        1. Mild, episodic constipation can usually be addressed by ensuring the diet contains adequate **soluble fibers** and by increasing the amount of water and sorbitol-containing juices.

        2. FFR management is based on **cleaning out the fecal mass, softening the stool,** and **educating** the patient and family.

           a. **Stool evacuation** is necessary to begin recovery and is performed using high-dose mineral oil, polyethylene glycol solutions, enemas, or manual disimpaction.

           b. **Maintenance therapy** most often includes **mineral oil** to soften and lubricate the stool.

           c. **Education is the most important intervention.** Emphasis is placed on identification and correction of triggers, creation of a regular toilet schedule, removal of negative reinforcements, and creation of a positive environment. Individual and family counseling may be helpful.

VIII. Diarrhea (see Chapter 7, section XI)

IX. Inflammatory Bowel Disease (IBD)

    A. **Definition.** This group of chronic, inflammatory gastrointestinal disorders includes **ulcerative colitis (UC)** and **Crohn's disease (CD)** and is characterized by exacerbations and remissions.

    B. **Epidemiology**

        1. The **age of onset is bimodal,** with a peak at 15–20 years of age and a second peak after 50 years of age.

           a. IBD is **increasing in frequency in children,** with 25–30% of all cases of CD and 20% of UC cases presenting before 20 years of age.

    b. Four percent of patients present before 5 years of age.

  2. Males and females appear equally affected by UC, but there is a 2:1 male-to-female ratio in CD.

  3. Positive family history for IBD is found in approximately 15–20% of patients.

C. Clinical Features

  1. Ulcerative colitis (Table 10-4)

    a. Inflammation is diffuse, limited to the **mucosa,** and **localized to the colon.** UC usually begins in the **rectum** and extends proximally in a **contiguous** fashion.

      (1) Disease of the rectum only is called **ulcerative proctitis.**

      (2) Disease affecting the entire colon is known as **pancolitis.**

    b. Severity

      (1) Mild disease, seen in 60% of cases, presents with rectal bleeding, diarrhea, and abdominal pain.

      (2) Moderate disease, seen in 30% of cases, presents with nocturnal stooling, cramping, and tenesmus. **Systemic symptoms** of weight loss, anorexia, fever, and anemia also occur.

      (3) Severe disease, seen in 10% of cases, presents with more than six stools per day, fever, anemia, leukocytosis, and hypoalbuminemia.

    c. Extraintestinal manifestations are less common during childhood (Table 10-4).

    d. Complications of severe UC

      (1) Toxic megacolon. This severe inflammation of the colon leads to decreased intestinal motility, disruption of the mucosal barrier which allows bacteria to enter, and colonic dilatation. Patients present with **fever, abdominal distension,** and **septic shock,** and they are at risk for perforation and hemorrhage.

      (2) Increased risk of colon cancer

  2. Crohn's disease (Table 10-4)

    a. CD may involve **any segment of the gastrointestinal tract,** from the mouth to anus.

      (1) Unlike UC, the inflammation is eccentric and **segmental** with **"skip lesions."**

      (2) Inflammation is **transmural** and may lead to sinus tracts, fistulas, and crypt abscesses.

      (3) Most children have disease involving the **terminal ileum.**

    b. Intestinal symptoms include abdominal pain, postprandial cramping, diarrhea, and anorexia.

      (1) Initial symptoms may be subtle, with abdominal pain or decreased growth the only findings.

      (2) Small bowel disease often leads to **malabsorption** with resultant iron, zinc, folate, and vitamin B_{12} deficiencies.

      (3) Perianal disease often precedes the development of intestinal disease and presents with skin tags, fissures, fistulas, and abscesses.

Table 10-4. Differentiation of Ulcerative Colitis and Crohn's Disease

Characteristic	Ulcerative Colitis	Crohn's Disease
Location	Colon	Any segment of gastro-intestinal tract, especially terminal ileum
Rectal bleeding	Frequent	Occasional
Rectal disease	Almost always	Occasional
Perianal disease (skin tags, fistulas, fissures, abscesses)	Rare	Common
Lesions	Contiguous lesions	Skip lesions
Transmural involvement	No	Yes
Extraintestinal manifestations	Uveitis, arthropathy, **pyoderma gangrenosum,** sclerosing cholangitis	FTT, delayed sexual development, oral aphthous ulcers, erythema nodosum, arthritis, renal stones
Serologic testing	**Antineutrophil cytoplasmic antibody** positive in 80%	**Anti-*Saccharomyces cerevisiae* antibody** positive in 70%
Complications	Toxic megacolon	Strictures, fistulas, abscesses
Risk of colon cancer	Significantly increased	Somewhat increased

FTT = failure to thrive.

    c. Extraintestinal complications are more common than in UC and are noted in **Table 10-4.**

    d. Complications are caused by the transmural nature of CD and include abscesses, fistulas, strictures, and adhesions.

    e. CD is a **chronic** disorder with high morbidity but low mortality. Patients are prone to **frequent exacerbations** despite treatment.

D. Evaluation. In addition to a history and physical examination, the following are generally indicated:

    1. Laboratory analyses

        a. CBC often shows anemia or leukocytosis.

        b. ESR is usually elevated.

        c. Serum albumin and **serum transaminases** to assess nutritional status and liver disease

        d. Serum antibody tests may help establish a diagnosis (see Table 10-4).

    2. Stool studies should be performed to rule out infectious enteropathies.

    3. Abdominal ultrasound and **CT imaging** can be used to visualize abscesses and thickened bowel walls. **UGI** with small bowel follow through can reveal mucosal ulcerations, narrowed lumens, thickened walls, and fistulas.

    4. Colonoscopy with biopsies of the colon and terminal ileum confirms the diagnosis.

E. Management. Treatment principles include controlling symptoms, reducing recurrences, and optimizing nutrition.

    1. Pharmacotherapy

    a. Sulfasalazine is effective for mild disease, especially for UC, and can also prevent relapses.

    b. Corticosteroids are often given to calm acute exacerbations and induce remission.

    c. Immunosuppressive agents are useful in inducing long-term remission.

    d. Metronidazole is used in the treatment of CD, especially for perianal involvement.

2. Surgery

    a. UC can be cured with a total proctocolectomy, but this is reserved for intractable colitis.

    b. Surgical therapy for CD is only considered for persistent bleeding, abscesses, and fistulas that do not respond to medical therapy. **Recurrence rate is high after bowel resection.**

3. Nutrition. Total parenteral nutrition may be necessary during flare-ups to ensure adequate growth and healing.

X. Gastrointestinal Bleeding

A. Definitions. Blood loss from the GI tract may occur in several ways, and the presentation may help determine origin of the bleeding.

    1. Hematemesis is the vomiting of fresh or old blood, which may have a "coffee ground" appearance from the denaturing of hemoglobin.

    2. Hematochezia is bright red blood passed per rectum, usually indicating a lower GI source or a significant rapid bleed from an upper lesion.

    3. Melena is dark, tarry stools and often indicates an upper GI bleed **proximal to the ligament of Treitz.**

B. Laboratory confirmation of GI bleeding. Occult bleeding from the GI tract is confirmed by positive guaiac testing of stool. Guaiac is a colorless dye that changes color from the peroxidase activity of hemoglobin in the presence of hydrogen peroxide developer.

    1. False-positive results may occur because of ingested iron, rare red meats, beets, and foods with a high peroxidase content, such as cantaloupe, broccoli, and cauliflower.

    2. False-negative results may occur as a result of large ingested doses of vitamin C.

C. Upper GI Bleeding

    1. Etiology

        a. Newborns may **swallow maternal blood** during delivery or while nursing from a bleeding nipple. Older children may swallow blood during an episode of **epistaxis** and can present with emesis that mimics a GI bleed.

        b. Gastritis or ulcers may occur as a result of severe stress of illness, surgery or burns, or from medications. Ulcers may also develop in children with *H. pylori* infection.

      c. Mechanical injury to the mucosa from vomiting (i.e., **Mallory-Weiss tear**) or from foreign body or caustic ingestion may cause upper GI bleeding.

      d. **Varices** as a result of portal hypertension or vascular malformations are less common causes.

  2. Evaluation

      a. Initial assessment must include a detailed **history and physical examination.**

         (1) Particular attention must be given to the patient's **hemodynamic status.**

         (2) Ongoing bleeding is assessed by obtaining a **nasogastric tube aspirate** for fresh blood.

         (3) **Nose and oropharynx** should be inspected for non-GI sources of bleeding.

      b. **Laboratory studies** should include hemoglobin and platelet counts, coagulation studies, serum transaminases, and a blood urea nitrogen (BUN) level (suggests GI bleed if elevated). Patients with active bleeding or hemodynamic changes should have blood sent for type and crossmatch.

      c. **Plain film radiography** has a **limited role** in diagnosis but may be useful if a foreign body or perforation is suspected.

      d. **Upper intestinal endoscopy** for diagnosis and management is indicated for active bleeding with hemodynamic changes.

  3. Management

      a. Initial **stabilization** of hypovolemia and anemia is essential. Intravenous access with two large-bore peripheral lines should be established, and a rapid **fluid bolus** of 20 mL/kg of normal saline solution should be given as needed. (See Chapter 20, section II.D for a discussion of the management of shock.)

      b. **Medical therapy** to control UGI bleeding may be useful. Octreotide (vasopressin) can be used to vasoconstrict varices. Ulcers associated with *H. pylori* should be treated with appropriate antibiotic therapy. Gastritis, esophagitis, and ulcers should also be treated with methods to decrease acid production, such as H_2-blockers or proton pump inhibitors.

      c. **Endoscopic therapy** (e.g., photocoagulation, banding, vessel ligation, injection with sclerosing agents) is indicated for active bleeding or if rebleeding is very likely.

      d. **Arteriographic embolization** may be used for serious bleeding from vascular malformations.

      e. **Surgical treatment** is usually indicated for duodenal ulcers with active arterial bleeding, perforation, or varices.

D. Lower GI Bleeding

  1. Etiology. Age is an important factor in determining the cause of lower GI bleeding (**Table 10-5**).

      a. **Necrotizing enterocolitis** should be considered in any newborn who presents with rectal bleeding, feeding intolerance, or abdominal distension (see Chapter 4, section XII.E).

Table 10-5. Differential Diagnosis of Lower Gastrointestinal Bleeding

Neonate (birth-1 month)	Infant/Young Child (1 month-2 years)	Preschool Age (2-5 years)	School Age (> 5 years)	Adolescent (10-21 years)
Swallowed maternal blood	Anal fissure	Infectious colitis	Infectious colitis	Infectious colitis
Allergic colitis	Allergic colitis	Juvenile polyp	Juvenile polyp	Juvenile polyp
Necrotizing enterocolitis	Infectious colitis	Meckel's diverticulum	Inflammatory bowel disease	Inflammatory bowel disease
Hirschsprung's disease	Hirschsprung's disease	Hemolytic uremic syndrome	Swallowed blood (e.g., epistaxis)	Mallory-Weiss tear
Volvulus	Intussusception	Henoch-Schönlein purpura	Mallory-Weiss tear	Peptic ulcer/gastritis
	Meckel's diverticulum	Swallowed blood (e.g., epistaxis)		
	Intestinal duplication	Mallory-Weiss tear		
	Vascular malformation			

    b. Juvenile polyps are the **most common cause** of significant lower GI bleeding beyond infancy. Bleeding is painless, intermittent, and often streaky. Colonoscopy with polypectomy is the definitive treatment.

    c. Hirschsprung's disease may present with colitis and abdominal distension.

    d. Allergic colitis from sensitization to protein antigens in cow's milk, soy milk, or breast milk may develop in neonates and infants.

    e. Infectious enterocolitis from bacterial pathogens such as *Salmonella, Shigella, Campylobacter, Yersinia,* and *E. coli* can occur at any age (see Chapter 7, Table 7-6).

    f. Meckel's diverticulum is an outpouching of the bowel in the terminal ileum that occurs in 2% of infants. It is an important cause of lower GI bleeding in infants and children. The diverticulum contains ectopic gastric mucosa that produces acid. This acid damages adjacent intestinal mucosa, causing the classic presentation of **painless, acute rectal bleeding** in an otherwise healthy child. A nuclear medicine scan identifies the **ectopic gastric mucosa,** and surgical resection is required.

    g. Ischemic diseases and vasculitis can also cause lower GI bleeding.

        (1) Hemolytic uremic syndrome is a vasculitis characterized by microangiopathic hemolytic anemia, thrombocytopenia, and acute renal failure. Intestinal ulceration and infarction of the bowel cause bleeding (see Chapter 11, section VI).

        (2) Henoch-Schönlein purpura is an IgA-mediated vasculitis that presents with a palpable, purpuric rash on the buttocks and lower extremities, large joint arthralgias, renal involvement, and GI bleeding from complications such as intussusception and bowel perforation (see Chapter 11, section IV.F.3 and Chapter 16, section I).

    h. Inflammatory bowel disease is an important cause of occult and frank GI bleeding.

  2. Evaluation and management. As with upper GI bleeding, assessment of hemodynamic status, monitoring for ongoing bleeding, and stabilization are essential. Laboratory studies, intravenous access, and fluid resuscitation are indicated as for upper GI bleeding. Specific management is based on the identified cause.

XI.   Liver Abnormalities and Hepatitis

A. General Concepts

  1. Hepatic injury

    a. Direct hepatocellular damage or damage to the biliary system results in derangements in the liver's synthetic ability, excretory function, or detoxification.

    b. Cellular damage also leads to the release of intracellular enzymes characteristic of the originating cell.

     c. Obstruction or damage to the biliary system causes retention of bile enzymes that damage the cells lining the biliary tree and hepatocytes.

B. Laboratory assessment of liver injury and function

  1. Hepatocellular enzymes

    a. Aspartate aminotransferase (AST) elevation is a **sensitive but nonspecific marker** of hepatocyte injury. AST is also found in skeletal muscle, red blood cells, and cardiac tissue.

    b. Alanine aminotransferase (ALT) elevation is a **very specific marker of liver disease.**

    c. Lactate dehydrogenase (LDH) elevation is nonspecific for liver disease, although it may serve as a marker for hepatocellular necrosis.

  2. Biliary enzymes

    a. Alkaline phosphatase may be elevated in biliary disease, although it may also be elevated in children because of rapid growth, in bone, kidney, and intestinal disease, and in trauma.

    b. Gamma glutamyl transpeptidase (GGTP) and 5′-nucleotidase (5NT) are also elevated in biliary disease. 5NT is more specific than GGTP for biliary tract damage.

  3. Bilirubin is derived from the breakdown of heme.

    a. Unconjugated (indirect) bilirubin is combined with glucuronide by the enzyme **UDP-glucuronyl transferase** in the liver to form mono- and di-conjugates (**conjugated or direct bilirubin**).

    b. Elevated bilirubin may be a consequence of **increased heme load** (e.g., hemolysis, polycythemia, hematoma), **decreased capacity for excretion** (e.g., hepatitis, liver failure), or **obstruction to bile flow** (e.g., biliary atresia, choledochal cyst).

  4. Synthetic function is assessed by evaluating protein production (e.g., **prealbumin, albumin,** and **prothrombin time**), serum chemistries (e.g., **glucose, cholesterol**), and toxin clearance (e.g., **lactate, ammonia**).

C. Infant Jaundice (Neonatal jaundice is discussed in Chapter 4, section X.)

  1. Definitions

    a. Infant jaundice is defined as elevated bilirubin after the neonate period and within the first year of life. Bilirubin collects in the skin, conjunctiva, and mucous membranes and becomes evident clinically when the total bilirubin level exceeds 3 mg/dL.

    b. Cholestatic jaundice is defined as **retention of bile within the liver** and occurs clinically when the **direct component of bilirubin is > 2 mg/dL or ≥ 15% of the total bilirubin.**

  2. Epidemiology

    a. As many as 50% of all neonates or infants experience transient jaundice, the majority of whom have **unconjugated (indirect) hyperbilirubinemia.**

    b. Conjugated (direct) hyperbilirubinemia is a marker for cholestasis. Cholestasis occurs in 1 in 10,000–15,000 live births, and more than **50% are caused by neonatal hepatitis or biliary atresia** (see section XI.D.2.3).

3. **Clinical features**

a. Jaundice typically **begins cranially and extends caudally** as bilirubin increases.

b. Infants often **appear otherwise well.**

4. **Evaluation.** It is important to focus on establishing whether cholestasis exists and whether the problem is isolated to the liver.

a. **History** should focus on timing of jaundice onset, associated symptoms (e.g., poor growth, bleeding, dark urine), feeding regimen (e.g., breast or bottle, frequency of feedings), and stool quality and color.

b. **Past medical history** should include prenatal history, medications, infections, and family history of liver disease or jaundice.

c. **Physical examination** should be comprehensive.

d. **Laboratory evaluation** should initially include CBC, electrolytes, and assessments of hepatic function. Further testing is directed on the basis of clinical suspicions. **It is difficult to predict the level of bilirubin from the extent of jaundice on physical examination. Measurement of direct and total bilirubin is therefore necessary in all patients with suspected jaundice.**

e. **Imaging** often includes abdominal ultrasound with Doppler evaluation of the hepatic vessels. Radionucleotide imaging (e.g., hepatobiliary iminodiacetic acid [HIDA] scan) of the biliary tree is warranted in suspected cholestasis.

f. **Liver biopsy** is invasive and is reserved for confirmation of diagnosis, assessment for hepatic injury, or when the evaluation remains inconclusive.

5. **Categories of jaundice**

a. The differential diagnosis of **unconjugated hyperbilirubinemia** is presented in **Chapter 4, section X.C** and **Figure 4-2.** Two additional causes of unconjugated hyperbilirubinemia are worth noting.

(1) **Inspissated bile syndrome** is associated with **hemolysis** (e.g., ABO incompatibility) or with a very large **hematoma.** In these cases, the biliary system becomes overwhelmed by the increased bilirubin load. Although unconjugated hyperbilirubinemia predominates early, conjugated hyperbilirubinemia eventually develops as hepatocellular function increases to meet demand.

(2) **UDP-glucuronyl transferase deficiency** can present in three distinct states.

(a) **Gilbert's syndrome,** in which **50% of enzyme activity is absent. Mild** unconjugated bilirubinemia occurs associated with stress or poor nutrition.

(b) **Crigler-Najjar type 1** is an **autosomal recessive** disorder in which **almost 100% of enzyme activity is absent.** Kernicterus caused by extremely high bilirubin levels occurs almost universally.

(c) **Crigler-Najjar type 2** is an **autosomal dominant** disorder in which **90% of enzyme activity is absent.** Bilirubin levels are more variable with a lower likelihood of kernicterus.

   b. The differential diagnosis of **conjugated hyperbilirubinemia** is presented in **Chapter 4, section X.D** and **Figure 4-3.**

D. Cholestatic Diseases of Infancy

  1. General concepts

    a. Cholestasis is characterized by retention of bile within the liver with **prolonged elevation of conjugated (direct) bilirubin.**

    b. Etiology

      (1) Infections (e.g., sepsis, hepatitis, viral infections)

      (2) Metabolic derangements (e.g., cystic fibrosis, hypothyroidism, galactosemia)

      (3) Extrahepatic mechanical obstruction (e.g., biliary atresia, bile duct stricture)

      (4) Intrahepatic mechanical obstruction (e.g., paucity of intrahepatic bile ducts, Alagille syndrome)

      (5) Idiopathic (e.g., neonatal hepatitis)

      (6) α_1-Antitrypsin deficiency

      (7) TPN-associated disease

    c. Clinical features of cholestasis

      (1) Jaundice

      (2) Acholic or light stools

      (3) Dark urine

      (4) Hepatomegaly

      (5) Bleeding (occurs as a result of prolongation of the prothrombin time as a result of diminished hepatic synthetic function)

      (6) FTT

  2. Neonatal hepatitis

    a. Definition. Neonatal hepatitis is **idiopathic hepatic inflammation** during the neonatal period. It is a **diagnosis of exclusion** and is the **most common cause of cholestasis in the newborn.**

    b. Epidemiology. Incidence is 1 in 5,000–10,000 live births, with a **male predisposition.**

    c. Clinical features

      (1) Symptoms may range from transient jaundice and acholic stools to liver failure, cirrhosis, and portal hypertension.

      (2) Presenting features in the first week of life include jaundice and hepatomegaly in 50% of patients. FTT and more significant liver disease occur later in infancy in 33% of patients.

      (3) The **course of disease is generally self-limited,** with full recovery during infancy in as many as 70% of patients.

    d. Diagnosis is on the basis of clinical presentation, results of liver biopsy, and exclusion of other causes of cholestasis.

    e. Management is supportive.

      (1) Decreased fat absorption may lead to growth failure and vitamin deficiencies. Increased **nutritional support** with concentrated calories, use of medium-chain triglyceride–containing formulas, and provision of **fat-soluble vitamins A, D, E, and K** are indicated. **TPN** may be needed if growth remains problematic.

(2) **Ursodeoxycholic acid,** a bile acid, is used to enhance bile flow and to reduce bile viscosity. Ursodeoxycholic acid is not used until biliary obstruction has been excluded as a possibility.

(3) **Liver transplantation** may be necessary in cases of severe liver failure.

3. **Biliary atresia (BA)**

   a. **Definition.** BA is a **progressive fibrosclerotic** disease that affects the **extrahepatic biliary tree.** Fifty percent of all pediatric liver transplants are performed for liver failure caused by BA.

   b. **Epidemiology.** Incidence is 1 in 10,000 live births.

   c. **Etiology is unknown.**

   d. **Clinical features**

      (1) **Two thirds of patients present between the ages of 4 and 6 weeks** with jaundice, dark urine, and pale or acholic stools. The remaining one third of patients present earlier, within the first 2 weeks of life, and therefore the presentation **can be confused with physiologic jaundice.**

      (2) **Bilirubin levels are moderately elevated.**

      (3) **Progression of disease is rapid,** with **bile duct obliteration and cirrhosis occurring by 4 months of age.**

      (4) Other signs and symptoms include **hepatosplenomegaly,** ascites, poor growth, steatorrhea, peripheral edema, and coagulopathy.

      (5) Some infants have an associated **polysplenia syndrome** with bilobed lungs, abdominal heterotaxia, and situs ambiguous. These patients present earlier and progress more rapidly.

   e. **Diagnosis** must be rapid to affect outcome.

      (1) Abdominal ultrasound, radionucleotide imaging, and liver biopsy are performed in rapid sequence to rule out other causes of cholestasis.

      (2) **Intraoperative cholangiogram with laparotomy to examine the biliary tree confirms the diagnosis.**

   f. **Management** focuses on supportive care and reestablishing bile duct continuity.

      (1) **Kasai portoenterostomy** (Roux-en-Y intestinal loop attached directly to the porta hepatis) is the **treatment of choice to establish bile flow;** however, its success diminishes rapidly with increasing patient age at presentation. **Success is highest if the procedure is performed by 50–70 days of age. Cholangitis** is a worrisome complication of the procedure that occurs in as many as 50% of patients, and repeated episodes can stop all bile flow.

      (2) **Liver transplantation** is indicated for liver failure and late clinical presentations.

(3) **Supportive care** includes nutrition, fat-soluble vitamin supplementation, and, once bile flow is reestablished, ursodeoxycholic acid.

4. **Alagille syndrome**

a. **Definition.** This **autosomal dominant** disorder is characterized by **paucity of intrahepatic bile ducts and multiorgan involvement.**

b. **Epidemiology.** Incidence is 1 in 70,000 live births. Two thirds of patients have an abnormality on chromosome 20 affecting the jagged 1 gene.

c. **Clinical features**

(1) Features of **cholestatic liver disease** are indistinguishable from neonatal hepatitis and BA. Of note, **pruritus in these patients can be debilitating.**

(2) **Unusual facial characteristics** include a broad forehead, deep-set and wide-spaced eyes, a saddle nose with a bulbous tip, pointed chin, and large ears.

(3) **Cardiac disease** often includes **pulmonary outflow obstruction** alone or as part of tetralogy of Fallot.

(4) **Renal disease** occurs in up to one half of patients.

(5) **Eye anomalies** include **posterior embryotoxon.**

(6) **Musculoskeletal anomalies** include butterfly vertebrae and broad thumbs.

(7) **Growth failure and short stature**

(8) **Pancreatic insufficiency**

(9) **Hypercholesterolemia**

d. **Diagnosis** is on the basis of clinical features and, sometimes, liver biopsy and radionucleotide imaging to exclude other causes of cholestasis, such as BA.

e. **Management** is supportive.

E. **Wilson's disease** may cause acute and chronic hepatitis and liver failure. Hepatic involvement is more common than neuropsychiatric symptoms during childhood. See Chapter 5, section XI.A.

F. **Viral Hepatitis**

1. **General concepts**

a. **Epidemiology.** Incidence varies with the specific virus. The **majority of infections in children and adolescents are caused by hepatitis A and B.**

b. **Pathophysiology**

(1) Liver inflammation associated with viral hepatitis is caused by either hepatotropic viruses (hepatitis A, B, C, D, and E [discussed below]) or other viruses that cause liver inflammation as part of a more widespread disease process (e.g., EBV, varicella-zoster virus, HIV, herpes simplex virus).

(2) Infection results in varying degrees of liver inflammation and

swelling. Although hepatocytes are primarily infected, hepatobiliary obstruction results from local swelling. Damage also occurs as a result of the host immune response.

   c. **Clinical features. Most infections during infancy and childhood are asymptomatic.**

      (1) If present, **symptoms** may include malaise, anorexia, vomiting, fever, diffuse or right upper quadrant abdominal pain, edema, and bruising or bleeding.

      (2) **Signs on examination** may include jaundice, hepatosplenomegaly, ascites, increased abdominal vascular markings, caput medusae, spider hemangiomas, and clubbing.

   d. **Management** is supportive in the acute phase with specific therapies for chronic disease.

   e. **Prevention** of hepatitis A and B is now possible through vaccination. See Chapter 1, sections III.C.1 and III.C.7 for discussions of these vaccinations.

  2. **Hepatitis A infection** is caused by hepatitis A virus (HAV), a picornavirus.

   a. **Epidemiology**

      (1) **Transmission** is by the **fecal-oral** route through contaminated foods and water or by contact with contaminated individuals (e.g., food handlers). **It is the most common hepatitis virus causing infection.**

      (2) Virus is shed in the stool 2–3 weeks before the onset of symptoms and 1 week after the onset of jaundice.

   b. **Clinical features**

      (1) **Incubation period** is **2–6 weeks,** with mean symptom onset at 28 days.

      (2) Infection is **asymptomatic in the majority of children (>70%). Jaundice occurs very rarely in symptomatic children.** Older children and adults are more likely to have symptomatic infection.

      (3) Chronic infection does not occur, although the disease may relapse with return of symptoms in up to 25%.

   c. **Diagnosis is based on serology.** Figure 10-2 describes the time course of infection and the presence of detectable antibodies to HAV.

      (1) **Elevated IgM anti-HAV** is present early and can persist for as long as 6 months after infection.

      (2) **Elevated IgG anti-HAV** also occurs early in infection and confers lifelong immunity.

   d. **Management** of symptomatic infection is supportive.

  3. **Hepatitis B infection** is caused by hepatitis B virus (HBV), a DNA virus.

   a. **Epidemiology. Transmission** is by **perinatal vertical** exposure from an infected mother to her fetus, by the **parenteral** route through exposure to infected blood products, tattooing needles, and intravenous drug use, or by exposure to infected **body secretions.**

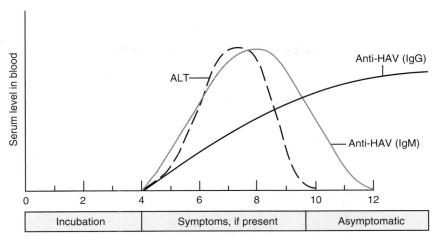

Figure 10-2. Time course of hepatitis A infection and the presence of detectable antibodies to hepatitis A. *IgM Anti-HAV* = IgM antibody to hepatitis A; *IgG Anti-HAV* = IgG antibody to hepatitis A; *HAV* = hepatitis A virus; ALT = alanine aminotransferase.

HBV is found in most body fluids, including blood, tears, saliva, semen, vaginal secretions, urine, feces, and breast milk.

  b. Clinical features

    (1) Incubation period is 45–160 days with mean symptom onset of 90 days.

    (2) Acute symptoms of hepatitis (see section XI E.1.d) occur in < 5% of infants, 5–15% of preschool children, and 30–50% of older children and adolescents. **Symptoms are extremely variable,** ranging from asymptomatic infection to nonspecific systemic illness to clinical hepatitis and fulminant liver failure.

    (3) Chronic HBV infection is most common in young infants who acquire the virus from perinatal exposure but is less common in older children. Chronic HBV infection may result in chronic liver disease with cirrhosis, hepatic fibrosis, portal hypertension, and **increased risk for hepatocellular carcinoma.**

  c. Diagnosis is on the basis of **serology** (see also **Figure 10-3,** which describes the time course of infection and the presence of detectable antigens and antibodies to HBV).

    (1) HBV surface antigen (HBsAg) is pathognomonic for active disease. It is the antigen used in the hepatitis B vaccine.

    (2) HBV surface antibody (HBsAb) is protective and can result from **vaccination** or **natural infection.**

    (3) HBV core antibody (HBcAb) results from natural infection (not vaccination) and persists lifelong.

    (4) HBV e antigen (HBeAg) rises very early in active infection and is therefore useful in diagnosing acute infection.

    (5) HBV e antibody (HBeAb) rises late in infection.

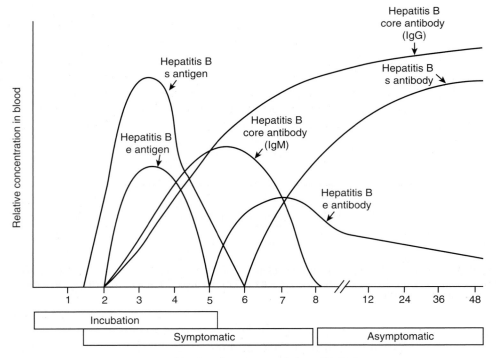

Months after exposure to hepatitis B virus

Figure 10-3. Time course of acute hepatitis B infection and the presence of detectable antigens and antibodies to hepatitis B.

  (6) HBV polymerase chain reaction (PCR) may be used for both diagnosis and assessing the response to therapy.

 d. **Management** includes supportive care for acute infection and consideration of interferon-α and antivirals for chronic infection.

4. **Hepatitis C infection** is caused by hepatitis C virus (HCV), an RNA virus in the flavivirus family.

 a. **Epidemiology**

  (1) Transmission is by perinatal vertical route from mother to fetus, or by parenteral exposure.

  (2) HCV accounts for 90% of transfusion-associated hepatitis and 50% of "non-A, non-B" hepatitis.

 b. **Clinical features.** Acute infection is **rarely symptomatic** (especially in children), although **chronic infection** may result in cirrhosis and hepatic fibrosis. Chronic infection occurs in 80% of infected patients.

 c. **Diagnosis** is by serology demonstrating HCV antibody in the blood. HCV PCR is used as a confirmatory test for chronic infection.

5. **Hepatitis D infection** is caused by hepatitis delta virus (HDV), an RNA virus that **requires HBsAg for replication.** Transmission is by parenteral exposure and infection can occur with or without active hepatitis

B infection. Infection may be inconsequential, may cause progression of hepatitis B infection, or may precipitate fulminant liver failure. Diagnosis is by serology demonstrating HDV antigen and antibody.

6. **Hepatitis E infection** is caused by hepatitis E virus (HEV), an RNA virus. Hepatitis E is responsible for **50% of acute hepatitis in young adults in developing countries** and is associated with **20% mortality in infected pregnant women.** Transmission is by **fecal-oral** route. Chronic disease does not occur. Diagnosis is by serology demonstrating HEV antibodies.

G. Autoimmune Hepatitis

1. **Definition.** This **destructive and progressive** liver disease is characterized by **elevated serum transaminases, hypergammaglobulinemia, and circulating autoantibodies.**

2. **Categories.** Two categories of autoimmune hepatitis are based on autoantibody types.
   a. **Type 1 disease** is characterized by the presence of **antinuclear antibody** (ANA) or **anti-smooth muscle antibody.** Type 1 disease is more common than type 2 disease.
   b. **Type 2 disease** is characterized by anti-liver kidney microsome antibody or anti-liver cytosol type 1 antibody.

3. **Epidemiology**
   a. Autoimmune hepatitis occurs predominantly in **females with presentation before puberty.**
   b. Other **nonhepatic autoimmune diseases** (e.g., UC, vasculitis, vitiligo) occur in 20–40% of patients.

4. **Clinical features**
   a. **Fifty percent** of patients present with **acute hepatitis,** mimicking viral hepatitis, and **50%** of patients present with **chronic liver disease.**
   b. **Jaundice** is usually mild to moderate.
   c. **Nonhepatic signs and symptoms** include fatigue, anorexia, arthritis, rash, nephritis, and vasculitis.

5. **Diagnosis** is on the basis of clinical presentation, typical laboratory findings, and exclusion of other liver diseases. A **high degree of suspicion** is required in patients with a family history of autoimmune disease, in those with nonhepatic autoimmune disease, and in those with chronic liver disease.
   a. **Laboratory studies** reveal **elevated serum transaminases, hypergammaglobulinemia, and circulating autoantibodies.**
   b. **Liver biopsy** is generally performed to evaluate for cirrhosis, to grade disease activity, and to exclude other diagnoses.

6. **Management** includes supportive care, **corticosteroids** for initial control of hepatic inflammation, and **immunosuppressive agents,** such as azathioprine or 6-mercaptopurine. Liver transplantation is indicated for severe liver disease.

Review Test

1. A 2-month-old infant presents with acute onset of crying and bilious vomiting. On examination, her abdomen is tender and distended. Upper intestinal contrast imaging demonstrates intestinal malrotation with midgut volvulus. Which of the following conditions is also associated with malrotation?

(A) Hypertrophic pyloric stenosis
(B) Ulcerative colitis
(C) Renal anomalies
(D) Down syndrome
(E) Heterotaxy

2. A 6-week-old male infant is admitted to the pediatric ward with vomiting and dehydration. The parents note that their child has been vomiting for the past 3 weeks with increasing severity and frequency. Initially, he would spit up a small amount after every other feeding. However, for the past week, he has vomited forcefully after each breastfeeding. To the parents, it seems like he vomits the entire feeding. He has remained hungry, is afebrile, and has no diarrhea. During the past 2 days, he has had only two wet diapers per day. After admission, serum electrolytes are drawn. Based on the most likely diagnosis, which of the following would be the most likely electrolyte pattern?

(A) Hypernatremic, hypokalemic metabolic acidosis
(B) Hypernatremic, hypokalemic metabolic alkalosis
(C) Hypochloremic, hypokalemic metabolic alkalosis
(D) Hyperchloremic, hypokalemic metabolic alkalosis
(E) Hypochloremic, hypokalemic, metabolic acidosis

3. You are called to evaluate a newborn in the nursery who has been vomiting after every feeding. The prenatal history is notable for polyhydramnios, and the physical examination is significant for a scaphoid abdomen and paucity of bowel sounds. Which of the following is the most likely diagnosis?

(A) Congenital diaphragmatic hernia
(B) Hypertrophic pyloric stenosis
(C) Intestinal malrotation
(D) Duodenal atresia
(E) Hirschsprung's disease

4. An 8-year-old girl is brought to the emergency department with a 3-day history of periumbilical abdominal pain that radiates to the back, as well as nausea, vomiting, and anorexia. The girl's mother denies any recent travel, ill contacts, and trauma to her abdomen. Laboratory assessment reveals an elevated white blood cell count, mild hyperglycemia, and elevated amylase and lipase. The clinical picture appears consistent with pancreatitis. Which of the following is the most likely underlying cause of her disorder?

(A) Idiopathic
(B) Sepsis
(C) Viral infection
(D) Drug or toxin exposure
(E) Congenital anomalies of the pancreas

5. A previously healthy 9-month-old girl is brought to the emergency department with an 18-hour history of intermittent, inconsolable crying interspersed with periods of lethargy. She has vomited twice and has had one bowel movement that the mother describes as bloody. Based on the clinical presentation, which of the following is the most appropriate diagnostic procedure at this time?

(A) Plain abdominal radiography
(B) Upper gastrointestinal imaging with small bowel follow through study
(C) Barium enema
(D) Surgical exploration
(E) Abdominal ultrasound

6. A 3-year-old boy is brought to the office by his parents, who are concerned because he has hard, painful stools. For the past 4 months, their son defecates every 3–4 days and cries during the stooling. The resulting stool is very hard. Physical examination of the child is normal. Which of the following is correct regarding his constipation?

(A) His constipation is unlikely to lead to encopresis.
(B) A barium enema should be ordered to evaluate for Hirschsprung's disease.
(C) His constipation likely resulted from a traumatic triggering event, such as a severe, painful diaper rash or painful diarrhea.
(D) Abdominal radiographs should be ordered to evaluate for an underlying organic cause of his constipation.
(E) The parents should be instructed to encourage their son to drink juice with each meal, and the boy should be reevaluated in 3–4 months.

7. A 4-week-old, formula-fed male infant has a history of blood-tinged stools with mucus for the past few days. His mother reports that he has been fussier than usual lately but has had no fever, vomiting, or cold symptoms. Physical examination reveals mild abdominal distension but is otherwise normal. You suspect cow's milk protein allergy. Which of the following is the most appropriate next step to confirm diagnosis?

(A) Abdominal radiographs
(B) Small bowel biopsy
(C) Allergen skin testing
(D) Stool-reducing substances and pH
(E) Change his diet to an alternative protein source

The response options for statements 8 and 9 are the same. You will be required to select one answer for each statement in the set.

(A) Celiac disease
(B) Crohn's disease
(C) Ulcerative colitis
(D) Irritable bowel syndrome
(E) Lactase deficiency

For each patient, select the likely diagnosis.

8. A 15-year-old girl presents with abdominal cramps and diarrhea for 2 weeks. Examination reveals two perianal skin tags and pubertal delay.

9. A 10-year-old boy presents with bloody diarrhea and abdominal pain. Serologic studies reveal the presence of anti-neutrophil cytoplasmic antibody.

10. A 4-year-old girl is brought to the urgent care center with an acute onset of vomiting blood. Her parents report that her symptoms began abruptly 3 hours ago, and since then she has had four episodes of bloody emesis. Vital signs reveal a heart rate of 152 beats/min and a blood pressure of 110/56 mm Hg. Which of the following is the most appropriate first step in management?

(A) Begin intravenous H_2-blockers.
(B) Order urgent upper endoscopy.
(C) Order a complete blood count to assess the patient's hemoglobin.
(D) Place two large-bore peripheral lines and administer a 20 mL/kg normal saline fluid bolus.
(E) Place a nasogastric tube and aspirate to assess for blood.

11. A 12-month-old female infant with failure to thrive is brought to the office. Her parents note that she is very fussy and often spits up after feedings. She also has two loose foul-smelling stools each day. Serologic testing reveals elevated serum tissue transglutaminase antibody. Which of the following foods can she eat safely without aggravating or inducing her symptoms?

(A) Rice
(B) Wheat
(C) Oats
(D) Barley
(E) Rye

12. A 4-month-old female infant has gastroesophageal reflux disease confirmed by pH probe. She has failed to respond to conservative management that included positioning and thickened feeds. Which of the following is the most appropriate next management step?

(A) Initiation of medical therapy
(B) Changing her diet to a hydrolyzed amino acid formula
(C) Nissen fundoplication
(D) Gastric antroplasty
(E) Gastrostomy tube feedings

13. A 5-week-old male infant has been brought to the clinic by his parents, who have concerns about jaundice. He was born at full-term, weighing 8 pounds, 9 ounces, and he had an uncomplicated delivery and neonatal course. Today, his weight is 9 pounds, 1 ounce, and his vital signs are normal. On examination, his liver is enlarged and 4 cm below the right costal margin. Jaundice is present. Laboratory evaluation reveals a total bilirubin of 12.9 mg/dL with a direct component of 5.9 mg/dL. Which of the following is the next most appropriate step in management?

(A) Begin phototherapy to treat the patient's jaundice.
(B) Refer the patient for a liver transplant.
(C) Begin ursodeoxycholic acid to enhance bile flow.
(D) Order an urgent abdominal ultrasound and radionucleotide imaging study of the liver.
(E) Reassure the parents that no treatment is required as he likely has neonatal hepatitis.

14. A 5-year-old girl has a 4-day history of nausea, vomiting, diarrhea, and loss of appetite. On physical examination, her conjunctiva are icteric, and the right upper quadrant of her abdomen is tender. You suspect hepatitis A infection. Which of the following is correct regarding this diagnosis?

(A) The presence of jaundice is unusual in a child of her age with hepatitis A infection.
(B) She should also be tested for hepatitis D infection, which may occur in association with hepatitis A.
(C) Chronic infection occurs in 25% of patients.
(D) She is likely to be noninfectious at this point in her illness.
(E) Serologic testing at this point in her illness will reveal elevated IgM antibody to hepatitis A only; IgG antibody to hepatitis A rises late in infection.

15. A 10-year-old girl is in the office for follow-up of abdominal pain that first occurred 5 months ago. The pain is periumbilical in location and is described vaguely as sometimes sharp, sometimes dull, and sometimes burning. The pain occurs only during the day; she denies waking up at night secondary to pain. She is able to participate in her soccer practice and games after school and on weekends. Fever, vomiting, diarrhea, and dysuria are all absent. Examination is normal, except for very mild abdominal tenderness on palpation of her periumbilical region. She is otherwise a very healthy-appearing girl with normal growth and development. You suspect functional abdominal pain. Which of the following is correct regarding this diagnosis?

(A) Almost all patients have resolution of their symptoms by adulthood.
(B) Most cases of chronic abdominal pain have an organic cause.
(C) Your counseling should include making sure the patient understands that her pain is not real, but imagined.
(D) Even though her pain is functional, she may also have a minor disturbance in her sympathetic or parasympathetic nervous system that has put her at risk for pain.
(E) Given the degree of pain, she should be given permission to miss school when the pain is present.

Answers and Explanations

1. The answer is E [IV.B.2]. Malrotation is the result of abnormal rotation and fixation of the intestines in utero. In heterotaxy, the intestines begin their rotation from an already abnormal position and this results in final fixation in a variable position. This variable rotation and final position can lead to twisting of the intestines and volvulus. Pyloric stenosis is a thickening of the pylorus muscle that results in projectile vomiting. Intestinal malrotation is not present in this disorder. Ulcerative colitis is a type of inflammatory bowel disease in which many intestinal manifestations may be present, including rectal bleeding, diarrhea, abdominal pain, and toxic megacolon, but not intestinal malrotation. Patients with Down syndrome may have duodenal atresia but are at no increased risk for malrotation. Renal anomalies are not associated with malrotation.

2. The answer is C [IV.A.4, IV.A.5]. The infant's symptoms are the classic presentation of hypertrophic pyloric stenosis. Forceful vomiting of stomach contents develops, and the vomiting persists unless it is corrected surgically. This persistent vomiting causes a progressive loss of hydrogen ions and chloride, resulting in hypochloremia and a metabolic alkalosis. If hydrogen ion loss is severe, hypokalemia often develops as well.

3. The answer is D [IV.C.1]. Duodenal atresia is a congenital anomaly that develops because of failure of the intestinal lumen to recanalize early in gestation. As a result, the fetus is unable to swallow significant amounts of amniotic fluid, and this may lead to polyhydramnios. Postnatally, duodenal atresia leads to vomiting, epigastric distension (proximal to the obstruction), and an absence of intestinal bowel gas that causes a scaphoid appearance to the abdomen. Although the abdomen may be scaphoid in appearance with congenital diaphragmatic hernia, polyhydramnios is not associated with this condition, and these infants present with severe respiratory distress at birth. Neither pyloric stenosis, malrotation, nor Hirschsprung's disease is associated with a scaphoid abdomen or polyhydramnios.

4. The answer is A [V.B.2.d]. In children, approximately 25% of cases of pancreatitis are idiopathic (without identifiable cause). Idiopathic pancreatitis is second only to blunt abdominal trauma, which is the leading cause of acute pancreatitis during childhood. Sepsis, viral infections, and drug or toxin exposure are other important causes of pancreatitis in children but are less common than trauma or the idiopathic category. Congenital anomalies of the pancreas and biliary tree are also less common causes.

5. The answer is C [IV.D.5]. This infant's history is consistent with intussusception, in which the intestine telescopes into itself, causing bowel wall edema, mucosal injury, and eventually necrosis. The child typically presents with colicky abdominal pain, often accompanied by vomiting, lethargy, and bloody stools. The most important diagnostic test is the contrast enema, which demonstrates the involved intestinal segment. In addition, the pressure from the contrast enema will usually reduce the intussusception. The contrast enema is therefore both diagnostic and therapeutic. Although ultrasound may demonstrate the intussusception, it is generally not the initial diagnostic study for a patient with presumed intussusception. Surgical exploration is indicated for intussusception that fails to reduce with contrast enema or if peritonitis is suspected. Plain radiography is not generally sensitive for diagnosis. Upper gastrointestinal imaging with small bowel follow through will not show most cases of intussusception, which most commonly occurs in the ileocolic location.

6. The answer is C [VII.D.1]. This patient's constipation is most likely functional or nonorganic (functional fecal retention). Functional constipation results from an inappropriate constriction of the external anal sphincter. Most commonly, toddlers retain stool purposely because of a traumatic event, such as a painful diaper rash, painful diarrhea, or even physical or sexual abuse. Encopresis is almost always associated with severe constipation and could eventually result in this patient. Organic causes of constipation (e.g., Hirschsprung's disease, hypothyroidism, infant botulism) account for less than 5% of constipation seen during childhood. Therefore, radiographic studies are not indicated unless suggested on the basis of history or physical examination. Because this patient's constipation is associated with pain, management should include stool evacuation using mineral oil, enemas, or other modalities. Recommendations for increased dietary fiber, water, and juice are important adjuncts to treatment but alone are insufficient for this patient whose constipation is significant and resulting in very hard stools and crying during defecation.

7. The answer is E [II.B.4]. Protein intolerance occurs in up to 8% of all infants and is usually caused by cow's milk protein or soy protein allergy. Protein intolerance may present with vomiting, diarrhea, irritability, rectal bleeding, and weight loss. Diagnosis of protein intolerance is made on resolution of symptoms after a complete withdrawal of the suspected antigen. Symptoms usually resolve within 1–2 weeks of stopping the offending protein. Because this approach to treatment and diagnosis is noninvasive and effective, abdominal radiographs, small bowel biopsy, and allergy testing are not necessary and are overly invasive for this 4-week-old. In addition, radiographs are not diagnostic, and this infant is too young for a response to allergy skin testing. Stool-reducing substances and an abnormal acidic pH are found in carbohydrate, not protein, malabsorption.

8 and 9. The answers are B and C, respectively [IX.C and Table 10-4]. Patients with Crohn's disease, like the girl in question 8, may present with diarrhea, abdominal cramping, and loss of appetite. Perianal skin disease, such as skin tags, fissures, and fistulas, may precede intestinal symptoms. Patients with Crohn's disease may also have poor growth and delayed puberty. Patients with ulcerative colitis, like the boy in question 9, often present with rectal bleeding, diarrhea, and abdominal pain. Eighty percent are positive for antineutrophil cytoplasmic antibody. In contrast, celiac disease presents with bloating, foul-smelling stools, diarrhea, and vomiting. Delayed sexual maturity is unusual, stools are nonbloody, and perianal disease is not usually present. Irritable bowel syndrome is associated with bloating, cramping, and alterations in stool patterns. Lactase deficiency is a disorder of carbohydrate absorption and presents with bloating and diarrhea.

10. The answer is D [X.C.3.a]. Before further investigation or definitive therapy, the most important step in any patient who may have hypovolemia or significant or worsening anemia is initial stabilization, including the ABCs (airway, breathing, and circulation). This includes placement of two large-bore intravenous lines for fluid resuscitation. Because the heart rate is elevated, suggesting hypovolemia, a normal saline solution bolus would also be an appropriate initial step in management. After stabilization, placement of a nasogastric tube to confirm upper gastrointestinal bleeding and ordering a complete blood count to assess the patient's hemoglobin are appropriate. Intravenous H_2-blockers are used if gastritis, esophagitis, or ulcer disease is suspected. Upper endoscopy would also likely be needed to diagnose the cause of the bleeding, but after the patient has been initially stabilized.

11. The answer is A [II.C.2.b, II.C.5]. This patient presents with the classic features of celiac disease (gluten-sensitive enteropathy). Signs and symptoms usually develop between 6 months and 2 years of age when gluten is introduced into the diet. The treatment of celiac disease is restriction of gluten from the diet. Wheat, barley, and rye all contain gluten. Oats also usually contain gluten because most oats are harvested in fields that also contain wheat. Rice is the only food listed that does not contain gluten and can be eaten safely by patients with celiac disease.

12. The answer is A [III.G.2]. Gastroesophageal reflux disease results from inappropriate transient lower esophageal sphincter relaxation that allows gastric contents to reflux into the esophagus, and manifests as vomiting, irritability, arching of the back, poor weight gain, and pulmonary symptoms (e.g., wheezing). After a trial of conservative management that includes positioning and thickened feeds, medical management with antacids, H_2-blockers, proton pump inhibitors, or motility agents is indicated. Dietary changes would be ineffective at this time. Nissen fundoplication with gastric antroplasty and gastrostomy tube feedings may be required should medical management fail.

13. The answer is D [XI.C.1, XI.C.4.e, XI.C.4.f]. This patient has cholestasis, or retention of bile within the liver, manifested by the elevated conjugated (direct) bilirubin. In addition, the findings of hepatomegaly and poor growth (he has only gained 8 ounces since birth) support the diagnosis of cholestasis. The causes of cholestasis are many, and biliary atresia and choledochal cyst must always be considered and rapidly ruled out in any infant who presents with conjugated hyperbilirubinemia. This evaluation includes an abdominal ultrasound, radionucleotide imaging, and liver biopsy in rapid sequence. Should biliary atresia not be identified promptly (by 50–70 days of age), liver transplantation may be the only treatment option. Phototherapy is not indicated for direct hyperbilirubinemia. Neonatal hepatitis is a possible cause of this patient's symptoms, but biliary atresia must first be ruled out. Ursodeoxycholic acid enhances bile flow, but it is recommended only once biliary obstruction has been excluded.

14. The answer is A [XI.F.2 and Figure 10-2]. Hepatitis A infection is the most common hepatitis virus infection and usually occurs through fecal-oral contamination. Only 30% of children infected with the hepatitis A virus have symptoms of hepatitis (the majority of hepatitis A infections are asymptomatic during childhood), but even those with hepatitis symptoms very rarely have jaundice. Hepatitis D infection requires the presence of hepatitis B surface antigen (HBsAg) for replication, not hepatitis A virus. Chronic hepatitis A infection does not occur, but up to 25% can have a relapse of symptoms at some point after recovery from the initial infection. Patients shed virus in the stool for 2–3 weeks before the onset of any symptoms and for 1 week after the onset of symptoms. Serologic testing confirms the diagnosis. Both IgM and IgG antibodies to hepatitis A virus rise early in infection.

15. The answer is D [VI.C.2]. Nonorganic or functional abdominal pain is much more common than organic abdominal pain in children. Yet, although the pain is nonorganic, some children do have minor disturbances in gastrointestinal motility or in their parasympathetic or sympathetic nervous systems that make them susceptible to the pain. It is important to understand that the pain is real to the patient, and therefore management should focus on empowering the child and family to overcome the discomfort. In addition, the child must resume and normalize all activities, including attending school even when pain is present. Although 50% of patients have resolution of symptoms during childhood, at least 25% still have pain as adults.

11

Nephrology and Urology

Elaine S. Kamil, M.D., and Lee Todd Miller, M.D.

I. Fluids, Electrolytes, and Dehydration

A. General Principles

1. The **most common cause of acute fluid and electrolyte imbalance is acute diarrhea with dehydration.**

2. Worldwide, acute diarrheal diseases are one of the leading causes of childhood morbidity and mortality, accounting for more than 5 million childhood deaths each year.

3. Patients with acute dehydration may be managed with both parenteral rehydration and oral rehydration therapy.

B. Total body fluid requirement is the sum of a patient's maintenance fluid needs, plus replacement of prior fluid losses (i.e., deficits), plus replacement of ongoing losses, if any.

1. **Maintenance water and electrolyte calculations** are designed to balance the usual daily losses of water and salts that occur as a result of normal daily metabolic activities. These losses take both measurable forms (**sensible losses**), such as urinary losses, and less readily measurable but still clinically significant forms (**insensible losses**), such as losses from the skin, lungs, and gastrointestinal (GI) tract.

   a. **Maintenance water requirement is** approximately **1,500 mL/m²/d** for children.

   b. **Maintenance water requirement may alternatively be calculated** from the patient's weight:

      (1) **100 mL/kg/day** for the first 10 kg of body weight

      (2) **50 mL/kg/day** for the second 10 kg of body weight

      (3) **20 mL/kg/day** for each kg above the first 20 kg of body weight

   c. **Maintenance fluids should be increased** if the patient has **increased insensible losses,** such as **respiratory distress and fever (i.e., a 12% increase for every degree of temperature above 38°C.**

   d. **Maintenance sodium (Na⁺) requirement is approximately 2–3 mEq/kg/d.**

e. **Maintenance potassium (K⁺) requirement** is approximately 2 mEq/kg/d during infancy but decreases with age.

2. **Deficit fluid calculations** are designed to replace **abnormal losses of water and salts** caused by pathologic states, such as diarrhea and vomiting.

3. **Ongoing loss calculations** are designed to replace additional losses of water and salts after the patient's initial evaluation (e.g., ongoing vomiting or diarrhea, nasogastric tube aspirate). These ongoing losses are replaced milliliter for milliliter.

C. **Dehydration may be classified** by both the **initial serum Na⁺ level and by the degree of dehydration.**

1. **Classification by serum sodium concentration**
   a. **Hyponatremic** dehydration **(Na⁺ < 130 mmol/L)**
   b. **Isonatremic** dehydration **(Na⁺ 130–150 mmol/L)**
   c. **Hypernatremic** dehydration **(Na⁺ > 150 mmol/L)**

2. **Classification by degree of dehydration**
   a. **Mild** dehydration (3–5%)
   b. **Moderate** dehydration (7–10%)
   c. **Severe** dehydration (≥ 12%)

D. **Parenteral rehydration** should occur in **two phases:**

1. **Emergency phase**
   a. **The goal of the emergency phase** is to restore or maintain the intravascular volume to ensure perfusion of vital organs.
   b. The emergency phase is **the same for all patients,** regardless of the patient's initial serum sodium level.
   c. **20 mL/kg boluses** of intravenous (IV) solutions with a high enough oncotic load (e.g., **normal saline** or **lactated Ringer's**) are commonly used.

2. **Repletion phase**
   a. The **goal of the repletion phase** is a more gradual correction of the patient's water and electrolyte deficits.
   b. Patients with the **acute onset of hyponatremic or isonatremic dehydration** generally have their fluid and electrolyte deficits replaced **over 24 hours.** Chronic hyponatremia should be corrected much more slowly.
   c. Patients with **hypernatremic dehydration** generally have their fluid and electrolyte deficits replaced more slowly, usually **over 48 hours,** to minimize the risk of **cerebral edema** that may accompany rapid fluid correction.

E. **Oral Rehydration Therapy (ORT)**

1. **ORT may be an effective, safe, and inexpensive alternative** to IV rehydration therapy.

2. **Oral rehydration salt (ORS) solutions** are **balanced mixtures of glucose and electrolytes** for use in treating and preventing dehydration, potassium depletion, and base deficits caused by diarrhea.

3. ORT is based on the principle that the intestinal absorption of sodium and other electrolytes is enhanced by the active absorption of glucose (**coupled co-transport mechanism**). This coupled co-transport process of intestinal absorption **continues to function normally during secretory diarrhea,** whereas other pathways of intestinal absorption of sodium are impaired.

4. **ORT is inappropriate** for patients with severe life-threatening dehydration, for patients with paralytic ileus or GI obstruction, and for patients with extremely rapid stool losses or repeated severe emesis losses.

II. Hematuria

A. **Definition.** Hematuria is defined as the presence of red blood cells (RBCs) in the urine. Hematuria may be seen on voiding (**gross hematuria**) or only on urinalysis (**microscopic hematuria**). **Microscopic** hematuria is defined as ≥ 6 RBCs per high-power field (HPF) detected on three or more consecutive samples.

B. **Epidemiology.** Between 4 and 5% of school children have microscopic hematuria detected on a single voided urine sample, but only 0.5–2% have persistent microscopic hematuria.

C. **Clinical significance.** Microscopic hematuria may be an indicator of a serious medical condition such as a tumor or chronic glomerulonephritis, or may be of no serious medical consequence. The **differential diagnosis of hematuria** is outlined in **Figure 11-1.**

D. **Evaluation (Figure 11-2).** Detection of hematuria may be by urinary dipstick or by microscopy. **Urinary dipstick** detects the presence of hemoglobin or myoglobin in the urine. **False-negative results** may occur with **ascorbic acid** (vitamin C) ingestion. **Urinalysis may also provide clues.** When RBCs are present on microscopic examination, **careful examination of RBC morphology and identification of other urine elements may be extremely helpful** in determining the cause of the hematuria.

1. **RBC casts** are diagnostic of glomerular bleeding, which usually occurs in acute or active glomerulonephritis.

2. **RBC morphology**
   a. RBCs originating in the glomerulus are dysmorphic in character, often with blebs in the RBC membrane.
   b. RBCs that appear to be normal biconcave disks usually originate in the lower urinary tract.

3. The presence of other clues in the urine may also point to a diagnosis.
   a. **Crystals** may be indicative of renal stone disease.
   b. Large numbers of RBCs (especially in the presence of dysuria) may indicate **acute hemorrhagic cystitis,** which may result from bacterial infections, viral infections (e.g., adenovirus), or chemotherapeutic agents (e.g., cyclophosphamide).

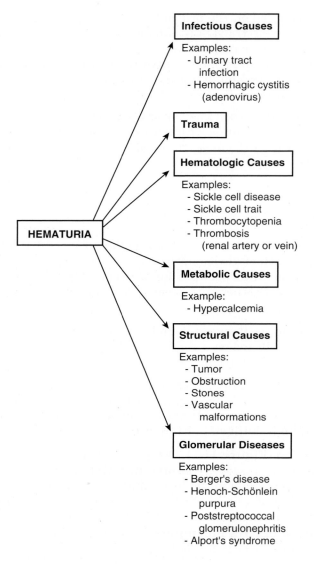

Figure 11-1. Differential diagnosis of hematuria.

III. Proteinuria

A. **Definition.** Whereas a small amount of protein is normally present in the urine, **proteinuria greater than 100 mg/m²/day** is considered pathologic.

B. **Detection**

1. **Urinary dipstick** is the most frequently used method of screening for proteinuria and detects variable levels of **albuminuria.**

   a. **False positives** may result if the urine is very concentrated (specific gravity > 1.025) or alkaline (pH ≥ 7.0), or if the patient has received certain medications (e.g., penicillin, aspirin, oral hypoglycemic agents).

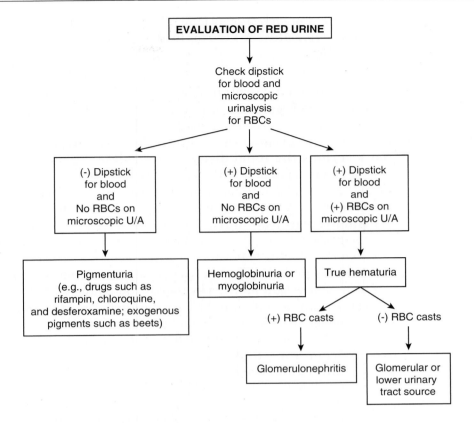

Figure 11-2. An approach to red urine. *RBC* = red blood cell; *U/A* = urinalysis.

    b. False negatives may result if the urine is very dilute.

  2. Twenty-four–hour urinary protein collection (normal is < 100 mg/m^2/day) **is the most accurate method of detecting proteinuria** but is very difficult to obtain in children. Instead, a **random spot urine total protein-to-creatinine ratio (TP/CR)** is usually performed. An early morning sample correlates well with 24-hour urinary protein excretion.

    a. Normal urine TP/CR for infants 6–24 months is < 0.5.

    b. Normal urine TP/CR for children > 2 years is < 0.2.

C. Epidemiology. Two to eleven percent of children have a single positive dipstick test for proteinuria at some point; however, $<1\%$ have persistent proteinuria on repeated dipstick evaluations.

D. Classification

  1. Benign transient proteinuria. Increased urinary protein excretion may sometimes be associated with vigorous exercise, fever, dehydration, and congestive heart failure.

  2. Orthostatic proteinuria

    a. Certain children and adults (especially athletic individuals) have increased urinary protein excretion while upright, but not while supine.

    b. Orthostatic proteinuria is usually a **benign condition** and its confirmation eliminates the need for further workup.

    c. The presence of orthostatic proteinuria is diagnosed with an elevated afternoon urine TP/CR and a normal first-morning urine TP/CR.

  3. Persistent pathologic proteinuria

    a. Persistent pathologic proteinuria may be associated with significant renal disease and is considered a marker for progression of renal disease.

    b. Generally, **the greater the magnitude of the proteinuria, the more serious the renal disease.** The highest amounts of proteinuria are seen in patients with nephrotic syndrome (see section V).

    c. Persistent pathologic proteinuria may have a **glomerular** origin or a **tubular** origin. Glomerular proteinuria is more common.

      (1) Glomerular proteinuria is caused by increased permeability of the glomerular capillaries to large molecular weight proteins, as seen in glomerulonephritis (see section IV).

      (2) Tubular proteinuria results from decreased reabsorption of low molecular weight proteins by the tubular epithelial cells.

        (a) Examples of tubular proteinuria include interstitial nephritis, ischemic renal injury (acute tubular necrosis), and tubular damage resulting from nephrotoxic drugs.

        (b) Laboratory findings include elevated levels of **urinary β_2-microglobulin,** a good marker for tubular proteinuria. This small molecule, which is freely filtered at the glomerulus, is normally almost completely reabsorbed by the tubular epithelial cells. Its presence therefore signifies tubular injury. **Glucosuria** and **aminoaciduria** may also accompany diffuse injury to the tubular epithelial cells.

  E. Evaluation of Proteinuria (Figure 11-3)

IV. Glomerulonephritis

  A. Definition. Glomerulonephritis refers to a group of diseases that cause inflammatory changes in the glomeruli.

  B. Etiology. Causes are varied, but generally involve **immune-mediated injury** to the glomerulus. Various antigens can stimulate immune complex deposition or formation within the glomerulus.

  C. Classification

    1. Primary glomerulonephritis refers to a disease process limited to the kidney.

    2. Secondary glomerulonephritis refers to a disease process that is part of a systemic disease (e.g., systemic lupus erythematosus).

  D. Clinical features. Presentation is variable.

    1. Some patients present with an **acute "nephritic" syndrome** characterized by **gross hematuria, hypertension, and occasionally signs of fluid overload from renal insufficiency.**

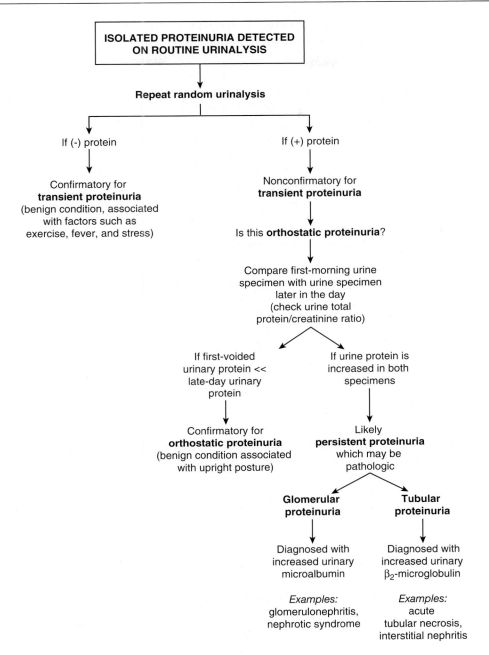

Figure 11-3. Evaluation of proteinuria.

2. Some patients may present with glomerulonephritis associated with **nephrotic syndrome** with heavy proteinuria, hypercholesteremia, and edema.

3. Some patients may be relatively **asymptomatic,** in whom glomerulonephritis is only detected as part of the evaluation of microscopic hematuria, proteinuria, or hypertension.

E. Laboratory Evaluation. Laboratory studies should be performed promptly to avoid missing key transient abnormalities (e.g., transient decrease in serum complement seen in poststreptococcal glomerulonephritis).

1. **Initial evaluation** should include **urinalysis** (to look for casts and to evaluate RBC morphology), **urinary TP/CR** (to quantify proteinuria), **blood chemistries** (including electrolyte panel, blood urea nitrogen [BUN], creatinine, serum albumin, liver enzymes, and cholesterol), **serum complement components, antibody testing** (antinuclear antibody [ANA], antistreptolysin O [ASO] and anti-DNase B [ADB]), and an **IgA level** if IgA nephropathy is suspected.

2. **Additional evaluation,** should the history be suggestive, may include HIV testing, hepatitis C and hepatitis B serologies to evaluate for other causes of postinfectious glomerulonephritis, and other autoimmune markers.

F. Common Types of Glomerulonephritis in Children

1. **Poststreptococcal glomerulonephritis**

   a. **Epidemiology. Poststreptococcal glomerulonephritis (PSGN)** is the **most common form of acute glomerulonephritis** that occurs in school-age children. (Note that other less common causes of postinfectious glomerulonephritis include HIV and hepatitis B and C.) PSGN is rare before 2 years of age.

   b. **Clinical features**

      (1) PSGN develops **8–14 days after an infection of the skin or pharynx** with a **nephritogenic strain of group A β-hemolytic streptococcus.** The latency period after impetigo may be as long as 21–28 days.

      (2) **Hematuria** (often gross hematuria), **proteinuria** (rarely of nephrotic proportion), and **hypertension** with signs of fluid overload (e.g., edema) are common clinical features.

      (3) **Low serum complement** (C3) is present but transient, and normalizes within 8–12 weeks.

      (4) Degree of impairment of renal function is variable and usually normalizes within 6–8 weeks. Severe renal failure is rare.

   c. **Diagnosis.** Diagnosis is on the basis of clinical features and laboratory findings, including evidence of prior streptococcal infection.

      (1) **Detection of prior streptococcal infection**

         (a) **ASO titer** is positive in 90% of children after streptococcal pharyngitis, but is positive in only 50% of patients with impetigo.

         (b) **ADB titer** is reliably positive after respiratory or skin infections with streptococcus.

      (2) **Other diagnostic tests** should include urinalysis, serum complement levels, renal ultrasound, tests of renal function, serum albumin, and serum cholesterol if the serum albumin is depressed.

      (3) **Renal biopsy** is indicated only if the patient has significant renal impairment or nephrotic syndrome, or if the serum complement fails to normalize within 8 weeks. **Biopsy** typically shows mesangial cell proliferation and increased mesangial matrix.

    d. Management. Treatment is supportive in most cases, and includes fluid restriction, antihypertensive medications, and dietary restriction of protein, sodium, potassium, and phosphorus.

    e. Prognosis is excellent with complete recovery in most patients.

    f. Prompt antibiotic treatment of infections with nephritogenic strains of group A β-hemolytic streptococcus does not reduce the risk of poststreptococcal glomerulonephritis, although it will reduce the risk of rheumatic fever (see Chapter 16, section VI and Chapter 7, section IX.A.5.f).

2. IgA nephropathy (Berger's disease)

    a. Epidemiology

        (1) IgA nephropathy is the **most common type of chronic glomerulonephritis worldwide.** It typically presents in the second or third decade of life.

        (2) It is more prevalent in **Asia** and **Australia** and in **Native Americans**, and it is rare in African Americans.

    b. Etiology. The cause is poorly understood but may relate to abnormal clearance or formation of IgA immune complexes.

    c. Clinical features. Clinical findings classically include **recurrent bouts of gross hematuria associated with respiratory infections.** Transient acute renal failure may occur in some patients. Microscopic hematuria is present in between the bouts of gross hematuria.

    d. Diagnosis. Renal biopsy, which shows mesangial proliferation and increased mesangial matrix on light microscopy, is the basis of diagnosis. Immunofluorescent microscopy reveals mesangial deposition of IgA as the dominant immunoglobulin. Approximately 50% of patients have elevated serum levels of IgA.

    e. Management. Treatment is supportive, and medications (angiotensin-converting enzyme [ACE] inhibitors, steroids, and immunosuppressants) usually are only recommended for patients with associated pathologic proteinuria or renal insufficiency.

    f. Prognosis is variable. Twenty to forty percent of patients eventually develop end-stage renal disease.

3. Henoch-Schönlein purpura (HSP) nephritis (see Chapter 16, section I)

    a. Definition. HSP is an **IgA-mediated vasculitis** characterized by **nonthrombocytopenic "palpable purpura" on the buttocks and thighs, abdominal pain, arthritis or arthralgias, and gross or microscopic hematuria.**

    b. Clinical features. Clinical findings related to renal involvement include:

        (1) If proteinuria is present, it may suggest severe glomerular inflammation. Renal biopsy is indicated for heavy or nephrotic-range proteinuria.

        (2) In the majority of patients, the renal features of HSP are self-limited with complete recovery within 3 months. One to five percent of patients develop chronic renal failure.

4. Membranoproliferative glomerulonephritis (MPGN)

a. Definition. MPGN is a term used for three forms of histologically distinct glomerulonephritis that share similar features. MPGN is characterized by lobular mesangial hypercellularity and thickening of the glomerular basement membrane.

b. Clinical features

(1) Patients typically present with nephritis, or with nephrotic syndrome accompanied by microscopic or gross hematuria.

(2) Hypertension is common.

(3) Seventy-five percent of patients have low serum complement levels.

(4) Clinical course is variable, although most patients ultimately develop end-stage renal disease.

c. Management. There is no definitive treatment for MPGN, although some patients may respond to corticosteroids. ACE inhibitors may slow disease progression.

5. Membranous nephropathy (MN) is a rare form of glomerulonephritis in young children, although it may be seen in adolescents. MN presents with heavy proteinuria and often progresses to renal insufficiency. MN is the most common cause of nephrotic syndrome in adults in the United States.

6. Systemic lupus erythematosus nephritis (see Chapter 16, section IV.D.8)

V. Nephrotic Syndrome (NS)

A. Definition. NS is a condition characterized by **heavy proteinuria (> 50 mg/kg/24 hours)**, hypoalbuminemia, hypercholesterolemia, and edema.

B. Epidemiology

1. Two thirds of cases present before 5 years of age.

2. In young children, the ratio of boys to girls is 2:1. By late adolescence, both sexes are equally affected.

C. Classification. There are **three categories of NS:**

1. **Primary NS,** which refers to cases that are not a consequence of systemic disease. Primary NS accounts for **90% of all childhood cases of NS. The most common cause of primary NS is minimal change disease (MCD),** which accounts for 95% of NS cases among young children and 50% of cases in older children and adolescents.

2. **NS that results from other primary glomerular diseases,** including IgA nephropathy, MPGN, and PSGN

3. **NS that results from systemic diseases,** including systemic lupus erythematosus and HSP

D. Pathophysiology

1. The basic physiologic defect is a loss of the normal charge- and size-selective glomerular barrier to the filtration of plasma proteins.

2. Excessive urinary protein losses lead to the hypoproteinemia of NS.

3. Hypercholesterolemia is a consequence of the hypoproteinemia.
    a. Reduced plasma oncotic pressure induces increased hepatic production of plasma proteins, including lipoproteins.
    b. Plasma lipid clearance is reduced because of reduced activity of lipoprotein lipase in adipose tissue.

E. Clinical Features

1. Most children present with **edema,** which can range from mild periorbital edema to scrotal or labial edema to widespread edema. The edema often **follows an upper respiratory infection (URI).** Pleural effusions and hypotension may also occur.

2. Patients may rarely be asymptomatic at the time of diagnosis. In these patients, NS is diagnosed during an evaluation for asymptomatic proteinuria.

3. Patients are **predisposed to thrombosis** secondary to hypercoagulability. Patients may present with stroke or other thrombotic events such as renal vein thrombosis, deep vein thrombosis, and sagittal sinus thrombosis.

4. Patients are also at an **increased risk** for infection with encapsulated organisms, such as *Streptococcus pneumoniae,* and therefore may present with **spontaneous bacterial peritonitis, pneumonia, or overwhelming sepsis.**

F. Diagnosis. Diagnosis is on the basis of clinical features and on the following studies:

1. **Urinalysis** typically reveals 3^+ to 4^+ protein, sometimes microscopic hematuria, and an elevated urinary TP/CR. The presence of RBC casts indicates a cause other than MCD.

2. **Complete blood count (CBC)** may show an elevated hematocrit as a result of hemoconcentration resulting from the hypoproteinemia. The platelet count may also be elevated.

3. **Routine chemistries** (electrolytes) may demonstrate metabolic acidosis, which may be caused by renal tubular acidosis. Hypoalbuminemia and elevated serum cholesterol are present. BUN and creatinine should be measured to assess for renal impairment.

4. **C3, ANA, and antistreptococcal antibodies** are indicated to rule out causes of NS other than MCD.

5. **Renal ultrasound** often shows enlarged kidneys.

6. **Renal biopsy** is rarely indicated in the child with typical NS unless the creatinine clearance is impaired or initial management with corticosteroids is ineffective.

G. Management. Treatment is dictated by the underlying cause of the NS, but supportive therapy is universally indicated.

1. Most children are hospitalized for initial treatment, although a relatively asymptomatic child with a reliable caregiver can be followed carefully as an outpatient.

2. If the child has widespread edema, scrotal or labial edema, hypotension, or symptomatic pleural effusions, IV infusions of **25% albumin** should be given to achieve a diuresis and to maintain the intravascular volume.

3. The **diet** should consist of meals with **no added salt**.

4. **Most patients with MCD respond to therapy with corticosteroids.** Steroid-dependent or steroid-resistant patients may respond to **cyclophosphamide** or **cyclosporine.**

5. **Because of the risk of pneumococcal infection, if the child is febrile,** evaluation should include blood culture, urine culture, and chest radiograph. If peritonitis is suspected, paracentesis for Gram stain, culture, and cell count of the ascites fluid is indicated. Empiric broad-spectrum IV antibiotic coverage should be initiated.

H. **Prognosis** varies according to the underlying cause.

1. **Mortality approaches 5%,** almost exclusively in children who are steroid-resistant, and almost always from **overwhelming infection** or **thrombosis.**

2. In the majority of children with steroid-sensitive NS, relapses typically occur with varying frequency but often disappear by the completion of puberty. Less than 10% of children who are initially steroid-sensitive develop end-stage renal disease (ESRD), resulting in **focal sclerosing glomerulosclerosis (FSGS).** In contrast, a majority of patients with steroid-resistant or steroid-dependent NS eventually develop ESRD.

VI. Hemolytic Uremic Syndrome (HUS) (see Chapter 13, section I.F.2.b.(3) and Chapter 7, Table 7-6)

A. **Definition.** HUS is a condition characterized by **acute renal failure in the presence of microangiopathic hemolytic anemia and thrombocytopenia.**

B. **Subtypes.** There are two different subtypes of HUS, which differ in their known etiology, treatments, and prognoses.

C. **Shiga toxin-associated HUS (Stx HUS)**

1. **Epidemiology.** Stx HUS is the most **common subtype seen in childhood.**

2. **Etiology**
   a. Stx HUS occurs as a result of intestinal infection with a **toxin-producing bacteria.** In North America, the most common pathogen is *Escherichia coli* **0157:H7.** Other pathogens include other strains of *E. coli* and *Shigella dysenteriae* type 1.
   b. Known sources of infection include undercooked beef, unpasteurized milk, and contaminated fruit juices. Human-to-human transmission has been described.

3. **Pathogenesis**
   a. **Vascular endothelial injury by the shiga toxin is the key to the pathogenesis of injury in Stx HUS.**

    b. The toxin binds to endothelial cells, causing endothelial cell injury, most especially in the renal vasculature, leading to platelet thrombi formation and renal ischemia.

  4. Clinical features. Clinical presentation is of a **diarrheal prodrome** (often bloody and may be severe) followed by the sudden onset of **hemolytic anemia, thrombocytopenia, and acute renal failure.**

  5. Management. Treatment is supportive.

    a. Transfusions are given as needed for severe anemia and thrombocytopenia.

    b. Acute renal failure is managed as described in section X.E.

    c. Antibiotics are not indicated for HUS. In addition, **antibiotic treatment of** *E. coli* **hemorrhagic colitis may increase the likelihood that the patient will eventually develop HUS.**

  6. Prognosis. The prognosis is generally **favorable** and depends on the severity of the presentation.

    a. Poor prognostic signs for renal recovery include a **high white blood cell (WBC) count** on admission and **prolonged oliguria.**

    b. A minority of patients die during the acute phase from the complications of colitis, such as **toxic megacolon,** or from central nervous system complications, such as cerebral infarctions.

D. Atypical HUS

  1. Epidemiology. Atypical HUS is much less common than Stx HUS.

  2. Etiology

    a. Drugs (e.g., oral contraceptives, cyclosporine, tacrolimus, and OKT3) may cause atypical HUS.

    b. Inherited atypical HUS has also been described, with both autosomal dominant and autosomal recessive inheritance patterns.

  3. Clinical features. Clinical findings are similar to those of Stx HUS, although diarrhea is absent and severe proteinuria and hypertension are more consistently present.

  4. Management. Treatment is supportive. Inciting medications, if any, must be stopped immediately.

  5. Prognosis. Some patients have a chronic relapsing course (**recurrent HUS**). All patients with atypical HUS have a higher risk of progression to ESRD than patients with Stx HUS.

VII. Hereditary Renal Diseases

A. General Concepts. Because many inherited renal diseases present in childhood, **a careful family history is critical** in all children with renal disease.

B. Alport's Syndrome

  1. Definition. Alport's syndrome is a form of **progressive hereditary nephritis** that is secondary to defects in the side chains of **type IV collagen** within the glomerular basement membrane.

2. **Etiology. Inheritance** is usually **X-linked dominant,** although autosomal dominant and autosomal recessive variants exist.

3. **Clinical features**
   a. **Renal manifestations** include hypertension and hematuria. ESRD may occur (most commonly in males).
   b. **Hearing loss** typically begins in childhood and progresses; approximately 50% of adults have some loss of hearing, ranging from mild to severe.
   c. **Ocular abnormalities** involving the lens and retina occur in 25–40% of patients.

4. **Management.** Therapy includes treatment of hypertension, use of ACE inhibitors to slow the progression of renal disease, and eventually renal transplantation.

C. **Multicystic Renal Dysplasia.** This condition is the **most common cause of a renal mass in the newborn,** occurring in 1 in 4,300 live births, and is most often unilateral. The inheritance is not clear, but it appears to be a sporadic occurrence. See section XI.D.2 for more details.

D. **Autosomal Recessive Polycystic Kidney Disease (ARPKD) or Infantile Polycystic Kidney Disease**

1. **Epidemiology.** ARPKD is uncommon, occurring in approximately 1 in 10,000 to 1 in 40,000 live births.

2. **Clinical features**
   a. The most severely affected infants have a maternal history of **oligohydramnios** secondary to nonfunctioning or poorly functioning kidneys. This leads to **pulmonary hypoplasia.**
   b. **Greatly enlarged cystic kidneys**
   c. **Severe hypertension** is common.
   d. **Liver involvement** of variable clinical severity is a constant finding, including cirrhosis with portal hypertension.

3. **Prognosis.** Whereas the degree of renal insufficiency in infancy may range from mild to severe, ARPKD is **progressive** and ultimately all patients require renal transplantation.

E. **Autosomal Dominant Polycystic Kidney Disease (ADPKD) or Adult Polycystic Kidney Disease**

1. **Epidemiology.** ADPKD is a common genetic disorder (affecting 1 in 600 individuals) that usually presents in **adulthood** (20–40 years of age).

2. **Clinical features.** Clinical findings are variable and include abdominal pain, flank masses, urinary tract infection (UTI), gross or microscopic hematuria, hypertension, or renal insufficiency. Associated cerebral aneurysms may occur, with early death.

3. **Prognosis.** Most patients develop severe hypertension and renal insufficiency, eventually requiring transplantation.

F. **Medullary Sponge Kidney.** This condition occurs sporadically or may have autosomal dominant inheritance. Patients may be asymptomatic or have hematuria, UTI, or nephrolithiasis.

G. **Nephronophthisis-Medullary Cystic Disease Complex (NPH-MCD).**
This histologic entity occurs in several forms. The **juvenile form** is auto-somal recessive and leads to ESRD in childhood, and the **adult form** is au-tosomal dominant and causes renal failure later in life.

VIII. Hypertension

A. **Definitions**

1. **Normal blood pressures** during childhood depend on the child's age, sex, height, and weight. Standards are based on upper arm blood pres-sures (blood pressures in the legs are generally higher than in the arms).

2. **Normal systolic and diastolic blood pressures** are defined as blood pressure **less than the 90th percentile** for age.

3. **Normal high blood pressures** are **between the 90th and 95th per-centiles** for age.

B. **Classification.** Hypertension is divided into categories based on severity and etiology.

1. **Significant hypertension** is defined as the average of three separate blood pressures that are **greater than the 95th percentile** for age.

2. **Severe hypertension** is defined as the average of three separate blood pressures that are **greater than the 99th percentile** for age.

3. **Malignant hypertension** is hypertension associated with evidence of end-organ damage, such as retinal hemorrhages, papilledema, seizures, and coronary artery disease (in adults).

4. **Essential hypertension** is defined as hypertension without a clear eti-ology.

5. **Secondary hypertension** is hypertension that has a recognizable cause (e.g., renal parenchymal disease, coarctation of the aorta). **Most hypertension in childhood is secondary hypertension.**

C. **Measurement**

1. **Blood pressure cuff size**
    a. It is critical to use the proper size cuff. A cuff that is **too small** will give **factitiously elevated blood pressures,** and a cuff that is **too large** will give **falsely depressed blood pressures.**
    b. The cuff bladder should measure two thirds of the length of the arm from the shoulder to the elbow.

2. **Position**
    a. Blood pressure in infants should be measured in the supine position.
    b. Blood pressure in children and adolescents should be measured in the seated position with the fully exposed right arm resting on a sup-portive surface at heart level.

D. **Etiology (Table 11-1).** Causes of hypertension vary with the child's age.

1. In **neonates and young infants,** the most common causes include re-nal artery embolus after umbilical artery catheter placement, coarctation of the aorta, congenital renal disease, and renal artery stenosis.

Table 11-1. Etiology of Hypertension in Children

Essential hypertension*	No identifiable cause, but heredity, salt sensitivity, obesity, and stress all may play a role
Renal diseases	Glomerulonephritis Reflux nephropathy Renal dysplasia Polycystic kidney disease Renal trauma Obstructive uropathy Hemolytic uremic syndrome
Renal vascular lesions	Renal artery stenosis or embolus Renal vein thrombosis Vasculitis Neurofibromatosis
Cardiac diseases	Coarctation of the aorta
Endocrine disorders	Neuroblastoma Pheochromocytoma Congenital adrenal hyperplasia Hyperthyroidism Hyperparathyroidism Hyperaldosteronism Cushing's syndrome
Central nervous system disorders	Increased intracranial pressure (e.g., hemorrhage, tumor) Encephalitis Familial dysautonomia
Drug-related causes	Corticosteroids Illicit drugs (e.g., amphetamines, cocaine, PCP) Anabolic steroids Cold remedies Oral contraceptives
Miscellaneous causes	Wilms' tumor Blood pressure cuff too small Anxiety Pain Fractures and orthopedic traction Hypercalcemia

*Essential hypertension is rare in young children. All children with hypertension should have a careful evaluation to determine the cause of the hypertension.
PCP = phencyclidine.

2. In **children 1–10 years of age,** the most common causes include renal diseases and coarctation of the aorta.

3. In **adolescents,** the most common causes include renal diseases and essential hypertension.

E. **Clinical features. Clinical presentations of hypertension** also vary with the child's age. **Some children, like some adults, are asymptomatic.**

1. **Infants** may present with nonspecific signs and symptoms including irritability, vomiting, failure to thrive, seizures, or even congestive heart failure (CHF) if the hypertension is severe.

2. **Children** with malignant hypertension, especially of **acute onset,** may develop headaches, seizures, and stroke.

3. **Children** with **chronic hypertension** may frequently have growth retardation and poor school performance.

F. **Evaluation.** Because most children with hypertension have secondary hypertension, the cause of the hypertension is usually identified through a careful history (including family history and birth history), physical examination, and diagnostic testing. Testing is guided by the most likely causes of hypertension on the basis of the child's age and clinical presentation.

1. **Physical examination**

   a. All children should undergo an assessment of growth and careful, accurate measurements of **four limb blood pressures** to evaluate for coarctation of the aorta (see Chapter 8, section III.F). In coarctation, hypertension is usually noted in the right arm with lower blood pressures in the legs.

   b. In children, a careful **funduscopic examination** may show retinal hemorrhages, papilledema, or, in long-standing hypertension, arterial-venous nicking.

   c. Other important physical findings include signs of CHF, café-au-lait spots as seen in neurofibromatosis, abdominal masses, abdominal bruits, or ambiguous genitalia.

2. **Laboratory evaluation and imaging**

   a. **Initial evaluation** should include a CBC, electrolyte panel, BUN and creatinine, urinalysis, plasma renin, chest radiograph, and renal ultrasound.

   b. If the initial evaluation is suggestive, further studies may include a thyroid panel, plasma catecholamines, measurement of plasma and urinary steroids, and echocardiography. Radioisotope renal scan with the administration of captopril or renal angiography identifies renal artery stenosis.

G. **Management.** The treatment of hypertension should be aimed at curative therapies, whenever possible. **In chronic hypertension, the ultimate goal is to maintain the child's blood pressure well below the 90th percentile for age.**

1. If a specific, treatable cause of hypertension is identified, directed management, such as surgical correction of a coarctation of the aorta, treat-

ment of hyperthyroidism, or removal of a catecholamine-secreting tumor, is performed as a cure.

2. If the child appears to have **essential hypertension,** the initial approach is conservative through implementation of a diet with no added salt, and if appropriate, weight loss. This approach requires frequent monitoring and encouragement.

3. If the child has **underlying renal disease** or severe hypertension, or if conservative hypertension treatment has failed, antihypertensive medications are used.

4. **Hypertensive emergencies** (e.g., seizures, severe headache, stroke, funduscopic changes, CHF) require prompt therapy with intravenous antihypertensives.

IX. Renal Tubular Acidosis (RTA)

A. **Definition.** Renal tubular acidosis refers to a group of congenital or acquired disorders that result from the **inability of the kidney to maintain normal acid-base balance because of defects in bicarbonate conservation or because of defects in the excretion of hydrogen ions.**

B. **Etiology** (Table 11-2)

1. **Congenital forms** of RTA are caused by mutations in various transporters in the proximal or distal tubular cells.

2. **Acquired forms** of RTA may be caused by nephrotoxic drugs (e.g., amphotericin) or systemic diseases (e.g., autoimmune disorders).

C. **Clinical Features** (see Table 11-2). **Symptoms vary with the type of RTA** and with the patient's **age.**

1. **Infants and young children** tend to present with **growth failure and vomiting,** and at times with life-threatening metabolic acidosis.

2. **Older children and adults** may have recurrent calculi, muscle weakness, bone pain, and myalgias.

3. Some forms of RTA result in **nephrocalcinosis,** which in turn may lead to polyuria from urinary concentrating defects.

4. **Classic electrolyte presentation** is a **hyperchloremic metabolic acidosis** with a **normal serum anion gap.**

D. **Types of RTA** (see Table 11-2)

E. **Evaluation.** RTA should be considered in patients who present with a non–anion gap hyperchloremic metabolic acidosis. Acidosis should be confirmed by a venous blood gas.

1. **Initial laboratory studies** should include serum potassium and phosphorus, urine pH, and urinalysis to evaluate for proteinuria and glucosuria. Calculation of the **urine anion gap** (urine Na^+ + urine K^+ − urine chloride) is important; a **positive urine anion gap is seen in distal RTA.**

2. If there are signs of a diffuse tubular disorder (manifested by hy-

Table 11-2. Types of Renal Tubular Acidosis (RTA)

Type of RTA	Characteristic Features	Causes or Associations	Clinical Presentation	Treatment
Distal RTA (Type I)	Inability of the distal renal tubular cells to excrete acid (H^+)	Isolated inherited defect Associated with nephrotic syndrome Associated with drugs (amphotericin)	Vomiting Growth failure Acidosis If untreated, nephrocalcinosis and nephrolithiasis	Small doses of oral alkali
Proximal RTA (Type II)	Impaired bicarbonate reabsorption by the proximal renal tubular cells	Isolated defect Intoxication (heavy metals) Drugs (gentamicin) Associated with more global defects in tubular reabsorption (Fanconi syndrome*)	Vomiting Growth failure Acidosis Muscle weakness	Large doses of oral alkali
Type III RTA	A variant of type I, complicated by proximal tubular bicarbonate wasting during infancy			Large doses of oral alkali
Type IV RTA	**Transient** acidosis in infants and children **Hyperkalemia is the hallmark**	Associated with renal disorders such as obstructive uropathy Associated with aldosterone deficiency states	Patients may be asymptomatic, or may present with failure to thrive	Furosemide to lower serum potassium; oral alkali

*Findings associated with Fanconi syndrome: proximal RTA, hyperphosphaturia, aminoaciduria, glucosuria, and potassium wasting.

pokalemia, hypophosphatemia, and aminoaciduria), the patient should be evaluated for **Fanconi syndrome** (see Table 11-2) by performing more extensive testing of other tubular functions.

X. Renal Failure

A. Definition. Acute renal failure (ARF) is defined as an abrupt decrease in the ability to excrete nitrogenous wastes.

B. Etiology (Table 11-3)

C. Clinical Features

  1. Systemic signs and symptoms depend on the cause and severity of the renal insult, but often include lethargy, nausea, vomiting, respiratory distress, hypertension, and sometimes seizures.

  2. The clinical presentation may be oliguric (diminished urine output) or nonoliguric (normal urine output). In children, **oliguria** is defined as a **urine output < 1 mL/kg/hr.**

D. Evaluation

  1. **Laboratory tests** should include serum electrolytes, BUN, creatinine, urinalysis, and urinary protein and creatinine levels.

  2. **Imaging studies** may include a renal or pelvic ultrasound and a nuclear renal scan to evaluate renal function.

E. Management

  1. If possible, the specific cause should be addressed (e.g., removal of a nephrotoxic drug).

  2. If the patient is intravascularly volume depleted, **the intravascular volume should be restored first, and then total fluid intake should be restricted to the patient's insensible losses (approximately 300 mL/m^2/day) plus output (urine, stool) replacement.**

  3. **Electrolyte intake should be matched to estimated electrolyte losses.** Typically, sodium, potassium, and phosphorus intake are restricted.

  4. **Protein intake should be restricted** to the recommended dietary allowance (RDA) of protein for age. Caloric intake should also be at the RDA for age.

  5. **Patient monitoring** should include daily weights, frequent blood pressure measurements, calculation of intake and output, and monitoring of electrolytes.

  6. **Dialysis therapy** (peritoneal dialysis or hemodialysis) is used when conservative management fails to maintain the patient in safe biochemical, nutritional, and fluid balance.

F. Chronic Renal Insufficiency and End-Stage Renal Disease (ESRD)

  1. **Etiology**

    a. The **most common causes** include glomerular diseases (e.g., FSGS), congenital or inherited kidney diseases (e.g., renal dysplasias or ob-

Table 11-3. Etiologies of Acute Renal Failure (ARF)

Categories of ARF	Causes of Renal Failure	Specific Examples	Laboratory Findings
Prerenal	Caused by a reversible ↓ in renal perfusion that leads to a ↓ in GFR	Dehydration Hemorrhage Congestive heart failure Septic shock Hypoproteinemic states	↑ BUN/Creat ratio > 20 ↑ Urine SG ≥ 1.030 Urine osmolality > 500 Urine Na$^+$ < 20 *FE$_{Na}$ < 1% in older children, < 2.5% in neonates
Renal parenchymal	Damage to glomerulus	PSGN Lupus nephritis HUS	Hematuria Proteinuria
	Damage to tubules (acute tubular necrosis)	Ischemic injuries from renal hypoperfusion	↑ Urinary β$_2$-microglobulin FE$_{Na}$ > 1% in children, > 2.5% in neonates
	Damage to interstitium (acute interstitial nephritis)	Drugs (semisynthetic penicillins)	Eosinophilia, eosinophiluria ↑ Urinary β$_2$-microglobulin
Postrenal	Obstruction of urine flow from either a solitary kidney, from both kidneys, or from the urethra	Stones Tumor Ureterocele Urethral trauma Neurogenic bladder Posterior urethral valves in males	Dilation of renal collecting system on renal ultrasound
Vascular	↓ Perfusion of the kidneys	Renal artery embolus (especially in the presence of an umbilical artery catheter) Renal vein thrombosis, presenting with sudden-onset gross hematuria and a unilateral or bilateral flank mass, with ↑ incidence in infants of diabetic mothers	↓ Renal blood flow on nuclear renal scan

*FE$_{Na}$ = $\dfrac{\text{(urine sodium) / (plasma sodium)}}{\text{(urine creatinine) / (plasma creatinine)}} \times 100\%$

HUS = hemolytic uremic syndrome; *PSGN* = poststreptococcal glomerulonephritis; *FE$_{Na}$* = fractional excretion of sodium; *SG* = specific gravity; *GFR* = glomerular filtration rate; *Creat* = creatinine; *BUN* = blood urea nitrogen.

structive uropathies), reflux nephropathy, collagen vascular diseases, cystic kidney diseases, interstitial nephritis, and HUS.

   b. The cause is unknown in up to 10% of cases.

   c. Determining the cause of the child's chronic renal insufficiency may have implications for the child and his or her family. Specific therapies may modify disease progression, some genetic diseases may occur in siblings or offspring, and some diseases may recur in transplanted kidneys.

2. Clinical features. Clinical findings may include short stature, anemia, failure to thrive, polyuria and polydipsia, lethargy, and rickets.

3. Evaluation

   a. Investigation for the causes of ARF (Table 11-3)

   b. Careful family history

   c. Assessment of growth and nutrition

   d. Evaluation for renal osteodystrophy (i.e., bone disease secondary to renal failure)

   e. Serologic testing for collagen vascular diseases

   f. Renal imaging to look for structural kidney abnormalities

   g. Renal biopsy (in some cases)

4. Management

   a. Medical

   (1) Nutritional management includes assurance of adequate caloric intake and avoidance of high phosphorus, high sodium, and high potassium foods. Patients are also given oral phosphate binders and vitamin D analogs to prevent renal osteodystrophy. Protein intake should be at the RDA for age.

   (2) Biochemical management includes monitoring and management of serum electrolytes, BUN, creatinine, calcium, and alkaline phosphatase.

   (3) Blood pressure monitoring and management are critical.

   (4) Anemia is treated with iron and recombinant erythropoietin therapy.

   (5) Growth is closely monitored, and patients may require recombinant human growth hormone if their growth fails to normalize with other medical interventions.

   b. Dialysis is initiated or **transplantation** is considered when the **glomerular filtration rate is 5–10% of normal.**

   (1) Peritoneal dialysis is generally the **preferred dialysis modality in infants and children.**

   (2) Chronic hemodialysis may also be performed in children and requires vascular access via an indwelling catheter or an arteriovenous fistula.

   (3) Kidney transplantation is the **preferred treatment for children with ESRD.**

   (a) Living-related donors and living-unrelated donors are preferred over cadaveric donors because of better kidney transplant outcome. Graft outcome varies with donor source. Approximately 80% of living donor kidneys and 65% of cadaveric kidneys remain functioning 5 years after transplant.

(b) Kidney transplantation requires lifelong immunosuppression with increased risks of infection and subsequent malignancies.

(c) The **most common causes of transplant loss** include acute and chronic rejection, noncompliance with medications, technical problems during surgery, and recurrent disease.

XI. Structural and Urologic Abnormalities

A. Structural and urologic abnormalities are **common,** occurring in 6–10% of children.

B. Congenital obstructive abnormalities may occur at any level in the urinary tract. Bilateral lesions may threaten renal function.

1. **Ureteropelvic junction obstruction** may occur as a result of kinks, fibrous bands, or overlying aberrant blood vessels.

2. **Ureterovesical junction obstruction** may occur as a result of ureteroceles, primary megaureters, or abnormal insertion of the ureter into the bladder.

3. **Bladder outlet obstruction** may occur as a result of **posterior urethral valves in males,** polyps, or **prune belly syndrome** (i.e., absence of rectus muscles, bladder outlet obstruction, and, in males, cryptorchidism). Bladder outlet obstruction is typically associated with impairment in renal function.

4. Any form of congenital obstruction, if severe in utero, may lead to abnormal renal development (**renal dysplasia**). Severe impairment of renal function from any in utero cause may lead to oligohydramnios, which results in pulmonary hypoplasia that may be incompatible with life.

C. Acquired obstruction may occur as the result of renal calculi (see section XII), tumors, or strictures.

D. Renal Abnormalities

1. **Renal agenesis** occurs as a result of the failure of development of the mesonephric duct or the metanephric blastema, and may be associated with severe congenital anomalies in other organ systems (e.g., heart and hearing).

   a. **Unilateral renal agenesis** occurs in 0.1–0.2% of children.

   b. **Bilateral renal agenesis** is very rare. Infants die in the perinatal period secondary to associated pulmonary hypoplasia.

2. **Renal dysplasia** is much more common than renal agenesis.

   a. **Pathologically,** renal dysplasia is associated with altered structural organization of the kidney, ranging in severity from mild to severe.

   b. **Functionally,** renal dysplasia is associated with concentrating defects, renal tubular acidosis, and varying degrees of renal insufficiency.

   c. Patients with relatively mild renal dysplasia and its associated renal functional abnormalities at birth may temporarily improve in later infancy and childhood, only to deteriorate in late childhood or adolescence.

    d. Severe renal dysplasia results in a nonfunctional kidney.

      (1) The most common abdominal mass discovered in newborns is the multicystic dysplastic kidney, which is usually associated with an atretic ureter.

      (2) If bilateral and severe, multicystic dysplastic kidneys are incompatible with life. These infants are usually born with the stigmata of Potter's syndrome (see Chapter 5, section III.E.1).

  3. Other structural abnormalities include **horseshoe kidney** (fusion of the lower poles of the kidneys), **renal ectopia** (kidney located outside of the renal fossa, such as in the pelvis), and **duplication anomalies.**

E. Vesicoureteral Reflux (VUR)

  1. Definition. VUR is defined as urine refluxing from the urinary bladder into the ureters and the renal collecting system.

  2. Epidemiology

    a. Approximately 0.5% of healthy infants have some degree of VUR.

    b. VUR is identified in 30–50% of infants and young children with UTIs.

  3. Etiology

    a. VUR is caused by **abnormalities of the ureterovesical junction,** most commonly a short submucosal tunnel in which the ureter inserts through the bladder wall.

    b. VUR has autosomal dominant inheritance with variable expression.

  4. Classification. VUR is graded from grade 1 to grade 5 **(Figure 11-4).**

  5. Clinical features

    a. Most children with lower grades of VUR eventually have spontaneous resolution of the reflux.

    b. VUR may predispose to episodes of pyelonephritis, and severe pyelonephritis in turn may lead to renal scarring, especially in infants and young children.

    c. Reflux nephropathy is the pathologic entity resulting from severe VUR. This may lead to ESRD and hypertension. Kidneys show segmental scars, contraction, and interstitial nephritis.

  6. Diagnosis. VUR is diagnosed by **voiding cystourethrogram (VCUG)** in which contrast is introduced into the urinary bladder via a urinary catheter. The bladder and kidneys are imaged under fluoroscopy during filling of the bladder and during voiding.

  7. Management

    a. Low-dose prophylactic antibiotics are prescribed to reduce the incidence of UTI until the child outgrows the VUR.

    b. Children with grade 4 or 5 reflux should be referred to a pediatric urologist for consideration of surgical reimplantation of the ureters.

XII. Urolithiasis

  A. Epidemiology. Renal stones are uncommon in children, and predisposing metabolic disorders should be sought in any child presenting with urinary calculi.

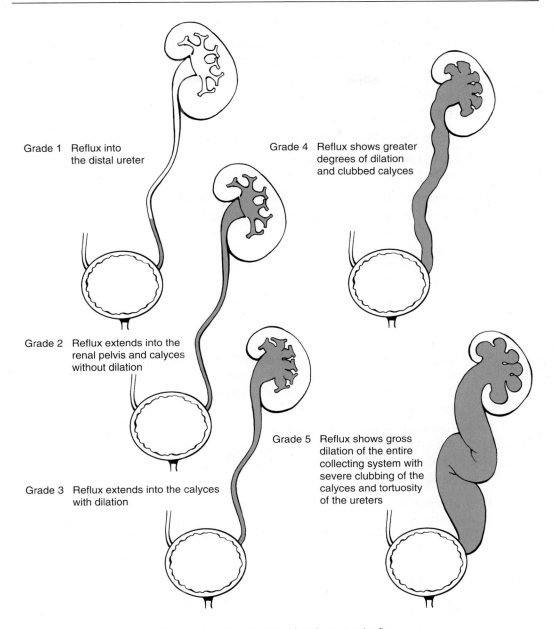

Figure 11-4. Classification of vesicoureteral reflux.

B. Etiology. The **most common stones seen in childhood** include stones of calcium salts, uric acid, cysteine, or magnesium ammonium phosphate (struvite). Conditions associated with urolithiasis that should be considered include the following:

    1. Hypercalciuria, which predisposes to calcium-containing stones. Hypercalciuria may be idiopathic, or caused by hypercalcemia, familial hypercalciuria, or furosemide use (especially in premature infants).

    2. Hyperoxaluria, which may be inherited or secondary to enteric malabsorption (e.g., inflammatory bowel disease)

3. **Distal RTA**

4. **Hyperuricosuria,** which may occur during the treatment of leukemia or lymphoma, with Lesch-Nyhan syndrome, or with primary gout

5. **Cystinuria,** which is an **autosomal recessive** disorder that may lead to radiopaque renal stones

6. **UTI,** especially with *Proteus mirabilis*

7. **Hyperparathyroidism**

C. **Clinical features.** Clinical findings include flank or abdominal pain, gross or microscopic hematuria, or symptoms of cystitis or pyelonephritis.

D. **Diagnosis and Evaluation.** Because of the possibility of an underlying metabolic disorder, children with urolithiasis should have a careful evaluation, including the following:

1. **Laboratory testing** should include electrolytes, BUN, creatinine, calcium, phosphorus, parathyroid hormone (PTH) level, uric acid level, and venous blood gas to rule out RTA.

2. **Urine testing** should include urinalysis with microscopy, urinary oxalate-to-creatinine ratio to identify hyperoxaluria, random first-morning urine for calcium-to-creatinine ratio to identify hypercalciuria and uric acid-to-creatinine ratio to identify hyperuricosuria, urine culture, and testing for cystinuria. Twenty-four–hour urine collections may also be necessary for creatinine, oxalate, uric acid, citrate (low urinary citrate predisposes to stone formation), calcium, phosphorus, magnesium, and cysteine.

3. **Imaging studies,** including a plain radiograph of the abdomen and renal ultrasound, are necessary to confirm and identify the stone(s). Sometimes a high-resolution abdominal CT scan can identify the stone.

4. **Stone fragment analysis,** if a fragment is collected.

E. **Management.** Treatment is aimed first at hydration and the relief of any obstruction, treatment of any associated UTI, and then specific therapy on the basis of the underlying predisposing cause of the urolithiasis.

XIII. Urinary Tract Infection (UTI)

A. **Epidemiology. UTI is one of the most common bacterial infections in children.**

1. **Incidence** of symptomatic UTI during infancy is 0.4–1%.

2. Until 6 months of age, UTIs are twice as common in infant boys than girls. After 6 months of age, UTIs are much more common in girls.

3. Before 6 months of age, UTIs are 10 times more common in **uncircumcised boys** as compared with boys who are circumcised.

B. **Etiology.** The vast majority of UTIs are caused by enteric bacteria, especially ***E. coli***. Other pathogens include *Klebsiella, Pseudomonas, Staphylococcus saprophyticus* (especially in adolescent females), *Serratia, Proteus* (associated with a high urinary pH), and *Enterococcus*.

C. **Pathogenesis**

1. Most bacteria enter the urinary tract by **ascending** through the urethra.

2. Bacterial properties that promote the adherence of bacteria to the urothelium increase the likelihood of UTI.

D. **Clinical Features. UTI symptoms vary with the age of the child.**

1. **In neonates,** symptoms are nonspecific and include lethargy, fever or temperature instability, irritability, and jaundice.

2. **In older infants,** symptoms include fever, vomiting, and irritability. **Pyelonephritis is difficult to diagnose in young nonverbal children, but should be suspected if fever or systemic symptoms are present.**

3. **In young children** who were previously toilet-trained or dry at night, UTI may present with nocturnal enuresis or daytime wetting.

4. **In older children, cystitis** (lower tract infection) is diagnosed when children present with only low-grade or no fever and with complaints of dysuria, urinary frequency, or urgency. **Pyelonephritis** (upper tract infection) is associated with back or flank pain, high fever, and other symptoms and systemic signs such as vomiting and dehydration.

E. **Diagnosis and Evaluation**

1. Diagnosis depends on the proper collection of the urine specimen.

   a. **In neonates and infants,** urine for culture must be collected by suprapubic aspiration of the urinary bladder or via a sterile urethral catheterization. A clean "bagged" urine sample is adequate for a screening urinalysis, but **not** for culture.

   b. **In older children** who can void on command, a careful "clean-catch" urine sample is adequate for culture.

   c. Because bacteria multiply exponentially at room temperature, it is crucial that the urine be cultured immediately, or at least refrigerated immediately until it can be cultured.

2. **Urinalysis findings suggestive of UTI** include the presence of leukocytes on microscopy (> 5–10 WBCs/HPF) and a positive nitrite or leukocyte esterase on dipstick.

3. **Urine culture** remains the **"gold standard"** for diagnosis. **Significant colony counts** depend on the culture method:

   a. Any growth on urine collected by suprapubic aspiration

   b. $\geq$ 10,000 colonies in samples obtained by sterile urethral catheterization

   c. $\geq$ 50,000–100,000 colonies of a single organism in urine collected by clean-catch technique

4. **Imaging**

   a. Imaging is indicated in selected children with UTI because children with UTI have a significant incidence of structural abnormalities of the urinary tract (e.g., vesicoureteral reflux).

   b. All children with pyelonephritis, all children with recurrent UTI, all males, and all girls younger than 4 years of age with cystitis should have an imaging evaluation, which should include a renal ultrasound and a VCUG.

F. **Management**

1. **Empiric antibiotic therapy** should be started in symptomatic patients with a suspicious urinalysis while culture results are pending. Commonly used oral antibiotics include trimethoprim–sulfamethoxazole or cephalexin.

2. **Neonates** with UTIs are admitted to the hospital for initial intravenous management, which commonly includes ampicillin and gentamicin.

3. **Toxic-appearing children** with high fever and children with dehydration should also be admitted to the hospital for initial intravenous antibiotics and hydration. Oral antibiotics are started once the child has shown initial improvement.

4. Duration of treatment for cystitis is usually 7–10 days, and for pyelonephritis, 14 days.

5. Because the risk of renal scarring after pyelonephritis is greatest in infants, they should receive low-dose prophylactic antibiotics for at least 3 months after an episode of pyelonephritis.

Review Test

1. A 3-week-old uncircumcised male infant presents with a 2-day history of very poor feeding. He now takes only 1 ounce of formula every 3 hours, instead of the usual 2–3 ounces. The parents state that their son has become increasingly irritable, and they deny fever, vomiting, or other symptoms. You perform a laboratory evaluation to look for evidence of infection. A urinalysis demonstrates 25–50 white blood cells per high-power field. You suspect that the infant has a urinary tract infection (UTI). Which of the following statements regarding UTI in this infant is correct?

(A) There would be no significant difference in his risk of UTI had he been circumcised.
(B) During infancy, the risk of this boy developing a UTI is greater than that of a girl, but after infancy, he has the same risk as a girl.
(C) A clean "bagged" urine sample is adequate for culture in this febrile infant with no obvious source of infection.
(D) If diagnosed with a UTI, this infant has an increased risk of having vesicoureteral reflux as compared with an infant without a UTI.
(E) This infant should be treated empirically with oral antibiotics on an outpatient basis, and reevaluated within 24 hours.

2. A 5-year-old boy is brought to your office by his parents, who noticed that when their son urinated earlier in the day, his urine appeared red. Dysuria, urinary frequency, and fever are absent, and he is well-appearing on examination. Which of the following statements regarding this patient's presentation and subsequent workup is correct?

(A) This patient may be diagnosed with microscopic hematuria if there are ≥ 10 red blood cells (RBCs) per high-power field on a single urine sample.
(B) On urinalysis, RBCs that appear as biconcave disks indicate that they originated in the glomerulus, and this suggests that he has glomerulonephritis.
(C) Because of his presentation with hematuria at a young age, this patient will likely have persistent microscopic hematuria.
(D) This patient's red-colored urine may have resulted from eating beets the previous day.
(E) This patient's urinary dipstick for blood may be falsely positive if he has recently ingested ascorbic acid (vitamin C).

3. A 4-year-old girl who recently returned from Southeast Asia presents with a history of watery diarrhea, vomiting, and decreased urine output. She is irritable and is crying, although she stops crying when held by her parents. Examination reveals tachycardia with a normal blood pressure, dry mucous membranes, and good peripheral perfusion with normal skin turgor. Which of the following statements regarding rehydration of this child is correct?

(A) The goal of the emergency phase of intravenous rehydration is to restore or maintain intravascular volume to ensure perfusion of the vital organs. The type of intravenous fluids administered depends on the serum level of sodium in the blood.

(B) Appropriate bolus fluids in the emergency phase of intravenous rehydration should include 20 mL/kg of one half–normal saline solution.

(C) If this patient is isonatremic or hypernatremic, her fluid deficits should be replaced over 24 hours, but if she is hyponatremic, her fluid deficits should be replaced over 48 hours.

(D) If stool losses continue, these losses should not be replaced until all the deficit fluids are replaced.

(E) Oral rehydration therapy may be effective even if this child has a secretory diarrhea.

4. A 5-year-old boy has a 3-day history of headache, "puffiness," and dark-colored urine. Physical examination reveals hypertension and periorbital and peripheral edema. Urinalysis reveals hematuria with red blood cell casts and 1+ proteinuria. The diagnosis of poststreptococcal glomerulonephritis is suspected pending further evaluation. Which of the following statements regarding this patient's diagnosis is correct?

(A) If diagnosed with poststreptococcal glomerulonephritis, this patient would be expected to have mild to moderate impairment of renal function and normal serum complement levels.

(B) This patient is likely to have had an infection of the skin or pharynx with a nephritogenic strain of group A β-hemolytic streptococcus 60–90 days before the current presentation.

(C) A negative antistreptolysin O titer would rule out the diagnosis of poststreptococcal glomerulonephritis in this patient.

(D) Antibiotic treatment with penicillin for streptococcal pharyngitis would have prevented this patient's glomerulonephritis.

(E) If the diagnosis of poststreptococcal glomerulonephritis is confirmed, the prognosis for this patient is excellent; complete recovery normally occurs.

5. A previously healthy 3-year-old girl presents with a 2-week history of progressive facial edema. You suspect nephrotic syndrome. Which of the following statements regarding this patient's presentation, evaluation, and management is correct?

(A) This patient's nephrotic syndrome is most likely a consequence of a primary glomerular disease, such as IgA nephropathy.

(B) This patient's age of presentation is atypical; the peak age of presentation of nephrotic syndrome is between 5 and 15 years.

(C) This patient should undergo renal biopsy to confirm the diagnosis and to establish an appropriate approach to management.

(D) If this patient develops a high fever, she should be empirically treated with antibiotics to cover possible pneumococcal peritonitis.

(E) Discovery of heavy proteinuria, hypoalbuminemia, and hypocholesterolemia on laboratory testing would confirm the diagnosis.

6. A previously healthy 3-year-old boy presents with lethargy, pallor, and bloody diarrhea. He has had bloody stools for 4 days, and in the past 2 days he has developed fatigue and pale skin. He is drinking less than normal, and his urine output is somewhat decreased. The parents deny any travel or medication use. Physical examination reveals mild hypertension, pale mucous membranes, abdominal tenderness, and a petechial skin rash on the trunk and extremities. Hemolytic uremic syndrome (HUS) is suspected. Which of the following statements regarding the suspected diagnosis is correct?

(A) Given the nature of this patient's symptoms and his young age, he is most likely to have atypical HUS.

(B) Parenteral antibiotic treatment with gentamicin is indicated for the treatment of suspected *Escherichia coli* hemorrhagic colitis.

(C) Although he has a petechial rash, his platelet count will be normal.

(D) The prognosis is poor; he will likely have a chronic relapsing course, with a high chance of end-stage renal disease.

(E) The renal impairment is caused by toxin binding to renal vascular endothelial cells.

7. A 14-year-old Japanese American boy has 3+ protein and 4+ blood with red blood cell casts on a routine screening urinalysis conducted as part of a health maintenance evaluation. Further questioning reveals two prior episodes of "brown-colored urine" concurrent with upper respiratory tract infections during the last 3 years. Which of the following is the most likely diagnosis?

(A) Membranous nephropathy
(B) Systemic lupus erythematosus nephritis
(C) IgA nephropathy
(D) Membranoproliferative glomerulonephritis
(E) Henoch-Schönlein purpura nephritis

8. A 9-month-old female infant has a 2-day history of fever, irritability, and emesis. Urine culture grows > 100,000 colonies/mL of *Escherichia coli*. She is treated with cephalexin and returns 10 days later for an imaging evaluation to rule out a structural abnormality of the urinary tract. A voiding cystourethrogram reveals grade 2 vesicoureteral reflux (VUR). Which of the following statements regarding VUR is correct?

(A) Inheritance of VUR is autosomal recessive.
(B) The chance of developing chronic renal insufficiency as a result of VUR is 50%.
(C) Referral to a pediatric urologist for ureteral reimplantation is appropriate.
(D) The VUR is likely caused by a short submucosal tunnel in which the ureter inserts through the bladder wall.
(E) Because this patient has only grade 2 VUR, she does not require low-dose prophylactic antibiotics; the risk of subsequent urinary tract infection is low.

9. A 1-year-old boy has a 2-day history of irritability, decreased oral intake, decreased urine output, occasional watery diarrhea, and tactile fever. On physical examination, he is nontoxic and moderately dehydrated, and has a temperature of 101°F (38.3°C). You admit him for intravenous rehydration because of his dehydration. Which of the following statements regarding his maintenance fluid and electrolyte requirements is correct?

(A) His maintenance sodium requirement is approximately 1 mEq/kg/day.
(B) His maintenance water requirement is 1,000 mL/m^2/day of body surface area.
(C) His fever will result in increased insensible losses, and maintenance fluids should therefore be increased by 5% for every degree of fever above 38°C (0° Fahrenheit).
(D) His maintenance fluid calculations need to be adjusted for increased ongoing losses should he develop protracted vomiting or profuse watery diarrhea.
(E) Maintenance fluid calculations for this child take into account both sensible and insensible losses.

10. A 4-day-old male infant has gross hematuria. His parents noticed the bleeding today when they changed his diaper. Perinatal history is remarkable for a term gestation complicated by gestational diabetes mellitus. Physical examination reveals hypertension and a right-sided flank mass. In addition, the infant appears very sleepy, and his mucous membranes are dry. Which of the following is the most likely explanation for his hematuria?

(A) Maternal systemic lupus erythematosus nephritis
(B) Adenovirus infection
(C) Sickle cell disease
(D) Hypercalciuria
(E) Renal vein thrombosis

11. A 6-month-old female infant with a 2-week history of vomiting is brought to your office by her parents. The vomiting occurs three to four times per day, and her parents report she has been very fussy. Review of her growth records reveals very poor growth consistent with failure to thrive. A complete blood count is normal, but an electrolyte panel shows metabolic acidosis. Which of the following laboratory findings would be most consistent with suspected renal tubular acidosis?

(A) Hypokalemia
(B) Hyperphosphatemia
(C) Hyperchloremia
(D) Elevated serum anion gap
(E) Hypocalcemia

The response options for statements 12–14 are the same. You will be required to select one answer for each statement in the set.

(A) Autosomal dominant
(B) Autosomal recessive
(C) Sporadic
(D) X-linked dominant
(E) X-linked recessive

For each patient, select the likely mode of inheritance of the disease.

12. A 6-month-old girl with bilateral abdominal masses and severe hypertension, whose older sister died as a neonate after being diagnosed with oligohydramnios.

13. A 12-year-old boy who has three renal cysts on a renal ultrasound that was performed for the evaluation of microscopic hematuria. The patient's paternal grandfather died of a stroke at 32 years of age, and the patient's father has hypertension.

14. A 15-year-old boy who has mild hearing loss, mild hypertension, hematuria, and proteinuria.

Answers and Explanations

1. The answer is D [XIII.A, XIII.E.1, XIII.F]. Infants with urinary tract infections (UTIs) have an increased risk of having underlying structural abnormalities, including vesicoureteral reflux. A structural abnormality of the urinary tract, such as vesicoureteral reflux, predisposes a child to developing a UTI. Before 6 months of age, UTIs are twice as common in boys, but after 6 months of age, UTIs are more common in girls. Before 6 months of age, UTIs are 10 times more common in uncircumcised boys as compared with circumcised boys. In neonates and infants, urine for culture must be collected by suprapubic aspiration of the urinary bladder or by a sterile urethral catheterization. Bagged specimens obtained from an infant are inappropriate for culture as they are highly likely to be contaminated. Outpatient management for older nontoxic children with suspected UTI may be appropriate. However, toxic-appearing children, neonates, and patients who have significant dehydration should be hospitalized and administered intravenous antibiotics initially.

2. The answer is D [Figure 11-2]. Patients may develop red-colored urine from the ingestion of exogenous pigments, such as those found in beets, and from medications, such as phenytoin and rifampin. Such patients have negative urine dipsticks for blood. Although 4–5% of school children may have microscopic hematuria on a single voided urine sample, only 0.5–2% have persistent microscopic hematuria on retesting. The diagnosis of microscopic hematuria may be made if ≥ 6 red blood cells (RBCs) are noted per high-power field on three or more consecutive urine samples. Patients with positive dipsticks for blood should have microscopic evaluations of fresh urine specimens. RBCs that appear as normal biconcave disks usually originate in the lower urinary tract, unlike dysmorphic RBCs, which are more likely to originate in the glomerulus. False-negative results on dipstick for blood may occur with ascorbic acid (vitamin C) ingestion.

3. The answer is E [I.D, I.E]. Oral rehydration therapy has been shown to be a safe and inexpensive alternative to intravenous rehydration, and effective even in the face of secretory diarrhea, such as would be seen in cholera. Patients with secretory diarrhea still maintain their ability to absorb fluid and electrolytes through an intact, coupled co-transport mechanism. However, oral rehydration therapy should not be used for patients with severe life-threatening dehydration, paralytic ileus, or gastrointestinal obstruction. In patients with these problems, parenteral rehydration is more appropriate. The goal of the first phase of parenteral rehydration (emergency phase) is to restore or maintain the intravascular volume to ensure perfusion of vital organs, and this phase is the same for all patients (regardless of the patient's initial serum sodium level). Appropriate fluids for use in the emergency phase include isotonic crystalloids, such as normal saline or lactated Ringer's solutions in boluses of 20 mL/kg. One quarter– or one half–normal saline is not an appropriate intravenous fluid for the emergency phase. The subsequent repletion phase, or the more gradual correction of fluid and electrolyte deficits, should occur over 24 hours for patients with isonatremic and hyponatremic dehydration, and over 48 hours for patients with hypernatremic dehydration. There is a risk of cerebral edema if deficit replacement occurs too quickly in patients with hypernatremic dehydration. Ongoing losses should be replaced on a "milliliter for milliliter basis" concurrent with the replacement of deficits.

4. The answer is E [IV.F.1]. The most common form of acute glomerulonephritis in school-age children is poststreptococcal glomerulonephritis. Patients usually present with hematuria, proteinuria, and hypertension after an infection of the skin (sometimes up to 28 days after impetigo) or pharynx with a nephritogenic strain of group A β-hemolytic streptococcus. The prognosis for children with poststreptococcal glomerulonephritis is excellent, and affected children usually recover completely; renal failure is rare. Laboratory features consistent with the diagnosis include transient low serum complement levels. The antistreptolysin O titer is positive in 90% of children after a respiratory infection but in only 50% of patients who have had skin infections. Antibiotic treatment of streptococcal pharyngitis or impetigo does not reduce the risk of poststreptococcal glomerulonephritis, although the risk of rheumatic fever is reduced.

5. The answer is D [V.A, V.B, V.E, V.G.5]. Nephrotic syndrome in children is defined as heavy proteinuria (> 50 mg/kg/24 hr), hypoalbuminemia, hypercholesterolemia, and edema. Patients with nephrotic syndrome are susceptible to infections with encapsulated organisms, such as pneumococcal infections, and are at risk for developing peritonitis, pneumonia, and overwhelming sepsis. Patients with nephrotic syndrome and fever should therefore be treated empirically with antibiotics. The most common form of nephrotic syndrome in children is minimal change disease, which comprises 90% of all cases. Primary glomerular disease (e.g., IgA nephropathy) and systemic diseases (e.g., systemic lupus erythematosus) are less common causes of nephrotic syndrome in children. Most cases of childhood nephrotic syndrome (two thirds) occur in children younger than 5 years of age. Renal biopsy to establish the diagnosis or to determine a management approach is not indicated for most patients with nephrotic syndrome. However, it is indicated for patients who have impaired creatinine clearance or those who do not respond to initial management with corticosteroids.

6. The answer is E [VI.C.3]. There are two subtypes of HUS, a shiga toxin-associated form (most common form in childhood) and an atypical form caused by medications or genetic inheritance. Shiga toxin-associated HUS occurs as a result of intestinal infection with a toxin-producing bacteria, most commonly *Escherichia coli* 0157:H7. The toxin binds to vascular endothelial cells, especially in the renal vasculature, causing platelet thrombi and resultant renal ischemia. Patients with HUS have a microangiopathic hemolytic anemia, renal impairment, and thrombocytopenia, which may result in visible petechiae on the skin. The prognosis for patients with shiga-toxin associated HUS is generally good, although poor prognostic signs include elevated white blood cell count on admission and prolonged oliguria. Antibiotic treatment of the *E. coli* hemorrhagic colitis is not indicated and may actually increase the likelihood that a patient will go on to develop HUS.

7. The answer is C [IV.F.2]. This patient's clinical presentation and ethnicity are consistent with IgA nephropathy (Berger's disease), the most common form of chronic glomerulonephritis in the world. Patients with IgA nephropathy typically present in the second or third decade of life with recurrent bouts of gross hematuria associated with respiratory infections. IgA nephropathy is most common in Asia and Australia, and in Native Americans. Membranoproliferative nephritis, membranous nephropathy, and nephritis as a result of systemic lupus erythematosus during childhood are all less common causes of glomerulonephritis in children. This patient's clinical presentation is not consistent with Henoch-Schönlein purpura, which is characterized by abdominal pain, palpable purpura on the buttocks and thighs, and joint symptoms.

8. The answer is D [XI.E]. Vesicoureteral reflux (VUR) is caused by abnormalities of the ureterovesical junction, most commonly a shortened submucosal tunnel in which the ureter inserts through the bladder wall. The inheritance pattern is most commonly autosomal dominant with variable expression. The majority of children with VUR eventually outgrow the reflux, although a minority develop severe renal impairment owing to reflux nephropathy from severe VUR. Patients with grade 4 or 5 VUR should be referred to a pediatric urologist for consideration of ureteral reimplantation. Patients with VUR of any grade are treated with low-dose prophylactic antibiotics to decrease the risk of urinary tract infection.

9. The answer is E [I.B, I.C]. Maintenance water and electrolyte calculations are designed to balance the usual daily losses of water and salts as a result of normal daily metabolic activities. These losses include both measurable forms (sensible losses), such as urinary losses, and less readily measurable but still clinically significant forms (insensible losses), such as losses from the skin, lungs, or gastrointestinal tract. The maintenance sodium requirement is approximately 2–3 mEq/kg/day for infants and children. When calculating maintenance fluids using the surface area method, the maintenance water requirement for children is 1,500 mL/m^2/day. Fever will result in increased insensible losses, and maintenance fluids should be increased by 12% for every degree of fever above 38°C. Maintenance fluid calculations should not be adjusted for increased ongoing losses, such as profuse watery diarrhea. Instead, any increased stool losses should be replaced on a "milliliter per milliliter" basis.

10. The answer is E [Figure 11-1 and Table 11-3]. This patient likely has a renal vein thrombosis, which presents in infancy with the sudden onset of gross hematuria and unilateral or bilateral flank masses. Acute renal failure may result. Infants of diabetic mothers have a greatly increased risk of renal vein thrombosis. Maternal systemic lupus erythematosus (SLE) does not result in hematuria in the infant; however, maternal SLE is associated with infant heart block. Adenovirus infection is a cause of hemorrhagic cystitis, which often causes hematuria; however, this would be unusual in a neonate. Similarly, although sickle cell disease also causes hematuria, it is an uncommon presentation in a neonate. Hypercalciuria is a common cause of hematuria; however, a flank mass would not be a presenting sign.

11. The answer is C [IX.E and Table 11-2]. The classic electrolyte presentation seen in renal tubular acidosis (RTA) is a hyperchloremic metabolic acidosis with a normal serum anion gap. Hypokalemia is not specifically associated with RTA; however, type IV RTA is associated with hyperkalemia. Patients with Fanconi syndrome may present with proximal (type II) RTA with glucosuria, aminoaciduria, and hyperphosphaturia (therefore low serum phosphorus levels, not high serum phosphorus levels). Hypocalcemia is not a feature of RTA.

12–14. The answers are B, A, and D, respectively [VII.D, VII.E, and VII.B]. Infantile polycystic kidney disease is an autosomal recessive disorder characterized by greatly enlarged cystic kidneys, severe hypertension, and variable degrees of liver involvement. Severe cases are associated with oligohydramnios, pulmonary hypoplasia, and early neonatal death. Although the family history may be negative in recessive disorders, there is a 25% risk of affected siblings in subsequent pregnancies. In contrast, adult polycystic kidney disease is inherited in an autosomal dominant pattern, and there is considerable variability in its severity, ranging from mild microscopic hematuria to severe hypertension and renal failure. Adult polycystic kidney disease is also associated with cerebral aneurysms and early death. Alport's syndrome is inherited in multiple patterns, but the X-linked dominant form is by far the most common. Alport's syndrome is characterized by renal manifestations, including hypertension and hematuria, as well as renal failure in males; hearing loss; and ocular abnormalities of the lens and retina.

12

Neurology

Charles E. Niesen, M.D.

I. The Hypotonic Infant

A. Definition. Hypotonia is the decreased resistance of movement during passive stretching of muscles. In contrast, **weakness** is the decreased or less than normal force generated by **active contraction** of muscles.

B. Classification of hypotonia

1. **Central hypotonia** is dysfunction of **upper motor neurons** (i.e., cortical pyramidal neurons and their descending corticospinal pathways).

2. **Peripheral hypotonia** is dysfunction of **lower motor neurons** (i.e., spinal motor neurons and distally to the muscle fibers).

C. Clinical features

1. **History** may reveal **antenatal or neonatal problems. Decreased fetal movements and breech presentation** may be associated with a peripheral hypotonia. **Seizures in the neonatal period** may be associated with a central hypotonia.

2. **Physical examination findings** in both central and peripheral hypotonia may include a **weak cry, decreased spontaneous movement, a frog-leg posture** (the hips are externally rotated and flexed), and **muscle contractures.** When lifted up from under the axillae, the infant slips easily through the examiner's hands.

   a. In **central hypotonia,** there is an **altered level of consciousness and increased deep tendon reflexes (DTRs), often with ankle clonus.**

   b. In **peripheral hypotonia, consciousness is unaffected, but muscle bulk and DTRs are decreased.**

   c. In addition to hypotonia, patients with **congenital neuromuscular disorders** may have additional findings such as bilateral ptosis, ophthalmoplegia, flat mid-face, fish-shaped mouth, high-arched palate, chest wall abnormalities (e.g., bell-shaped chest, pectus excavatum or carinatum), and bilateral cryptorchidism.

D. Etiology. Hypotonia may be caused by systemic pathology (e.g., sepsis, electrolyte abnormalities, hepatic or renal encephalopathy) or by neural pathology that may occur anywhere along the transmission route of a neural impulse (Figure 12-1).

E. Evaluation

1. **Acute life-threatening causes,** such as sepsis, meningitis, or an acute metabolic disorder, must be ruled out.

2. **When central hypotonia is suspected,** it is necessary to consider:

   a. **Head computed tomography (CT) scan** to rule out acute central nervous system (CNS) injury or congenital malformation

   b. **Serum electrolytes**, calcium and magnesium levels, and ammonia, lactate, and pyruvate levels to rule out metabolic disorders

   c. **High-resolution chromosome studies** and fluorescent in situ hybridization (FISH) tests for suspected genetic disorders (e.g., Prader-Willi syndrome)

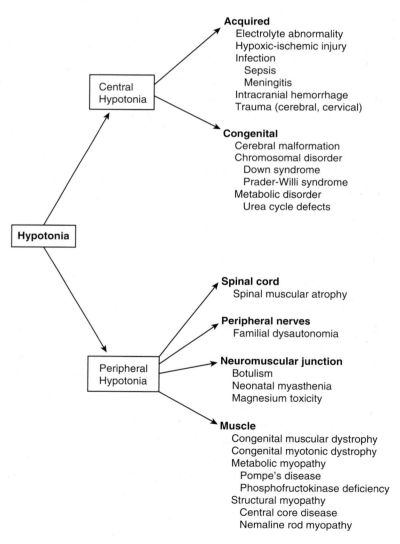

Figure 12-1. Differential diagnosis of hypotonia.

3. **When peripheral hypotonia is suspected,** it is necessary to **consider:**
    a. **Serum creatine kinase (CK)** levels
    b. **DNA tests** for spinal muscular atrophy (see section F.1)
    c. Electromyography (**EMG**). **Nerve conduction studies** are crucial to identify myasthenic disorders.
    d. **Muscle biopsy**

F. **Specific peripheral hypotonic disorders** are described in more detail in the following discussion.

1. **Spinal muscular atrophy (SMA)**
    a. **Definition.** SMA is anterior horn cell degeneration that presents with hypotonia, weakness, and tongue fasciculations.
    b. **Epidemiology.** Incidence is 1 in 10,000–25,000 live births. SMA is the **second most common hereditary neuromuscular disorder** after Duchenne muscular dystrophy.
    c. **Classification**
        (1) **Type 1** or **infantile form** with onset < 6 months of age (also known as **Werdnig-Hoffman disease**)
        (2) **Type II** or **intermediate form** with onset at 6–12 months of age
        (3) **Type III** or **juvenile form** with onset > 3 years of age
    d. **Etiology**
        (1) **Autosomal recessive inheritance**
        (2) All three forms of SMA are caused by mutations in the **survival motor neuron gene (*SMN1*)** on **chromosome 5.**
        (3) **Pathology** of the spinal cord shows **degeneration and loss of anterior horn motor neurons** and infiltration of microglia and astrocytes.
    e. **Clinical features**
        (1) **Weak cry, tongue fasciculations,** and difficulty sucking and swallowing
        (2) **Bell-shaped chest**
        (3) **Frog-leg posture** when in supine position, generalized hypotonia, weakness, and areflexia
        (4) **Normal extraocular movements** and **normal sensory** examination
    f. **Diagnosis**
        (1) **DNA testing** for the abnormal gene is **diagnostic in $> 90\%$ of cases.**
        (2) **Muscle biopsy** shows a characteristic atrophy of groups of muscle fibers that were innervated by the damaged axons.
    g. **Management. Treatment is supportive.** There is **no cure** for this degenerative neuronal disorder. Supportive care includes **gastrostomy tube feeding** to ensure adequate nutrition, **diligent surveillance** and therapy of respiratory infections, and **physical therapy** to maintain range of motion and prevent contractures.
    h. **Prognosis. For SMA type I,** survival beyond the first year of life is unusual. Death occurs as a result of respiratory insufficiency or pneu-

monia. **For SMA types II and III,** survival until adolescent and adult years, respectively, is common.

2. Infantile botulism

a. **Definition.** Infantile botulism is **bulbar weakness and paralysis** that develops in infants during the first year of life **secondary to ingestion of *Clostridium botulinum* spores and absorption of botulinum toxin.**

b. **Etiology.** The source of the botulinum toxin is infected foods, such as contaminated **honey,** or spores unearthed from the ground. **The toxin prevents the presynaptic release of acetylcholine.**

c. **Clinical features**

   (1) **Onset of symptoms** occurs **12–48 hours** after ingestion of spores.

   (2) **Constipation is the classic first symptom of botulism.**

   (3) **Neurologic symptoms follow, including weak cry and suck, loss of previously obtained motor milestones, ophthalmoplegia, and hyporeflexia.**

   (4) **Paralysis is symmetric and descending,** and, at times, diaphragmatic paralysis may occur.

d. **Diagnosis.** Diagnosis is based on suggestive history, neurologic examination, and identification of the toxin or bacteria in the stool. **EMG** is sometimes performed and shows brief, small-amplitude muscle potentials with **an incremental response during high-frequency stimulation.**

e. **Management. Treatment is supportive** with nasogastric feeding and assisted ventilation as needed.

   (1) **Botulism immune globulin** improves the clinical course.

   (2) **Antibiotics are contraindicated** and may worsen the clinical course.

f. **Prognosis.** The outlook is **excellent,** and complete recovery is expected. However, recovery may take weeks or even months.

3. Congenital myotonic dystrophy

a. **Definitions**

   (1) **Myotonia is the inability to relax contracted muscles.**

   (2) **Congenital myotonic dystrophy** is an **autosomal dominant** muscle disorder that presents in the newborn period with weakness and hypotonia.

b. **Epidemiology.** Incidence is 1 in 30,000 live births.

c. **Etiology.** Myotonic dystrophy is a **trinucleotide repeat disorder with autosomal dominant inheritance** and variable penetrance. The gene has been identified on chromosome 19. Transmission to affected infants is **through the affected mother** in more than 90% of cases. The earlier the onset of the disease in the mother, the more likely she will have affected offspring.

d. **Clinical features**

   (1) **Antenatal history** may reveal polyhydramnios caused by poor swallowing in utero and decreased fetal movements.

(2) **Neonatal history** is often significant for **feeding and respiratory problems.**

(3) **Physical examination** of the neonate is notable for facial diplegia (bilateral weakness), hypotonia, areflexia, and arthrogryposis (multiple joint contractures).

(4) **Myotonia is not present in the newborn,** but develops later, almost always by 5 years of age.

(5) **In adulthood,** typical myotonic features include **myotonic facies** (atrophy of masseter and temporalis muscles), ptosis, a stiff, straight smile, and an **inability to release the grip after handshaking (myotonia).**

(6) **Additional problems** include mental retardation, cataracts, cardiac arrhythmias, and infertility.

e. **Diagnosis**

(1) **This disorder should be suspected in all infants with hypotonia.** The child's **mother should also be examined;** she will have the typical features of myotonic dystrophy.

(2) **DNA testing** to identify the gene can be performed to confirm the diagnosis. Because of the availability of DNA testing, EMG and muscle biopsy are no longer indicated.

f. **Management. Treatment is supportive.** Infants may require assisted ventilation and gastrostomy tube feedings.

g. **Prognosis. Outlook is guarded.** Infant mortality can be as high as 40% because of respiratory problems.

(1) All survivors have **mental retardation (average intelligence quotient [IQ] of 50–65).**

(2) Feeding problems tend to subside with time.

II. Hydrocephalus

A. **Definition.** Hydrocephalus is **increased cerebrospinal fluid (CSF) under pressure** within the ventricles of the brain. Hydrocephalus results from **blockage of CSF flow, decreased CSF absorption,** or, rarely, **increased CSF production.**

B. **Types of Hydrocephalus**

1. **Noncommunicating hydrocephalus** refers to enlarged ventricles caused by obstruction of CSF flow through the ventricular system (e.g., aqueductal stenosis).

2. **Communicating hydrocephalus** refers to enlarged ventricles as a result of increased production of CSF (e.g., tumors) or decreased absorption of CSF (e.g., bacterial meningitis).

3. **Hydrocephalus ex vacuo** is not true hydrocephalus, but rather a term used to describe ventricular enlargement caused by brain atrophy.

C. **Etiology**

1. **Congenital causes**

a. **Chiari type II malformation** is characterized by downward displacement of the cerebellum and medulla through the foramen magnum, blocking CSF flow. This malformation is often associated with a lumbosacral myelomeningocele.

    b. Dandy-Walker malformation, a combination of an absent or hypoplastic cerebellar vermis and cystic enlargement of the fourth ventricle, which blocks the flow of CSF.

    c. Congenital aqueductal stenosis (some cases of aqueductal stenosis are inherited as an **X-linked trait** and these patients may have thumb abnormalities and other CNS anomalies such as spina bifida)

  2. Acquired causes include **intraventricular hemorrhage** (most common in preterm infants), **bacterial meningitis,** and **brain tumors.**

D. Clinical Features

  1. Increasing head circumference that crosses percentile lines, or head circumference > 97% for age.

  2. Infants with open cranial sutures have the following clinical signs:

    a. Large anterior and posterior fontanelles and split sutures

    b. Sunset sign, a tonic downward deviation of both eyes caused by pressure from the enlarged third ventricles on the upward gaze center in the midbrain

  3. Older children with closed cranial sutures have the symptoms and signs of **increased intracranial pressure:**

    a. Headache

    b. Nausea and vomiting

    c. Unilateral sixth nerve palsy

    d. Papilledema

    e. Brisk DTRs but with a usually downward plantar response.

E. Evaluation. Increasing head circumference and signs or symptoms of increased intracranial pressure mandate an **urgent head CT scan.**

F. Management. Hydrocephalus requires the surgical placement of a **ventriculoperitoneal shunt** to divert the flow of CSF. Complications of ventriculoperitoneal shunts include **shunt infection** and **shunt obstruction.**

G. Prognosis. Outcome varies depending on the cause of the hydrocephalus.

  1. Patients with aqueductal stenosis have the best cognitive outcome.

  2. Patients with Chiari type II malformation may have low-normal intelligence and language disorders.

  3. Patients with X-linked hydrocephalus may have severe mental retardation.

III. Spina Bifida

A. Definitions

  1. Spina bifida (SB) is a general term that refers to **any failure of bone fusion** in the posterior midline of the vertebral column.

2. **Neural tube defect** is a broad term that includes all forms of failure of neural tube closure, from anencephaly to sacral meningocele.

3. **Myelomeningocele** is the **herniation of spinal cord tissue and the meninges** through a bony cleft, most commonly in the lumbosacral region. Myelomeningocele is 20 times more common than meningocele.

4. **Meningocele** is the **herniation of the meninges only** through a bony cleft, most commonly in the lumbosacral region. Meningocele is **usually not associated with any neural deficits.**

5. In **SB occulta,** there is **no herniation** of tissue through the vertebral cleft.

B. **Epidemiology.** Incidence of neural tube defects varies with geographic location. The **highest incidence is in Ireland** (1 in 250 live births), and the **lowest is in Japan** (1 in 3,000 live births).

C. **Etiology.** The **multifactorial etiology includes environmental, genetic, nutritional, and teratogenic factors.**

1. Mothers taking a multivitamin preparation that includes **folic acid** have decreased incidence of SB. The mechanism of action of folic acid is uncertain.

2. **Teratogens** that cause SB include **valproate,** phenytoin, colchicine, vincristine, azathioprine, and methotrexate.

D. **Clinical Features**

1. **SB occulta.** The skin on the back (usually lumbosacral region) is epithelialized and a hairy patch or dimple often covers the area. No neurologic deficits are present.

2. **Meningocele.** A fluctuant midline mass is present overlying the spine. The mass is filled with CSF and can be transilluminated. Neurologic deficits are usually not present or are only very mild.

3. **Myelomeningocele**

   a. A **fluctuant midline** mass is present anywhere along the spine, but most commonly in the lumbosacral region.

   b. **Neurologic defects are present and depend on the level of the lesion,** varying from complete paraplegia (above L3) to preserved ambulation and variable bladder or bowel incontinence (S3 and below).

   c. **Associated anomalies and complications**

      (1) **Hydrocephalus. Ninety percent of lumbosacral myelomeningoceles are associated with Chiari type II malformation and hydrocephalus.** Cervical and thoracic myelomeningoceles are not associated with hydrocephalus.

      (2) **Cervical hydrosyringomyelia** (accumulation of fluid within the central spinal cord canal and with the cord itself)

      (3) **Defects in neuronal migration** (e.g., gyral anomalies, agenesis of the corpus callosum)

      (4) **Orthopedic problems (e.g., rib anomalies, deformities of the lower extremities, lower extremity fractures from loss of sensation)**

      (5) **Genitourinary defects**

E. Diagnosis

1. **Prenatal diagnosis is common.**

    a. **α-Fetoprotein (AFP),** the main serum protein in fetal life, is elevated in amniotic fluid and maternal serum in open neural tube defects and, when measured in maternal serum at 16–18 weeks gestation, **detects 80% of spinal defects.**

    b. **Fetal sonography** is highly sensitive in detecting spinal defects.

2. **Diagnosis after birth**

    a. **SB occulta** is suggested by finding any skin abnormality overlying the spine and is confirmed by spinal radiographs.

    b. **Meningocele** is suggested by physical examination findings and is confirmed by magnetic resonance imaging (MRI) of the spinal cord and spine.

    c. **Myelomeningocele** is a clinical diagnosis based on physical examination at birth.

F. Management

1. **SB occulta** does not require treatment.

2. **Meningocele** requires surgical repair.

3. **Myelomeningocele** requires urgent surgical repair within 24 hours of birth to reduce the morbidity and mortality from infection and to prevent further trauma to the exposed neural tissue.

G. Prognosis.

1. **SB occulta and meningocele have excellent prognoses** as a result of the absence of neurologic deficits.

2. **Myelomeningocele.** Ninety percent of patients survive to adolescence, but many are handicapped. Associated problems include **wheelchair dependency, bladder or bowel incontinence, mental retardation, seizures, precocious puberty, pressure sores, and fractures.**

IV. Approach to the Comatose Patient

A. Definition.
Coma is a state of unawareness of self and environment in which the patient lies with the eyes closed and is unarousable by external stimuli.

B. Etiology (Table 12-1)

1. In children younger than 5 years of age, **nonaccidental trauma and near-drowning are the most common causes of coma.**

2. In older children, **drug overdose and accidental head injury are the most common causes of coma.**

C. Assessment.
The **goal** of assessment of the comatose patient is to determine the depth of coma, to identify the neurologic signs that indicate the site and cause of the coma, and to monitor the patient's recovery.

Table 12-1. Causes of Coma in Childhood and Adolescence

Focal lesions (abnormal neuroimaging studies)
  Supratentorial lesions
    Vascular: subarachnoid hemorrhage, multiple infarcts, thalamic infarct
    Trauma: subdural hematoma, nonaccidental trauma
    Tumors
    Demyelination (e.g., postinfectious encephalitis)
  Infratentorial lesions
    Vascular: cerebellar hemorrhage
    Trauma
    Tumors

Diffuse lesions (often with normal neuroimaging studies)
  Ingestion
    Drugs:*   Atropine, scopolamine
                  Benzodiazepines, barbiturates
                  Ethanol, lithium
                  Opiates
                  Tricyclic antidepressants
    Toxins: Lead, mercury
  Infection
    Encephalitis
  Hypoxemia
    Near-drowning, carbon monoxide
  Abnormal metabolites
    Metabolic: Hypo- or hyperglycemia
                  Hypo- or hypernatremia
                  Thiamine deficiency
    Endocrine: Hypo- or hyperthyroidism
                  Hypo- or hypercortisolism
  Organ failure
    Cardiac arrest, hepatic failure, uremia
  Seizures
    Nonconvulsive status epilepticus
  Reye syndrome

*Amphetamine, cocaine, and hallucinogens (lysergic acid diethylamide [LSD], mescaline, phencyclidine hydrochloride [PCP]) cause agitation, confusion, delirium, and hallucinations but *not* coma.

1. **Glasgow Coma Scale** provides a standard measure to monitor the level of consciousness (see **Chapter 20, Table 20-1**).

2. **Head and neck exam.** The patient should be assessed for **scalp injuries**, **breath odors** (for alcohol intoxication or ketosis caused by diabetic ketoacidosis), and **nuchal rigidity** (caused by meningitis). **CSF or blood draining** from the nose or auditory canal may indicate a basilar skull fracture.

3. **Abnormal motor responses** to stimuli can indicate the location of brain damage.

   a. **Flaccidity or no movement** suggests severe spinal or brainstem injury.

   b. **Decerebrate posturing (extension of arms and legs)** indicates subcortical injury.

   c. **Decorticate posturing (flexion of arms and extension of legs)** suggests bilateral cortical injury.

   d. **Asymmetric responses** suggest hemispheric injury.

4. **Abnormal respiratory responses** may indicate the location of brain injury or its cause.

   a. **Hypoventilation** suggests opiate or sedative overdose.

   b. **Hyperventilation** suggests metabolic acidosis (Kussmaul respirations, or rapid, deep breathing, may occur), neurogenic pulmonary edema, or midbrain injury.

   c. **Cheyne-Stokes breathing** (alternating apneas and hyperpneas) suggests bilateral cortical injury.

   d. **Apneustic breathing** (pausing at full inspiration) indicates pontine damage.

   e. **Ataxic or agonal breathing** (irregular respirations with no particular pattern) indicates medullary injury and impending brain death.

5. **Pupillary size and reactivity** may provide clues:

   a. Unilateral dilated nonreactive pupil suggests **uncal herniation.**

   b. Bilateral dilated nonreactive pupils suggest topical application of a dilating agent, a postictal state, or irreversible brainstem injury.

   c. Bilateral constricted reactive pupils suggest opiate ingestion or pontine injury.

6. **Other brainstem reflexes** should be assessed to determine the extent of injury to the brainstem.

   a. **Oculocephalic maneuver (doll's eyes).** When turning the head of an unconscious patient, the eyes normally look straight ahead and then slowly drift back to midline position because the intact vestibular apparatus senses a change in position. In an **injured brainstem**, movement of the head does not evoke any eye movement. This is termed a **negative oculocephalic maneuver** or negative doll's eyes.

   b. **Caloric irrigation.** When the oculocephalic response is negative or cannot be performed because of possible cervical cord injury, caloric testing should be performed. This involves angling the head at 30° and irrigating each auditory canal with 10–30 mL of ice water. An intact (normal) cold caloric response is reflected by eye deviation to the irrigated side. An abnormal response suggests pontine injury.

   c. **Abnormal corneal and gag reflexes** indicate significant brainstem injury.

D. **Evaluation.** Once the airway, breathing, and circulation are stable, further diagnostic workup may begin.

   1. **Glucose should be checked immediately** in any comatose patient.

   2. **Urine toxicology screen, serum electrolytes, and metabolic panel** should also be evaluated.

   3. **Head CT scan** should be performed to identify mass lesions or trauma.

   4. **Lumbar puncture to rule out meningoencephalitis should be considered** if the CT scan is negative.

   5. **Urgent electroencephalography (EEG) should be considered,** even in patients without a history of clinical seizures.

V. Seizure Disorders of Childhood

A. Definitions

1. A **seizure** is a transient, involuntary alteration of consciousness, behavior, motor activity, sensation, or autonomic function caused by an excessive discharge from a population of cerebral neurons.

2. **Epilepsy** is the occurrence of two or more spontaneous seizures without an obvious precipitating cause.

3. **Status epilepticus** is a seizure that lasts $\geq$ 30 minutes during which the patient does not regain consciousness.

B. Epidemiology

1. Four to six percent of children have a single afebrile seizure before 16 years of age.

2. Fewer than one third of children who have a single seizure go on to develop epilepsy, which has an incidence of 0.5–0.8% during childhood.

C. Etiology

1. The seizure discharge is caused by an imbalance between excitatory and inhibitory input within the brain or abnormalities in the membrane properties of individual neurons.

2. In some children, the cause of seizures is known (**Table 12-2**).

3. In **60–70%** of cases, the **cause is unknown.**

D. Classification of Seizures. Criteria for classification are the presence or absence of fever, the extent of brain involvement, whether consciousness is impaired, and the nature of the movements (Figure 12-2).

1. **Febrile seizures** are a common but benign type of seizure associated with fever (see section V.K).

2. **Afebrile seizures** are either generalized or partial, depending on whether both sides or one side of the brain are involved.

   a. **Generalized seizures** are caused by the discharge from a group of neurons in **both cerebral hemispheres.** Two common types are tonic-clonic and absence seizures.

Table 12-2. Causes of Acute Seizures During Childhood

Head trauma	Cerebral contusion, subdural hematoma
Brain tumor	Astrocytoma, meningioma
Toxins	Amphetamines, cocaine
Infections	Meningitis, encephalitis, brain abscess, neurocysticercosis
Vascular	Cerebral infarction, intracranial hemorrhage
Metabolic disturbances	Hypocalcemia, hypoglycemia, hypomagnesemia, hypo- or hypernatremia, pyridoxine deficiency
Systemic diseases	Hypertension, hypoxic-ischemic injury, inherited metabolic disorder, liver disease, renal failure, neurocutaneous disorders (tuberous sclerosis)

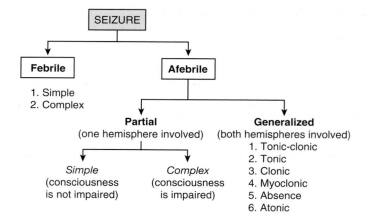

Figure 12-2. Classification of seizures.

    (1) Tonic-clonic seizures are the **most common type of generalized seizure.** These seizures are characterized by increased thoracic and abdominal muscle tone, followed by clonic movements of the arms and legs, eyes rolling upward, incontinence, decreased consciousness, and a **postictal state** of variable duration.

    (2) Absence seizures are brief staring spells that occur without loss of posture and with only minor motor manifestations (e.g., eye blinking or mouthing movements). The seizure lasts < 15 seconds, and there is **no postictal state.**

  b. Partial (focal) seizures are caused by the discharge from a group of neurons in **one hemisphere.** Seizure symptoms may have predominately **motor, sensory, or psychomotor features.** There are two types, simple and complex.

    (1) In **simple partial seizures,** consciousness is **not** impaired.

    (2) In **complex partial seizures, consciousness is decreased.**

E. Classification of epilepsy. Classification may be based on either the **predominant seizure type** or **the site of origin of the epileptic discharge.** For example, a child may have generalized or complex partial epilepsy, or it may be more convenient to refer to the site of the seizure discharge (e.g., frontal lobe epilepsy).

F. Differential diagnosis of seizurelike events (Table 12-3)

G. Diagnosis. Epilepsy is diagnosed on the basis of **history** and **physical examination.** Other studies may be useful.

  1. EEG identifies the focus and particular pattern of the epileptic discharge. **However, an abnormal EEG is not required for the diagnosis of epilepsy** (i.e., a normal EEG does not exclude the diagnosis of seizures or epilepsy).

  2. Video-EEG monitoring is a useful tool when clinical information is inadequate or incomplete (e.g., when patients are < 3 years of age, when

Table 12-3. Differential Diagnosis of Seizurelike Events

Breath-holding spells (in infants)
Gastroesophageal reflux disease (Sandifer syndrome)
Syncope
Migraine
Vertigo
Movement disorder (e.g., tics, chorea)
Sleep disturbances (e.g., night terrors, somnambulism)
Transient ischemic attack
Rage attacks
Psychogenic seizures

seizurelike events occur during sleep, or when parents are poor historians).

3. **Neuroimaging studies** should be performed in all children with epilepsy, except those with absence seizures or benign rolandic epilepsy (see sections V.L.4 and V.L.5).

H. Evaluation

1. Initial treatment starts with assessment of the patient's airway, breathing, and circulation (**ABCs**).

2. **Laboratory studies** are based on the patient's age, clinical features, and the physical examination.

   a. A **first-time afebrile seizure** in an otherwise healthy child with a **normal neurologic examination** does not warrant further investigation.

   b. **Serum electrolytes and neuroimaging** should be performed in a child who has had prior afebrile seizures.

   c. **In a febrile seizure, CNS infection must be ruled out** clinically or by examination of CSF. Other studies may include complete blood count (CBC), chest radiograph, and urine and blood cultures (see section V.K).

I. Management

1. **Treatment of status epilepticus requires intravenous anticonvulsants,** such as a **short-acting benzodiazepine (e.g., lorazepam or diazepam)** followed by a loading dose of either **phenobarbital or phenytoin.**

2. **Treatment of epilepsy**

   a. **Pharmacotherapy.** Once the type of seizure has been determined, **single-drug therapy** is started with the antiepileptic drug that has the best combination of high efficacy and low toxicity. **Recommended drugs** include:

      (1) Generalized epilepsy: valproic acid or phenobarbital

      (2) Absence epilepsy: ethosuximide

      (3) Partial epilepsy: carbamazepine or phenytoin

   b. **Surgery**

(1) **For medically intractable epilepsy,** surgery to remove epileptic tissue may be an option.

(2) The best prognosis is for patients with temporal lobe lesions, 75% of whom have complete seizure control or remission after surgery.

c. **Alternative treatments.** Patients with poorly controlled seizures for whom surgery is not an option have two additional choices.

(1) **Vagal nerve stimulator** is a pacemaker-sized device that sends an electrical impulse to the vagus nerve. A common side effect is hoarseness.

(2) **Ketogenic diet (a high-fat, low-carbohydrate diet)** is thought to suppress seizure activity by producing a **state of ketosis.**

J. **Prognosis. Epilepsy is not a lifelong disorder.** About 70% of epileptic children can be weaned off their medications after a 2-year seizure-free period and normalization of the EEG.

K. **Febrile Seizures**

1. **Definition.** A febrile seizure is any seizure that is accompanied by a fever owing to a non-CNS cause in patients from **6 months to 6 years of age.**

2. **Epidemiology.** Febrile seizures are **common, occurring in 3%** of all children.

3. **Etiology**

a. The **pathophysiologic mechanism is unknown.**

b. Febrile seizures can be inherited, and several gene mutations have been found.

4. **Classification**

a. **A simple febrile seizure lasts less than 15 minutes and is generalized.**

b. **A complex febrile seizure lasts more than 15 minutes, has focal features, or recurs within 24 hours.**

5. **Diagnosis**

a. **The diagnosis of a febrile seizure is based on history, a normal neurologic examination, and the exclusion of any CNS infection.**

b. **A lumbar puncture** is necessary only if meningitis is suspected.

c. **Neither neuroimaging nor EEG is needed** unless the neurologic examination is abnormal.

6. **Management**

a. **First-time or occasional febrile seizures** are not treated with anticonvulsants.

b. Aggressive antipyretic treatment of subsequent febrile illnesses may help prevent febrile seizures.

c. **Frequent, recurrent febrile seizures** do pose a risk and may require additional treatment, including:

(1) **Daily anticonvulsant prophylaxis** with valproic acid or phenobarbital

(2) **Abortive treatment with rectal diazepam**

7. **Prognosis. Approximately 30% of patients with one febrile**

seizure will have a recurrence. Recurrence risk decreases with increasing patient age. The risk of epilepsy is low (2%).

L. Epileptic Syndromes

1. **Definition.** Epileptic syndromes are epileptic conditions characterized by a specific age of onset, seizure characteristic, and EEG abnormality.

2. **Classification.** More than 15 epileptic syndromes are recognized. Each syndrome has its own seizure severity and outcome. Three of the most common are **infantile spasms, absence epilepsy of childhood,** and **benign rolandic epilepsy.**

3. **Infantile spasms (West syndrome)**

   a. **Epidemiology. Age of onset** is typically 3–8 months. Infantile spasms are rare in children older than 2 years of age.

   b. **Etiology. Tuberous sclerosis is the most commonly identified cause** of infantile spasms. Other inherited and acquired causes include phenylketonuria, hypoxic-ischemic injury, intraventricular hemorrhage, meningitis, and encephalitis.

   c. **Clinical features**

      (1) Brief, myoclonic jerks, lasting 1–2 seconds each, occurring in clusters of 5–10 seizures spread over 3–5 minutes.

      (2) The jerks consist of sudden arm extension or head and trunk flexion (also known as **jackknife seizures** or **salaam seizures**).

   d. **Diagnosis.** The EEG **shows the characteristic hypsarrhythmia pattern,** a highly disorganized pattern of high amplitude spike and waves occurring in both cerebral hemispheres.

   e. **Management**

      (1) **Adrenocorticotropic hormone (ACTH)** intramuscular injections for a 4- to 6-week period are effective in more than 70% of affected patients.

      (2) **Valproic acid** is the second-line drug of choice.

      (3) **Vigabatrin** is the most effective drug for patients with infantile spasms associated with tuberous sclerosis.

   f. **Prognosis. Outlook is poor.** Despite the success of these different medications in suppressing seizures, children often develop moderate to severe mental retardation.

4. **Absence epilepsy of childhood**

   a. **Epidemiology. Age of onset** is between 5 and 9 years of age. There is a female-to-male predominance of 3:2.

   b. **Etiology.** Inheritance is **autosomal dominant with age-dependent penetrance.**

   c. **Clinical features**

      (1) Absence seizures last 5–10 seconds.

      (2) They occur frequently—tens to hundreds of times per day.

      (3) They are often accompanied by automatisms, such as eye blinking and incomprehensible utterances.

      (4) **Loss of posture, urinary incontinence, and a postictal state do not occur.**

    d. **Diagnosis.** The **EEG** shows the characteristic **generalized 3-Hz spike and wave discharge** arising from both hemispheres.

    e. **Management. Treatment includes ethosuximide** (first-line drug) or **valproic acid.**

    f. **Prognosis. Outlook is very good;** the seizures usually resolve by adolescence without cognitive impairment.

5. **Benign rolandic epilepsy (benign centrotemporal epilepsy)**

    a. **Definition.** Benign rolandic epilepsy involves nocturnal partial seizures with secondary generalization.

    b. **Epidemiology**

       (1) Benign rolandic epilepsy is the **most common partial epilepsy during childhood,** accounting for 15% of epilepsy.

       (2) It commonly presents at 3–13 years of age. Peak incidence is at 6–7 years. Boys are more likely to be affected.

    c. **Etiology.** Inheritance is **autosomal dominant** with variable penetrance.

    d. **Clinical features**

       (1) Seizures occur in the **early morning hours** when patients are asleep with **oral-buccal manifestations** (i.e., moaning, grunting, pooling of saliva).

       (2) Seizures spread to face and arm, then generalize into **tonic-clonic seizures.**

    e. **Diagnosis. The EEG** shows biphasic **spike and sharp wave disturbance in the mid-temporal and central regions.**

    f. **Management.** Treatment includes valproic acid (first-line drug) or carbamazepine.

    g. **Prognosis. Outcome is excellent.** Seizures remit spontaneously during adolescence with no adverse effects on development or cognition.

VI. Headaches in Childhood

  A. **Etiology.** Headaches may have intracranial or extracranial causes (Figure 12-3).

    1. **Intracranial causes**

      a. **Primary headaches** are caused by a primary dysfunction of **neurons** (e.g., migraine headaches) or **muscles** (e.g., tension headaches).

      b. **Secondary headaches** are caused by increased intracranial pressure (ICP; e.g., hydrocephalus) or meningeal irritation (e.g., meningitis, subarachnoid hemorrhage).

    2. **Extracranial causes**

      a. **Local causes** include sinusitis, perioral abscess, toothache, chronic otitis media, or refractive errors.

      b. **Systemic causes** include anemia and hypoglycemia in children, and depression and hypertension in adolescents.

  B. **Important clinical information** about a patient's headache helps determine the cause.

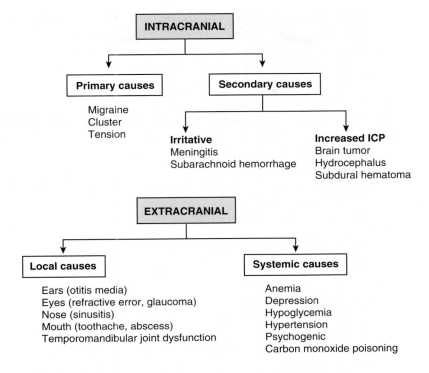

Figure 12-3. Causes of headache. *ICP* = intracranial pressure.

1. **Quality of pain.** Throbbing or pounding pain suggests migraine headaches, whereas an aching feeling of pressure is more common in tension headaches.

2. **Site and radiation.** Migraine headaches are usually unilateral and may begin in the periorbital area and spread to the forehead and occiput, whereas tension headaches are often generalized or bitemporal.

3. **Time of onset.** Tension headaches occur toward the end of the day, whereas headaches from increased ICP occur in the morning.

4. **Duration.** The shorter the headache duration, the less likely a serious disorder is responsible.

C. **Migraine Headaches**

1. **Definition.** Migraine headaches are prolonged (often > 1 hour), unilateral headaches that are associated with nausea, vomiting, or visual changes and are caused by changes in cerebral blood flow.

2. **Epidemiology**
   a. Migraines are the **most common cause of headaches in children and adolescents,** occurring in up to 5% of school-age children.
   b. **Age of onset** is younger than 5 years in 20% of patients.
   c. Before puberty, incidence is higher in males; after puberty, incidence is higher in females.

3. **Etiology**

    a. Inheritance is **autosomal dominant.** More than 80% of children with migraines have at least one affected parent.

    b. **Changes in cerebral blood flow** are secondary to release of **serotonin (5-HT),** substance P, and vasoactive intestinal peptide from changes in neuronal activity.

  4. **Classification**

    a. **Migraine without aura is the most common form of migraine in children.** Headaches occur in the absence of any warning symptoms.

    b. **Migraine with aura.** The onset of the headache is preceded by transient visual changes (e.g., blurred vision, small areas of decreased vision [scotomata], streaks of light, or hemianopsia) or unilateral paresthesias or weakness.

    c. **Migraine equivalent.** In young children, the headache itself may be absent, but there is a prolonged, albeit transient, alteration of behavior that manifests as cyclic vomiting, cyclic abdominal pain, or paroxysmal vertigo.

    d. Migraines associated with focal neurologic signs.

      (1) **Ophthalmoplegic migraine.** Unilateral ptosis or cranial nerve III palsy accompanies this headache.

      (2) **Basilar artery migraine.** Vertigo, tinnitus, ataxia, or dysarthria may precede the onset of this headache.

  5. **Precipitating factors.** There is **no obvious precipitating cause,** although many migraine sufferers are sensitive to vasoactive substances in certain wines, cheeses, preserved meats, and chocolate. Some patients note that stress, fatigue, menstruation, or exercise induce the headache.

  6. **Clinical features**

    a. **A prolonged, throbbing, unilateral headache** starts in the supraorbital area and radiates to the occiput. In young children, the headache is often bifrontal.

    b. **Nausea and vomiting** may occur. A history of motion sickness is common.

    c. **Visual disturbances** include blurred vision, scotomata, and jagged streaks of light that take on the outline of old forts (**fortifications**).

    d. **Photophobia or phonophobia** occurs. Many patients treat themselves by lying in a dark, quiet room.

    e. Over-the-counter analgesics are often ineffective.

    f. **Symptoms are improved by sleep.**

    g. **Neurologic examination is normal.**

  7. **Diagnosis.** Diagnosis is made by history and the presence of a normal neurologic examination.

  8. **Management.** Treatment includes rest and elimination of known triggers. Medications may be very helpful:

    a. **Abortive treatment** includes **sumatriptan,** a **selective 5-HT agonist,** available in injectable, intranasal, and oral forms.

    b. **Propranolol is the drug of choice for prophylactic treatment** of frequent migraines.

9. **Prognosis.** Migraines can be a lifelong disorder with a waxing and waning course.

D. **Tension Headaches**

1. **Definition.** Tension headaches are bifrontal or diffuse, dull, aching headaches that are often associated with muscle contraction.

2. **Epidemiology.** Tension headaches are unusual during childhood and extremely rare in children younger than 7 years of age.

3. **Clinical features**

a. Pain is described as **dull, aching, and rarely throbbing,** and it increases in intensity during the day.

b. The pain is usually bifrontal but may be diffuse.

c. **Isometric contraction** of the temporalis, masseter, or trapezius muscle often accompanies the headache.

d. **No vomiting, visual changes, or paresthesias occur.**

4. **Diagnosis.** Clinical presentation provides a clue to the diagnosis, although no laboratory or imaging study is diagnostic. **Tension headaches are very rare in childhood, and therefore other diagnoses (e.g., migraines) should be preferentially considered.**

5. **Management.** Treatment includes reassurance and pain control (e.g., acetaminophen, ibuprofen). Stress and anxiety reduction may provide long-term relief.

E. **Cluster Headaches.** These headaches are extremely rare during childhood. They are characterized by **unilateral frontal or facial pain, accompanied by conjunctival erythema, lacrimation, and nasal congestion.** The headaches usually last < 30 minutes but may recur several times in a day and then not occur again for weeks or months (hence the term "cluster"). Treatment includes abortive therapy with oxygen or sumatriptan. Prophylactic treatments include calcium-channel blockers and valproic acid.

VII. Approach to Unsteady Gait

A. **Definition.** Ataxia is the **inability to coordinate muscle activity during voluntary movement.** It can involve the trunk or limbs and is caused by cerebellar or proprioceptive dysfunction.

B. **Differential diagnosis.** A variety of neurologic problems can give the appearance of an unsteady gait.

1. **Cerebellar dysfunction.** Children with a **cerebellar gait** have **an unsteady, wide-based stance with irregular steps and veering** to one side or the other. See **Table 12-4** for the causes of cerebellar ataxia.

2. **Weakness.** Any cause of muscle weakness, such as spinal cord lesions or acute disorders of the motor unit (e.g., **Guillain-Barré syndrome,** see section VII.D), can lead to an unsteady gait.

3. **Encephalopathy as a result of infection, drug overdose, or recent head trauma** may cause decreased levels of consciousness, which may affect gait.

Table 12-4. Differential Diagnosis of Cerebellar Ataxia

Brain tumors	Cerebellar astrocytoma
	Cerebellar primitive neuroectodermal tumor (medulloblastoma)
	Neuroblastoma
Trauma	Cerebellar contusion
	Subdural hematoma
Toxins	Ethanol
	Anticonvulsants
Vascular	Cerebellar infarction or hemorrhage
Infections	Meningitis
	Encephalitis
Inflammatory	Acute cerebellar ataxia of childhood
Demyelination	Acute disseminated encephalomyelitis
	Multiple sclerosis

    4. Seizures. During a **seizure or while in the postictal period,** the patient's gait is irregular and unsteady.

    5. Vision problems can mimic the appearance of an unsteady gait.

    6. Vertigo from migraines, acute labyrinthitis, and brainstem tumors may lead to unsteady walking.

C. Acute Cerebellar Ataxia of Childhood

    1. Definition. Acute cerebellar ataxia is an unsteady gait secondary to a presumed autoimmune or postinfectious cause.

    2. Epidemiology

        a. Acute cerebellar ataxia is the **most common cause of ataxia in children.**

        b. Age of onset is between 18 months and 7 years. Acute cerebellar ataxia rarely occurs in children older than 10 years of age.

    3. Etiology

        a. Common preceding infections include **varicella, influenza, Epstein-Barr virus (EBV), and mycoplasma.** The ataxia usually follows a viral illness by 2–3 weeks.

        b. The postulated cause is immune complex deposition in the cerebellum.

    4. Clinical features

        a. Truncal ataxia with deterioration of gait is characteristic. Young children may refuse to walk for fear of falling.

        b. Slurred speech and nystagmus are often present, although hypotonia and tremors are less common.

        c. Fever is absent.

    5. Diagnosis. Diagnosis is by history and physical examination and by exclusion of other causes of ataxia. **An urgent neuroimaging study is necessary in all patients suspected of cerebellar ataxia** to rule out acute life-threatening causes, such as tumors or hemorrhage in the posterior fossa. **Head CT scan is normal in this disorder.**

    6. Management. Treatment is supportive. Complete resolution of symptoms may take as long as 2–3 months. Physical therapy may be useful.

D. Guillain-Barré Syndrome (acute inflammatory demyelinating poly-neuropathy)

1. **Definition.** Guillain-Barré syndrome is a demyelinating polyneuritis characterized by ascending weakness, areflexia, and normal sensation.

2. **Etiology.** The **most commonly associated infectious agent is *Campylobacter jejuni,*** which causes a prodromal gastroenteritis. Many other infectious agents have been associated with Guillain-Barré syndrome, such as cytomegalovirus, EBV, herpes zoster virus, influenza, varicella, and coxsackievirus.

3. **Pathophysiology**
   a. The **principal sites of demyelination** are the ventral spinal roots and peripheral myelinated nerves.
   b. Injury is triggered by a **cell-mediated immune response** to an infectious agent that cross-reacts to antigens on the Schwann cell membrane.

4. **Clinical features**
   a. **Ascending, symmetric paralysis** may progress to respiratory arrest.
   b. **No sensory loss occurs,** although low back or leg pain may be present in 50% of patients.
   c. **Cranial nerve involvement.** Facial weakness occurs in 40–50% of patients.
   d. **Miller-Fisher syndrome,** a **variant** of Guillain-Barré syndrome, is characterized by ophthalmoplegia, ataxia, and areflexia.

5. **Diagnosis**
   a. **Lumbar puncture** shows **albuminocytologic dissociation** (i.e., increased CSF protein in the absence of an elevated cell count), which is usually evident 1 week after symptom onset.
   b. **EMG** demonstrates decreased nerve conduction velocity or conduction block.
   c. **Spinal MRI** may be necessary in children younger than 3 years of age to rule out compressive lesions of the spinal cord because the sensory examination in children of this age is often difficult to evaluate.

6. **Management.** Treatment should be initiated as soon as the diagnosis is established because of the risk of respiratory muscle paralysis.
   a. **Intravenous immune globulin (IVIG),** given for 2–4 days, is the **preferred treatment for children** because of its relative safety and ease of use. The mechanism of action of IVIG is unknown.
   b. **Plasmapheresis** removes the patient's plasma along with the presumed anti-myelin antibodies and is performed over a 4- to 5-day period.

7. **Prognosis. Complete recovery is the rule in children** but depends on the severity and extent of the weakness. Physical therapy may be necessary for several weeks or longer to aid recovery.

VIII. Movement Disorders

A. Sydenham chorea (St. Vitus' dance)

1. **Definition.** Sydenham chorea is a self-limited **autoimmune disorder** associated with **rheumatic fever (see Chapter 16, section VI)** that

presents with chorea (uncontrolled, restless proximal limb movements) and emotional lability.

2. **Epidemiology**
   a. Sydenham chorea occurs in approximately **25% of patients with rheumatic fever.**
   b. **Onset is most common between 5 and 13 years of age.**

3. **Pathophysiology.** Sydenham chorea occurs secondary to **antibodies that cross-react with membrane antigens on both group A β-hemolytic streptococcus and basal ganglia cells.**

4. **Clinical features**
   a. **Immunologic response** usually follows the streptococcal pharyngitis by **2–7 months.**
   b. **Children appear restless.** The face, hands, and arms are mainly affected, and the movements appear continuous, quick, and random. The chorea may begin as clumsiness of the hands.
   c. **Speech is also affected** and can be jerky or indistinct.
   d. Patients are unable to sustain protrusion of the tongue (**chameleon tongue**).
   e. The wrist is held flexed and hyperextended at the metacarpal joints (**choreic hand**). On gripping the examiner's fingers, patients are unable to maintain the grip (**milkmaid's grip**).
   f. **Emotional lability** is common.
   g. **Gait and cognition are not affected.**

5. **Differential diagnosis. Other conditions that may cause chorea** include many acquired and congenital conditions, including encephalitis, kernicterus, systemic lupus erythematosus, Huntington's disease, and Wilson's disease.

6. **Diagnosis.** There is **no single confirmatory test for Sydenham chorea.** The diagnosis rests on presumptive evidence of rheumatic fever and the exclusion of other likely causes of chorea.
   a. **Elevated antistreptolysin O (ASO) or anti-DNase B (ADB) titer** may indicate a recent streptococcal infection.
   b. **Neuroimaging**
      (1) **Head MRI** may show **increased signal intensity in the caudate and putamen** on T_2-weighted sequences.
      (2) **Single-photon emission computed tomography (SPECT)** may demonstrate **increased perfusion** to the thalamus and striatum.

7. **Management.** Treatment involves the use of **haloperidol, valproic acid, or phenobarbital.**

8. **Prognosis.** Symptoms **may last from several months to 2 years.** Generally, all patients recover.

B. **Tourette Syndrome**

1. **Definitions**
   a. **Tourette syndrome is a chronic, lifelong movement disorder** that presents with **motor and phonic tics before 18 years of age.**

  b. Tics are brief, stereotypical behaviors that are initiated by an unconscious urge that can be temporarily suppressed.

2. **Epidemiology.** The prevalence of Tourette syndrome is 1 in 1,000 live births. However, tics occur in 3% of children.

3. **Etiology.** The cause of Tourette syndrome is unknown. In some patients, there is a genetic predisposition.

4. **Clinical features**

  a. Motor tics can be simple (e.g., eye blinking, head or shoulder shaking) or complex (e.g., bouncing, jumping, kicking).

  b. Phonic tics can be simple (e.g., coughing, groaning, barking) or complex (e.g., echolalia, which is the repetition of heard words or phrases).

  c. Tics must be present ≥ 1 year, although their severity and frequency waxes and wanes.

  d. Absence of any signs of a neurodegenerative disorder

  e. Coprolalia, the utterance of obscene words, is a dramatic symptom that occurs in 15% of patients but is rare at initial presentation.

  f. Associated findings include learning disabilities, attention deficit/hyperactivity disorder, and obsessive-compulsive traits.

5. **Differential diagnosis. Disorders that may cause tics** include Wilson's disease, Sydenham chorea, partial seizures, pediatric autoimmune neuropsychiatric disorders associated with streptococcal infection (**PANDAS**) (see Chapter 7, section IX.A.5.f.(4)), or simple habits. (**Habits differ from tics** in that habits are situation-dependent and are under voluntary control.)

6. **Diagnosis**

  a. Tourette syndrome is **a clinical diagnosis based on history and neurologic findings.**

  b. No laboratory or imaging tests confirm the diagnosis.

7. **Management**

  a. Pimozide is the drug of choice because it is effective with minimal extrapyramidal side effects.

  b. Clonidine is less effective than pimozide. The major side effect is sedation.

  c. Haloperidol was the first drug used to treat Tourette syndrome, but the risk of tardive dyskinesia has limited its use.

  d. Hypnotherapy has been effective in some patients.

8. **Prognosis**

  a. Tics tend to **decrease in adulthood.**

  b. Pharmacotherapy is generally successful, but side effects from the medications may be limiting.

IX. Duchenne and Becker Muscular Dystrophies (DMD, BMD)

 A. Definition. DMD and BMD are progressive, **X-linked myopathies** characterized by myofiber degeneration. **DMD is more severe than BMD.**

B. Epidemiology

1. These worldwide disorders occur in all ethnic groups.

2. Prevalence is 1 in 25,000 live births.

3. **Onset** of symptoms is between 2 and 5 years of age.

C. Etiology. These X-linked disorders are caused by a **deletion in the dystrophin gene.**

D. Pathophysiology

1. **Dystrophin** is a high molecular weight cytoskeletal protein that associates with actin and other structural membrane elements.

2. The **absence of dystrophin** causes weakness and eventually rupture of the plasma membrane, leading to injury and degeneration of muscle fibers.

E. Pathology. Both DMD and BMD have the same appearance on light microscopy.

1. **Degeneration and regeneration** of muscle fibers

2. **Infiltration of lymphocytes** into the injured area and **replacement** of damaged muscle fibers **with fibroblasts and lipid deposits**

F. Clinical Features

1. **Slow, progressive weakness affecting the legs first**

2. **In DMD, children lose the ability to walk by 10 years of age. In BMD, patients lose the ability to walk by 20 or more years of age.**

3. **Pseudohypertrophy of calves** is present because of the excess accumulation of lipids, which replace the degenerating muscle fibers. This is more common in DMD than in BMD.

4. **Gowers' sign is present.** Because of the weakness of pelvic muscles, patients arise from the floor in a characteristic manner by extending each leg and then "climbing up" each thigh until they reach an upright position.

5. **Cardiac involvement** (e.g., cardiomegaly, tachycardia, or cardiac failure) occurs in 50% of patients.

6. Mild cognitive impairment occurs in DMD, but normal intelligence is present in BMD.

G. Diagnosis

1. **The presence of enlarged calf muscles in a young boy with muscle weakness suggests the diagnosis.**

2. **CK levels are very high.**

3. **EMG** shows small, polyphasic muscle potentials with normal nerve conductions.

4. **Muscle biopsy** shows the typical dystrophic pattern.

5. **Absent or decreased dystrophin levels** are present on immunocytochemistry or Western blot assay of muscle.

6. **DNA testing** may reveal the gene deletion in > 90% of patients.

H. Management. There is no cure but oral steroids can improve strength transiently when the disease is in the early stages. Gene replacement, myoblast transplantation, and dystrophin replacement have not been successful in clinical trials.

I. Prognosis

1. **In DMD,** patients are wheelchair dependent by 10 years of age and often die in their late teens from respiratory failure. Assisted ventilation may help individuals live longer.

2. **In BMD,** patients become wheelchair dependent in their twenties. Life expectancy is in the fifties.

X. Myasthenia Gravis

A. Definition. Myasthenia gravis is an **autoimmune disorder** that presents with progressive weakness or diplopia.

B. Etiology. Myasthenia gravis is caused by **antibodies against the acetylcholine receptor (AChR) at neuromuscular junctions.**

C. Classification

1. **Neonatal myasthenia** is a **transient weakness** in the newborn period secondary to transplacental transfer of maternal AChR antibodies from a mother affected with myasthenia gravis.

2. **Juvenile** myasthenia gravis presents in childhood secondary to AChR antibody formation.

D. Epidemiology. Juvenile myasthenia gravis affects **girls** two to six times more frequently than boys.

E. Clinical Features

1. **In neonatal myasthenia, hypotonia, weakness, and feeding problems** are the most common findings.

2. **In juvenile MG,** several findings are characteristic.
   a. **Bilateral ptosis is the most common presenting sign.**
   b. **Characteristic increasing weakness** occurs later in the day and with repetitive or sustained muscle activity.
   c. **Diplopia** secondary to decreased extraocular movements may be the only manifestation.
   d. **DTRs are preserved.**
   e. **Other autoimmune disorders,** including juvenile rheumatoid arthritis, diabetes mellitus, and thyroid disease, may coexist.

F. Diagnosis. Diagnosis is made by the following:

1. **Tensilon test. Intravenous injection of edrophonium chloride,** a rapidly acting cholinesterase inhibitor, produces transient improvement of ptosis.

2. **Decremental response** to low-frequency (3–10 Hz) repetitive nerve stimulation

3. **Presence of AChR antibody titers**

G. **Management**

1. **In neonatal myasthenia, treatment is often symptomatic,** because the disorder is self-limited. If respiration is compromised, cholinesterase inhibitors or IVIG may be indicated.

2. **In juvenile myasthenia gravis,** treatment involves the following:

   a. **Cholinesterase inhibitors** are the mainstay of treatment. **Pyridostigmine bromide** is the drug of choice.

   b. **Immunotherapy**

      (1) **Corticosteroids** are used when cholinesterase inhibitors fail.

      (2) **Plasmapheresis lowers the level of AChR antibodies.** It is useful when symptoms worsen, when respiratory effort is compromised, or when the patient is unresponsive to other therapies.

      (3) **IVIG** also may be effective.

   c. **Thymectomy** is often performed.

H. **Prognosis**

1. **In neonatal myasthenia, symptoms are mild and generally resolve within 1–3 weeks.**

2. **In juvenile myasthenia gravis,** remission of symptoms can be as high as 60% after thymectomy.

Review Test

1. You are called to the nursery to examine a "floppy" female infant born within the past 24 hours. The neonate is hypotonic with diminished deep tendon reflexes. There are no tongue fasciculations. When you greet the baby's mother, she is anxious and has difficulty releasing her grip after shaking your hand. Which of the following is the most likely diagnosis?

(A) Muscular dystrophy
(B) Congenital myotonic dystrophy
(C) Neonatal myasthenia gravis
(D) Spinal muscular atrophy, type 1
(E) Infantile botulism

2. A 10-year-old girl is being evaluated for "weakness" of 3 days' duration. Medical history is significant for a 4-day episode of diarrhea 2 weeks before her current presentation. She is otherwise well with no chronic medical conditions and is taking no medications. Physical examination reveals symmetric weakness at the ankles and knees, with normal strength at the hip joints. Deep tendon reflexes are absent in the distal lower extremities. Sensory examination is normal. Which of the following statements is most consistent with the most likely diagnosis?

(A) This patient is most likely to have had a prodromal gastroenteritis with *Salmonella typhi*.
(B) Electromyography would be expected to show normal nerve conduction.
(C) Management should include intravenous immune globulin.
(D) This patient is likely to have elevated antistreptolysin O or anti-DNase B titers.
(E) The prognosis for complete recovery is poor.

3. A 6-month-old male infant is evaluated for lethargy and poor feeding. Recent dietary changes include the introduction of cereals, fruits, and herbal tea with honey. Physical examination reveals an afebrile infant with normal vital signs. Neurologic examination is notable for decreased muscle tone and a weak suck. Which of the following statements regarding this infant's most likely diagnosis is most accurate?

(A) Infants typically present with ascending paralysis.
(B) Antibiotics should be administered immediately.
(C) Infants present with brisk deep tendon reflexes.
(D) Electromyography is not helpful in making the diagnosis.
(E) Constipation is the classic initial symptom in infants.

4. An 8-year-old girl is noted by her teacher to have brief staring spells throughout the day. She is referred to you for further evaluation. Neurologic examination is normal. You order an electroencephalogram, which shows a generalized 3-Hz spike and wave discharge pattern arising from both hemispheres. Which of the following statements regarding the most likely diagnosis is most accurate?

(A) Further questioning would probably reveal that this patient loses control of her bladder during the event.
(B) This patient's condition is inherited in an autosomal recessive pattern.
(C) This patient's staring spells would be expected to last less than 10 seconds each.
(D) This patient is likely to have prolonged postictal periods.
(E) Phenobarbital is the drug of choice for this patient's condition.

5. A 4-month-old female infant is brought to your office by her parents, who are concerned about some behaviors they have witnessed. They note that during the past week, she has had brief jerking episodes, lasting 1–2 seconds each, with sudden arm extension followed by flexion of the head. You order an electroencephalogram, which reveals a highly disorganized pattern of high-amplitude spike and waves in both cerebral hemispheres, consistent with a hypsarrhythmia pattern. Which of the following is the most commonly identified cause of the patient's disorder?

(A) Prior episode of bacterial meningitis
(B) Perinatal asphyxia
(C) Shaken baby syndrome
(D) Tuberous sclerosis
(E) Neurofibromatosis type 1

6. A 6-year-old boy complains of a 4-day history of low back pain and difficulty walking. On examination, you note weakness in his lower extremities and absent lower extremity deep tendon reflexes. Sensation in the lower extremities is intact. A magnetic resonance imaging scan of the spine is normal. Which of the following is the most likely diagnosis?

(A) Duchenne muscular dystrophy
(B) Myasthenia gravis
(C) Acute cerebellar ataxia of childhood
(D) Guillain-Barré syndrome
(E) Becker muscular dystrophy

7. A 2-year-old boy is brought to the office by his parents, who note that their son has had weakness in his legs for the past several months that appears to be getting worse. On examination, you note that the calf muscles are enlarged. Which of the following statements regarding this patient's likely condition is correct?

(A) DNA testing is normal.
(B) Dystrophin levels are normal.
(C) Progressive weakness leads to loss of ambulation before 10 years of age.
(D) Electromyography reveals delayed nerve conduction.
(E) Treatment with intravenous immune globulin can transiently improve symptoms.

8. A previously healthy 3-year-old girl is brought to the emergency department with a 2-day history of unsteady gait and one episode of vomiting. Parents deny any history of trauma, medications, or ingestion. She has no other symptoms, and her last illness was an upper respiratory infection with cough 3 weeks ago. On examination, she is well appearing and afebrile and has normal deep tendon reflexes but refuses to walk. Which of the following is the next step in management?

(A) Obtain a complete blood count, serum electrolytes, and glucose.
(B) Perform a lumbar puncture.
(C) Order a head computed tomography scan.
(D) Order an electroencephalogram.
(E) Reevaluate her the next day to monitor her progress.

9. Two hours ago a 2-year-old boy had a 5-minute episode of whole body shaking associated with a temperature of 103°F (39.4°C). The boy's parents state that their son has had runny nose and cough for the past 24 hours. He now acts normal except for his cold symptoms, according to his parents. The parents remind you that this is his second febrile seizure. Physical examination is normal, revealing no focal neurologic signs. Which of the following would be the most appropriate recommendation at this time?

(A) Order a stat head computed tomography scan.
(B) Order an electroencephalogram.
(C) Begin treatment with phenobarbital.
(D) Reassure the parents that no workup or medications are necessary at this point.
(E) Admit the patient to the hospital for overnight observation.

10. A 12-year-old girl is brought to see you for evaluation of frequent headaches. She has had headaches three times per week for the past several months, and her parents are concerned that she may be having migraines. Which of the following statements would support this diagnosis?

(A) The headaches are bilateral, throbbing, and bitemporal in location.
(B) The neurologic examination is abnormal during the headache.
(C) The headaches awaken the patient in the early morning hours.
(D) The duration of the headache is > 1 hour.
(E) This patient is likely to have an aura with her headache.

11. Examination of a comatose 13-year-old boy in the emergency department is significant for bilaterally nonreactive and dilated pupils. An oculocephalic maneuver is negative. Which of the following is the most likely diagnosis?

(A) Postictal state from status epilepticus
(B) Brainstem injury
(C) Subdural hematoma with herniation
(D) Opiate overdose

12. A 2-month-old boy is brought to your office for evaluation with a 2-day history of poor feeding and vomiting. Parents deny fever, cold symptoms, or diarrhea. On physical examination, the child is well hydrated but has a large anterior and posterior fontanelle and a persistent downward deviation of both eyes. This patient's presentation is most consistent with which of the following diagnoses?

(A) Cerebral infarct
(B) Congenital myotonic dystrophy
(C) Myasthenia gravis
(D) Becker muscular dystrophy
(E) Infantile hydrocephalus

The response items for statements 13–15 are the same. You will be required to select one answer for each statement in the set.

(A) Dandy-Walker malformation
(B) X-linked hydrocephalus
(C) Infantile botulism
(D) Spinal muscular atrophy type 1 (Werdnig-Hoffman disease)
(E) Juvenile myasthenia gravis
(F) Congenital myotonic dystrophy

For each patient, select the most likely diagnosis.

13. A 4-month-old male infant has generalized weakness, hypotonia, areflexia, and tongue fasciculations.

14. An 8-month-old female infant with a 5-day history of constipation presents with a weak cry, hyporeflexia, ophthalmoplegia, and an inability to sit without support when she previously had been able to do so.

15. A 6-month-old male has had hypotonia, facial weakness, areflexia, and a history of feeding problems since birth.

Answers and Explanations

1. The answer is B [I.F.3]. This patient most likely has congenital myotonic dystrophy. Patients present with hypotonia and often have feeding and respiratory problems. Facial weakness and hyporeflexia are common. Infants acquire the disorder through autosomal dominant inheritance, most commonly from an affected mother. Mothers of infants with congenital myotonic dystrophy have myotonia, an inability to relax contracted muscles, which manifests as difficulty releasing a hand grip during a firm handshake. Muscular dystrophy rarely presents during infancy. Infants with botulism have constipation, hypotonia, problems with suck and swallow, and progressive weakness that may lead to paralysis. Neonatal myasthenia is a transient muscle disorder caused by the transplacental passage of acetylcholine receptor antibodies. Weakness and hypotonia may be present, but deep tendon reflexes are preserved. Infants with spinal muscular atrophy have hypotonia but also have characteristic tongue fasciculations.

2. The answer is C [VII.D]. This patient's presentation is most consistent with Guillain-Barré syndrome. The diagnosis of Guillain-Barré syndrome should be considered in any child with ascending symmetric weakness or paralysis, absence of deep tendon reflexes, and a normal sensory examination. Management should be initiated as soon as the diagnosis is established because of the risk of respiratory muscle paralysis. Intravenous immune globulin is the preferred treatment in children. Many infectious agents have been associated with Guillain-Barré syndrome, but the most common infectious agent is *Campylobacter jejuni,* which causes a prodromal gastroenteritis. Electromyography would be expected to demonstrate decreased nerve conduction velocity or conduction block. There is no known association between Guillain-Barré syndrome and prior group A β-hemolytic streptococcal infection. The prognosis for children with Guillain-Barré syndrome is excellent, and complete recovery is likely.

3. The answer is E [I.F.2]. Infantile botulism is caused by the ingestion of *Clostridium botulinum* spores and the release of botulinum toxin within the intestine. The toxin prevents the release of acetylcholine at peripheral cholinergic synapses, initially causing constipation, which is followed by a weak suck and swallow, cranial nerve palsies, and weakness. Patients with infantile botulism have a symmetric descending paralysis. Contaminated honey is a common source of the toxin. Physical examination is notable for diffuse weakness, hypotonia, and hyporeflexia (i.e., diminished deep tendon reflexes). The diagnosis is suggested by the history and physical examination findings and confirmed by the identification of the toxin or bacteria within the stool. Electromyography may also be helpful in diagnosis and may show brief, small-amplitude muscle potentials with an incremental response during high-frequency stimulation. Treatment includes supportive care and botulism immune globulin. Antibiotics are not helpful.

4. The answer is C [V.L.4]. This patient's clinical presentation and electroencephalogram (EEG) are consistent with absence epilepsy of childhood. Patients usually present with multiple absence seizures, which are brief staring spells that occur without warning and are not followed by postictal drowsiness. Urinary continence and loss of posture are also not seen in absence seizures. Absence seizures last less than 10 seconds and have a very characteristic EEG pattern, showing a generalized 3-Hz spike and wave abnormality. Absence epilepsy of childhood is inherited in an autosomal dominant pattern with age-dependent penetrance. The antiepileptic medication of choice is ethosuximide.

5. The answer is D [V.L.3]. This clinical presentation is consistent with infantile spasms (West syndrome). Patients with infantile spasms typically present with brief, myoclonic jerks, lasting 1–2 seconds each, occurring in clusters of 5–10 seizures spread out over 3–5 minutes. Patients may have sudden extension of the arms and sudden flexion of the head (jackknife or salaam seizures). A variety of different prenatal, perinatal, and postnatal insults to the central nervous system may result in infantile spasms. Tuberous sclerosis is the most commonly identified cause of this disorder. Perinatal asphyxia, intraventricular hemorrhage, and meningitis are other causes of infantile spasms. Neurofibromatosis type 1 is not typically associated with infantile spasms.

6. The answer is D [VII.D]. Guillain-Barré syndrome (acute inflammatory demyelinating polyneuropathy) typically presents with ascending paralysis without sensory loss. Despite this finding, about 50% of children complain of low back pain or discomfort in their legs. Deep tendon reflexes are absent, and spinal magnetic resonance imaging is normal. The diagnosis is based on the findings of albuminocytologic dissociation in the cerebrospinal fluid and by decreased nerve conduction velocity on electrophysiologic studies. In both Duchenne and Becker muscular dystrophy, the onset of weakness is slow and progressive. Myasthenia gravis, which is more common in girls, presents with weakness that increases during the day and normal deep tendon reflexes. Acute cerebellar ataxia of childhood presents with ataxia (unsteady gait or truncal unsteadiness) rather than weakness.

7. The answer is C [IX.B, IX.E, IX.I.1]. This patient's presentation with increasing weakness in the lower extremities and calf enlargement is consistent with Duchenne muscular dystrophy, an X-linked progressive degenerative muscle disorder for which there is no cure. Children typically present between 2 and 5 years of age with gait problems and weakness, and they are often wheelchair dependent by their 10th birthday. On examination, patients have enlarged calf muscles as a result of fatty infiltration of the degenerating muscles, and laboratory studies reveal elevated creatine kinase levels. The diagnosis can be made by DNA testing of the dystrophin gene, which shows a deletion in more than 90% of patients. Electromyography shows small, polyphasic muscle potentials but normal nerve conduction velocities. Intravenous immune globulin has no role in the management of Duchenne muscular dystrophy.

8. The answer is C [VII.C.2, VII.C.5]. Acute cerebellar ataxia of childhood is the most common cause of ataxia during childhood and is therefore the most likely diagnosis in this patient. However, because there are no diagnostic laboratory tests or imaging studies to confirm this diagnosis, acute cerebellar ataxia of childhood is a diagnosis of exclusion. Therefore, all patients who present with ataxia require an urgent neuroimaging study to rule out potentially life-threatening disorders of the posterior fossa, such as cerebellar tumors or hemorrhage. Electrolyte abnormalities do not cause gait disturbances. A lumbar puncture should be considered to evaluate for meningoencephalitis, but the absence of fever in this patient makes this diagnosis unlikely. Patients who have had seizures may have an unsteady gait after the seizure, and an electroencephalogram should therefore be a future consideration. Waiting to reevaluate this child may delay the diagnosis of significant underlying pathology.

9. The answer is D [V.K.6]. Febrile seizures are defined as any seizure that accompanies a fever owing to a non-CNS cause in patients between the ages of 6 months and 6 years. Febrile seizures are benign events that are not generally associated with serious acute or long-term neurologic sequelae. A computed tomography scan is not indicated in the absence of papilledema or focal neurologic deficits. An electroencephalogram is useful when the diagnosis of epilepsy is being considered but not in recurrent febrile seizures. Anticonvulsant treatment is usually not initiated until a patient has multiple febrile seizures. Febrile seizures do not require inpatient observation.

10. The answer is D [VI.B, VI.C]. Migraines are characterized by unilateral, or sometimes bilateral, frontal throbbing headaches that last for at least 1 hour. The neurologic examination of patients with migraines is usually normal. Headaches that occur on awakening in the morning are more characteristic of headaches resulting from increased intracranial pressure. Migraine without aura is the most common form of migraine in children.

11. The answer is B [IV.C.6]. The physical examination of this patient's eyes, including both the negative oculocephalic test and bilateral dilated nonreactive pupils, is most consistent with brainstem injury. The oculocephalic maneuver is also termed doll's eyes, and an abnormal response (when the head is turned, the eyes follow the head and continue to look straight ahead rather than drifting to midline) suggests a damaged vestibular system. Pupils may also be dilated during and immediately after a seizure or after topical ophthalmic application of a dilating agent, but the vestibular nerve is usually unaffected in these situations (the oculocephalic maneuver would be positive). An enlarging subdural hematoma can cause uncal herniation with a unilateral dilated, nonreactive pupil. Opiate ingestion causes constricted pupils.

12. The answer is E [II.D]. This patient's eye findings are termed the sunset sign, or a tonic downward deviation of the eyes. The sunset sign is suggestive of hydrocephalus. Increased pressure in the third ventricle from noncommunicating hydrocephalus injures the upward gaze center in the mid-brain, causing this downward deviation of the eyes. In contrast, patients with myasthenia commonly present with ptosis. There are no specific eye abnormalities in congenital myotonic dystrophy, muscular dystrophy, or cerebral infarcts.

13–15. The answers are D, C, and F, respectively [I.F.1–3]. The 4-month-old infant has spinal muscular atrophy type 1 (Werdnig-Hoffman disease), an autosomal recessive disorder that presents with hypotonia, weakness, problems with suck and swallow, and tongue fasciculations. It presents within the first 6 months of life. The 8-month-old infant has infantile botulism, an environmentally acquired disorder of the neuromuscular junction in which botulinum neurotoxin blocks release of acetylcholine at the neuromuscular junction. The toxin is released from the spores of *Clostridium botulinum,* which are found in contaminated honey or soil. Constipation is often the presenting symptom, followed by weakness, cranial nerve findings, poor abilities to feed, and paralysis. The 6-month-old infant has congenital myotonic dystrophy, an autosomal dominant disorder presenting in infancy with hypotonia, facial weakness, and feeding problems. The diagnosis may be missed if the mother of the patient is not seen or examined because the typical myotonia (i.e., inability to relax contracted muscles) is most apparent in adults.

13

Hematology

Annette B. Salinger, M.D., and Lloyd J. Brown, M.D.

I. Anemia

A. General Concepts

1. **Definition.** Anemia is a reduction in red blood cell (RBC) number or in the hemoglobin (Hgb) concentration to a level that is more than two standard deviations below the mean.

2. **Hgb and age**

   a. The Hgb is **high at birth** in most newborns and normally declines, reaching the **physiologic lowest point (nadir)** between **2 and 3 months of age in the term infant** and between **1 and 2 months of age in the preterm infant.** Hgb values reach adult levels after puberty.

   b. **Fetal hemoglobin (Hgb F)** is a major constituent of Hgb during fetal and early postnatal life. It declines and gradually disappears by 6–9 months of age.

3. **Epidemiology.** Anemia is one of the **most common laboratory abnormalities** during childhood. Approximately 20% of all children in the United States and 80% of children in developing nations have anemia at some time during childhood.

B. Classification

1. Classification is made on the basis of the **mean corpuscular volume (MCV) and the morphologic appearance of the RBC** (i.e., size, color, shape). Terms used include the suffix *-cytic,* referring to size, and the suffix *-chromic,* referring to color. Primary classifications include:

   a. **Microcytic, hypochromic anemia** (small, pale RBCs; low MCV)

   b. **Macrocytic anemia** (large RBCs, high MCV)

   c. **Normocytic, normochromic anemia** (normal RBCs in size, color, and shape, normal MCV)

2. Classification based on **reticulocyte count** is also helpful. The reticulocyte count reflects the number of immature RBCs in the circulation and, therefore, the activity of the bone marrow in producing RBCs. The

usual percentage of RBCs that are reticulocytes is 1% (normal absolute count = 40,000 cells/mm³). In most anemias, reticulocyte counts should rise. **Low reticulocyte counts indicate bone marrow failure or diminished hematopoiesis.**

3. **Figure 13-1** presents the differential diagnosis of anemia on the basis of the previously discussed classification schemes. Descriptions of the more common forms of anemia in childhood follow.

C. **Clinical Features of Anemia (Table 13-1)**

D. **Microcytic, Hypochromic Anemias.** The two most common types of microcytic, hypochromic anemia during childhood are **iron deficiency anemia** and **β-thalassemia trait.**

1. **Iron deficiency anemia** is the **most common blood disease during infancy and childhood.**

    a. **Etiology.** The majority of cases are caused by **inadequate iron intake.**

        (1) **Nutritional iron deficiency** is most common in two age groups.

            (a) **Nine to twenty-four months of age:** owing to inadequate intake and inadequate iron stores (iron stores are typically

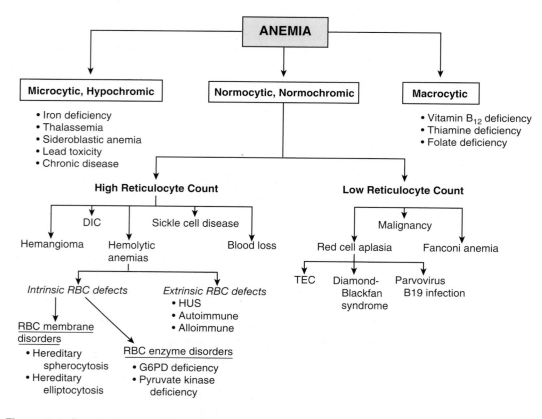

Figure 13-1. Classification and differential diagnosis of anemia. *DIC* = disseminated intravascular coagulation; *HUS* = hemolytic uremic syndrome; *TEC* = transient erythroblastopenia of childhood; *G6PD* = glucose-6-phosphate dehydrogenase; *RBC* = red blood cell.

Table 13-1. Clinical Features of Anemia

Mild
    Pallor (noted especially on skin and on mucous membranes)

Moderate
    Weakness and fatigue
    Decreased exercise tolerance
    Irritability
    Tachycardia
    Tachypnea
    Anorexia
    Systolic heart murmur

Severe
    Congestive heart failure
    Cardiac dilation
    Shortness of breath
    Hepatosplenomegaly

depleted by 6–9 months of age). Blood loss during birth may contribute to the anemia. The typical toddler's diet consists of large quantities of iron-poor cow's milk. Iron-rich foods (e.g., iron-fortified cereal) are therefore recommended beginning at 4–6 months of age to prevent anemia.

    (b) Adolescent girls: because of poor diet, rapid growth, and loss of iron in **menstrual blood**

    (2) Occult blood loss with resultant iron deficiency may be secondary to polyps, Meckel's diverticulum, inflammatory bowel disease (IBD), peptic ulcer disease, and the early ingestion of whole cow's milk before 1 year of age.

b. Clinical features. The signs and symptoms of anemia are listed in Table 13-1. Infants are often pale and may be underweight (suggestive of malnutrition), and older children may have **spoon-shaped nails** and **diminished attention and ability to learn.**

c. Laboratory findings

    (1) Because iron stores disappear first, an **early finding of iron deficiency anemia** is **low serum ferritin.** Ferritin can be a useful assessment of iron stores; however, because ferritin is also an acute-phase reactant, it may be increased in infection, disease states, and stress.

    (2) As **serum iron decreases,** iron binding capacity increases, manifested as **increased transferrin** and **decreased transferrin saturation.**

    (3) Increased free erythrocyte protoporphyrin may be noted.

    (4) Other findings include a normal or increased reticulocyte count.

d. Management

    (1) Elemental iron (4–6 mg/kg/day) is prescribed orally for mild to moderate anemia. Iron is given with vitamin C (e.g., orange juice) to enhance intestinal iron absorption.

    (2) Dietary counseling to increase nutritional iron

(3) Slow and careful RBC transfusion may be required for severe anemia that results in congestive heart failure (CHF).

(4) Further evaluation to rule out other causes of anemia is necessary in patients with anemia unresponsive to iron.

2. **α- and β-Thalassemia**

a. **Definition.** Thalassemia is a group of inherited anemias characterized by defective synthesis of one of the Hgb chains.

b. **Pathophysiology**

(1) **Normally,** the major Hgb in RBCs is hemoglobin A_1, a tetramer of two α chains and two β chains. $HgbA_2$ and Hgb F may also be present in small amounts.

(2) **α-Thalassemia** results from **defective α-globin chain synthesis** and **β-thalassemia** results from **defective β-globin chain synthesis.**

(3) Both types of thalassemia result in hemolysis that leads to increased bone marrow activity. As marrow activity increases, the marrow spaces enlarge, increasing the size of bones in the face, skull, and other bones.

c. **α-Thalassemia** is caused by a genetically mediated deletion of the **α-globin chain** and occurs predominantly in Southeast Asians. There are four disease states categorized on the basis of the number of α-globin genes deleted (normally there are four α-globin genes per diploid cell).

(1) **Silent carrier.** One α-globin gene is deleted. Patients have **no anemia** and are **asymptomatic.**

(2) **α-Thalassemia minor.** Two α-globin genes are deleted. Patients have **mild anemia.**

(3) **Hgb H disease.** Three α-globin genes are deleted. Patients have **severe anemia at birth** with an elevated **Hgb Bart's** (Hgb Bart's is a type of Hgb that binds oxygen very strongly and does not release it to tissue). Anemia is lifelong and severe.

(4) **Fetal hydrops.** Four α-globin genes are deleted. Only Hgb Bart's are formed, and in utero, this causes profound anemia, CHF, and death.

d. **β-Thalassemia** is caused by a genetically mediated deletion of the **β-globin chain.** Because there are only two β-globin genes in each cell, there are only two disease states:

(1) **β-Thalassemia major** (Cooley's anemia or homozygous β-thalassemia) may be caused by either **total absence of the β-globin chains or deficient β-globin chain production.**

(a) **Epidemiology.** β-Thalassemia major occurs predominantly among patients of Mediterranean background.

(b) **Clinical features.** Clinical findings include profound hemolytic anemia beginning in infancy, marked **hepatosplenomegaly,** and, if untreated, **bone marrow hyperplasia** in sites that result in a characteristic **"thalassemia facies"** (frontal bossing, maxillary hyperplasia with prominent cheekbones, and skull deformities). Delayed growth and puberty may also be present.

        (c) Laboratory findings. Studies show **severe hypochromia and microcytosis,** target cells and poikilocytes on the blood smear, and elevated unconjugated bilirubin, serum iron, and lactate dehydrogenase (LDH). Electrophoresis demonstrates low or absent Hgb A and elevated Hgb F.

        (d) Management. Treatment includes **lifelong transfusions** and often splenectomy. Bone marrow transplant is a potential option.

        (e) Complications. Hemochromatosis (iron accumulation within the heart, liver, lungs, pancreas, and skin) is a major complication and is caused by increased iron absorption from the intestine and from iron in transfused RBCs. Chelation of iron with the drug deferoxamine promotes iron excretion and may help delay hemochromatosis.

     (2) β-Thalassemia minor (heterozygous β-thalassemia or β-thalassemia trait) causes a **mild asymptomatic anemia** with Hgb levels 2–3 g/dL below age-appropriate norms.

        (a) Laboratory findings include hypochromia and microcytosis with target cells and anisocytosis (excessive variation of size of RBCs) on smear.

        (b) No treatment is required.

        (c) It is important to note that patients with β-thalassemia minor may be very easily misdiagnosed as having iron deficiency anemia and treated inappropriately with iron. However, the iron level in β-thalassemia minor is normal or elevated.

   3. Sideroblastic anemia is a group of anemias characterized by the presence of **ring sideroblasts** in the bone marrow. Ring sideroblasts result from the accumulation of iron in the mitochondria of RBC precursors. Sideroblastic anemia may be inherited or may be acquired as a result of drugs or toxins (e.g., isoniazid, alcohol, lead poisoning, chloramphenicol).

   4. Lead poisoning (see Chapter 1, section IV.J) and **chronic diseases,** such as malignancy, infections, and kidney disease (termed *anemia of chronic disease*), may demonstrate a microcytic, hypochromic anemia.

E. Macrocytic (Megaloblastic) Anemias. These anemias are characterized by **large RBCs with MCV > 95.** The two major causes in children are folic acid and vitamin B_{12} deficiencies.

   1. Folic acid deficiency

     a. Etiology. Causes include **decreased folic acid intake** (i.e., from a diet lacking uncooked fresh fruits and vegetables or from **exclusive feedings with goat's milk** as the sole source of milk protein) and **decreased intestinal absorption of folic acid** (i.e., from diseases affecting the small intestine, such as celiac disease, chronic infectious enteritis, Crohn's disease, or medications, such as anticonvulsants and oral contraceptives).

     b. Clinical features. In addition to the characteristic signs and symptoms of anemia, patients may have failure to thrive, chronic diarrhea, and irritability.

    c. Diagnosis. Documentation of **low serum folic acid** is diagnostic.

    d. Management. Treatment includes **dietary folic acid** and identification and treatment of the underlying cause.

2. **Vitamin B$_{12}$ deficiency**

    a. Normal physiology. To be absorbed, dietary vitamin B$_{12}$ must first combine with a glycoprotein (**intrinsic factor**) secreted by the gastric parietal cells. Absorption then occurs in the terminal ileum.

    b. Etiology. Causes include **inadequate dietary intake** (e.g., from a strict vegetarian [vegan] diet), an inherited **inability to secrete intrinsic factor** (juvenile pernicious anemia), or an **inability to absorb vitamin B$_{12}$** (e.g., Crohn's disease).

    c. Clinical features. In addition to the characteristic features of anemia, patients may also have anorexia, **a smooth red tongue,** and **neurologic manifestations** (ataxia, hyporeflexia, positive Babinski responses).

    d. Diagnosis. Documentation of **low serum vitamin B$_{12}$ level** is diagnostic.

    e. Management. Treatment is by **monthly intramuscular vitamin B$_{12}$ injections.**

F. Normocytic, Normochromic Anemias. These anemias are characterized by normal size (normal MCV) and shape of the RBCs.

1. **General concepts**

    a. Common causes include hemolytic anemias (premature destruction of RBCs), red cell aplasias, and sickle cell anemia.

    b. Reticulocyte count may be used to differentiate among the disorders (see Figure 13-1).

        (1) Low reticulocyte count reflects bone marrow suppression or failure and is consistent with red cell aplasias, pancytopenia, and malignancy.

        (2) High reticulocyte count reflects high bone marrow production of RBCs as seen in hemolytic anemias and sickle cell anemia.

2. **Hemolytic anemias**

    a. Intrinsic RBC defects include RBC membrane disorders and RBC enzyme disorders.

        (1) Hereditary spherocytosis is the **most common inherited abnormality of the RBC membrane** and occurs predominantly in persons of Northern European ancestry.

            (a) Etiology. There is a deficiency or abnormality of the structural RBC membrane protein **spectrin** that causes the RBC to assume its spherical shape. Inheritance is usually **autosomal dominant.**

            (b) Clinical features. Clinical findings are related to increased RBC destruction and the diminished ability of the RBC to pass through small blood vessels. Signs and symptoms include **splenomegaly** by 2–3 years of age (spherocytes are trapped in the spleen and destroyed), pallor, weakness, **pigmentary gallstones,** and **aplastic crises,** most commonly associated with parvovirus B19 infection. Infants may present with jaundice and anemia.

    (c) Laboratory findings. Studies show an elevated reticulocyte count, hyperbilirubinemia, **spherocytes** on blood smear, and **abnormal RBC fragility with osmotic fragility studies.**

    (d) Management. Treatment includes transfusions. Splenectomy cures the disorder. To decrease the incidence of invasive disease caused by encapsulated bacteria, splenectomy is generally delayed until after 5 years of age.

(2) Hereditary elliptocytosis is another **autosomal dominant** defect in the structure of **spectrin** that may or may not result in hemolysis. Clinical features are more variable than in hereditary spherocytosis. The **majority of patients are asymptomatic,** although 10% have jaundice at birth and, later, splenomegaly and gallstones. **Elliptical RBCs** are found on blood smear in older children. Treatment includes splenectomy for patients with chronic hemolysis. No treatment is needed for patients without hemolysis.

(3) Glycolytic enzymatic defects of RBCs include **pyruvate kinase deficiency** and **glucose-6-phosphate dehydrogenase deficiency.**

    (a) Pyruvate kinase (PK) deficiency is an **autosomal recessive** disorder that results in decreased production of PK isoenzyme leading to ATP depletion and decreased RBC survival.

        (i) Clinical features include pallor, jaundice, and splenomegaly. Kernicterus has been reported in neonates.

        (ii) Laboratory findings include varying degrees of anemia and a blood smear showing **polychromatic RBCs.**

        (iii) Diagnosis is by finding decreased PK activity in the RBCs.

        (iv) Management includes transfusions and splenectomy for severe disease.

    (b) Glucose-6-phosphate dehydrogenase deficiency (G6PD) is the most common RBC enzymatic defect. It may occur as an **acute** hemolytic disease induced by infection or medications, or as a **chronic** hemolytic disease. The epidemiology, etiology, clinical findings, and treatment are described in **Table 13-2.**

b. Defects extrinsic to the RBC

(1) Autoimmune hemolytic anemia (AIHA) occurs when **antibodies are misdirected against the RBCs.**

    (a) Etiology

        (i) Primary AIHA is generally **idiopathic,** in which no underlying disease is identified. Viral infections and occasionally drugs may be causal in some patients.

        (ii) Secondary AIHA is associated with an **underlying disease process,** such as lymphoma, systemic lupus erythematosus (SLE), or immunodeficiency disease.

Table 13-2. Features of Glucose-6-Phospate Dehydrogenase (G6PD) Deficiency

Epidemiology	Mediterranean, Arabic, Asian, and African ethnic groups
Pathophysiology	G6PD enzyme is critical for protecting the RBC from oxidative stress. Deficiency results in RBC damage when the RBC is exposed to oxidants.
Triggers of hemolysis	Infection Fava beans Drugs (e.g., sulfa, salicylates, antimalarials)
Clinical features	Symptoms occur 24–48 hours after exposure to oxidant. Hemolysis occurs, resulting in abdominal pain, V/D, fever, and hemoglobinuria followed by jaundice. HSM may be present.
Laboratory findings	Hemoglobinuria ↑ Reticulocyte count Smear shows "bite" cells and "hemighosts"; Heinz bodies
Diagnosis	Low levels of G6PD in RBCs
Treatment	Transfusions as needed; splenectomy not beneficial

V/D = vomiting, diarrhea; *RBC* = red blood cell; *HSM* = hepatosplenomegaly.

    (b) Clinical features

        (i) Fulminant acute type AIHA occurs in infants and young children and is preceded by a respiratory infection. Presenting features include acute onset of pallor, jaundice, hemoglobinuria, and splenomegaly. A **complete recovery is expected.**

        (ii) Prolonged type AIHA is characterized by a protracted course and high mortality. Underlying disease is frequently present.

    (c) Laboratory findings. Studies show severe anemia, spherocytes on blood smear, prominent reticulocytosis, and leukocytosis. A **direct Coombs test is positive** (detects coating of antibodies on the surface of RBCs or complement).

    (d) Management. Treatment may include transfusions that unfortunately may provide only transient benefit. **Corticosteroids** are often used for severe anemia and are continued until hemolysis diminishes. The acute form responds well to steroids.

  (2) Alloimmune hemolytic anemia most commonly involves newborn Rh and ABO hemolytic diseases.

    (a) Rh hemolytic disease occurs when the mother, who has no Rh antigen (Rh negative), produces antibodies to the Rh antigen on her fetus's RBCs (Rh positive). In **subsequent pregnancies,** antibodies pass from the mother to the fetus causing hemolysis that presents as severe jaundice (which can lead to kernicterus), anemia, hepatosplenomegaly, and **hydrops fetalis.** A direct Coombs test is **strongly positive.**

    (b) ABO hemolytic disease occurs when the mother is blood group O and her fetus is blood group A, B, or AB. The mother produces antibodies to either the A or B blood group antigen that then pass to the fetus, causing hemolysis with resultant jaundice. A direct Coombs test is **weakly positive.** Of note, ABO disease can occur in the **first pregnancy,** unlike Rh hemolytic disease.

    (c) Management. Treatment may include phototherapy for mild to moderate jaundice and exchange transfusion for severe jaundice.

  (3) Microangiopathic hemolytic anemia

    (a) Definition. This form of anemia results from mechanical damage to RBCs caused by passage through an injured vascular endothelium.

    (b) Etiology. Causes include severe hypertension, **hemolytic uremic syndrome** (HUS), artificial heart valves, a giant hemangioma, and disseminated intravascular coagulation (DIC).

    (c) Clinical features. Signs and symptoms are those characteristic of anemia and thrombocytopenia.

    (d) Laboratory findings. Studies show RBC fragmentation seen as "burr" cells, "target" cells, and irregularly shaped cells on the blood smear, and thrombocytopenia.

    (e) Management. Therapy includes supportive care and treatment of the underlying cause.

3. Sickle cell (SS) hemoglobinopathies

  a. Epidemiology. SS disease occurs in 1 in 800 black newborns in the United States. Eight percent have SS trait.

  b. Etiology and pathophysiology

    (1) SS disease is caused by a **single amino acid substitution** of **valine for glutamic acid** on the **number 6 position of the β-globin chain** of Hgb.

    (2) The mutation results in polymerization (stacking) of Hgb within the RBC membrane when the RBC is exposed to low oxygen or acidosis.

    (3) Polymerization of Hgb results in a **distorted RBC shape** (sickled) that leads to decreased RBC lifespan (**hemolysis**) and **occlusion of small vessels,** resulting in distal ischemia, infarction, and organ dysfunction.

    (4) SS disease is the result of having **two genes for Hgb S** (homozygous).

    (5) SS trait is defined as having only **one gene for Hgb S** (heterozygous). Persons with SS trait have both Hgb A (50–60%), Hgb S (35–45%), and a small percentage of Hgb F. Patients are usually **asymptomatic without anemia** unless exposed to severe hypoxemia. Some patients have an inability to concentrate the urine or hematuria (5%) during adolescence.

  c. Diagnosis. Diagnosis of SS disease is now usually made at birth through state newborn screening programs. Hgb electrophoresis is a highly sensitive and specific test that demonstrates Hgb S and Hgb F (fetal hemoglobin) in the newborn with SS disease.

  d. Clinical features. Clinical characteristics are not generally present until protective Hgb F declines (by 6 months of age). Clinical episodes are often termed *crises* because they occur suddenly. **Table 13-3** de-

Table 13-3. Clinical Features and Management of Crises Occurring in Sickle Cell Disease

Crisis	Clinical Features	Management
Vasoocclusive crisis Painful bone crisis	Most common crisis Ischemia/infarction of bone or marrow Deep, gnawing, or throbbing pain lasting 3–7 days Subtype: **acute dactylitis**—painful swelling of digits of the hands and feet DDx: **osteomyelitis**	Pain control Intravenous fluids at 1.5–2× maintenance Incentive spirometry to decrease the risk of ACS Severe, unremitting pain may respond to partial exchange transfusion. (Simple transfusion of RBCs is not indicated. It increases viscosity of blood and may worsen crisis.)
Acute abdominal crisis	Abdominal pain and distension Often caused by sickling within mesenteric artery DDx: cholecystitis, appendicitis, splenic sequestration	Low threshold for imaging abdomen Same management as for painful bone crisis
Stroke	Dysarthria, hemiplegia; may be asymptomatic Occurs in up to 11% of patients (subclinical stroke occurs in up to 20% of patients)	Same management as for painful bone crisis Urgent exchange transfusion Patient should be started on chronic transfusion program to prevent recurrence, which occurs in 60–90%
Priapism	Painful, sustained erection **Always consider SS disease in any patient presenting with priapism.**	Same management as for painful bone crisis
Acute chest syndrome (ACS)	Definition: new pulmonary infiltrate associated with respiratory symptoms (e.g., cough, shortness of breath, chest pain) Hypoxemia May be severe and may cause up to 25% of deaths in patients with SS disease Causes include infection (e.g., viral, *Mycoplasma pneumoniae, Chlamydia pneumoniae, Streptococcus pneumoniae*), sickling, atelectasis, fat embolism, painful bone crisis involving the ribs, and pulmonary edema from fluid overload	Careful hydration and pain management Oxygen Appropriate antibiotics (usually cefuroxime and azithromycin) Incentive spirometry Early use of partial exchange transfusion in a patient who does not improve rapidly
Sequestration crisis	Rapid accumulation of blood in spleen (or less commonly, liver) Occurs in patients < 6 years of age Abdominal distension, abdominal pain, shortness of breath, tachycardia, pallor, fatigue, and shock. Mortality can be high. Labs: ↓ Hgb; ↑ reticulocytes	Supportive care Transfusion of RBCs Splenectomy recommended by some practitioners because recurrence occurs in up to 50%

(continues)

Table 13-3. Clinical Features and Management of Crises Occurring in Sickle Cell Disease (Continued)

Crisis	Clinical Features	Management
Aplastic crisis	Temporary cessation of RBC production often caused by parvovirus B19 or other infectious agent Pallor, fatigue, tachycardia Labs: ↓ Hgb; ↓ reticulocytes	Supportive care Transfusion of RBCs
Hyperhemolytic crisis	Rapid hemolysis. Often occurs in patients with other hemolytic diseases (e.g., G6PD deficiency). Pallor, fatigue, tachycardia, jaundice Labs: ↓ Hgb; ↑ reticulocytes; ↑ bilirubin	Supportive care Transfusion of RBCs

DDX = differential diagnosis; *RBCs* = red blood cells; *SS* = sickle cell disease; *G6PD* = glucose-6-phosphate dehydrogenase; *Hgb* = hemoglobin.

scribes the clinical features and management of the common SS disease crises.

e. **Laboratory findings (Table 13-4)**

f. **Management**

(1) **Infection is the leading cause of death** from SS disease, and up to **30% of patients develop sepsis or meningitis** in the first 5 years of life.

(a) Infection is a result of **decreased splenic function.** Patients are at risk for infection with **encapsulated bacteria (i.e., *Haemophilus influenzae* type b, *Streptococcus pneumoniae*, *Salmonella*, *Neisseria meningitidis*).**

(b) **Fever** in any patient with SS disease is managed with urgent assessment and appropriate cultures (blood and urine), chest radiograph to rule out pneumonia, and parenteral antibiotics until bacterial infection can be safely excluded.

(c) **Osteomyelitis** may occur and **may mimic a painful bone crisis.** Infection is most commonly caused by *Salmonella* species acquired through the gastrointestinal (GI) tract, although *Staphylococcus aureus* may also cause osteomyelitis.

Table 13-4. Usual Laboratory Findings in Sickle Cell Anemia

Red blood cell lifespan	10–50 days
Hemoglobin	6–9 g/dL
Hematocrit	18–27%
Reticulocyte count	5–15%
White blood cell count	12,000–20,000 cells/mm^3
Platelet count	Increased, often > 500,000 platelets/μL
Bilirubin	Increased
Blood smear	Sickled cells, target cells, Howell-Jolly bodies
Bone marrow	Erythroid hyperplasia

Clinical features include fever and pain, induration, tenderness, warmth, and erythema of the involved area. Treatment includes appropriate intravenous antibiotics.

g. **Preventive care**

(1) **Hydroxyurea,** a chemotherapeutic agent that increases Hgb F, has been shown to decrease the incidence of vasoocclusive crises.

(2) **Daily oral penicillin prophylaxis** is started in the first few months of life to decrease the risk of *S. pneumoniae* infection.

(3) **Daily folic acid** is given to prevent folic acid deficiency.

(4) **Routine immunizations** and also yearly influenza vaccination, 23-valent polysaccharide pneumococcal vaccine at 2 years of age, and meningococcal vaccine should be given.

(5) **Serial transcranial Doppler ultrasound or magnetic resonance angiography** is recommended beginning at 2 years of age to identify patients at risk for stroke.

h. **Prognosis**

(1) Median life expectancy is in the forties.

(2) **Long-term complications** include delayed growth and puberty, cardiomegaly, hemochromatosis, cor pulmonale, gallstones, poor wound healing, avascular necrosis of the femoral and humeral heads, and diminished cognition and school performance.

i. **Other SS diseases** include **sickle cell–thalassemia disease** (with clinical features similar to SS disease) and **sickle cell–hemoglobin C disease** (Hgb SC disease) caused by the inheritance of both Hgb S and Hgb C genes. Clinical features of sickle cell–hemoglobin C disease are less severe than SS disease.

4. **Red blood cell aplasias** are a group of congenital or acquired blood disorders characterized by anemia, reticulocytopenia, and a paucity of RBC precursors in the bone marrow. The clinical features of the three most common disorders occurring in childhood, **congenital hypoplastic anemia (Diamond-Blackfan anemia), transient erythroblastopenia of childhood, and parvovirus B19–associated red cell aplasia,** are presented in Table 13-5.

II. Pancytopenia

A. **Definition.** Pancytopenia is defined as **bone marrow failure** with decreased RBCs, leukocytes, and platelets.

B. **Pancytopenia** may be **congenital or acquired.**

1. **Congenital aplastic anemia** is also known as **Fanconi anemia.**

a. **Etiology.** Inheritance is **autosomal recessive.**

b. **Clinical features**

(1) Onset of bone marrow failure occurs at a **mean age of 7 years.** Typical presentation is with ecchymosis and petechiae.

(2) **Skeletal abnormalities,** which include **short stature** in almost all patients, and **absence or hypoplasia of the thumb and radius**

Table 13-5. Characteristics of the Red Blood Cell Aplasias

Aplasia	Etiology	Clinical Features	Laboratory Findings	Treatment
Congenital hypoplastic anemia (Diamond-Blackfan anemia)	Unknown Autosomal recessive or autosomal dominant inheritance	Anemia within first year of life Rapid onset One fourth to one third have physical findings: craniofacial, renal, cardiac anomalies; short stature; triphalangeal thumbs Signs and symptoms of anemia	↓ Hgb ↓ Reticulocytes ↑ Hgb F ↓ or normal platelet count Marrow: ↓ RBC precursors; other marrow elements normal	RBC transfusion Corticosteroids (up to 70% respond) Bone marrow transplant if no response to corticosteroids
TEC	Unknown Possible postviral autoimmune reaction	Anemia begins > 1 year of age Slow in onset Signs and symptoms of anemia	↓ Hgb ↓ Reticulocytes Normal platelet count Marrow: ↓ RBC precursors	Spontaneous recovery within several weeks No treatment required
Parvovirus B19–associated pure RBC aplasia*	Parvovirus B19 infection	Anemia generally not symptomatic May have associated URI symptoms and facial rash ("slapped cheeks") of fifth disease Aplastic crisis in patients with SS disease	↓ Hgb ↓ Reticulocytes Normal platelet count	Spontaneous recovery within 2 weeks RBC transfusions may be required for patients with aplastic crisis associated with SS disease

TEC = transient erythroblastopenia of childhood; *URI* = upper respiratory infection; *Hgb* = hemoglobin; *RBC* = red blood cells.
*Note that **Epstein-Barr virus, cytomegalovirus, HIV, and drugs (e.g., chloramphenicol) may cause an acquired RBC aplasia similar to parvovirus B19.**

(3) Skin hyperpigmentation

(4) Renal abnormalities

c. **Laboratory findings.** Studies show pancytopenia, RBC macrocytosis, low reticulocyte count, elevated Hgb F, and bone marrow hypocellularity.

d. **Management.** Treatment includes transfusions of RBCs and platelets as needed, and bone marrow transplant from an HLA-compatible donor, if available. Immunosuppressive therapy (e.g., corticosteroids, cyclosporin) may also help.

2. **Acquired aplastic anemia**

a. **Etiology.** Causes include **drugs** (e.g., sulfonamides, anticonvulsants, chloramphenicol), **infections** (e.g., human immunodeficiency virus [HIV], Epstein-Barr virus [EBV], cytomegalovirus [CMV]), **chemicals,** and **radiation.** These all may damage bone marrow stem cells directly or may induce autoimmune destruction. Acquired aplastic anemia may also be **idiopathic.**

b. **Clinical features.** Signs and symptoms include bruising, petechiae, pallor, or serious infection as a result of neutropenia.

c. **Laboratory findings.** Studies show pancytopenia, low reticulocyte count, and hypocellular bone marrow.

d. **Management.** Treatment includes identifying and stopping the causative agent, transfusions as needed, bone marrow transplant, and immunosuppressive therapy.

III. Polycythemias

A. **Definition.** Polycythemia is defined as an **increase in RBCs relative to total blood volume.** It may also be defined as a hematocrit (Hct) > 60%, or as an Hgb or Hct more than two standard deviations above normal values for age.

B. **Primary polycythemia (polycythemia vera)** is an extremely rare cause of polycythemia during childhood. It is a **malignancy** involving the RBC precursor.

C. **Secondary polycythemia** is caused by **increased erythropoietin production.** Production may be appropriate or inappropriate.

1. **Appropriate polycythemia** may be caused by chronic **hypoxemia** as a result of **cyanotic congenital heart disease (most common cause of polycythemia in childhood)**, pulmonary disease, or residence at high altitudes.

2. **Inappropriate polycythemia** may be caused by benign and malignant tumors of the kidney, cerebellum, ovary, liver, and adrenal gland; excess hormone production (e.g., corticosteroids, growth hormone, androgens); and kidney abnormalities such as hydronephrosis.

3. **Clinical features** include a ruddy facial complexion with a normal size liver and spleen.

4. **Laboratory findings** reveal elevated Hgb and Hct but normal platelet and white blood cell (WBC) counts. Erythropoietin levels are high.

5. **Management** is directed toward identifying and treating the underlying cause. Phlebotomy is also used to keep the Hct < 60%.

D. **Relative polycythemia** refers to an **apparent increase in RBC mass** caused by a **decrease in plasma volume.** The most common cause is **dehydration,** and this should be considered in every patient with a high Hgb or Hct. Appropriate fluid management normalizes the Hct.

E. **Complications** of polycythemia include **thrombosis** (vasoocclusive crisis, stroke, myocardial infarction) and **bleeding.**

IV. Disorders of Hemostasis

A. **General Concepts**

1. **Hemostasis** requires normal function of three important elements: **blood vessels, platelets, and soluble clotting factors. Hemorrhage** may result from deficiency or dysfunction of any of these elements. **Thrombosis** may also occur but is rare during childhood.

2. **See Figure 13-2 for a depiction of the clotting cascade.**

3. **Clinical features suggesting abnormal hemostasis include:**
   a. **Cutaneous bleeding** (e.g., ecchymoses, petechiae)
   b. **Spontaneous epistaxis** that is **severe and recurrent** without an obvious cause
   c. **Prolonged bleeding** after simple surgical procedures, circumcision, trauma, or dental extraction
   d. **Recurrent hemarthroses**
   e. **Deep venous thrombosis,** pulmonary embolism, or **stroke**

4. **Diagnostic studies. Evaluation** for clotting abnormality typically includes these screening tests:
   a. **Complete blood count (CBC)**
   b. **Platelet count**
   c. **Blood smear to evaluate platelet morphology**
   d. **Activated partial thromboplastin time (aPTT)**
   e. **Prothrombin time (PT)**
   f. **Platelet function assay.** Bleeding time (assesses platelet function and platelet interaction with the vessel wall) is less commonly performed now; it is painful and sometimes inaccurate.
   g. **Table 13-6 summarizes the laboratory and clinical findings of coagulation disorders.**

5. **Differential diagnosis (Figure 13-3)**

B. **Congenital Clotting Factor Disorders.** These disorders include deficiency of factor VIII, deficiency of factor IX, and von Willebrand's disease.

1. **General considerations. Factor VIII disorders** includes two inherited disorders, **hemophilia A** and **von Willebrand's disease.** These two diseases involve different regions and different functions of the factor VIII molecule.

Table 13-6. Laboratory and Clinical Findings in Coagulation Disorders

Disorder	aPTT	PT	Bleeding Time	Platelet Count	Petechiae	Hemarthroses
Factor VIII, IX deficiency	Prolonged	Normal	Normal	Normal	No	Yes
von Willebrand's	Prolonged	Normal	Prolonged	Normal	No	Rare
Thrombocytopenia	Normal	Normal	Prolonged	Low	Yes	No
Platelet function defect	Normal	Normal	Prolonged	Normal	Yes	No
Vitamin K deficiency	Prolonged	Prolonged	Normal	Normal	Yes	Yes
DIC	Prolonged	Prolonged	Prolonged	Low	Yes	Sometimes

aPTT = activated partial thromboplastin time; *PT* = prothrombin time; *DIC* = disseminated intravascular coagulation

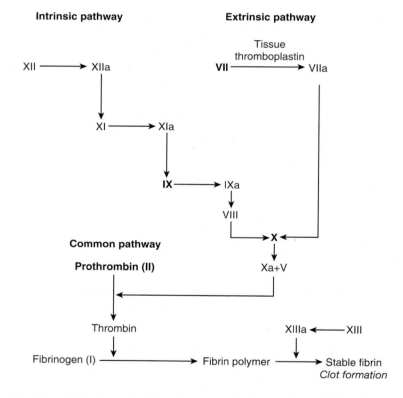

Figure 13-2. Coagulation cascade. Activated partial thromboplastin time measures the function of the intrinsic pathway and the extrinsic pathway, except for factor VII; the prothrombin time measures the function of the extrinsic pathway (factors VII, X, and V), fibrinogen, and prothrombin (factor II). Factors in bold type are vitamin K–dependent coagulation factors.

    a. Hemophilia A represents a defect in factor VIII procoagulant activity (antihemophilic factor; factor VIII protein). Platelet function is normal.

    b. In **von Willebrand's disease,** factor VIII procoagulant activity is variable but platelet function is defective because of a decrease or de-

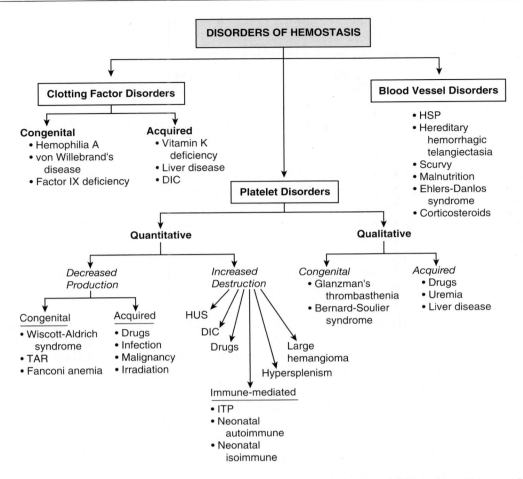

Figure 13-3. Overview of the differential diagnosis of disorders of hemostasis. *DIC* = disseminated intravascular coagulation; *HUS* = hemolytic uremic syndrome; *HSP* = Henoch-Schönlein purpura; *TAR* = thrombocytopenia absent radius syndrome; *ITP* = immune thrombocytopenic purpura.

fect in **von Willebrand's factor,** a substance necessary for platelet adhesion to blood vessel walls and maintenance of a normal bleeding time. See also section IV.B.3.

2. **Factor VIII deficiency—hemophilia A**

   a. **Etiology.** Inheritance is **X-linked** and occurs in 1 in 5,000–10,000 Caucasian male births. More than 200 different mutations or deletions have been identified in the factor VIII gene.

   b. **Clinical features**

      (1) **Hemarthroses** (involving the knees, elbows, and ankles most commonly) **and deep soft-tissue bleeding** are the **hallmarks.** Bleeding into the iliopsoas muscle may be especially severe as a result of delayed recognition of the bleeding and the potential for significant blood accumulation. **Risk of serious and life-threatening hemorrhage is lifelong.**

      (2) **Severe, moderate, and mild forms** exist based on the activity level of factor VIII protein.

      (a) Severe: spontaneous bleeding (< 1% factor VIII protein activity)

      (b) Moderate: bleeding only with trauma (1–5% factor VIII protein activity)

      (c) Mild: bleeding only after surgery or major trauma (> 5% factor VIII protein activity)

    (3) Central nervous system (CNS) bleeding is the most dreaded complication and is usually the result of head trauma.

  c. Laboratory findings

    (1) Prolonged aPTT (in mild form, aPTT may be normal)

    (2) Normal PT, bleeding time, platelet count, and **platelet function assay**

    (3) Low factor VIII protein activity in the presence of normal von Willebrand's factor assay

  d. Management. Treatment includes prevention of trauma and replacement of factor VIII. Desmopressin acetate (DDAVP) may cause the release of stored factor VIII from the patient's own cells and may be useful in mild hemophilia.

3. von Willebrand's disease. This group of disorders involves defects or deficiency in the von Willebrand's factor (vWf) portion of the factor VIII complex and is the **most common hereditary bleeding disorder.**

  a. Etiology. Inheritance is **autosomal dominant.**

  b. Categories

    (1) Type I (classic type): mild quantitative deficiencies of vWf and factor VIII protein. It is the **most common form.**

    (2) Type II: qualitative abnormality in vWf

    (3) Type III: absence of vWf; the most severe type

  c. Clinical features

    (1) Most patients have mild to moderate bleeding, usually involving mucocutaneous surfaces. More profound bleeding occurs in type III disease.

    (2) Common signs and symptoms include epistaxis, **menorrhagia,** bruising, and bleeding after dental extraction or tonsillectomy. Excessive bleeding after trauma may occur.

    (3) Hemarthroses are unusual.

  d. Laboratory findings

    (1) Prolonged bleeding time and **prolonged aPTT may be present, but not always** (they are always present in type III disease).

    (2) Quantitative assay for vWf antigen and activity (ristocetin cofactor assay) are diagnostic.

  e. Management. DDAVP induces vWf release from endothelial cells and is used for mild to moderate bleeding and for prophylaxis before surgery. DDAVP is most useful in type I disease and is sometimes effective in type II disease. Cryoprecipitate, which contains intact vWf, may be used for serious bleeding, for extensive surgeries, or for type III disease.

4. **Factor IX deficiency—hemophilia B (Christmas disease).** This **X-linked disorder** has clinical features similar to those of hemophilia A. aPTT is prolonged and low factor IX activity is found. PT and platelet count are normal. Management includes factor IX replacement.

C. **Acquired Clotting Factor Disorders**

1. **Vitamin K deficiency**

   a. **Vitamin K,** a fat-soluble vitamin, is essential for the synthesis of both procoagulant and anticoagulant factors, such as **factors II, VII, IX, and X** and **proteins C and S.**

   b. **Etiology**

      (1) **Dietary deficiency is unusual,** except during early infancy.

      (2) Pancreatic insufficiency, biliary obstruction, and prolonged diarrhea may result in diminished ability to absorb vitamin K.

      (3) **Medications** may interfere with vitamin K metabolism (e.g., cephalosporins, rifampin, isoniazid, warfarin).

      (4) **Hemorrhagic disease of the newborn** is a special type of vitamin K deficiency. It may occur early (within 24 hours after birth), within the first week of life (**classic form**), or late (1–3 months after birth).

   c. **Clinical features.** Clinical manifestations include bruising, oozing from skin puncture wounds (e.g., previous blood draw sites), and bleeding into organs. **Hemorrhagic disease of the newborn is characterized by serious bleeding in the early and late forms,** but classic disease generally presents only with cutaneous bleeding, hematemesis, and bleeding from the circumcision site or umbilical cord. CNS bleeding may occasionally occur.

   d. **Laboratory findings. Prolonged aPTT and PT** occur.

   e. **Management.** Treatment includes administration of vitamin K. **Intramuscular administration of vitamin K after birth prevents hemorrhagic disease of the newborn.** In severe disease, fresh-frozen plasma (FFP) may be needed.

2. **Liver disease**

   a. The liver is the major site of production of most coagulation factors. Therefore, with liver disease, synthesis of clotting factors is often diminished, with the vitamin K–dependent factors most severely affected (see IV.C.1.a). Consumption of clotting factors and platelets may also occur.

   b. **Laboratory findings.** Laboratory results are the same as those seen in DIC (see section IV.C.3), including **prolonged PT and aPTT, increased fibrin degradation products, and thrombocytopenia.**

   c. **Management.** Treatment includes vitamin K, FFP, and platelets as needed.

3. **Disseminated intravascular coagulation (DIC)**

   a. **Definition.** DIC is a group of laboratory and clinical features indicative of both accelerated fibrinogenesis and fibrinolysis. The initiating event is clotting that leads to consumption of procoagulant factors and resultant hemorrhage.

b. Etiology. DIC is a secondary phenomenon that occurs in response to local factors (e.g., large hemangiomas as seen in Kasabach-Merritt syndrome) and systemic factors (e.g., sepsis, hypothermia, malignancy, heat stroke, snake bite, burns).

c. Clinical features. Signs include cutaneous and internal organ bleeding.

d. Laboratory findings. Studies show **thrombocytopenia, prolongation of PT and aPTT, reduction in clotting factors** (especially **fibrinogen** and factors II, V, and VIII), **elevated fibrin degradation products** (positive D-dimer assay), and fragmented and helmet-shaped RBCs on blood smear.

e. Management. Therapy includes treatment of the underlying cause and transfusions of fibrinogen, FFP, and platelets as needed. Heparin may be useful if the underlying defect cannot be corrected.

D. Disorders of Blood Vessels. These diseases affect the integrity of blood vessels and may present with bleeding.

1. **Henoch-Schönlein purpura,** an IgA-mediated vasculitis, presents with **palpable purpura** on the lower extremities and buttocks, renal insufficiency, arthritis, and abdominal pain. Platelet count is normal. (See also Chapter 16, section I.)

2. **Hereditary hemorrhagic telangiectasia** is an **autosomal dominant** disorder characterized by locally dilated and tortuous veins and capillaries of the skin and mucous membranes.

3. **Scurvy** is **vitamin C deficiency** and causes impaired collagen synthesis that results in weakened blood vessels.

4. **Inherited disorders of collagen synthesis** (e.g., Ehlers-Danlos syndrome) may result in capillary fragility.

5. **Malnutrition and corticosteroids** may weaken the collagen supporting vessels.

E. Platelet Abnormalities

1. **General concepts**

   a. Platelet abnormalities may be quantitative (i.e., decreased or increased in number) or **qualitative** (i.e., intrinsic abnormality in function).

   b. Thrombocytopenia is defined as a decreased number of platelets, generally < 100,000/μL. It is the **most common cause of bleeding.**

2. **Quantitative disorders** may be secondary to diminished platelet production or to increased platelet destruction or sequestration (within the spleen). They may also be congenital or acquired.

   a. Decreased platelet production

      (1) Congenital disorders

         (a) Wiskott-Aldrich syndrome is an **X-linked** disorder characterized by **thrombocytopenia** with unusually small platelets, **eczema,** and defects in T- and B-cell immunity.

         (b) Thrombocytopenia–absent radius syndrome (TAR) is an **autosomal recessive** disorder characterized by thrombocytopenia and limb abnormalities, especially absence of the radius (note that the thumb is present, in contrast to Fanconi anemia, in which the thumb is absent; see section II.B.1). Cardiac and renal disease may be present. Thrombocytopenia improves in the second or third year of life.

(2) Acquired disorders are generally those that cause pancytopenia (see section II.B.2).

b. Increased platelet destruction

(1) Immune-mediated thrombocytopenias

(a) Immune thrombocytopenic purpura (ITP) is the most common acquired platelet abnormality in childhood.

(i) Etiology. ITP may be viral, drug-induced, or **idiopathic** (most common).

(ii) Pathophysiology. Because ITP often follows a viral infection, it is thought that the virus triggers antibodies that cross-react with platelets, causing their destruction and removal by the spleen.

(iii) Clinical features. Illness typically occurs 1–4 weeks **after a viral infection.** It begins abruptly with cutaneous bleeding (e.g., petechiae, bruising) or mucous membrane bleeding (e.g., epistaxis, gum bleeding). Internal bleeding into the brain (occurs in < 1%), kidneys, or GI tract may occur but is rare.

(iv) Laboratory findings. Studies reveal thrombocytopenia and a blood smear showing few large "sticky" platelets.

(v) Management. Treatment includes supportive care. Very low platelet counts (< 20,000/μL) or active bleeding warrant treatment with intravenous immunoglobulin (**IVIG**) or corticosteroids. Anti-D immunoglobulin is a second-line agent that may also be effective. This immunoglobulin binds to erythrocyte D antigen (Rh) on RBCs (patients must be Rh-positive). These antibody-coated RBCs are cleared by the spleen, preferentially allowing platelets to escape destruction. Platelet transfusions are generally avoided because transfused platelets are rapidly destroyed.

(vi) Prognosis. Most cases (70–80%) resolve spontaneously within months. Chronic ITP, which occurs in 10–20%, is diagnosed if ITP lasts > 6 months. Chronic ITP results in long-lasting or relapsing thrombocytopenia and is more common in adults and in children older than 10 years of age. Splenectomy results in a normal platelet count in 75% of patients with chronic ITP, but because of the risk of infection after spleen removal, there is a reluctance to offer it to children.

(b) Neonatal immune-mediated thrombocytopenia

(i) Passive autoimmune thrombocytopenia occurs when the mother has ITP, and antibodies against her own platelets cross the placenta and destroy the fetus's platelets. **The mother has thrombocytopenia.**

    (ii) Isoimmune thrombocytopenia occurs when the mother produces antibodies against her fetus's platelets as a result of sensitization to an antigen that her own platelets lack. **The mother's platelet count is normal.**

   (2) Drugs, DIC, and an enlarged spleen may all cause platelet destruction.

   (3) Hemolytic uremic syndrome is characterized by thrombocytopenia (see Chapter 11, section VI).

   (4) Large hemangiomas may sequester and destroy platelets (e.g., **Kasabach-Merritt syndrome** characterized by an enlarging hemangioma, microangiopathic hemolytic anemia, thrombocytopenia, and consumptive coagulopathy).

  3. Qualitative platelet disorders (i.e., defect in platelet function despite normal number) may be **congenital** or **acquired.**

   a. Congenital disorders

    (1) Glanzmann's thrombasthenia is an **autosomal recessive** disorder characterized by diminished ability of platelets to aggregate and form a clot as a result of deficient adhesive glycoprotein IIb/IIIa on the platelet cell membrane.

    (2) Bernard-Soulier syndrome is an **autosomal recessive** disorder characterized by decreased platelet adhesion as a result of absence of platelet membrane glycoproteins. Severe hemorrhage may occur, and large unusual platelets are seen on blood smear.

   b. Acquired disorders are usually caused by **drugs** (e.g., **aspirin,** valproic acid) that impair platelet function. **Uremia** and severe **liver disease** may also decrease platelet function.

 F. Hypercoagulability

  1. Inherited coagulation abnormalities leading to hypercoagulability most commonly include deficiencies of **proteins C and S or antithrombin III,** or mutations in **factor V** (factor V Leiden).

   a. Protein C deficiency

    (1) Protein C is a vitamin K–dependent factor that is the most potent anticoagulant protein known. Homozygous and heterozygous deficiency states have been described, and inheritance may be either autosomal recessive or dominant.

    (2) Clinical features

     (a) Homozygotes usually have no protein C activity and are detected soon after birth. **Purpura fulminans,** a nonthrombocytopenic purpura, is often the initial presentation. It is characterized by fever, shock, and rapidly spreading skin bleeding and intravascular thrombosis.

     (b) Heterozygotes often present later with **deep venous or CNS thrombosis.**

    (3) Diagnosis is by careful family history and specific testing for protein C.

    (4) Management. Treatment may include heparin, FFP, and warfarin. Purified concentrates of protein C have been used.

b. **Protein S, antithrombin III, and factor V Leiden deficiencies** present similarly to protein C deficiency. Specific testing for levels and function of each factor is diagnostic.

2. **Disease states** associated with thrombosis include SS disease, malignancy, inflammatory diseases (e.g., ulcerative colitis), liver disease, kidney disease (e.g., nephrotic syndrome), dehydration, vasculitis (e.g., Kawasaki disease), diabetes mellitus, and homocystinuria. Pregnancy and contraceptive use may also be associated with thrombosis.

V. Neutropenia

A. General Concepts

1. **Definition.** Neutropenia is a **low absolute number of neutrophils** and is often expressed as the **absolute neutrophil count (ANC;** percentage of WBCs that are neutrophils, bands, and immature myeloid cells).

2. **Risk of infection is directly related to the ANC.**
   a. **Mild neutropenia** is an ANC of 1,000–1,500 cells/mm^3.
   b. **Moderate neutropenia** is an ANC of 500–1,000 cells/mm^3. Infection generally involves the mucous membranes and skin (e.g., stomatitis, cellulitis, gingivitis).
   c. **Severe neutropenia** is an ANC < 500 cells/mm^3. Severe infections may result, such as pneumonia, sepsis, and meningitis. *S. aureus* and Gram-negative bacteria (e.g., *Klebsiella, Serratia, Escherichia coli,* and *Pseudomonas*) are typical organisms.

B. Neutropenia caused by decreased production

1. **Infections are the most common cause of neutropenia during childhood.** Viruses (e.g., HIV, EBV, CMV, hepatitis A and B, influenza A, parvovirus B19), bacteria (e.g., typhus, Rocky Mountain spotted fever), and protozoans (e.g., malaria) may all suppress the bone marrow, marginate neutrophils, or exhaust marrow reserves, resulting in neutropenia.

2. **Chronic benign neutropenia of childhood (CBN),** a common cause of neutropenia in children younger than 4 years of age, refers to a group of acquired and inherited disorders with **noncyclic neutropenia** as the only abnormality.
   a. **Clinical features.** CBN has a **variable course,** with most children having an increased incidence of **mild infections,** such as otitis media, sinusitis, pharyngitis, and cellulitis. Severe infections may occur but are uncommon. Children are otherwise healthy, with normal appearance and growth.
   b. **Laboratory findings.** Studies show a low ANC with a normal or slightly low WBC. Bone marrow demonstrates immature neutrophil precursors (development of mature neutrophils is arrested).
   c. **Prognosis.** In most children, CBN resolves spontaneously within months to years.

3. **Severe congenital agranulocytosis (Kostmann syndrome)** is an **autosomal recessive** disorder with frequent and life-threatening pyogenic bacterial infections beginning in infancy. ANC is usually < 300 cells/mm^3.

4. **Cyclic neutropenia**
   a. **Clinical features. Cyclic alterations in neutrophil counts** result in **regular episodes of neutropenia** with resultant infections. Fever, oral ulcers, and stomatitis may occur during the neutropenia. Cycles last an average of 21 days in 70% of patients. Some cases are inherited in an autosomal dominant pattern.
   b. **Diagnosis** is made by documenting the cyclic nature of the neutropenia by obtaining **serial neutrophil counts** during a 2- to 3-month period.

5. **Genetic syndromes**
   a. **Chédiak-Higashi syndrome** is an autosomal recessive disorder characterized by **oculocutaneous albinism,** large blue-gray granules in the cytoplasm of neutrophils, neutropenia, and **blond or brown hair with silver streaks.** Patients are at high risk for serious infection.
   b. **Cartilage-hair hypoplasia syndrome** is an autosomal recessive disorder characterized by **short stature, immunodeficiency, fine hair,** and **neutropenia.**

6. **Schwachman-Diamond syndrome** is characterized by **exocrine pancreatic insufficiency** with malabsorption, **short stature** caused by **metaphyseal chondrodysplasia, and neutropenia.** Failure to thrive and recurrent infections (especially otitis media) are common.

7. **Drugs** (e.g., antibiotics, anticonvulsants, aspirin), environmental toxins, radiation, and chemotherapy may all cause neutropenia.

8. **Metabolic diseases,** such as hyperglycinemia, methylmalonic acidemia, and Gaucher's disease, may result in neutropenia.

C. **Neutropenia caused by increased destruction**

1. **Infections** (especially viral)

2. **Drugs**

3. **Hypersplenism**

4. **Autoimmune neutropenia** describes a disorder in which **antineutrophil antibodies** are produced in response to infection (e.g., EBV), drugs, SLE, and juvenile rheumatoid arthritis (JRA), or for unknown reasons.

5. **Isoimmune neutropenia** describes the passive transfer of antineutrophil antibodies from the mother to her fetus after maternal sensitization by antigens on the fetal neutrophils. Infants are initially susceptible to infection, but neutropenia resolves by 8 weeks of life.

Review Test

1. You are evaluating a 2-month-old healthy full-term male infant at a routine health care maintenance visit. His mother is concerned because he seems pale. Although your examination is normal, you draw a hemoglobin (Hgb) level to reassure the parents. Which of the following statements is correct regarding the expected Hgb concentration?

(A) Evidence of nutritional iron deficiency anemia is likely.
(B) The Hgb is likely at its physiologic lowest point.
(C) Fetal Hgb has disappeared by now, and the Hgb level will be slightly lower than at birth.
(D) The Hgb was likely low at birth and is now increasing.
(E) Evidence of macrocytic anemia is likely.

2. A 2-year-old boy is brought to your office with a history of multiple bacterial infections, including six episodes of otitis media, three episodes of sinusitis, and one episode of periorbital cellulitis. He is normal appearing with normal growth and development. Biweekly laboratory assessments for the past 3 months have revealed consistently low white blood cell counts at 2,000–2,500 cells/mm^3, with an absolute neutrophil count of 500–1,000 cells/mm^3. Which one of the following is the most likely diagnosis?

(A) Chédiak-Higashi syndrome
(B) Schwachman-Diamond syndrome
(C) Chronic benign neutropenia of childhood
(D) Cyclic neutropenia
(E) Kostmann syndrome

3. A 3-year-old girl is brought to the office with petechiae and bruising on the face, chest, back, and lower extremities, which her mother noticed early this morning. The mother states that her daughter has been healthy except for a viral upper respiratory illness 2 weeks ago. Laboratory assessment reveals a platelet count of 25,000/μL. Which of the following statements regarding the likely diagnosis is correct?

(A) Hemarthroses commonly occur in this disorder.
(B) Spontaneous recovery within several weeks to months is expected.
(C) Platelet transfusion should be urgently performed.
(D) Prothrombin time and activated partial thromboplastin time are prolonged.
(E) Considering the girl's young age, this disorder will likely become chronic.

4. A 15-month-old girl has a hypochromic, microcytic anemia (hemoglobin of 10.6 g/dL) on a routine anemia screen performed in the office. History reveals a diet consisting of six 8-ounce glasses of whole cow's milk per day since the age of 9 months. Which of the following statements regarding the likely diagnosis is correct?

(A) The anemia is caused by a benign disorder, and there are no physical or intellectual effects.
(B) Low serum ferritin is a late finding.
(C) The reticulocyte count is low, considering the impact of this disorder on the bone marrow.
(D) Transferrin saturation is low.
(E) Free erythrocyte protoporphyrin is low.

5. You are evaluating a term newborn female infant during a routine health maintenance evaluation at 2 weeks of age. You receive the results of a routine newborn screen performed on the second day of life. The results of the newborn screen are normal, with the exception of the sickle cell screen, which reveals that the infant has hemoglobin (Hgb) A, Hgb S, and Hgb F. Which of the following is correct regarding the diagnosis?

(A) Mild anemia is expected.
(B) A vasoocclusive crisis involving the hands and feet is likely by 6 months of age.
(C) Splenic function is expected to decrease by 3 years of age.
(D) Penicillin prophylaxis should be started immediately.
(E) Hematuria may be the only manifestation of this disorder.

6. An 8-year-old boy with sickle cell anemia presents with severe right arm pain that began today. His pain has been unresponsive to oral acetaminophen. His mother states that he has been afebrile, and she denies he suffered any injury. On examination, his right arm is mildly tender and is minimally warm along the humerus. Range of motion of the upper extremity is normal. There is no fever. Which of the following is the appropriate initial management?

(A) Administration of maintenance intravenous fluids
(B) Red blood cell transfusion
(C) Administration of hydroxyurea
(D) Intravenous pain control
(E) Magnetic resonance imaging (MRI) to rule out osteomyelitis

7. A 17-year-old girl presents with concerns about her menstrual periods. Menarche occurred at 13 years of age, and for the past 2 years, her menstrual cycles have been regular but characterized by extremely heavy bleeding lasting 7–8 days. She also has a history of frequent nosebleeds since early childhood. She denies bleeding into her joints and has been otherwise healthy. She also denies medications, including aspirin. Based on her history, which of the following is the most likely diagnosis?

(A) Hemophilia A
(B) Hemophilia B
(C) Vitamin K deficiency
(D) Immune thrombocytopenic purpura (ITP)
(E) von Willebrand's disease

8. A 7-year-old girl comes to your office for the first time. Her parents bring her to see you because she has had widespread bruising for 3 days. They also believe that she is abnormally pale. On examination, you note that she is pale and has multiple areas of ecchymosis on her arms, legs, and trunk. Her past medical history is remarkable for being born with absence of her right thumb and right radius. Laboratory studies reveal a hemoglobin of 7 g/dL, platelet count of 30,000/μL, and white blood cell count of 800 cells/mm^3. Which of the following statements regarding the likely diagnosis is correct?

(A) The reticulocyte count is elevated.
(B) Spontaneous recovery from this disorder is likely.
(C) The growth chart likely reveals short stature.
(D) Intravenous immunoglobulin should be administered for immune thrombocytopenic purpura (ITP).
(E) Causes of the disorder include drugs, radiation, or chemical exposure.

9. A 10-year-old Italian boy has had chronic anemia since infancy that is characterized by severe hypochromia and microcytosis. Examination reveals a short child, an enlarged liver and spleen, and prominent facial bones, especially the maxilla, forehead, and cheekbones. Which of the following statements regarding the likely diagnosis is correct?

(A) Management should include supplemental iron.
(B) Hemochromatosis is a likely future complication.
(C) His hemoglobin (Hgb) electrophoresis will reveal Hgb S and Hgb F.
(D) The cause of his disorder is deletion of the α-globin chain.
(E) His blood smear will show spherocytes.

10. A 2-year-old girl has anemia with a hemoglobin of 9.8 g/dL on routine laboratory screening. History reveals a diet consisting of large amounts of goat's milk. Which of the following statements regarding the anemia is correct?

(A) The cause of the anemia is diminished intake of vitamin B$_{12}$.
(B) Spoon-shaped nails may be seen on examination.
(C) Smooth red tongue may be seen on examination.
(D) The anemia is normochromic and normocytic.
(E) Management includes administration of folic acid.

The response items for questions 11–13 are the same. You will be required to select one answer for each item in the set.

(A) Thrombocytopenia–absent radius (TAR) syndrome
(B) Fanconi anemia
(C) Wiskott-Aldrich syndrome
(D) Immune thrombocytopenic purpura
(E) Hemolytic uremic syndrome
(F) Kasabach-Merritt syndrome
(G) Glanzmann's thrombasthenia
(H) Bernard-Soulier syndrome

For each patient, select the likely diagnosis.

11. 2-year-old boy with thrombocytopenia and a large hepatic hemangioma.

12. 5-year-old boy with thrombocytopenia, moderate eczema, and both humoral and cell-mediated immunodeficiency.

13. Newborn girl with thrombocytopenia, ventricular septal defect, and absence of a radius. The girl's thumb is present.

The response items for questions 14–15 are the same. You will be required to select one answer for each question in the set.

(A) Transient erythroblastopenia of childhood
(B) Diamond-Blackfan anemia
(C) Parvovirus B19 red blood cell aplasia

For each clinical description, select the likely diagnosis.

14. A 6-month-old male infant presents with rapid onset of anemia. He has triphalangeal thumbs on examination. Corticosteroids improve his anemia.

15. A 2-year-old girl develops the gradual onset of significant anemia 2 weeks after a viral upper respiratory infection. Her anemia improves spontaneously.

The response items for questions 16–19 are the same. You will be required to select one answer for each item in the set.

(A) Hemophilia B
(B) Platelet function defect
(C) Vitamin K deficiency
(D) Disseminated intravascular coagulation (DIC)
(E) von Willebrand's disease
(F) Immune thrombocytopenic purpura

For each patient, select the most likely diagnosis.

16. A 6-year-old boy with prolonged diarrhea lasting 2 weeks develops a hemarthrosis involving the knee. He has a prolonged prothrombin time and prolonged activated partial thromboplastin time with a normal bleeding time.

17. A 2-year-old boy with newly diagnosed acute lymphocytic leukemia presents with fever, petechiae, and ecchymoses. He has thrombocytopenia, prolonged prothrombin time, prolonged activated partial thromboplastin time, and a prolonged bleeding time.

18. A 5-year-old boy presents with a hemarthrosis involving the knee. He has a normal prothrombin time, prolonged activated partial thromboplastin time, and normal bleeding time.

19. An 8-year-old boy develops severe bleeding following tonsillectomy. He has a normal prothrombin time, prolonged activated partial thromboplastin time, and prolonged bleeding time.

Answers and Explanations

1. The answer is B [I.A.2]. The hemoglobin of a healthy full-term infant is high at birth and decreases during the next several months, reaching its nadir, or physiologic lowest point, by 2–3 months of age. The hemoglobin of a preterm infant is at its physiologic low point at 1–2 months of age. Iron deficiency anemia does not generally appear until 9–24 months of age as a result of inadequate iron intake and depletion of iron stores acquired during fetal life. Fetal hemoglobin, a major constituent of red blood cells during early postnatal life, gradually declines and disappears by 6–9 months of age. Macrocytic anemia, caused most commonly by folic acid or vitamin B_{12} deficiency, would not normally occur at 2 months of age.

2. The answer is C [V.B.2]. This patient's clinical presentation and age are most consistent with chronic benign neutropenia of childhood (CBN). This noncyclic neutropenia is most common in children younger than 4 years of age. CBN is characterized by normal appearance and growth and a history of mild infections, such as sinusitis, cellulitis, and otitis media. Absolute neutrophil count (ANC) and white blood cell counts are low. Chédiak-Higashi and Kostmann syndromes are characterized by more severe infections, and Chédiak-Higashi syndrome is also notable for the presence of oculocutaneous albinism. Kostmann syndrome (severe congenital agranulocytosis) is an autosomal recessive disorder with frequent severe infections and a very low ANC. Schwachman-Diamond syndrome is characterized by poor growth, pancreatic insufficiency, and metaphyseal chondrodysplasia. Cyclic neutropenia, as its name suggests, is characterized by regular cycles of neutropenia occurring on average every 21 days.

3. The answer is B [IV.E.2.b.(1) and Table 13-6]. The most likely diagnosis is immune thrombocytopenic purpura (ITP) based on the acuteness of the presentation and the classic history of signs and symptoms after a viral infection. Spontaneous recovery is the rule, occurring in 70–80% of patients. Clinical features of ITP most commonly include cutaneous or mucous membrane bleeding, rather than bleeding into joints (hemarthroses). Platelet transfusions are generally not recommended because transfused platelets will be destroyed by the patient's antibodies. Patients with ITP have low platelet counts but normal activated partial thromboplastin time and prothrombin time. Treatment includes supportive care, intravenous immune globulin, or corticosteroids, and sometimes anti-D immunoglobulin. Chronic ITP occurs more commonly in patients older than 10 years of age.

4. The answer is D [I.D.1]. The history of excessive intake of iron-poor cow's milk and the presence of a microcytic, hypochromic anemia at 15 months of age are both consistent with iron deficiency anemia. In iron deficiency anemia, findings include increased free erythrocyte protoporphyrin, increased transferrin, and decreased transferrin saturation. Significant physical and intellectual effects may occur in iron deficiency anemia and include poor weight gain, diminished attention, and diminished abilities to learn. One of the earliest laboratory findings is a low serum ferritin. Reticulocyte count is often elevated, reflecting increased bone marrow activity.

5. The answer is E [I.F.3.d]. The presence of both hemoglobin (Hgb) A and Hgb S indicate that this patient has sickle cell trait (all children also have Hgb F at birth). The presence of Hgb A excludes sickle cell disease; affected patients with sickle cell disease have only Hgb S and Hgb F. Patients with sickle cell trait are generally asymptomatic, although during adolescence they may have an inability to concentrate the urine or hematuria. Patients do not have anemia; they are generally free of crises unless they have severe hypoxemia, and have normal splenic function. Prophylactic penicillin is unnecessary given the normal splenic function.

6. The answer is D [Table 13-3]. Extremity pain in patients with sickle cell disease may be caused by trauma, osteomyelitis, or a vasoocclusive crisis. Because there is no trauma or fever, a painful bone crisis (type of vasoocclusive crisis) is most likely. Appropriate management includes pain control (including intravenous morphine sulfate) and high-volume intravenous fluids at 1.5–2× maintenance. Red blood cell transfusion is contraindicated because it will lead to increased blood viscosity that may result in increased vasoocclusion. Hydroxyurea is most effective in prevention of painful bone crises, not in treatment. Because osteomyelitis is less likely given the acute onset of the pain and the absence of fever, magnetic resonance imaging would not be an appropriate initial management step.

7. The answer is E [IV.B.3]. von Willebrand's disease is characterized by mild to moderate bleeding in most patients. Common signs and symptoms include bruising, epistaxis, menorrhagia (i.e., prolonged or excessive uterine bleeding occurring at regular intervals), and bleeding after surgical procedures or dental extraction. Hemarthroses are unusual and are more typical in hemophilia A and B, in which deep soft tissue bleeding occurs. In addition, these bleeding disorders occur in males; they have X-linked inheritance. Vitamin K deficiency in an adolescent would likely be caused by medications or disorders that cause diminished vitamin K absorption, such as pancreatic insufficiency, biliary obstruction, or prolonged diarrhea. Symptoms would also likely be more severe. Immune thrombocytopenic purpura may present with petechiae, bruising, or nosebleeds. However, the onset of symptoms is generally acute.

8. The answer is C [II.B.1]. The patient most likely has Fanconi anemia, or congenital aplastic anemia, on the basis of pancytopenia, her age at presentation, and her history of absence (hypoplasia may also occur) of the thumb and radius. Fanconi anemia is an inherited lifelong disorder that results in bone marrow failure. Almost all patients have short stature, and many also have skin hyperpigmentation and kidney anomalies. Management includes transfusions and bone marrow transplant. Because Fanconi anemia is characterized by bone marrow failure, the reticulocyte count would be expected to be very low. Because the hemoglobin and white blood cell count are also low, this girl does not have immune thrombocytopenic purpura.

9. The answer is B [I.D.2.d]. This patient's anemia and physical features suggest β-thalassemia. β-Thalassemia occurs most commonly in patients of Mediterranean background and is caused by deletion of the β-globin chain. If untreated, β-thalassemia results in bone marrow hyperplasia (often noted within the facial bones), delays in growth and puberty, and hepatosplenomegaly. Many children suffer from hemochromatosis (iron overload) as a complication, and therefore iron is contraindicated in these patients. The presence of both hemoglobin S and hemoglobin F is not consistent with β-thalassemia and would instead suggest sickle cell anemia. Spherocytes are not present on blood smear.

10. The answer is E [I.E.1]. Feedings exclusively with goat's milk as a sole source of milk protein can lead to folic acid deficiency and a macrocytic anemia. Dietary folic acid is the treatment. Spoon-shaped nails are seen in iron deficiency anemia, and a smooth red tongue is seen in vitamin B_{12} deficiency.

11-13. The answers are F, C, and A, respectively [IV.E.2.b.(4), IV.E.2.a.(1)(a), IV.E.2.a.(1)(b)]. The 2-year-old boy has a large hemangioma that sequesters and destroys platelets, which is termed Kasabach-Merritt syndrome. The 5-year-old boy has Wiskott-Aldrich syndrome, which is characterized by eczema, defects in T- and B-cell immunity, and low platelet counts. The newborn girl has thrombocytopenia–absent radius (TAR) syndrome, which is characterized by thrombocytopenia, at times cardiac and renal disease, and absence of the radius. The thumb is present in TAR syndrome, in contrast to Fanconi anemia (pancytopenia with hypoplasia or absence of the radius and thumb).

14-15. The answers are B and A, respectively [Table 13-5]. The 6-month-old infant has Diamond-Blackfan anemia, which is characterized by rapid onset of anemia within the first year of life and physical abnormalities, including triphalangeal thumbs, short stature, and cardiac and renal anomalies, in one fourth to one third of patients. Treatment includes transfusions and corticosteroids. The 2-year-old girl has transient erythroblastopenia of childhood, which is characterized by the slow onset of anemia after the first year of life. The cause is likely a postviral autoimmune reaction, and no treatment is generally required. Parvovirus B19 red blood cell aplasia generally results in no symptoms of anemia in healthy children. Associated features may include a "slapped cheek" red facial rash and upper respiratory symptoms.

16–19. The answers are C, D, A, and E, respectively [Table 13-6]. The clinical characteristics and laboratory abnormalities can differentiate the causes of bleeding in pediatric patients. The 6-year-old boy has vitamin K deficiency, which can occur with pancreatic insufficiency, biliary obstruction, and prolonged diarrhea. Vitamin K deficiency affects the vitamin K–dependent coagulation factors (II, VII, IX, and X) and therefore results in hemarthroses, a prolonged prothrombin time (PT) and activated partial thromboplastin time (aPTT), and normal bleeding times. The 2-year-old boy has disseminated intravascular coagulation (DIC), which may be caused by malignancy, sepsis, snakebite, heat stroke, and burns. DIC is characterized by abnormalities in all coagulation constituents, including low platelet counts and prolonged aPTT, PT, and bleeding time. Both petechiae and hemarthroses may be present. The 5-year-old boy has hemophilia B, or factor IX deficiency. Hemophilia B is characterized by hemarthroses and prolonged aPTT, but normal PT and bleeding time. The 8-year-old boy has von Willebrand's disease, which can present with epistaxis, menorrhagia, and bleeding after tonsillectomy or dental surgery. von Willebrand's disease is characterized by prolonged aPTT and prolonged bleeding time, but normal PT. Hemarthroses may sometimes occur.

14

Oncology

Carole Hurvitz, M.D., Liliana Sloninsky, M.D., Margaret Sanford, M.D., and Lloyd J. Brown, M.D.

I. General Considerations

    A. Incidence. Approximately 6,000–7,000 children between 1 and 15 years of age develop cancer each year.

        1. Cancer is the **leading cause of death from disease** in childhood.

        2. Unlike adult cancers, most childhood cancers are not carcinomas. The **most common childhood cancers,** in order of declining incidence, are leukemia, brain tumors, lymphoma, neuroblastoma, soft tissue sarcomas, Wilms' tumor, and bone tumors.

    B. Etiology. The **cause of childhood cancers is often unknown.** However, genetic disorders, immunodeficiency diseases, infections, and environmental factors may predispose to certain cancers.

        1. Ten to fifteen percent of cancers have a familial association or are associated with a genetic disorder. **Table 14-1** lists common genetic syndromes and their associated cancer(s).

        2. Immunodeficiency diseases may predispose to cancer.

            a. Wiskott-Aldrich syndrome, characterized by B- and T-cell dysfunction, atopic dermatitis, and thrombocytopenia, is associated with lymphoma and leukemia.

            b. X-linked lymphoproliferative disease, associated with Epstein-Barr virus (EBV) infection, may result in lymphoma.

        3. Infectious diseases, such as EBV and HIV, are associated with Burkitt's lymphoma and Kaposi's sarcoma, respectively.

        4. Environmental factors, such as prior chemotherapy and ionizing radiation, may result in malignancy.

    C. Typical presenting features of childhood cancer

        1. Persistent fever, especially if associated with weight loss or night sweats, may be associated with leukemia, lymphoma, and other cancers.

        2. Palpable or visible mass

Table 14-1. Genetic Disorders and Their Association with Childhood Cancer

Genetic Disorder	Type of Cancer
Down syndrome	Leukemia (ALL or AML)
Turner syndrome	Gonadoblastoma
Trisomy 13	Leukemia, teratoma
Trisomy 18	Wilms' tumor, neurogenic tumors
Klinefelter syndrome	Leukemia, germ cell tumors, breast cancer
Fanconi anemia	Leukemia
Xeroderma pigmentosa	Basal and squamous cell carcinoma, melanoma
Ataxia telangiectasia	Hodgkin's and non-Hodgkin's lymphoma, leukemia, sarcomas
Bloom syndrome	Leukemia, lymphomas, gastrointestinal malignancies, solid tumors
Beckwith-Wiedemann syndrome	Wilms' tumor, hepatoblastoma, rhabdomyosarcoma, adrenocortical carcinoma
Neurofibromatosis type I	Brain tumors, lymphoma, leukemia, malignant schwannoma
Neurofibromatosis type II	Acoustic neuroma

ALL = acute lymphocytic leukemia; *AML* = acute myelogenous leukemia

   a. **Abdominal mass** should be considered malignant until proven otherwise. Wilms' tumor and neuroblastoma are the two most common malignant abdominal tumors that may present with an abdominal mass.

   b. **Mass on the trunk or extremities** may be caused by rhabdomyosarcoma or bone tumor.

3. **Bone pain** may reflect metastatic cancer, primary tumors of bone or connective tissue, or leukemic infiltration of bone marrow.

4. **Supraclavicular lymphadenopathy,** nontender, firm lymph nodes, or enlarging lymph nodes may be caused by leukemia, lymphoma, or metastatic disease.

5. **Early morning headache** and **vomiting,** or change in gait, may be caused by a space-occupying tumor within the central nervous system (CNS).

6. **Bruising, petechiae, and pallor** may be caused by tumor infiltration of bone marrow.

7. **Leukocoria** (i.e., white reflex in the pupillary area) may be caused by retinoblastoma (see Chapter 18, section VIII.B).

8. **Hypertension** may be caused by neuroblastoma, Wilms' tumor, or pheochromocytoma.

II. Leukemias

   A. **Acute Lymphocytic Leukemia (ALL)** [acute lymphoblastic leukemia]
      1. **Epidemiology**

a. **ALL is the most common childhood cancer.**

b. **ALL** represents **80–85%** of childhood leukemias.

c. **Peak incidence** occurs at **2–6 years of age.** ALL is more common in **males** and in Caucasians.

2. **Etiology.** The cause is generally unknown; however, ALL may be associated with ionizing radiation, chemotherapy, genetic syndromes (e.g., Down syndrome, Bloom syndrome), chemical agents, and immunodeficiency diseases (e.g., ataxia telangiectasia).

3. **Classification** is based on morphology and immunophenotype of the leukemic cells (i.e., lymphoblasts).

   a. **Cell morphology** is classified as L1, L2, or L3, with **L1 being the most common in childhood.** L1 lymphoblasts are small with little cytoplasm and indistinct nucleoli, whereas L3 lymphoblasts are large with one or more nucleoli.

   b. **Immunophenotype**

      (1) **T-cell phenotype: 25%**

      (2) **B-cell phenotype: <5%**

      (3) **Pre–B-cell phenotype: 70%.** Pre–B-cell ALL may be further subdivided on the basis of the presence of common acute lymphocytic leukemia antigen (**CALLA**).

         (a) CALLA-positive (**70%**)

         (b) CALLA-negative (**30%**)

4. **Clinical features**

   a. **Fever** and **bone or joint pain** are the **most common symptoms.** Bone or joint pain often manifests as refusal to bear weight.

   b. **Pallor, bruising, hepatosplenomegaly, and lymphadenopathy** are the **most common signs.**

   c. Epistaxis, anorexia, fatigue, testicular pain and swelling, and abdominal pain may also be present.

5. **Diagnosis**

   a. ALL is **suggested** by a complete blood count (CBC) that demonstrates **anemia** and **thrombocytopenia. The white blood cell (WBC) count is variable.**

      (1) **WBC is high in one third** of cases (> 50,000 cells/mm^3), **normal in one third** of cases, and **low in one third** of cases (< 10,000 cells/mm^3).

      (2) **Leukemic blasts** (i.e., lymphoblasts) are often seen.

      (3) **Note: A normal CBC does not rule out leukemia.**

   b. **Confirmation** is by **bone marrow evaluation** demonstrating **marrow replacement by lymphoblasts.** Other normal marrow elements are decreased or absent. Cytogenetics to evaluate for translocations and immunophenotyping must be performed.

   c. **Prognostic factors** for ALL at time of diagnosis are listed in **Table 14-2.** Most patients have disseminated disease at presentation, so there is no staging system for ALL.

6. **Management.** The best treatment for ALL remains under investigation,

Table 14-2. Prognostic Factors for ALL at Time of Diagnosis

Prognostic Factor	Favorable	Unfavorable
Age	1–9 years of age	< 1 or > 9 years of age
Sex	Female	Male
Race	White	Black
WBC	< 50,000 cells/mm^3	> 50,000 cells/mm^3
Ploidy	Hyperploidy (more than 53 chromosomes within leukemic cells)	Low ploidy (fewer than 53 chromosomes within leukemic cells)
Organ involvement	None	Organomegaly, central nervous system involvement, mediastinal mass
Immunophenotype	CALLA (+)	CALLA (−)
Chromosomal translocation	None	t(9,22)

ALL = acute lymphocytic leukemia; *CALLA* = common acute lymphocytic leukemia antigen; *WBC* = white blood cell count.

and patients should be encouraged to participate in a national clinical trial. Management involves **three stages: induction, consolidation, and maintenance.**

a. **Induction** aims to destroy as many cancer cells as possible to induce remission.

   (1) Drugs vary based on study protocol but typically include corticosteroids, vincristine, and L-asparaginase. **Intrathecal methotrexate** is given to all children during induction. Other agents are added on the basis of expected prognosis.

   (2) Remission is induced in 95% of patients.

b. **Consolidation** involves a continuation of systemic chemotherapeutic agents and prophylactic regimens to prevent CNS involvement because systemic chemotherapy poorly penetrates the blood-brain barrier.

   (1) **Intrathecal methotrexate** is continued during consolidation.

   (2) **Cranial irradiation** may be given to high-risk children. Radiation should generally be avoided in children younger than 5 years of age, if possible, because of the risk of subsequent neuropsychological effects.

c. **Maintenance** therapy involves daily and periodic chemotherapy during remission for up to 3 years. Chemotherapy is usually discontinued after 2–3 years if the patient remains disease-free.

d. **Bone marrow transplant** may be performed for very high-risk children and for those who have relapsed. (The bone marrow is the most common site of relapse.)

e. **Complications** during treatment often occur. **Supportive care** is important and includes management of anemia and thrombocytopenia with appropriate blood products, and therapy for the following common complications:

   (1) **Infection associated with neutropenia is potentially life-threatening. Children with fever and severe neutropenia**

(absolute neutrophil count < 500 cells/mm³) must be assumed to have a serious bacterial infection, such as sepsis, until proven otherwise.** Common infectious agents include *Staphylococcus aureus, Staphylococcus epidermidis, Pseudomonas aeruginosa,* and *Escherichia coli.* It is necessary to give **empiric treatment with intravenous broad-spectrum antibiotics after appropriate cultures** of blood and urine and any other noticeable sources of infection, are obtained.

(2) Opportunistic infections with organisms, such as herpes simplex virus, *Pneumocystis carinii* pneumonia (PCP), and fungi (*Candida albicans, Aspergillus*), may occur as a result of immunosuppression associated with chemotherapy. Fungal infection should be considered in patients with fever lasting longer than 1 week while on intravenous antibiotics. Prophylaxis with trimethoprim-sulfamethoxazole is generally effective in preventing PCP infection.

(3) Metabolic complications from spontaneous or therapy-induced cell lysis (**tumor lysis syndrome**)

(a) Hyperuricemia may result in renal insufficiency.

(b) Hyperkalemia may result in cardiac dysrhythmias.

(c) Hyperphosphatemia may result in hypocalcemia with tetany.

(4) Other complications include medication-induced pancreatitis (L-asparaginase and corticosteroids), cardiomyopathy (doxorubicin), and cystitis (cyclophosphamide). Cranial irradiation may result in mental retardation, learning problems, stroke, hormonal problems (e.g., growth delay, hypothyroidism, hypopituitarism), and secondary malignancy.

7. Prognosis. The outlook for patients with ALL is generally good. Overall long-term survival occurs in 85% of patients.

B. Acute Myelogenous Leukemia (AML)

1. Epidemiology. AML represents **15–20% of childhood leukemias.**

2. Etiology. The **cause of AML is unknown.** AML is associated with **Down syndrome,** Fanconi anemia, Kostmann syndrome, and neurofibromatosis. It may also be associated with ionizing radiation and occur as a secondary malignancy resulting from chemotherapy.

3. Classification is based on cell morphology and histochemical characteristics. There are seven types of AML: M1, M2, M4, and M5 together account for 90% of childhood AML.

a. M1: acute myeloblastic leukemia (no maturation)

b. M2: acute myeloblastic leukemia (some maturation)

c. M3: acute promyelocytic leukemia (Auer rods common)

d. M4: acute myelomonocytic leukemia

e. M5: acute monocytic leukemia

f. M6: erythroleukemia

g. M7: acute megakaryocytic leukemia (associated with Down syndrome)

4. **Clinical features** are similar to those of ALL. However, **CNS involvement** occurs more commonly in AML than in ALL.

  a. **Symptoms and signs include fever, hepatosplenomegaly,** bruising and bleeding, **gingival hypertrophy,** and bone pain. Lymphadenopathy and testicular involvement are uncommon.

  b. **Laboratory findings** may include pancytopenia or leukocytosis, and disseminated intravascular coagulation (DIC).

5. **Diagnosis** is **suggested** by clinical features and blood smear demonstrating **leukemic myeloblasts.** Blasts containing **Auer rods** are consistent with myeloid leukemia. **Confirmation** is by morphologic analysis and immunophenotyping of cells obtained by bone marrow biopsy.

6. **Management.** AML, unlike ALL, requires very intensive myeloablative therapy to induce remission. **Bone marrow transplant** is recommended once patients are in remission, if they have an HLA-matched donor.

7. **Prognosis.** Aggressive chemotherapy is effective in 50% of patients. Bone marrow transplant from a matched sibling is curative in 70% of patients. AML associated with Down syndrome is very responsive to therapy, for unknown reasons.

C. **Chronic Myelogenous Leukemia (CML)**

  1. **Epidemiology.** CML is the **least common** type of leukemia, representing 3–5% of childhood leukemia. Males are more commonly affected.

  2. **Classification.** Two forms of CML occur in children.

    a. **Adult-type CML**

      (1) **Twice as common as the juvenile form**

      (2) Occurs predominantly in **older children and adolescents**

      (3) Characterized by the presence of the **Philadelphia chromosome** (reciprocal translocation between the long arms of chromosomes 9 and 22, leading to the fusion gene *BCR/ABL1* that produces the BCR-ABL fusion protein)

    b. **Juvenile chronic myelogenous leukemia** (juvenile myelomonocytic leukemia [**JMML**])

      (1) Occurs predominantly in **infants and children** younger than 2 years of age

      (2) Sometimes characterized by abnormalities of chromosome 7 or 8. The Philadelphia chromosome is absent.

  3. **Clinical features.** Signs and symptoms vary based on the type of CML.

    a. **Adult-type CML**

      (1) Nonspecific symptoms such as fatigue, weight loss, and pain

      (2) **Massive splenomegaly** leading to abdominal distension. CML is typically discovered after an incidental finding of splenomegaly on examination.

      (3) **Extremely high WBC (often > 100,000 cells/mm^3)**

    b. **JMML**

      (1) **Fever**

      (2) **Chronic eczemalike facial rash**

(3) Suppurative lymphadenopathy

(4) Petechiae and purpura

(5) Moderate leukocytosis (< 100,000 cells/mm³), anemia, and thrombocytopenia

4. **Management.** Treatment of both adult-type CML and JMML is **bone marrow transplantation,** either HLA-matched (ideally) or unmatched. Radiation therapy is not effective; however, the newer chemotherapeutic agent, imatinib mesylate has been shown to induce remission in adult-type CML.

5. **Prognosis**
   a. **Adult-type CML** may have a **biphasic course.** During the initial chronic phase, chemotherapy controls the leukocytosis. During the subsequent acute phase resembling acute leukemia, the patient deteriorates and is unresponsive to therapy.
   b. **JMML** is often fatal. Relapse occurs in 50% of cases, even with bone marrow transplantation.

III. Lymphomas. Lymphomas account for 10–15% of childhood cancers.

A. **Hodgkin's disease** is a cancer of the antigen-processing cells found within the lymph nodes or spleen.

1. **Epidemiology**
   a. Hodgkin's disease is **associated** with **EBV infection.** Patients with EBV-associated mononucleosis have a two to four times greater risk of developing Hodgkin's disease later in life.
   b. Hodgkin's disease is more common in older children and adolescents.

2. **Clinical features.** Most children with Hodgkin's disease present with **painless lymphadenopathy,** most commonly in the supraclavicular or cervical regions. **Signs and symptoms** of Hodgkin's disease are listed in **Table 14-3.**

3. **Diagnosis.** The basis of diagnosis is histologic review of tissue obtained

Table 14-3. Clinical Features of Hodgkin's Disease and Non-Hodgkin's Lymphoma

Clinical Feature	Hodgkin's Disease	Non-Hodgkin's Lymphoma
Symptom onset	Slow, indolent	Rapid
Common location	Cervical and supraclavicular nodes	Abdominal, mediastinal, and supraclavicular nodes
Systemic symptoms*	Relatively common (30%)	Uncommon
Abdominal findings†	Rare	Common
Painless adenopathy	Common	Common
SVC syndrome	Rare	Common
Airway compression	Rare	Common

*Systemic symptoms include fever, drenching night sweats, and weight loss.
†Abdominal findings include abdominal pain, intussusception, abdominal mass, and obstruction.
SVC = superior vena cava.

by **lymph node biopsy.** The hallmark histologic feature is the **Reed-Sternberg cell,** a large multinucleated cell with abundant cytoplasm.

4. **Staging.** Classification by the **Ann Arbor system** is the basis for treatment and provides prognostic information. There are four basic stages, and **each stage is subclassified** into "A" or "B," reflecting clinical symptoms. **A** refers to lack of systemic symptoms. **B** refers to the presence of systemic symptoms, such as fever, night sweats, or > 10% weight loss.

   a. **Stage I:** involvement of a single lymph node or extralymphatic site

   b. **Stage II:** involvement of two or more lymph node regions on the same side of the diaphragm, or extension to an extralymphatic site and one or more lymph node regions on the same side of the diaphragm

   c. **Stage III:** involvement of lymph nodes on both sides of the diaphragm (in this case, the spleen is considered a lymph node)

   d. **Stage IV:** diffuse or disseminated involvement of one or more extralymphatic organs or tissues

5. **Management.** Treatment is based on the child's age, disease stage, and tumor burden. Treatment most commonly includes chemotherapy and radiation therapy. **Late complications of therapy** include the following:

   a. **Growth retardation** as a result of radiation therapy

   b. **Secondary malignancies**, including breast cancer, AML, and non-Hodgkin's lymphoma

   c. **Hypothyroidism** (10–20%)

   d. **Male sterility (very common)**

6. **Prognosis.** Overall, prognosis of stages I and II disease is excellent, with ≥ 80% long-term survival. More advanced disease carries a long-term survival rate of 60–70%.

B. **Non-Hodgkin's lymphoma** is a **very aggressive** cancer and is 1.5 times more common than Hodgkin's disease.

   1. **Epidemiology**

      a. **Male predominance**

      b. Associated with **immunodeficiency states,** such as HIV, Wiskott-Aldrich syndrome, ataxia telangiectasia syndrome, and prior EBV infection.

      c. **Increasing incidence after 5 years of age**

   2. **Classification.** There are three major categories of non-Hodgkin's lymphoma. (The more **uncommon categories** include anaplastic large cell and large cell, noncleaved immunoblastic lymphoma.)

      a. **Lymphoblastic lymphoma** is histologically similar to the lymphoblast of ALL. It is generally **T-cell** in origin.

      b. **Small, noncleaved cell lymphoma** includes **Burkitt's lymphoma, the most common lymphoma in childhood.** Burkitt's lymphoma is **B-cell** in origin.

      c. **Large cell lymphoma** is generally **B-cell** in origin.

   3. **Clinical features (see Table 14-3). Painless lymphadenopathy is the most common presenting feature.**

      a. **Lymphoblastic lymphoma** commonly presents with an **anterior**

mediastinal mass, and the patient may develop **superior vena cava syndrome** or **airway obstruction** as a result.

   b. **Small, noncleaved cell lymphoma**

   (1) **Intussusception,** abdominal pain, or mass. **Lymphoma must be considered as a possible cause (lead point) in any child older than 3 years of age presenting with intussusception.**

   (2) **Burkitt's lymphoma** is endemic in Africa, where it presents as a **jaw mass.**

   c. **Large cell lymphoma** commonly presents as enlargement of lymphoid tissue in the tonsils, adenoids, or Peyer's patches.

4. **Diagnosis and staging.** The basis of diagnosis is pathologic examination of tissue obtained by biopsy. Evaluation for dissemination is the basis of staging. This evaluation often includes chest radiograph or chest computed tomography (CT) scan, abdominal and pelvis CT scan, bone scan or gallium scan, measurement of hepatic transaminases, bone marrow biopsy, and cerebrospinal fluid analysis.

5. **Management. Treatment must be rapid** because of the aggressiveness of this cancer. Management includes surgery to remove or debulk the tumor, chemotherapy specific for the tumor type, prophylaxis for CNS disease, and treatment of tumor lysis syndrome, should it occur.

6. **Prognosis.** Outlook is **best for localized lymphoma,** with a cure rate > 90%. Prognosis is poorest for patients with disseminated disease.

IV. Brain Tumors

A. Epidemiology

1. Brain tumors are the **second most common childhood cancer** after leukemia and are the **most common solid tumors.**

2. They account for 20% of all childhood cancers.

3. Brain tumors may be associated with underlying diseases such as neurofibromatosis, tuberous sclerosis, and von Hippel-Lindau disease.

B. Classification is by histology, grade, and location.

1. **Histology**

   a. **Glial cell tumors are most common** (40–60% of brain tumors) and include astrocytomas. High-grade (i.e., aggressive) tumors often arise in the supratentorial region, and low-grade (i.e., less aggressive) tumors arise in the infratentorial region.

   b. **Primitive neuroectodermal tumors (PNETs)** are the second most common tumor and include medulloblastomas arising from the cerebellum.

   c. **Ependymomas** are the third most common tumor.

   d. **Craniopharyngiomas** are the fourth most common tumor.

2. **Grade.** The grade of the tumor refers to its aggressiveness.

   a. **High grade:** aggressive, proliferative cells

   b. **Low grade:** less aggressive, more-differentiated cells

3. **Location. Infratentorial tumors are more common** than supratentorial tumors, except at age extremes of < 1 or > 12 years of age.

    a. **Medulloblastoma** is the **most common infratentorial tumor,** followed by cerebellar astrocytoma and brainstem glioma.

    b. **Astrocytoma** is the **most common supratentorial tumor.**

C. **Clinical features.** Signs and symptoms are typically based on the location of the tumor and the child's age.

    1. **Key point: Even benign tumors can be lethal if their location interferes with brain function.**

    2. **Initial nonspecific symptoms** are caused by increased intracranial pressure (and are often **worse during sleep** or **on awakening**). Symptoms commonly subside during the day as venous return from the head improves with upright posture.

        a. **Headache:** diffuse, occipital, or frontal

        b. **Vomiting:** often resolves the accompanying headache

        c. **Drowsiness or irritability**

        d. **Abnormal behavior**

        e. **Ataxia:** associated with cerebellar tumors

        f. **Seizure:** associated with supratentorial tumors

        g. **Head tilt**

    3. **Physical examination findings**

        a. **Enlarged** or **bulging fontanelle** in infants, or enlarged head circumference

        b. **Nystagmus**

        c. **Papilledema**

        d. **Cranial nerve abnormalities,** especially sixth nerve palsy

        e. **Lethargy or irritability**

    4. **Features associated with specific tumors**

        a. **Optic glioma** is associated with diminished vision, visual field deficits, and strabismus.

        b. **Craniopharyngioma** is associated with growth retardation, delayed puberty, visual changes, diabetes insipidus, and other hormonal problems because of involvement of the hypothalamic-pituitary axis.

D. **Diagnosis**

    1. **Neuroimaging** by CT or magnetic resonance imaging (MRI) is critical for diagnosis and management. MRI is generally preferred because it is better able to visualize the temporal lobes, cranial base, and brainstem. MRI is also able to image the tumor in multiple planes, allowing for operative planning.

    2. **Cerebrospinal fluid** obtained at surgery is useful for staging and assessment of tumor markers (i.e., α-fetoprotein or β-human chorionic gonadotropin for germ cell tumors; homovanillic acid [HVA], vanillylmandelic acid [VMA], and polyamines for medulloblastoma).

   E. **Management**
   1. **Surgery.** Resection or debulking the tumor is the **principal treatment.**
   2. **Radiation therapy.** Almost all brain tumors are radiosensitive. However, radiation should be reserved, if possible, for children older than 5 years of age because of the risk of adverse effects (see Chapter 14, section II.A.6.e.(4)).
   3. **Chemotherapy.** This method is effective for many tumors and is often used together with radiation therapy and surgery.
   F. **Prognosis.** Outlook depends on tumor grade, size, and type.
   1. **Astrocytomas.** Low-grade, completely resectable astrocytomas have a good prognosis (> 75% survival). High-grade astrocytomas have a poor prognosis (35% survival at 3 years) because of their infiltrative nature.
   2. **PNETs.** Survival is > 75% if the majority of the tumor can be resected and there are no metastases or extension. Prognosis is worse in children younger than 4 years of age.
   3. **Brainstem gliomas.** The prognosis is poorest with brainstem gliomas. It is not possible to resect these tumors, and chemotherapy is ineffective.

V. Renal and Suprarenal Tumors

   A. **Neuroblastoma.** This malignant tumor of neural crest cells may arise anywhere along the sympathetic ganglia chain and within the adrenal medulla.
   1. **Epidemiology**
      a. Neuroblastomas are the **second most common solid tumors,** after brain tumors.
      b. Neuroblastomas are responsible for 8–10% of all childhood cancers.
      c. **Peak incidence is in the first 5 years of life.** Median age at time of diagnosis is 2 years.
      d. Approximately **75% occur in the abdomen or pelvis,** 20% occur in the posterior mediastinum, and 5% occur in the neck.
   2. **Etiology.** The cause is unknown; however, chromosomal abnormalities have been detected. Such abnormalities include a deletion on the short arm of chromosome 1, an unbalanced translocation between 1p and 17q, and anomalies on chromosomes 14q and 22q.
   3. **Clinical features.** Signs and symptoms are presented in **Figure 14-1.**
   4. **Diagnosis**
      a. Urine excretion of **excessive catecholamines,** including VMA and HVA, is characteristic (found in 90% of patients). **Definitive diagnosis** is by positive bone marrow biopsy plus elevated urine catecholamines, or by results of tissue biopsy.
      b. CT or MRI is generally used to assess tumor spread.
      c. Skeletal survey or technetium 99m bone scan is used to assess for metastasis to bone.

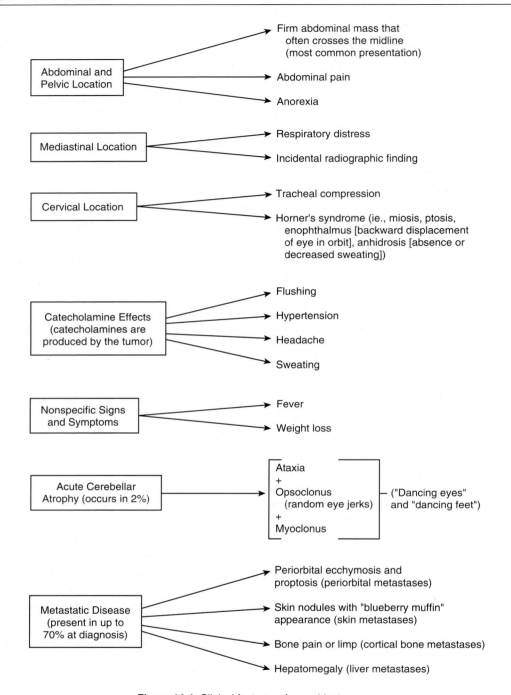

Figure 14-1. Clinical features of neuroblastoma.

5. **Staging.** Several systems may be used. The most commonly used system, the Evan's system, has five stages.

   a. **Stage I:** localized tumor confined to the structure of origin

   b. **Stage II:** tumor extends beyond structure of origin but does not cross midline

   c. **Stage III:** tumor extends past midline
   d. **Stage IV:** metastasis to bone, lymph nodes, bone marrow, or soft tissue
   e. **Stage IVS:** localized tumor at stage I or II but with distant metastasis to any organ but bone

6. **Management**
   a. **Surgery alone may be curative for stage I and II disease.**
   b. **Chemotherapy** is used, especially for metastatic disease (stage IV and sometimes IVS) and for locally advanced disease.
   c. **Radiation therapy** is used for advanced disease.

7. **Prognosis**
   a. **Good** prognosis occurs in children younger than 1 year of age and in patients with stage I and II disease. **Spontaneous regression without treatment may occur in young infants with stage IVS disease.**
   b. **Poor** prognosis is associated with stage III and IV disease, amplification of the oncogene **N-*myc*** (found on chromosome 2), tumor cell diploidy, and high levels of the serum markers ferritin, lactic dehydrogenase, and neuron-specific enolase.

B. **Wilms' tumor** (nephroblastoma) is a tumor of the kidney.

1. **Epidemiology**
   a. Wilms' tumor is the **most common childhood renal tumor.** It is responsible for 7% of childhood cancers.
   b. Seventy-five percent of cases occur in children **younger than 5 years of age** (median age at diagnosis is 3 years).
   c. Associated **genetic findings or syndromes** include Beckwith-Wiedemann syndrome (hemihypertrophy, macroglossia, visceromegaly), deletion of the short arm of chromosome 11, and WAGR syndrome (Wilms' tumor, aniridia, genitourinary abnormalities, and mental retardation).

2. **Clinical features**
   a. **Abdominal mass,** generally found on routine evaluation, is the **most common presentation.** The mass is smooth and firm, and rarely crosses the midline.
   b. **Abdominal pain** (50% of patients) with or without vomiting
   c. **Hematuria** (25% of patients)
   d. **Hypertension** (25% of patients) secondary to pressure on the renal artery or increased renin secretion by the tumor
   e. **Nonspecific** findings including fever, anorexia, and weight loss.
   f. Associated congenital anomalies in 15% of cases
      (1) **Genitourinary malformations**
      (2) **Hemihypertrophy**
      (3) **Sporadic aniridia**

3. **Diagnosis.** Wilms' tumor should be considered in any child who presents with hematuria or abdominal mass. Wilms' tumor is bilateral in 5% of cases. Confirmation is by imaging with abdominal CT or MRI scan and by histologic evaluation of tissue. Evaluation for distant metastasis to lung, liver, bone, and brain should also be completed.

4. **Staging.** The National Wilms' Tumor Study Group classification is used to stage Wilms' tumor.
   a. **Stage I:** tumor limited to kidney and completely excised intact without rupture
   b. **Stage II:** tumor extends locally but can still be completely excised without residual disease
   c. **Stage III:** residual tumor remains in abdomen or spillage of tumor occurs during resection
   d. **Stage IV:** distant metastasis to lung (most common), liver, bone, and brain
   e. **Stage V:** bilateral renal involvement

5. **Management.** Treatment includes prompt surgery for staging and to remove as much tumor as possible. Chemotherapy is used for all stages. Radiation therapy is also used for advanced disease (stages III and IV).

6. **Prognosis.** Outcome is usually **excellent,** with an overall cure rate > 90%. Prognosis is dependent on staging and histology. Favorable histology and stage I, II, or III disease results in a 2-year survival > 95%. Unfavorable histology accounts for 12% of cases but 90% of deaths.

VI. Soft Tissue Tumors. Rhabdomyosarcoma is the most common soft tissue sarcoma in childhood and is a malignant tumor of the same embryonic mesenchyme that gives rise to skeletal muscle.

A. **Epidemiology. Two thirds** of rhabdomyosarcomas occur in children **younger than 10 years of age.**

B. **Etiology.** The cause is generally unknown. Patients with neurofibromatosis are at higher risk.

C. **Clinical features.** Signs and symptoms depend on the site of involvement. Any part of the body may be affected. The initial presentation is usually a **painless soft tissue mass.**

1. **Head and neck,** including the orbit, are the **most common sites** of involvement (40% of cases).
   a. **Orbital tumors** typically present with proptosis, chemosis (i.e., conjunctival edema), eyelid swelling and cranial nerve palsies.
   b. **Nasopharyngeal tumors** typically present with epistaxis, airway obstruction and chronic sinusitis.
   c. **Laryngeal tumors** typically present with hoarseness.

2. **Genitourinary tract** is the 2nd most common site of involvement (20% of cases). Tumors in this location typically present with hematuria, urinary tract obstruction, vaginal bleeding, and/or an abdominal mass.

3. **The extremities** are the 3rd most common site of involvement (18% of cases). Tumors in this location present with a painless growing mass.

    4. Other sites of involvement include the trunk, retroperitoneum, medi-astinum, and paratesticular and perianal regions.

D. Diagnosis. Rhabdomyosarcoma should be considered in any patient presenting with a painless enlarging mass. Imaging studies (CT or MRI) are performed to determine the extent of local extension and to prepare for surgical excision. Histologic evaluation of tissue obtained by biopsy provides a definitive diagnosis.

E. Management. Most importantly, treatment includes an attempt at complete surgical resection. Chemotherapy and radiation therapy are used (1) to treat local disease and distant metastases and (2) to prevent tumor recurrence.

F. Prognosis. Tumors of the head and neck and the genitourinary tract have the best prognosis, with a cure rate > 90%. Poor prognosis is associated with metastases (20% have metastatic disease at time of diagnosis), tumor recurrence, and tumors at sites other than the head and neck or the genitourinary tract.

VII. Bone Tumors

A. Osteogenic sarcoma is a malignant tumor that forms osteoid, or new bone.

    1. Epidemiology

        a. Osteogenic sarcoma is the **most common malignant bone tumor.**

        b. The incidence of this tumor **peaks during the rapid growth spurt** of adolescence. **Males** are more commonly affected.

    2. Etiology. The cause is unknown; however, it is associated with previous retinoblastoma, Paget's disease of bone, radiation therapy for cancer, and fibrous dysplasia.

    3. Clinical features. About **50% of tumors occur near the knee. Other**

Table 14-4. Clinical and Radiographic Features of Osteogenic Sarcoma and Ewing's Sarcoma

Feature	Osteogenic Sarcoma	Ewing's Sarcoma
Site	**Metaphysis** of tubular long bones 50% occur near the knee Most common sites (in order): distal femur, proximal tibia, proximal humerus, proximal femur	**Flat bones and diaphysis** of tubular bones; occasionally extraosseous Most common sites (in order): axial skeleton (especially pelvis), humerus, femur
Local and systemic findings	Pain, swelling, and soft tissue mass Systemic symptoms uncommon	Pain, swelling, and soft tissue mass Fever, malaise, and weight loss Leukocytosis and ↑ ESR
Radiographic findings	Periosteal reaction with **"sunburst"** appearance Lytic; or mixed lytic and destructive changes	Periosteal reaction with **"onion skin"** appearance Destructive changes
Metastases	Occurs in 15% at presentation Lungs (90%) and bone (10%)	Occurs in 25% at presentation Lungs (50%), bone (25%), and bone marrow (25%)

ESR = erythrocyte sedimentation rate.

signs and symptoms are listed in **Table 14-4,** which compares osteogenic sarcoma with Ewing's sarcoma.

4. **Diagnosis.** Diagnosis is suggested by findings on radiographs and MRI. Definitive diagnosis is by tissue biopsy. Bone scan and chest CT scan are performed to evaluate for metastatic disease.

5. **Management**
   a. **Surgery** to remove the primary tumor is performed by limb amputation or limb salvage procedures.
   b. **Chemotherapy** improves survival. Drugs used include high-dose methotrexate, cisplatin, doxorubicin, ifosfamide, and cyclophosphamide.
   c. **Pulmonary metastases** identified at the time of diagnosis are usually removed surgically.

6. **Prognosis.** Outcome has improved with the addition of chemotherapy, and survival is now > 60%.

B. **Ewing's sarcoma** is a sarcoma characterized as a small, round, blue cell tumor (undifferentiated, monomorphous cell appearance).

1. **Epidemiology**
   a. Ewing's sarcoma is the **second most common malignant bone tumor.**
   b. It **most commonly occurs during adolescence. Males** are more commonly affected.
   c. It is **rare** in Asians and African Americans.

2. **Etiology.** The cause is unknown. However, 95% have a **chromosomal translocation** between chromosomes 11 and 21 (a similar translocation to that noted in PNET brain tumors).

3. **Clinical features.** Signs and symptoms are listed in **Table 14-4,** which compares Ewing's sarcoma and osteogenic sarcoma. Ewing's sarcoma may occasionally develop in soft tissue instead of bone.

4. **Diagnosis**
   a. **Diagnosis is suggested** by radiographic findings; however, similar findings are found in osteomyelitis, lymphoma, osteogenic sarcoma, and Langerhans cell histiocytosis.
   b. **MRI** of affected bone can better delineate the tumor and its local extension.
   c. **Definitive diagnosis** is by histologic evaluation of tissue obtained by open biopsy.
   d. Bone scan, chest CT scan, chest radiograph, and bone marrow aspiration are generally performed to assess for metastases.

5. **Management.** Treatment includes multiagent chemotherapy followed by surgical excision, when possible. Chemotherapy is important because of the high risk of metastasis. Radiation therapy is used when complete surgical excision is impossible. Late complications of radiation therapy include pathologic fractures at the tumor site, retarded bone growth, limb length discrepancy, functional impairment, and secondary malignancy.

6. **Prognosis.** Outcome is good for local disease, with a 3- to 5-year survival rate of 80%. Prognosis is especially poor if metastases are present.

VIII. Liver Tumors. Liver tumors include **hepatoblastoma** and **hepatocellular carcinoma.**

A. Epidemiology

1. **Hepatoblastoma** is the **most common** type of liver tumor in childhood. It almost always occurs in children younger than 3 years of age. It is also associated with Beckwith-Wiedemann syndrome.

2. **Hepatocellular carcinoma** may occur in both young children and in adolescents. It is associated with **chronic active hepatitis B infection,** biliary atresia, glycogen storage disease type I, α_1-antitrypsin deficiency, and hereditary tyrosinemia.

B. Clinical features. Signs and symptoms both are similar in liver tumors and include presentation with a **right upper abdominal mass,** loss of appetite, and weight loss. Jaundice is generally absent.

C. Diagnosis. Diagnosis is made by abdominal imaging with CT or MRI scan and finding elevation of the serum tumor marker α-fetoprotein.

D. Management. Treatment includes surgical resection, if possible, and chemotherapy. Chemotherapy may convert a previously unresectable tumor to one that is amenable to surgery.

E. Prognosis. Outcome depends on surgical resectability. However, most tumors are unresectable and metastasize to the lungs, brain, and lymph nodes. Although the overall prognosis for both hepatoblastoma and hepatocellular carcinoma is very poor, hepatocellular carcinoma is generally less curable.

IX. Retinoblastoma. See Chapter 18, section VIII.B.

X. Germ Cell Tumors (germinomas) are malignancies derived from the cellular precursors of sperm and eggs.

A. Classification is by location and degree of cell differentiation. Germ cell tumors may be located in the **gonadal** region (i.e., testis, ovary) or in **extragonadal** regions (i.e., anterior mediastinum, sacrococcygeal area, retroperitoneum, neck). Types of germ cell tumors include seminoma (in males), dysgerminoma (in females), teratoma, yolk sac tumor, embryonal cell carcinoma, and choriocarcinoma.

B. Specific Tumors

1. **Teratomas** are tumors containing more than one of the three primary germ cell layers (i.e., ectoderm, mesoderm, and endoderm). Mature teratomas often contain skin, hair, or teeth, whereas immature teratomas contain fetal or embryonal type structures. Teratomas may be benign or

malignant. Malignant potential is based on the amount of immature tissue and the presence or absence of other germ cell tumor cells within the teratoma.

   a. Sacrococcygeal teratoma is the **most common teratoma during the first year of life.** The majority (75%) occur in **females.** The tumor arises from the coccyx and presents as a **soft tissue mass.** Almost all (95%) are **benign.** Treatment includes surgical excision of both the tumor and the coccyx to prevent recurrence.

   b. Anterior mediastinal teratomas are generally **benign** and may present with signs and symptoms of **airway obstruction.**

   c. Ovarian teratomas are the **most common ovarian tumor** and are generally **benign.** The teratoma is suggested by the presence of calcium within the tumor on abdominal radiograph.

  2. Testicular tumors may be derived from germ cells or stromal cells; 70% of childhood testicular tumors are germinomas.

   a. Epidemiology

    (1) The most common of these germinomas are yolk sac tumors (60%), followed by teratomas (15%) and, rarely, seminomas and embryonal carcinoma. (See also Chapter 3, section IX.C.1)

    (2) Peak ages are younger than 5 years and during adolescence.

    (3) There is an association with **cryptorchid testes.**

    (4) One third of testicular tumors in childhood are benign, unlike in adults, in whom almost all testicular tumors are malignant.

   b. Clinical features. Signs and symptoms include a solid, firm, painless testicular mass or generalized testicular swelling. Serum **α-fetoprotein is elevated** in yolk sac tumors. Malignant tumors may extend locally or may metastasize to retroperitoneal lymph nodes, lung, or liver.

   c. Management. Treatment is based on the tumor type and size. Treatment of yolk sac tumors involves radical orchiectomy and, if necessary, retroperitoneal lymph node dissection.

  3. Ovarian tumors most commonly include yolk sac tumors, teratomas, and dysgerminomas.

   a. Epidemiology

    (1) One third are malignant. The younger the child, the more likely it is that the tumor will be malignant.

    (2) Tumors increase in frequency during puberty.

   b. Clinical features. Signs and symptoms include abdominal mass, abdominal pain caused by torsion of the tumor together with the ovary, and vaginal bleeding. Serum **α-fetoprotein is elevated** in yolk sac tumors.

   c. Management. Treatment is based on tumor type and typically includes surgical resection, chemotherapy, and, sometimes, radiation therapy.

XI. Langerhans Cell Histiocytosis (LCH)

  A. Definition

   1. LCH is a diverse group of disorders characterized by the uncontrolled growth of the **Langerhans cell.**

2. **LCH** includes the disorders **eosinophilic granuloma, Hand-Schüller-Christian disease, and Letterer-Siwe disease,** which range from more localized bony changes (eosinophilic granuloma) to more disseminated disease (Letterer-Siwe). LCH was also formerly known as histiocytosis X.

B. **Etiology.** The cause is unknown. LCH is probably not a true malignancy but rather a severe immune dysregulation disease.

C. **Clinical features** are highly variable.

1. **Skeletal involvement** occurs in 80% of patients.
   a. **The skull is most commonly involved.**
   b. **Single or multiple bony lesions** may be present and may be painful, palpable, and associated with swelling.
   c. Pathologic fractures may occur.
   d. **Chronic draining ears** may indicate LCH involving the mastoid.

2. **Skin involvement** occurs in 50% of patients. It typically manifests as **seborrheic dermatitis of the diaper area and scalp** (it mimics cradle cap).

3. **Pituitary** or **hypothalamic involvement** may lead to growth retardation, diabetes insipidus, hypogonadism, and panhypopituitarism.

4. Other features include lymphadenopathy, hepatosplenomegaly, exophthalmos, anemia, and pulmonary infiltrates.

5. **Nonspecific systemic features** include weight loss, fatigue, fever, and failure to thrive.

D. **Diagnosis** is by identifying the typical histologic features on biopsy of skin or bone lesions.

E. **Management**

1. If a single lesion or organ is involved, local curettage or low-dose radiation is used to stop disease progression. Corticosteroids or single-agent chemotherapy (e.g., vinblastine) may be used instead of radiation.

2. If multiple lesions or organs are involved, multiagent chemotherapy is used.

F. **Prognosis** varies with the extent of disease. Single lesions may spontaneously resolve. Response rate to current treatments is high if the diagnosis is made rapidly. Long-term complications include growth impairment, learning problems, hearing loss, orthopedic deformities, and chronic lung disease.

Review Test

1. A 3-year-old Caucasian girl is brought to your office with a 3-week history of bruising, left elbow pain, and fever. Her white blood cell (WBC) count is 25,000 cells/mm^3. You refer her to a pediatric oncologist who performs a bone marrow aspirate, which confirms your suspicion that she has acute lymphocytic leukemia (ALL). Immunophenotyping reveals that the leukemic cells have pre–B-cell phenotype and are common acute lymphocytic leukemia antigen (CALLA) negative. In addition, the leukemic cells demonstrate hyperploidy (> 53 chromosomes). Which of the following characteristics predict an unfavorable prognosis in this patient?

(A) Leukemic cells that are CALLA(−)
(B) WBC count at diagnosis < 50,000 cells/mm^3
(C) Female sex
(D) Leukemic cells that demonstrate hyperploidy
(E) Age of 3 years

2. A 10-year-old girl has started induction chemotherapy for acute lymphocytic leukemia (ALL). Which of the following statements regarding the treatment of childhood ALL and its complications is correct?

(A) Remission is induced in 25% of patients.
(B) Fever associated with neutropenia is an anticipated complication of treatment and may be managed with acetaminophen alone.
(C) Intrathecal methotrexate is used only for children with an unfavorable prognosis at the time of diagnosis.
(D) Intracranial radiation is generally safe and free from side effects in children older than 1 year of age.
(E) Tumor lysis syndrome may include hyperkalemia, hyperphosphatemia, and hyperuricemia.

3. A 4-year-old boy has fever of unknown origin, enlargement of the spleen and liver, and gingival hypertrophy. A complete blood count shows leukemic myeloblasts. Which of the following statements regarding this patient's diagnosis is correct?

(A) Further examination would likely reveal generalized lymphadenopathy and testicular swelling.
(B) A blood smear may demonstrate Auer rods within his leukemic blasts.
(C) Evaluation of the chromosomes would reveal the Philadelphia chromosome.
(D) Bone marrow transplant is usually not necessary for treatment, given the high cure rate with standard chemotherapy.
(E) If this boy had Down syndrome, his leukemia would be very difficult to treat and would likely be fatal.

4. A 15-year-old boy has a 3-month history of fever and weight loss. Physical examination reveals posterior cervical and supraclavicular lymphadenopathy. You refer the patient to a pediatric general surgeon, who performs a lymph node biopsy. The diagnosis is Hodgkin's disease. Which of the following statements regarding this diagnosis is correct?

(A) The cancer would be classified as stage IA.
(B) Airway obstruction is a common complication of this type of cancer.
(C) Associated sterility is rare.
(D) Prognosis is poor.
(E) The biopsy likely shows Reed-Sternberg cells.

5. A 6-year-old girl has a 1-month history of vomiting in the early morning on awakening, occipital headache, and an unsteady gait. Physical examination is normal with the exception of a noticeable wide-based gait with ataxia. Although you were unable to view her optic discs to determine whether papilledema is present, you suspect that she may have a brain tumor. Which of the following statements regarding her probable diagnosis and her evaluation is correct?

(A) She most likely has a high-grade astrocytoma.
(B) She likely has a medulloblastoma in the infratentorial region.
(C) A head CT is the best imaging modality for diagnosis.
(D) Combination chemotherapy and radiation therapy are the principal treatments for suspected brain tumor.
(E) The cerebrospinal fluid tumor markers homovanillic acid and vanillylmandelic acid will be absent on evaluation.

6. A 15-year-old boy has a routine health maintenance examination. A firm, painless right testicular mass is found. Which of the following statements regarding a testicular tumor in this boy is correct?

(A) The tumor is most likely benign.
(B) Teratoma is the most common type of testicular tumor.
(C) Metastasis most commonly occurs to bone.
(D) A history of unilateral cryptorchid testes has put this patient at higher than usual risk for a testicular tumor.
(E) Chemotherapy and radiation therapy are the most appropriate initial treatments.

7. A 7-year-old boy with a history of biliary atresia managed with a Kasai portojejunostomy performed at 5 weeks of age now presents with a 10-pound weight loss during a 4-month period. His parents state that his appetite has been very poor. Physical examination shows a mass in the right upper quadrant of the abdomen. You suspect hepatocellular carcinoma given his prior history of biliary atresia. Which of the following statements regarding this type of cancer in childhood is correct?

(A) The malignancy is also associated with chronic active hepatitis B infection.
(B) Careful examination of the conjunctiva would likely reveal evidence of jaundice.
(C) A liver transplant is recommended because of the poor prognosis associated with this malignancy.
(D) Urine catecholamines are elevated.
(E) Human chorionic gonadotropin is elevated and diagnostic.

The response items for statements 8–11 are the same. You will be required to select one answer for each statement in the set.

(A) Acute myelogenous leukemia
(B) Retinoblastoma
(C) Burkitt's lymphoma
(D) Wilms' tumor
(E) Neuroblastoma
(F) Brain tumor
(G) Acoustic neuroma

For each patient with a genetic syndrome or infection, select the associated malignancy.

8. A 7-year-old African boy with a history of Epstein-Barr virus infection.

9. A 2-year-old girl with Down syndrome.

10. A 6-year-old boy with Beckwith-Wiedemann syndrome.

11. A 10-year-old boy with neurofibromatosis type II.

The response items for statements 12–16 are the same. You will be required to select one answer for each statement in the set.

(A) Osteogenic sarcoma
(B) Ewing's sarcoma
(C) Rhabdomyosarcoma
(D) Langerhans cell histiocytosis
(E) Yolk sac tumor
(F) Teratoma
(G) Non-Hodgkin's lymphoma

For each patient, select the most likely diagnosis.

12. A 4-year-old boy with a painless, growing, soft tissue mass within the orbit, with accompanying proptosis and eyelid swelling.

13. A 14-year-old boy with a painful, growing, soft tissue mass at the distal femur. Radiography reveals periosteal elevation with a "sunburst" appearance.

14. A 5-month-old girl with a soft tissue mass in the lower portion of the back near the coccyx.

15. A 5-year-old boy with a painful, growing mass behind the right ear with chronic right ear discharge.

16. A 16-year-old girl with a painful, growing, soft tissue mass involving the right pelvis. Radiography reveals periosteal elevation with an "onion-skin" appearance.

Answers and Explanations

1. The answer is A [Table 14-2]. Factors at the time of diagnosis that predict a favorable prognosis include female sex, age between 1 and 9 years, Caucasian race, white blood cell (WBC) count < 50,000 cells/mm³, hyperploidy of leukemic cells, absence of chromosomal translocation, and lack of involvement of the central nervous system, liver, spleen, and other organs. However, a common acute lymphocytic leukemia antigen (CALLA) negative immunophenotype is an unfavorable prognostic indicator, whereas CALLA (+) is a favorable prognostic indicator.

2. The answer is E [II.A.6.e]. Many complications may result from therapy for leukemia. Tumor lysis syndrome occurs when cells break apart spontaneously or after chemotherapy and release uric acid, potassium, and phosphate into the circulation. Therefore, hyperuricemia, hyperkalemia, and hyperphosphatemia may be seen. Induction chemotherapy induces remission in approximately 95% of patients. Fever associated with neutropenia is a feared complication that mandates immediate therapy with intravenous antibiotics because of the higher than usual risk of serious bacterial infection in immunosuppressed patients. Intrathecal methotrexate is administered to all patients, regardless of prognosis, during induction as prophylaxis against central nervous system involvement and to all patients during the consolidation phase of chemotherapy. Intracranial radiation is associated with many long-term complications and should generally be avoided, if possible, in children younger than 5 years of age.

3. The answer is B [II.B.5–7]. This patient's clinical presentation and the finding of leukemic myeloblasts are consistent with the diagnosis of acute myelogenous leukemia (AML). Auer rods found within the leukemic blast cells are consistent with the diagnosis of AML. AML is generally more difficult to treat than acute lymphocytic leukemia (ALL), and remission occurs with aggressive chemotherapy in only approximately 50% of patients. Bone marrow transplant is one of the mainstays of therapy in AML. Patients with AML may present with fever, hepatosplenomegaly, bruising, bone pain, and gingival hypertrophy, but testicular involvement and lymphadenopathy are not common clinical features. The Philadelphia chromosome is found in adult-type chronic myelogenous leukemia, rather than in AML. AML associated with Down syndrome is highly treatable.

4. The answer is E [III.A.2–4, Table 14-3]. Patients with Hodgkin's disease most commonly present with painless lymphadenopathy, generally in the cervical or supraclavicular regions. Systemic features, such as weight loss, night sweats, and fever, may also be present. Diagnosis is proven on the basis of the finding of Reed-Sternberg cells on lymph node biopsy. From the involvement of two lymph node regions on the same side of the diaphragm and systemic features in this patient, his cancer would be classified as stage IIB, rather than stage IA (in stage IA, only one lymph node region is involved and there would be no systemic manifestations such as fever and weight loss). Airway obstruction caused by involvement of anterior mediastinal nodes is more common in non-Hodgkin's lymphoma. Male sterility is very common in Hodgkin's disease. Prognosis for stage II disease is excellent.

5. The answer is B [IV.B–D]. The clinical presentation is consistent with a brain tumor. Between 1 and 12 years of age, infratentorial brain tumors are most common. In addition, the ataxia suggests an infratentorial tumor. Medulloblastoma, a primitive neuroectodermal tumor, is the most common infratentorial tumor and would therefore be the most likely tumor in this patient. Astrocytoma is the second most common infratentorial tumor, and brainstem glioma is the third most common infratentorial tumor. Although astrocytomas are possible tumors in the infratentorial region, they tend to be low-grade, rather than high-grade, tumors. Magnetic resonance imaging is the preferred diagnostic imaging study because of the likely cerebellar location of the medulloblastoma. The principal treatment is surgical resection, if it is possible. The tumor markers, homovanillic acid and vanillylmandelic acid, which are secreted by medulloblastomas, are detectable in the cerebrospinal fluid.

6. The answer is D [X.B.2]. Cryptorchid testes (testes that fail to descend into the scrotum) are at much higher than usual risk for malignancy. Two thirds of testicular tumors in childhood are malignant, and one third are benign. Teratomas account for approximately 15% of testicular tumors. In contrast, yolk sac tumors account for 60% of testicular tumors and are the most common testicular tumor. Management of testicular tumors is based on the tumor type, size, and presence of metastases that may involve the retroperitoneal lymph nodes, liver, or lung. Metastasis to bone is more unusual. Treatment of yolk sac tumors involves radical orchiectomy and retroperitoneal lymph node dissection, if necessary.

7. The answer is A [VIII.A.2]. Hepatocellular carcinoma is associated with chronic active hepatitis B infection, biliary atresia, α_1-antitrypsin deficiency, and glycogen storage disease type I. Typical presentation includes a right upper quadrant abdominal mass, weight loss, and anorexia; however, jaundice is generally absent. Although the prognosis is poor for all types of liver tumors, hepatocellular carcinoma has the worst prognosis. Liver transplant is not curative because of the high rate of metastatic disease. Diagnosis is based on findings on abdominal imaging and elevation of the serum marker α-fetoprotein. Urine catecholamines are not present, and human chorionic gonadotropin is not elevated.

8–11. The answers are C, A, D, and G, respectively [Table 14-1, II.B.2, I.B.2.b, I.B.3]. Genetic syndromes and infections may predispose to childhood cancers. Epstein-Barr virus infection may predispose to both Hodgkin's disease and non-Hodgkin's lymphoma, including Burkitt's lymphoma, which is endemic in Africa. Down syndrome may predispose to both acute myelogenous leukemia and acute lymphocytic leukemia. Beckwith-Wiedemann syndrome may predispose to Wilms' tumor, rhabdomyosarcoma, and hepatoblastoma. Neurofibromatosis type II may predispose to acoustic neuroma, while neurofibromatosis type I may predispose to brain tumors and lymphoma.

12–16. The answers are C, A, F, D, and B, respectively [VI.C.1.a, Table 14-4, XI.C.1.d, X.B.1.a]. Rhabdomyosarcoma is the most common soft tissue sarcoma and typically presents as a painless soft tissue mass. The head and neck are involved 40% of the time, and if the orbit is involved, the patient may present with proptosis, eyelid swelling, or cranial nerve palsies. Both osteogenic sarcoma and Ewing's sarcoma present as painful soft tissue masses. Osteogenic sarcoma generally involves the metaphysis of tubular long bones, especially the distal femur and proximal tibia. Ewing's sarcoma more commonly involves flat bones and the diaphysis of tubular bones. The axial skeleton, including the pelvis, is most commonly involved. Radiographic appearances of both osteogenic sarcoma and Ewing's sarcoma reveal periosteal elevation; however, osteogenic sarcoma has a more typical "sunburst" appearance (question 13), whereas Ewing's sarcoma has a more typical "onion skin" appearance (question 16). Langerhans cell histiocytosis often presents as bony lesions. If the mastoid bone is involved, a child may present with a mass behind the ear and chronic ear drainage. Sacrococcygeal teratoma, the most common teratoma in infancy, occurs as a soft tissue mass in the area of the coccyx. The majority (75%) of these teratomas occur in females.

15

Allergy and Immunology

Elizabeth A. Mumper, M.D., and Frank T. Saulsbury, M.D.

I. Anaphylaxis

A. Definition. Anaphylaxis is a potentially life-threatening, acute **systemic IgE-mediated reaction.** Antigen binding to IgE on the surface of mast cells and basophils results in the release of potent mediators that affect vascular tone and bronchial reactivity.

B. Etiology. Anaphylaxis is a rare reaction that occurs most commonly to **drugs, insect venom, foods, latex, and biologic agents.**

C. Clinical Features

    1. Pruritus, flushing, urticaria, and angioedema

    2. Dyspnea and wheezing

    3. Nausea, vomiting, diarrhea, and crampy abdominal pain

    4. Cardiovascular symptoms, ranging from mild hypotension to shock

D. Diagnosis is on the basis of the presence of **clinical signs and symptoms** that appear **within 30 minutes** after exposure to the offending agent.

E. Management

    1. Epinephrine is the principal treatment for acute respiratory and cardiovascular complications.

    2. Systemic antihistamines, corticosteroids, and β-adrenergic agonists are also used to treat the signs and symptoms of anaphylaxis.

II. Allergic Rhinitis

A. Definition. Allergic rhinitis is an **IgE-mediated inflammatory response** in the nasal mucosa to inhaled antigens.

B. Epidemiology. Allergic rhinitis affects 10–20% of children. It is one of the most common allergic conditions of childhood (Figure 15-1).

C. Etiology. Allergic rhinitis may be seasonal or perennial.

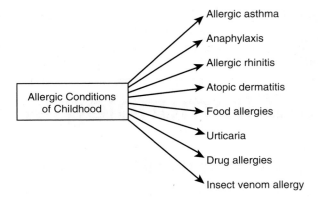

Figure 15-1. Allergic conditions of childhood.

1. **Seasonal rhinitis** occurs in specific seasons in response to **tree, grass, or weed pollens** (e.g., grass pollen in the spring, ragweed pollen in the fall).

2. **Perennial rhinitis** occurs across seasons in response to **indoor allergens,** most commonly dust mites and animal dander. Molds may also be allergens and are associated with high-humidity indoor environments.

D. **Pathophysiology**

   1. **Sensitization** to airborne allergens induces IgE formation.

   2. **Allergen-specific IgE** binds to receptors on **mast cells** and basophils in the nasal mucosa.

   3. **Subsequent exposure** produces an **IgE-mediated inflammatory response,** which occurs within minutes. **Mast cells degranulate** and release histamine, leukotrienes, kinins, and prostaglandins.

E. **Clinical Features**

   1. **Signs and symptoms** include sneezing, nasal congestion, rhinorrhea, nasal itching, and pale nasal mucosa.

      a. **Allergic shiners** are dark circles under the eyes caused by venous congestion.

      b. **Dennie's lines** are creases under the eyes as a result of chronic edema.

      c. **Allergic salute** occurs when the patient uses the palm of the hand to elevate the tip of the nose to relieve itching.

   2. **Allergic rhinitis is commonly associated with** asthma, chronic sinusitis, otitis media with effusion, and nasal polyps.

F. **Diagnosis.** The diagnosis of allergic rhinitis is on the basis of **clinical signs and symptoms.**

   1. **Medical history** may include **multiple episodes of otitis media, sinusitis, atopic dermatitis (eczema), and food or drug allergies.**

   2. **Laboratory evaluation**

      a. **Total IgE concentration** may be elevated.

      b. **Allergen skin testing (prick or intradermal testing)**

(1) Skin tests using purified allergens are the **most effective method** to diagnose allergic rhinitis.

(2) To avoid false-negative results, patients must discontinue antihistamines 4–7 days before skin testing.

c. **Nasal smear for cytology** may be helpful in differentiating allergic rhinitis from other disorders.

(1) More than 10% eosinophils suggests allergic rhinitis.

(2) A preponderance of polymorphic leukocytes suggests an infectious cause.

G. **Management**

1. **Allergen avoidance** is the first step in the management of allergic rhinitis.

a. **Avoidance measures**

(1) The **child's bedroom** should be free of allergens to the extent possible.

(2) Remove pets or keep them outdoors.

(3) Dust mite control measures include the use of plastic mattress covers and the removal of carpets and stuffed animals.

(4) Reduce humidity to inhibit growth of dust mites and mold.

(5) Avoid open windows during pollen season.

b. **IgE antibody** production may decrease with time in the absence of continual antigen exposure.

2. **Pharmacotherapy**

a. **Intranasal steroids** are the **most effective** class of drugs for controlling rhinitis symptoms. Side effects include local irritation, which may be minimized by careful technique of administration. Systemic absorption is minimal. The hypothalamic-pituitary-adrenal axis is not measurably affected at recommended doses.

b. **Antihistamines**

(1) First-generation antihistamines (over-the-counter products [e.g., diphenhydramine]) are often first-line therapy; however, they may cause sedation and impair academic performance.

(2) Second-generation antihistamines (e.g., cetirizine, fexofenadine, loratadine) are **safer and better tolerated than first-generation agents but no more effective.**

(3) Intranasal antihistamines may be effective.

c. **Intranasal cromolyn sodium prevents mast cell degranulation** and can be helpful.

d. **Decongestants** (e.g., pseudoephedrine) cause vasoconstriction and relieve nasal congestion. Because **side effects include insomnia, nervousness, and rebound rhinitis, decongestants** should be used judiciously and only for short periods of time.

e. Leukotriene receptor antagonists are emerging as effective therapy.

3. **Immunotherapy is effective** for allergic rhinitis, allergic asthma, and insect venom allergy.

a. **The principle of immunotherapy is that repeated injections of**

> **allergens with time lead to better tolerance of the allergen by the patient.**
>
> b. **Indications**
>
>   (1) Other therapy is ineffective in controlling symptoms.
>
>   (2) Environmental controls have been tried and failed, or exposure is unavoidable.
>
> 4. **Patient education** should include written instructions to enhance compliance.

III. Atopic Dermatitis

A. **Definition.** Atopic dermatitis is a chronic **inflammatory dermatitis** (also known as **eczema**) characterized by **dry skin** and **lichenification** (i.e., thickening of the skin). The skin is overly sensitive to many stimuli that produce **pruritus,** which leads to scratching, which causes many of the skin manifestations.

B. **Epidemiology**

1. **Atopic dermatitis affects 5–8% of children.**

2. Atopic dermatitis typically begins in early infancy, and 85% of patients have signs and symptoms before 5 years of age.

3. Atopic dermatitis is often worse in winter, or with extremes of temperature.

4. **Family history** commonly reveals family members with atopic dermatitis, asthma, or other allergic diseases.

C. **Clinical Features**

1. **Pruritus is universal.**

2. **Skin manifestations** may be acute or chronic (Table 15-1).

   a. **Acute changes** include **erythema, weeping and crusting,** and secondary bacterial (*Staphylococcus aureus*) or viral (herpes simplex virus) infection.

   b. **Chronic changes** include **lichenification,** dry scaly skin, and **pigmentary changes** (most commonly, hyperpigmentation; less commonly, hypopigmentation).

3. **Clinical presentation varies with age.**

   a. **Infantile form. Truncal and facial areas, along with the scalp,** are involved. **Extensor surfaces** are more involved than flexural surfaces.

Table 15-1. Acute Versus Chronic Manifestations of Atopic Dermatitis

Acute	Chronic
Erythema	Lichenification
Weeping and crusting	Dry, scaly skin
Secondary bacterial or viral infection	Pigmentary changes

    b. Early childhood. Flexural surfaces are more severely involved, and **lichenification,** the **hallmark of chronic itching,** is seen.

    c. Late childhood. Disease may be more localized, or there may be a tendency toward remission.

D. Diagnosis

  1. Three of four major criteria should be present.

    a. Pruritus

    b. Personal or family history of atopy

    c. Typical morphology and distribution

    d. Relapsing or chronic dermatitis

  2. Minor criteria, such as xerosis (i.e., abnormal dryness), pruritus with sweating, wool intolerance, dermatographism (stroking of the skin with a dull instrument that produces a pale wheal with a red flare), or skin infections, are also helpful in making the diagnosis.

E. Management

  1. Known triggers, which may include wool, foods (especially eggs, milk, and peanuts), excessive heat or cold, and harsh chemicals or soaps, should be avoided.

  2. Low- to medium-potency corticosteroids are indicated as needed on affected areas, except on the face. Systemic corticosteroids are used in severe cases.

  3. Antihistamines may be used at bedtime to decrease the itch-scratch cycle.

  4. Baths should be in tepid water. After bathing, the patient should blot the skin dry with absorbent towels, and skin lubricants should be applied.

IV. Food Allergy

A. Definition. Food allergy is an **IgE-mediated** response to food antigens.

B. Etiology

  1. Most allergic reactions to food (85–90%) are caused by **egg, milk, peanut, soy, wheat, and fish.**

  2. Exclusive breastfeeding for 6 months may decrease food allergies (as well as atopic dermatitis) in the infant.

C. Clinical Features

  1. Oral symptoms such as itching and swelling of the lips, tongue, or throat

  2. Gastrointestinal symptoms such as nausea, vomiting, diarrhea, and abdominal pain

  3. Respiratory symptoms such as nasal congestion, rhinorrhea, sneezing, and wheezing

  4. Atopic dermatitis

  5. Acute urticaria and angioedema

  6. Anaphylaxis

D. Diagnosis

1. **History** should elicit the types of symptoms, the timing of symptoms in relation to food ingestion, and the reproducibility and severity of symptoms. Histories are often not specific, and there may be confusion between an allergic reaction and an intolerance to a food.

2. **Laboratory evaluation**
   a. **Skin tests** may be helpful in identifying foods responsible for IgE-mediated hypersensitivity reactions.
   b. **Radioallergosorbent (RAST) tests** identify serum IgE antibodies to specific food antigens.

3. **Provocative oral food challenge** is necessary to determine whether a patient has true food hypersensitivity. **Double-blind placebo-controlled food challenge is the definitive test.**

E. Management

1. **Strict avoidance** of the responsible food allergen is the best therapy.

2. **Injectable epinephrine** should be carried by food-allergic patients who have a history of severe reactions to foods.

V. Insect Venom Allergy

A. **Definition.** Insect venom allergy is an **IgE-mediated** response to the venom of stinging or biting insects.

B. **Etiology.** The venom of many insects, including yellow jackets, hornets, wasps, bees, and fire ants, may cause allergic reactions.

C. **Clinical features** range from localized erythema and swelling to urticaria or anaphylaxis.

D. **Management**

1. **Local skin reactions** can be treated with cold compresses, analgesics, and antihistamines.

2. **Diffuse urticaria** can be treated with antihistamines, but may require treatment with systemic steroids.

3. **Anaphylaxis** can be treated as described in **section I.E.**

4. **Immunotherapy** is effective.

VI. Urticaria (Hives)

A. **Definition.** Urticaria is **circumscribed, raised, evanescent (vanishing) areas of edema that are almost always pruritic.** Hives are usually symmetric and migratory.

B. **Etiology.** The **causes of urticaria** are extensive, and some are listed in Table 15-2.

C. **Classification.** There are two types of urticaria.

Table 15-2. Causes of Urticaria

Acute	Chronic
Drugs	Malignancy
Penicillin	Rheumatologic disease
Aspirin	Systemic lupus erythematosus
Nonsteroidal anti-inflammatory drugs	Rheumatoid arthritis
Foods and food additives	IgG antibodies to IgE receptors
Eggs	Idiopathic
Shellfish	Thyroid disease
Milk	
Nuts	
Contactants	
Animal dander	
Latex	
Idiopathic	
Infection	
Group A β-hemolytic streptococcal pharyngitis	
Infectious mononucleosis	
Mycoplasma pneumoniae	
Hepatitis	
Coxsackievirus	
Insect venoms	
Transfusion reaction	
Heat and cold	
Skin pressure	
Exercise	

1. **Acute urticaria** is often precipitated by exercise, heat, cold, pressure, occupational exposure, medications, insect bites, foods, or recent infections. Health-care workers and patients with **myelomingocele** (who are commonly exposed to latex because of the need for repeated urinary catheterization) are at risk for **latex allergy,** which can present as urticaria.

2. **Chronic urticaria** (urticaria that lasts > 6 months) may be associated with **underlying conditions** such as malignancy and rheumatologic diseases. A substantial proportion of patients with chronic urticaria have an **IgG antibody to the IgE receptor.**

D. **Management.** The **precipitating factor should be avoided,** if it can be identified.

1. **Antihistamines** are the mainstays of therapy.

2. **Further evaluation** for underlying systemic disease is indicated in patients with chronic urticaria, especially if the urticaria is associated with other symptoms such as fever, arthralgias, weight loss, or abdominal pain.

VII. Drug Allergy

A. **Definition.** Reactions to drugs are **mediated by IgE or by direct mast cell degranulation.**

B. **Etiology. Many pharmaceutical agents** have been documented to cause allergic reactions or anaphylaxis. The most common offending agents include **penicillin,** sulfonamides, cephalosporins, **aspirin and other nonsteroidal anti-inflammatory drugs, and narcotics.**

C. **Clinical features include urticaria, angioedema, and anaphylaxis.** (Angioedema is a vascular reaction of the deep dermis or subcutaneous tissue, associated with localized edema from dilated capillaries with increased permeability and characterized by giant wheals.)

D. **Diagnosis** is made by clinical features and history of drug ingestion.

E. **Management**

1. **Antihistamines** may be effective.

2. **Anaphylaxis** should be treated as described in section I.E.

3. **Medic alert bracelets** should be worn by patients with previously identified significant drug reactions.

VIII. Asthma. Asthma (see Chapter 9, section IV.A) may have an allergic cause in some patients.

IX. Immunology Overview

A. **Main components of the immune system.** The immune system is a complex organization of cells and molecules that serves to protect the host from infection. The components of the immune system can be divided functionally into innate and adaptive components.

1. **Innate responses** are the first defense against infection. The cells and molecules of the innate system include **phagocytic cells, natural killer cells, toll-like receptors, mannose-binding protein, and the alternative pathway of complement.**

2. **Adaptive responses** develop more slowly, are highly specific, and improve with repeated exposure to an antigen. The adaptive system includes **T cells, B cells, and immunoglobulin molecules.**

B. **Immunodeficiency states may be primary or secondary** (Table 15-3).

C. In the evaluation of a patient with a suspected immunodeficiency, there is

Table 15-3. Categories of Immunodeficiency States

Primary	B-cell defects (disorders of humoral immunity)
	T-cell defects (disorders of cell-mediated immunity)
	Disorders of granulocytes
	Complement deficiencies
Secondary	Acquired immunodeficiency syndrome (AIDS)
	Medications (steroids, chemotherapy)
	Malnutrition
	Nephrotic syndrome

Table 15-4. Laboratory Evaluation of Primary Immunodeficiency States

Evaluation	Diagnostic Tests
Humoral immunity	Quantitative immunoglobulins B-cell enumeration Antibody titers to immunization (diphtheria, tetanus) Isohemagglutinin titers
Cell-mediated immunity	Peripheral smear (to look for lymphopenia) Anergy panel (delayed type hypersensitivity skin testing) T-cell subsets (CD3, CD4, CD8) In vitro T-cell proliferative responses to mitogens and antigens
Phagocyte function	Peripheral smear (to look for neutropenia) Nitroblue tetrazolium test Measurements of neutrophil chemotaxis
Complement	Total hemolytic complement (CH_{50}) Assays of specific components of complement

a variety of diagnostic tests used to identify the type of primary immuno-deficiency state (Table 15-4).

X. Disorders of Lymphocytes (Figure 15-2).
Abnormalities of B cells and T cells may lead to **deficiencies of antibody production, T-cell function, or both.** Whereas pure B-cell defects are uncommon, **hypogammaglobulinemia** is a feature of most disorders involving lymphocyte function. Thus, 75% of all primary immunodeficiency diseases involve abnormalities of antibody concentration or function.

A. IgA Deficiency

1. **Definition.** Selective IgA deficiency is characterized by **serum IgA concentrations < 7 mg/dL** but usually normal levels of other immunoglobulin isotypes. However, IgA deficiency may be associated with other defects in many patients. Fifty percent of patients with IgA deficiency have IgE deficiency and 20–30% have IgG_2 and IgG_4 subclass deficiencies.

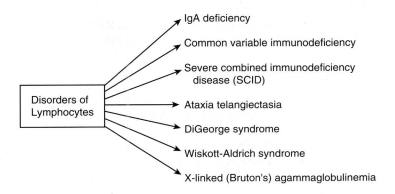

Figure 15-2. Disorders of lymphocytes.

2. **Epidemiology. IgA deficiency is the most common immune deficiency,** with a prevalence of 1 in 500–1,000.

3. **Etiology.** A genetic basis for IgA deficiency is sometimes present, but for most patients, the precise cause usually is unclear.

4. **Clinical features**
   a. **Respiratory infections,** such as sinusitis, pneumonia, otitis media, and bronchitis
   b. **Gastrointestinal manifestations,** such as chronic diarrhea and infection with *Giardia lamblia*
   c. **Autoimmune and rheumatic diseases,** such as systemic lupus erythematosus, juvenile rheumatoid arthritis, and celiac disease may be associated with IgA deficiency.
   d. **Atopic diseases,** such as allergic rhinitis, eczema, urticaria, and asthma, may occur in up to 50% of patients with IgA deficiency.

5. **Diagnosis. Quantitative measurement of serum immunoglobulins,** which reveals the deficiency of IgA (< 7 mg/dL), is the basis of diagnosis.

6. **Management.** IgA cannot be replaced, thus **management of infections and other complications** are the mainstays of therapy. Intravenous immunoglobulin (IVIG) is not indicated (it contains almost all IgG).

B. **Common Variable Immunodeficiency**

1. **Definition.** This heterogeneous group of disorders is characterized by **hypogammaglobulinemia.** Most patients have normal numbers of B and T cells but have variable degrees of T-cell dysfunction.

2. **Epidemiology.** Most cases are sporadic, with prevalence between 1 in 10,000 and 1 in 100,000.

3. **Etiology.** A variety of defects in B-cell function or in B cell–T cell interaction can produce the clinical picture of common variable immunodeficiency. The genetic basis of this disorder is largely unknown, but a number of genetic defects have recently been elucidated.

4. **Clinical features**
   a. **Respiratory infections** (frequently caused by *Haemophilus influenzae, Moraxella catarrhalis,* and *Streptococcus pneumoniae*) and **gastrointestinal infections** accompanied by chronic diarrhea (often caused by *G. lamblia* and *Campylobacter jejuni*)
   b. **Autoimmune disorders,** such as rheumatoid arthritis, autoimmune thyroiditis, autoimmune thrombocytopenia, and autoimmune hemolytic anemia
   c. **Increased risk of malignancy**

5. **Diagnosis**
   a. **Quantitative immunoglobulin measurement** shows decreased serum immunoglobulin concentrations.
   b. **Diminished antibody function** may be assessed by measuring titers generated in response to childhood immunizations (i.e., diphtheria and tetanus).
   c. T-cell proliferation to mitogens (nonspecific stimulators of lymphocyte production) may be diminished.

6. Management

   a. Monthly **IVIG** replacement.

   b. Aggressive management of infections with antibiotics.

   c. Chronic diarrhea management including nutritional support.

C. Severe Combined Immunodeficiency Disease (SCID)

1. Definition. SCID is a group of inherited disorders characterized by profoundly **defective T-cell and B-cell function.**

2. Etiology. More than 12 distinct genetic abnormalities that produce SCID have been identified.

   a. X-linked SCID, caused by deficiency of the common gamma chain of the receptor for cytokines interleukin (IL)-2, IL-4, IL-7, IL-9, and IL-15, accounts for about 50% of all cases of SCID.

   b. Autosomal recessive SCID is caused by a variety of genetic defects involving T-cell ontogeny or function. Adenosine deaminase deficiency accounts for approximately 30% of cases of autosomal recessive SCID.

3. Clinical features

   a. Increased susceptibility to **infection within the first few months of life** with common pathogens and with opportunistic organisms such as *Candida albicans* and *Pneumocystis carinii*

   b. Chronic diarrhea and **failure to thrive** are common.

4. Diagnosis

   a. Persistent lymphopenia (< 1,500 lymphocytes/mL) is a nearly constant feature in patients with SCID.

   b. Enumeration of lymphocyte populations by flow cytometry shows decreased numbers of T cells.

   c. Quantitative measurement of serum immunoglobulins shows severe hypogammaglobulinemia.

   d. T-cell responses to mitogens and antigens are severely depressed.

5. Management

   a. Supportive care with appropriate antibiotics, nutritional interventions, and psychosocial support is necessary.

   b. Blood products should be irradiated to prevent graft-versus-host disease.

   c. Monthly IVIG replacement is administered to maintain a normal serum IgG level.

   d. *P. carinii* **pneumonia (PCP) prophylaxis** with trimethoprim-sulfamethoxazole is indicated.

   e. Bone marrow transplant can be curative. Complications include graft-versus-host disease, infection, and medication toxicity. Other options include cord blood stem cell or peripheral blood stem cell transplant.

   f. Gene therapy is a potential future cure.

D. Ataxia Telangiectasia

1. Definition. Ataxia telangiectasia is an **autosomal recessive** disorder

characterized by **combined immunodeficiency, cerebellar ataxia, oculocutaneous telangiectasias, and predisposition to malignancy.**

2. **Etiology.** Ataxia telangiectasia results from a mutation of a gene on the long arm of **chromosome 11.** The gene product is involved in cell cycle control, DNA recombination, and cellular responses to DNA damage.

3. **Clinical features**

   a. **Variable immunodeficiency** that most commonly manifests as chronic sinopulmonary infections

   b. **Severe progressive cerebellar ataxia** that results in a need for wheelchair assistance by early adolescence in most patients

   c. **Telangiectasias** that appear on the bulbar conjunctiva between 2 and 5 years of age, and later on exposed skin and areas of trauma

   d. **High risk of malignancy,** particularly lymphoma and carcinoma, owing to defects in DNA repair

   e. **Other clinical features** such as café-au-lait spots, vitiligo, prematurely gray hair, and multiple endocrine abnormalities

4. **Diagnosis**

   a. **Quantitative measurement of serum immunoglobulins** reveals IgE deficiency in 85% of patients and IgA deficiency in 75% of patients.

   b. **Evaluation of T-cell function** may reveal skin test anergy and diminished T-cell proliferation to mitogens.

5. **Management**

   a. **Treat the neurologic complications.**

   b. **Aggressively treat infections.**

   c. **Monitor for malignancies.**

   d. **Avoid ionizing radiation,** which exacerbates DNA breakage and repair, thus increasing the risk of malignancy.

E. **DiGeorge syndrome** is a congenital immunodeficiency syndrome characterized by **c**ardiac defects, **a**bnormal facies, **t**hymic hypoplasia, **c**left palate, and **h**ypocalcemia because of a **submicroscopic deletion** on **chromosome arm 22q11 (mnemonic: CATCH-22).** See Chapter 5, section III.A.5.

F. **Wiskott-Aldrich syndrome**

1. **Definition.** Wiskott-Aldrich syndrome is an **X-linked** disorder characterized by **combined immunodeficiency, eczema, and congenital thrombocytopenia** with small platelets.

2. **Etiology.** Wiskott-Aldrich syndrome is caused by the mutation of a gene on the **short arm of the X chromosome.** The gene product is important in T-cell receptor signaling and cytoskeletal organization.

3. **Clinical features**

   a. **Susceptibility to infections with encapsulated organisms such as *H. influenzae* and *S. pneumoniae,*** because patients do not produce antibodies to polysaccharide antigens

   b. **Thrombocytopenia characterized by small defective platelets.** Bleeding episodes are frequent and are associated with a risk of intracranial hemorrhage.

    c. Eczema, which predisposes to skin infections

  4. Diagnosis

    a. Complete blood count reveals **thrombocytopenia and small platelets.**

    b. Decreased IgM is demonstrated by measurement of immunoglobulins.

    c. Antibody response to polysaccharide antigens (i.e., polysaccharide vaccines) **is defective.**

    d. Cellular immune function is defective and **anergy** is present. Patients have near-normal numbers of T cells, but they respond poorly to antigens and **do not develop antigen-specific cytotoxic T cells.**

  5. Management

    a. Human leukocyte antigen (HLA)–matched bone marrow transplantation is the therapy of choice.

    b. IVIG is administered for hypogammaglobulinemia.

    c. Splenectomy cures the thrombocytopenia in more than 90% of patients. Quality of life is improved, and medical management is simplified. **Prophylactic antibiotics or IVIG must be administered regularly after splenectomy.**

G. X-Linked (Bruton's) Agammaglobulinemia

  1. Definition. X-linked agammaglobulinemia is characterized by **severe hypogammaglobulinemia and a paucity of mature B cells (< 1% B cells in peripheral blood) with normal T-cell number and function.**

  2. Etiology. X-linked agammaglobulinemia is due to mutations in the **Bruton's tyrosine kinase (*BTK*) gene** on the X chromosome. The *BTK* gene is critical to normal B-cell ontogeny. Mutations lead to a block in the development from pre–B cell to mature B cell.

  3. Clinical features. Increased susceptibility to **infections with encapsulated bacteria** (*S. pneumoniae, H. influenzae*), *S. aureus,* and chronic enteroviral infection may occur.

  4. Diagnosis

    a. Quantitative immunoglobulin measurement reveals profound decreases in all immunoglobulin isotypes.

    b. B cells are absent or greatly diminished.

    c. T cells are present, and cell-mediated functions are preserved.

    d. Mutations in the *BTK* gene are demonstrated by mutation analysis.

  5. Management. Treatment includes **monthly IVIG replacement** to prevent infection.

XI. Disorders of Granulocytes (Figure 15-3)

A. Chronic Granulomatous Disease (CGD)

  1. Definition. CGD is a group of disorders characterized by **defective neutrophil oxidative metabolism** as a result of defects in the multicomponent reduced nicotinamide-adenine dinucleotide phosphate

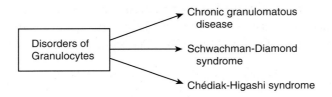

Figure 15-3. Disorders of granulocytes.

(NADPH) oxidase system. Defective oxidative metabolism results in **severely impaired intracellular killing of catalase-positive bacteria and some fungal pathogens.**

2. **Etiology. The inheritance of CGD** is predominantly X-linked (70%).

3. **Clinical features**

   a. **Increased susceptibility to infections** involving the lungs, lymph nodes, liver, spleen, bones, and skin. **Abscess formation** is characteristic.

   b. **Major pathogens** include *S. aureus, Pseudomonas aeruginosa, Salmonella* species, *Klebsiella pneumoniae, Serratia marcescens, Escherichia coli, C. albicans,* and *Aspergillus* species.

4. **Diagnosis.** Tests demonstrate defective neutrophil oxidative burst. The **nitroblue tetrazolium (NBT)** test is the classic test and is still widely used. The NBT test is being replaced by the **flow cytometric assay.**

5. **Management**

   a. **Abscesses** often require surgical drainage and antibiotics.

   b. **Prophylactic trimethoprim-sulfamethoxazole** reduces the incidence of serious infections.

   c. **Prophylactic itraconazole** reduces the incidence of *Aspergillus* infections.

   d. **Interferon-γ** is given prophylactically.

   e. **Bone marrow transplantation** is curative.

   f. **Gene therapy** is a potential future cure.

B. **Disorders of adherence and motility**

   1. **Schwachman-Diamond syndrome.** This syndrome is an autosomal recessive condition characterized by **decreased neutrophil chemotaxis, cyclic neutropenia, and pancreatic exocrine insufficiency.** Patients present with **recurrent soft tissue infection, chronic diarrhea, and failure to thrive.** (See also Chapter 13, section V.B.6.)

   2. **Chédiak-Higashi syndrome.** This syndrome is characterized by variable **neutropenia and thrombocytopenia** and giant lysosomal granules in neutrophils. Neutrophils and monocytes have functional defects, and natural killer cell function is impaired. *S. aureus* causes the majority of infections. Patients also have **partial oculocutaneous albinism** (see also Chapter 13, section V.B.5.a).

C. **Neutropenia** is discussed in Chapter 13, section V.

XII. Disorders of the Complement System. The complement system is composed of **plasma proteins and cellular receptors** functioning in an integrated series of reactions to prevent infection.

    A. Definition. These disorders involve absence or dysfunction of individual complement components or regulatory proteins.

    B. Etiology. Complement deficiencies are genetically determined. **Most are autosomal recessive.**

    C. Clinical features are **variable** and depend on the biologic function of the components that are deficient.

        1. Deficiencies of the early components of the classic pathway (C1q, C2, and C4) are associated with autoimmune diseases, such as systemic lupus erythematosus.

        2. Deficiencies of the late components of the classic pathway (C5, C6, and C8) are associated with increased susceptibility to disseminated **meningococcal and gonococcal infections.**

        3. Deficiency or dysfunction of C1 esterase inhibitor causes hereditary angioedema. Patients may experience episodic swelling of various body parts, especially the hands and feet. The bowel wall may also swell, leading to severe abdominal pain. Angioedema affecting the airway can be fatal.

    D. Diagnosis

        1. Quantitative. Specific assays measure levels of specific components.

        2. Qualitative. A normal **total serum hemolytic complement (CH_{50})** indicates that all components of the classic complement pathway are present and functional.

    E. Management

        1. Prompt diagnosis and treatment of bacterial infections.

        2. Management of autoimmune disease.

        3. Therapy with fibrinolysis inhibitors and attenuated androgens (such as danazol) for hereditary angioedema.

Review Text

1. An 8-year-old boy presents to the emergency department in acute severe respiratory distress after being stung by a bee. Vital signs are notable for a respiratory rate of 60 breaths/min, heart rate of 120 beats/min, and a blood pressure of 70/50 mm Hg. Physical examination shows severe respiratory distress, wheezing, and a diffuse urticarial eruption on the trunk and extremities. Which of the following is the best initial treatment for this patient?

(A) Antihistamines
(B) Systemic corticosteroids
(C) Epinephrine
(D) β-Adrenergic agonists
(E) Inhaled corticosteroids

2. A 10-year-old girl presents with a history of chronic rhinorrhea, nasal itchiness, and sneezing. Physical examination reveals dark circles under her eyes and pale boggy nasal mucosa. Which of the following categories of medications is the most effective for controlling this patient's signs and symptoms?

(A) First-generation antihistamines
(B) Second-generation antihistamines
(C) Intranasal steroids
(D) Intranasal cromolyn sodium
(E) Decongestants

3. During a routine health maintenance visit, the mother of a 1-year-old girl is particularly concerned about the family's history of food allergies. Which of the following foods are the most likely to cause food allergic reactions?

(A) Soy
(B) Citrus fruits
(C) Chocolate
(D) Tomatoes
(E) Cruciferous vegetables

4. The parents of a 5-year-old boy are concerned that their son may have food allergies. On two separate occasions, he exhibited a transient erythematous papular itchy rash and a stuffy nose within several hours after eating fish. Which of the following is the most definitive method for diagnosis of food allergy?

(A) Skin tests using extracts from the suspected offending food
(B) Radioallergosorbent testing (RAST) to identify IgE-specific food antibodies
(C) Double-blind, placebo-controlled provocative oral food challenges
(D) Total serum IgE measurements
(E) Parental reports of the suspected food allergy

5. A 12-year-old girl presents with a 9-month history of chronic diarrhea and an increased susceptibility to infections. During this period, she has had two episodes of pneumonia and multiple prolonged episodes of diarrhea. Physical examination is normal. You suspect an immunodeficiency disorder. Laboratory evaluation reveals normal numbers of B cells and platelets, decreased serum concentrations of IgG, IgA, and IgM, low antibody titers in response to immunizations, and poor T-cell function. The total serum hemolytic complement (CH_{50}) is normal. Which of the following is the most likely diagnosis?

(A) Severe combined immunodeficiency disease
(B) Common variable immunodeficiency disease
(C) Chronic granulomatous disease
(D) Complement deficiency
(E) Wiskott-Aldrich syndrome

6. A 4-year-old boy presents with a one-day history of fever to 103°F (39.4°C), a stiff neck, and altered mental status. Gram stain of the cerebrospinal fluid shows Gram-negative bacteria. His parents are concerned because he was also hospitalized with meningococcal sepsis at 2 months of age. Which of the following immunodeficiency disorders is the most likely diagnosis?

(A) Chédiak-Higashi syndrome
(B) Chronic granulomatous disease
(C) Selective IgA deficiency
(D) Ataxia telangiectasia
(E) Complement deficiency

7. A 1-year-old boy has a history of multiple episodes of otitis media, sinusitis, and pneumonia. He has not had any fungal, protozoan, or mycobacterial infections. You suspect a disorder of humoral immunity. Which of the following is the best initial screening test?

(A) Nitroblue tetrazolium test (NBT)
(B) Quantitative serum immunoglobulins
(C) Examination of the peripheral blood smear
(D) Total hemolytic complement (CH_{50})
(E) Anergy panel

8. A 10-year-old boy presents with rhinorrhea, sneezing, and an early morning cough, which is present throughout the year. He sleeps with a collection of stuffed monkeys, and his bedroom is carpeted. There are no pets in the household. Physical examination reveals Dennie's lines and an allergic salute. Nasal smear shows 90% eosinophils. Which of the following is the most likely cause of his allergies?

(A) Dust mites
(B) Tree pollens
(C) Weed pollens
(D) Molds
(E) Grasses

9. A 1-year-old girl has erythema and dry patches on her trunk, face, scalp, and extensor surfaces. She scratches frequently and seems sensitive to wool. Her parents also note that at times her cheeks get red, cracked, and weepy. Which of the following is the most likely diagnosis?

(A) Early childhood eczema
(B) Infantile eczema
(C) Idiopathic urticaria
(D) Drug allergy

The response options for statements 10–13 are the same. You will be required to select one answer for each statement in the set.

(A) Ataxia telangiectasia
(B) Deficiencies of the early components of the complement cascade
(C) Deficiencies of the late components of the complement cascade
(D) Adenosine deaminase deficiency
(E) Schwachman-Diamond syndrome
(F) DiGeorge syndrome
(G) Chronic granulomatous disease
(H) Wiskott-Aldrich syndrome

For each patient, select the most likely diagnosis.

10. A 1-year-old boy with a history of recurrent pneumonia, chronic diarrhea, and failure to thrive has a white blood cell count of 1,200 cells/mm^3.

11. A 2-year-old boy with a history of recurrent cervical adenitis and pneumonia presents with a perianal abscess.

12. An 18-month-old girl has a history of recurrent pneumococcal pneumonia, severe eczema, and a petechial rash on her trunk and face.

13. A 3-month-old boy with a history of chronic diarrhea and failure to thrive presents with *Pneumocystis carinii* pneumonia.

Answers and Explanations

1. The answer is C [I.E]. This patient's clinical presentation is consistent with anaphylaxis, a rare life-threatening, acute IgE-mediated reaction that occurs within 30 minutes after exposure to an offending agent. The most common causative agents are drugs, insect venoms, foods, latex, and biologic agents. Immediate administration of epinephrine is the principal initial treatment indicated for the hypotension, wheezing, and respiratory distress. Antihistamines, systemic corticosteroids, and β-adrenergic agonists are additional treatments for anaphylaxis. Inhaled corticosteroids are not helpful.

2. The answer is C [II.G.2]. The diagnosis of allergic rhinitis is made on the basis of the clinical signs and symptoms, which often include sneezing, nasal congestion, rhinorrhea, nasal itchiness, pale nasal mucosa, and allergic shiners (dark circles under the eyes caused by venous congestion). Intranasal steroids are the most effective therapy for allergic rhinitis. First-generation antihistamines (sedating) and second-generation antihistamines (nonsedating) are frequently also very effective. Intranasal cromolyn sodium is an alternative therapeutic option. Decongestants may cause insomnia, agitation, and rebound rhinitis; therefore, they should only be used for short periods.

3. The answer is A [IV.B.1]. Egg, milk, peanut, soy, wheat, and fish cause 85–90% of food allergies in children. Although allergies to citrus fruits, chocolate, and tomatoes may occur, these foods do not commonly induce allergy. Cruciferous vegetables are unlikely to cause food allergy reactions.

4. The answer is C [IV.D]. Provocative food challenges, which should be double-blinded and placebo-controlled, are the most definitive tests to confirm the cause of food allergy reactions. Skin tests and radioallergosorbent tests (RAST) can be helpful in evaluating food allergy but are not definitive. Total serum IgE is not specific and is therefore not helpful. Parental reports of suspected food allergy are helpful but are neither specific nor definitive. Parents may confuse food allergy with food intolerance.

5. The answer is B [X.B.1, X.B.4, X.B.5]. This patient's clinical presentation and laboratory findings are most consistent with common variable immunodeficiency disease. Patients with common variable immunodeficiency disease have increased susceptibility to respiratory and diarrheal infections. Laboratory evaluation shows variable degrees of hypogammaglobulinemia and T-cell dysfunction. Most have normal B-cell and T-cell numbers. Patients with severe combined immunodeficiency disease tend to present early in infancy with repeated infections, chronic diarrhea, and failure to thrive. Chronic granulomatous disease is a disorder of neutrophils and involves defective oxidative metabolism. It classically presents with abscesses and multiple infections. Complement deficiency is ruled out by the normal total hemolytic complement (CH_{50}). Wiskott-Aldrich syndrome is characterized by thrombocytopenia and is therefore ruled out by the normal platelet count.

6. The answer is E [XII.C.2]. This patient's clinical presentation suggests complement deficiency, particularly a deficiency of one of the late components of the classic complement pathway (C5, C6, C8). Patients with deficiencies of late complement components often present with meningococcal sepsis or meningitis. Chédiak-Higashi syndrome is characterized by neutropenia, thrombocytopenia, and partial oculocutaneous albinism. The majority of infections are associated with *Staphylococcus aureus*. Patients with chronic granulomatous disease tend to present with infections of the skin, bone, lymph nodes, and liver as a result of *S. aureus, Aspergillus,* and Gram-negative enteric organisms. Selective IgA deficiency presents with respiratory and gastrointestinal illnesses. Patients with ataxia telangiectasia present with cerebellar ataxia, telangiectasias on the bulbar conjunctiva and later on the skin, and chronic sinopulmonary infections.

7. The answer is B [Table 15-4, X.A.5]. Most primary immunodeficiency diseases involve abnormalities of immunoglobulin concentration or function (humoral immunity). The hallmark of immunoglobulin deficiency is increased susceptibility to sinopulmonary infections caused by encapsulated bacteria. Serum immunoglobulin concentrations should be measured in such patients. The NBT test is used to diagnose chronic granulomatous disease, a disorder of phagocyte oxidative metabolism. Examination of the peripheral smear can yield valuable information about neutropenia, lymphopenia, or thrombocytopenia. This information is useful adjunctive information, but it does not provide a definitive diagnosis. Total hemolytic complement assays are useful to exclude isolated deficiencies of complement components. Sinopulmonary infections are generally not associated with complement deficiency. Anergy panels are used to evaluate cell-mediated immune function.

8. The answer is A [II.C.2, II.G.1]. Allergic rhinitis symptoms that are present throughout the year (perennial rhinitis) suggest indoor allergens; the most common are dust mites and animal dander. This patient would benefit from allergy control measures in his bedroom, such as removing the stuffed animals and carpet. Tree pollen, weed pollen, and grasses are associated with seasonal allergies. Molds are associated with high-humidity indoor environments.

9. The answer is B [III.C.3]. Involvement of extensor surfaces and cheeks is characteristic of the infantile presentation of eczema. Common triggers include wool, foods, harsh chemicals, and extremes of temperature. Early childhood eczema typically involves the flexural surfaces, especially the elbows and knees. Urticaria is well-circumscribed, raised transient itchy areas of edema. Drug allergy is usually related to pharmaceutical agents such as penicillins and nonsteroidal anti-inflammatory drugs. Urticaria, angioedema, and anaphylaxis are the major clinical manifestations.

10–13. The answers are E, G, H, and D, respectively [XI.B.1, XI.A, X.F, X.C.2.b]. Schwachman-Diamond syndrome is an autosomal recessive condition characterized by decreased neutrophil activity and by cyclic neutropenia. Patients with Schwachman-Diamond syndrome have recurrent soft tissue infections as a result of the neutropenia, and also have pancreatic exocrine insufficiency with failure to thrive. Chronic granulomatous disease (CGD) refers to a group of disorders characterized by defective neutrophil oxidative metabolism resulting in severely impaired intracellular killing of catalase-positive bacteria and some fungal pathogens. CGD is predominantly X-linked. Patients with CGD have an increased susceptibility to infections of the lungs, liver, skin, lymph nodes, and skin, characteristically with abscess formation. Wiskott-Aldrich syndrome is an X-linked disorder characterized by combined immunodeficiency, eczema, and congenital thrombocytopenia (with small platelets). Patients typically present with recurrent infections with encapsulated organisms, thrombocytopenia, and eczema. Adenosine deaminase deficiency is a subtype of severe combined immunodeficiency disease (SCID) that is inherited in an autosomal recessive manner. SCID refers to a group of inherited disorders characterized by profoundly defective B-cell and T-cell function. Patients with adenosine deaminase deficiency usually present within the first few months of life with persistent lymphopenia, chronic diarrhea, failure to thrive, and infections with both common pathogens and opportunistic organisms (e.g., *Candida albicans, Pneumocystis carinii*).

16

Rheumatology

Jerome K. Wang, M.D., Lee Todd Miller, M.D.,
and Frank T. Saulsbury, M.D.

I. Henoch-Schönlein Purpura

A. Definition. A systemic **IgA-mediated vasculitis** involving the skin, joints, gastrointestinal (GI) tract, and kidneys.

B. Epidemiology

1. Henoch-Schönlein purpura is a disease of young children; 75% of cases occur in children younger than 10 years of age. The **median age of onset is 5 years.**

2. **Males** are more likely to be affected (male-to-female ratio is 2:1).

C. Clinical Features

1. **A viral syndrome or upper respiratory infection precedes** Henoch-Schönlein purpura in most patients. Twenty percent of patients have concomitant or prior group A β-hemolytic streptococcal infection.

2. Distinctive **skin, GI,** and **joint manifestations** follow the prodrome.

   a. Skin manifestations

   (1) Classically, urticarial or erythematous maculopapular lesions progress to **petechiae and palpable purpuric lesions concentrated on the buttocks and lower extremities.**

   (2) Children may also present with **edema** of hands, feet, scrotum, and scalp. (Infants may also present with a facial rash in addition to edema.)

   (3) GI and joint symptoms may precede the diagnostic rash by days or weeks in 30% of patients.

   b. Joint manifestations occur in **80%** of patients and manifest as arthralgia or arthritis. The knees and ankles are most commonly involved.

   c. GI manifestations occur in 67% of patients.

   (1) **Colicky abdominal pain** that may be severe

   (2) **GI bleeding** (either occult blood or grossly bloody stool)

   (3) Increased risk of **intussusception**

3. **Renal manifestations** (see Chapter 11, section IV.F.3)

    a. Presentations range widely, from mild hematuria and trace proteinuria to gross hematuria, nephrotic syndrome, chronic renal insufficiency, and end-stage renal disease (1% of cases).

    b. Renal manifestations may not become clinically apparent for up to 3 months after initial presentation in 25% of patients who develop nephritis.

D. Diagnosis

1. **History and characteristic physical examination** establish a clinical diagnosis.

2. Routine laboratory tests are neither specific nor diagnostic.

3. **Increased serum IgA** levels are present in 50% of patients.

4. Circulating IgA immune complexes in serum and IgA deposition in skin and glomeruli are suggestive of the diagnosis.

5. **Platelet counts are normal** despite the presence of petechiae and purpura (i.e., **the skin rash is a nonthrombocytopenic purpura**).

E. Management. Treatment is based on **relief of symptoms**, including pain control and hydration. **Steroids** may be effective for relief of abdominal pain and arthritis.

F. Prognosis

1. Most patients recover within 4 weeks.

2. Henoch-Schönlein purpura recurs at least once in 50% of patients.

3. Long-term morbidity is dependent on the severity of nephritis.

II. Kawasaki Disease (Mucocutaneous Lymph Node Syndrome)

A. Definition. An **acute febrile vasculitis of childhood,** of unknown origin, involving multiple organ systems, including the heart, skin, mucous membranes, GI tract, central nervous system (CNS), joints, and peripheral vascular bed.

B. Epidemiology

1. Kawasaki disease is the **most common cause of acquired heart disease** in children in the United States.

2. **Males** are slightly more commonly affected than females (male-to-female ratio is 3:2).

3. Most common in **children of Asian ethnicity**

4. The **mean age** at presentation is **18–24 months** (80% of cases occur in children younger than 5 years of age).

C. Diagnostic Criteria (Table 16-1)

1. **Fever > 102°F (38.9°C) lasting ≥ 5 days**

2. The patient must also have four of the following five clinical manifestations:

    a. **Bilateral conjunctivitis:** bulbar injection with limbic sparing and **without exudate**

Table 16-1. Diagnostic Criteria of Kawasaki Disease

I.   Fever for at least 5 days
             AND
II. Four of the following features:
     Conjunctivitis
     Oropharyngeal changes
     Cervical adenopathy
     Rash
     Changes in distal extremities
             AND
III. The illness may not be explainable by any other disease process (i.e., exclusion of known infectious etiologic factors, drug reactions, and other rheumatologic conditions, such as juvenile rheumatoid arthritis)

---

      b. Oropharyngeal changes: pharyngitis, strawberry tongue, or, most commonly, **red, cracked, swollen lips**

      c. Cervical adenopathy: a unilateral nonsuppurative cervical lymph node ≥ 1.5 cm in diameter

      d. Rash: primarily on the trunk. The rash may assume many forms (polymorphous), including erythematous maculopapular, morbilliform, or scarlatiniform.

      e. Changes in distal extremities

          (1) Early (first 7–10 days of illness): brawny edema and induration of the hands and feet with erythematous palms and soles

          (2) Later (7–10 days after the start of fever): peeling around the nail beds or of the distal extremities

   3. It is important that **the illness must not be explainable by any other disease process.** Known infectious causes (including bacterial, viral, and rickettsial infections), rheumatologic conditions (including juvenile rheumatoid arthritis), and drug reactions must be excluded to make the diagnosis of Kawasaki disease.

D. Other Clinical Features (*not* diagnostic criteria)

   1. Cardiovascular manifestations

      a. Coronary artery aneurysms occur in **20%** of untreated patients, usually around days 7–14 (most commonly in the subacute phase of the disease).

      b. Low-grade myocarditis is common.

      c. Congestive heart failure

      d. Arrhythmias

      e. Aneurysms of the brachial arteries

   2. Urethritis (sterile pyuria)

   3. Aseptic meningitis

   4. Hydrops of the gallbladder, which may occur in 10% of patients and should be considered in patients with acute right upper quadrant abdominal pain

   5. Arthritis (sterile) or arthralgias

   6. Anterior uveitis

E. **Time Course of Disease.** The clinical course is **triphasic** (see **Table 16-2**).

1. Phase I: **acute phase** (1–2 weeks)

2. Phase II: **subacute phase** (weeks to months)

3. Phase III: **convalescent phase** (weeks to years)

F. **Laboratory Findings. No laboratory tests** are **pathognomonic** for Kawasaki disease. Laboratory findings are not specific but include the following (see Table 16-2):

1. Acute phase: ↑ erythrocyte sedimentation rate (ESR), ↑ C-reactive protein (CRP)

2. Subacute phase: ↑ platelet count and a decreasing ESR and CRP

3. Convalescent phase: Laboratory findings usually normalize within 6–8 weeks.

G. **Management.** Treatment includes anti-inflammatory therapy and assessment for coronary artery disease with serial echocardiography.

1. **Intravenous immune globulin (IVIG).** High-dose (2 g/kg) IVIG, in combination with aspirin (ASA), initiated within 10 days of onset of fever substantially decreases the prevalence of coronary artery dilation and aneurysms detected 2 and 7 weeks later.

2. **ASA**
   a. Acute phase: **high-dose ASA** for its **anti-inflammatory** effect
   b. Subacute phase: **low-dose ASA** for its **antiplatelet** effect

3. **Steroids.** The use of these agents is controversial. Steroids have been contraindicated in the treatment of Kawasaki disease because of a find-

Table 16-2. Clinical Manifestations, Laboratory Findings, and Treatment of Kawasaki Disease

	Phase I Acute Phase	Phase II Subacute Phase	Phase III Convalescent Phase
Time Course	1–2 Weeks	**Weeks to Months**	**Weeks to Years**
Clinical manifestations	Fever Conjunctivitis Oropharyngeal changes Cervical adenopathy Rash Swollen hands	Defervescence of inflammation Peeling from nailbeds or distal extremities **Coronary artery aneurysms**	Gradual resolution of aneurysms
Laboratory findings	↑ ESR ↑ CRP	↓ ESR and ↓ CRP ↑ **Platelet count**	Normalization of all laboratory findings
Treatment	High-dose IVIG **High-dose** aspirin	**Low-dose** aspirin	Continue low-dose aspirin only if aneurysms remain

ESR = erythrocyte sedimentation rate; *CRP* = C-reactive protein; *IVIG* = intravenous immune globulin.

ing of increased morbidity associated with their use. However, steroids may be useful in some patients who are unresponsive to IVIG.

H. Prognosis

1. If coronary artery disease is absent, **no** long-term sequelae occur.

2. Even if coronary artery disease is present, mortality is < 1%, and aneurysms, even large ones, commonly regress.

3. Long-term prognosis is unclear. Increased risk of atherosclerotic heart disease in adulthood is possible.

III. Juvenile Rheumatoid Arthritis (JRA)

A. Definition. JRA is a disorder characterized by chronic joint inflammation in children, with or without extra-articular involvement.

B. Epidemiology

1. JRA is the **most common pediatric rheumatic disease with arthritis** as the distinguishing manifestation.

2. The mean age of onset is **1–3 years**; presentation before 6 months of age is unusual.

3. JRA most commonly occurs in **females,** with two exceptions. Males are **equally likely to have systemic-onset JRA,** and they are much more likely to have **late-onset pauciarticular JRA (male-to-female ratio is 10:1).**

C. Classification. The classification of JRA is determined on the basis of the **clinical features** present during the first 6 months of disease (**Table 16-3**). There are three categories of JRA: pauciarticular, polyarticular, and systemic. Regardless of type, all patients have arthritis during their clinical course.

D. Clinical Features

1. **Pauciarticular JRA (≤ four joints involved)** accounts for approximately 40% of cases.

   a. **Subtypes.** Two subtypes of pauciarticular JRA are recognized on the basis of the age of onset.

   (1) **Early-onset pauciarticular JRA** is **female** predominant. Patients usually present at 1–5 years of age. Seventy-five percent of patients have a **positive antinuclear antibody (ANA).** These patients are at **high risk for developing chronic uveitis** (50%), which is defined as inflammation of the iris and ciliary body. Uveitis must be monitored by regular slit-lamp evaluations.

   (2) **Late-onset pauciarticular JRA,** unlike all other JRA types and subtypes, is **male** predominant. Patients almost always present when older than 8 years of age. As in ankylosing spondylitis, the typical patient with late-onset pauciarticular JRA is male and is **HLA-B27 positive,** with involvement of the **hips and sacroiliac joints.** Uveitis is less common.

Table 16-3. Distinguishing Features of Juvenile Rheumatoid Arthritis Subtypes

Feature	Pauciarticular (≤ 4 joints)		Polyarticular (> 4 joints)		Systemic
Percentage of cases	~40%		~40%		~20%
Systemic inflammation	Absent		Mild or absent		**Severe**
Subtypes	**Early onset**	Late onset	**RF−**	**RF+**	**None**
Sex predominance	**Female**	**Male**	Female	Female	**Male = female**
Serologic markers	ANA+	**HLA-B27+**	RF−	RF+	−
Uveitis	**Common**	Uncommon	Rare		Rare
Joints	Hips and sacroiliac joints spared	**Hips and sacroiliac joints involved**	Multiple large and small joints		Multiple large and small joints
Prognosis	Risk of blindness if uveitis is untreated	Risk of spondylo-arthropathy	Children may suffer from deforming arthritis		50% recover completely 50% develop chronic destructive arthritis

RF = rheumatoid factor.

    b. Articular involvement may present with swelling of one or two joints, not necessarily symmetric. The most common joints involved are the knees and hips.

  2. Polyarticular JRA (> four joints involved) accounts for approximately 40% of cases, with systemic involvement and extra-articular features generally mild or absent.

    a. Subtypes. As in pauciarticular disease, polyarticular JRA can also be divided into two subtypes. Subtypes are based on the absence or presence of **serum rheumatoid factor (RF),** which is an IgM molecule directed against IgG. Both rheumatoid factor–negative (RF−) and rheumatoid factor–positive (RF+) polyarticular JRA affect **females** more frequently than males.

      (1) RF-negative disease presents both early and late in childhood.

      (2) RF-positive disease presents in children older than 8 years of age and is generally **more severe than RF-negative disease,** with **higher risk of severe arthritis** and rheumatoid nodules.

    b. Articular involvement is characterized by a symmetric polyarthritis that typically involves both small joints (hands and feet) and large joints (knees, ankles, and hips).

  3. Systemic-onset JRA (Still's disease) accounts for approximately 20% of cases. At presentation, severe systemic symptoms may overshadow joint symptoms.

    a. High spiking fevers (temperatures > 39°C [102.2°F]) occur most commonly in the late afternoon or evening and subsequently return quickly to baseline or subnormal levels. **Still's disease is therefore typically included in the differential diagnosis of "fever of unknown origin."**

    b. Transient salmon-colored rash is most commonly found on the trunk and proximal extremities, especially during febrile episodes. The rash is **evanescent** (occurs with fever spikes and then fades) and **nonpruritic.**

   c. **Hepatosplenomegaly**

   d. **Lymphadenopathy**

   e. Other features:

   (1) **Fatigue, anorexia, weight loss, and failure to thrive** are common.

   (2) **Serositis,** including pericarditis and pleuritis, is also common.

   (3) **CNS involvement,** including meningitis and encephalopathy, may occasionally be present.

   (4) **Myositis and tenosynovitis** can also be seen in addition to the arthritis.

E. **Diagnosis** is generally on the basis of history and clinical features. **Diagnostic criteria** are listed in **Table 16-4.**

F. **Laboratory findings.** Laboratory results are **nonspecific;** if present, they reflect the existence or extent of inflammation.

   1. **Anemia** is usually **microcytic and hypochromic,** consistent with anemia of chronic disease.

   2. **Acute-phase reactants** are **elevated,** including ESR, CRP, and platelet count.

   3. **Rheumatoid markers**

   a. **RF** is negative in the majority of patients with JRA.

   b. **ANA** is present in 75% of patients with early-onset pauciarticular JRA and in 50% of patients with polyarticular JRA. ANA is not present in children with systemic-onset JRA and late-onset pauciarticular disease.

G. **Management.** The goal of treatment is to decrease joint inflammation and preserve function.

   1. **Control of inflammation**

   a. Nonsteroidal anti-inflammatory drugs (NSAIDs) ease pain and inflammation.

   b. Immunomodulatory medications (e.g., glucocorticoids, methotrexate, sulfasalazine, hydroxychloroquine) are commonly used for more severe symptoms.

   2. **Mechanical and physical measures** include physical and occupational therapy, as well as selective splinting to minimize joint contractures.

Table 16-4. Diagnostic Criteria for Juvenile Rheumatoid Arthritis

---

Age of onset ≤ 16 years of age
Arthritis in ≥ 1 joint defined as:
   Swelling or effusion OR
   Limitation of motion, tenderness, increased warmth
Duration of disease > 6 weeks
Exclusion of other causes of arthritis

---

3. **Surgery** is generally reserved for patients who have recalcitrant joint contractures or destruction.

4. **Psychosocial support**

H. **Prognosis.** The outlook is generally good with current therapy. However, the incidence of complications depends on the type and subtype of JRA (see Table 16-3).

IV. Systemic Lupus Erythematosus (SLE)

A. **Definition.** This multisystem autoimmune disorder is characterized by widespread inflammation of the connective tissues and immune complex–mediated vasculitis.

B. **Epidemiology**

1. There is a **female** predominance (female-to-male ratio is 8:1).

2. **Age of onset** is rare before 10 years of age and peaks in **adolescence.**

C. **Etiology.** The cause of SLE is **unknown,** but the disease may be triggered by drug reactions, excessive sun exposure, infections, or hormonal changes (menarche, menopause, pregnancy).

D. **Clinical features.** Signs and symptoms are variable and may involve multiple organ systems.

1. **Constitutional symptoms** such as fever, weight loss, and malaise are common.

2. **CNS** involvement includes headache, encephalopathy, seizures, psychosis, and transverse myelitis.

3. **Skin findings** may include a **malar rash** ("butterfly distribution" covering the nasal bridge and upper cheeks) and **photosensitivity,** both common at presentation or during an illness flare. Other common skin findings include **alopecia** and **Raynaud's phenomenon.**

4. **Arthralgias and arthritis** are typically migratory and transient. SLE, unlike rheumatoid arthritis, **rarely causes joint deformity or erosion**. Myositis may also occur.

5. **GI involvement** may manifest as hepatosplenomegaly, splenic infarction, mesenteric thrombosis (secondary to vasculitis), and sterile peritonitis.

6. **Cardiovascular involvement** is variable, with **pericarditis** as the most frequent manifestation. Congestive heart failure, arrhythmias, and sterile valvular vegetations (**Libman-Sacks** endocarditis) may also occur. **Neonates** born to mothers with SLE may have **congenital heart block** secondary to transplacental passage of maternal antibodies.

7. **Pulmonary involvement** may include **pleuritis,** pulmonary hemorrhage, and interstitial fibrosis.

8. **Renal involvement** is nearly **universal,** although lupus nephritis may be subclinical. Glomerulonephritis, nephrotic syndrome, hypertension, and subsequent renal failure are common.

9. **Hematologic** manifestations typically include low white blood cell counts. In addition to leukopenia, anemia of chronic disease, thrombocytopenia, and Coombs-positive hemolytic anemia are also common findings.

E. **Diagnostic Criteria for SLE (Table 16-5)**

F. **Laboratory Findings**

1. Elevated ESR and CRP

2. Anemia of chronic disease or anemia secondary to hemolysis

3. Leukopenia

4. Thrombocytopenia

5. Urinalysis may show proteinuria depending on the extent of renal disease.

6. **Rheumatologic markers**

a. **ANA** is almost **universally elevated** ($>$ 95%) in SLE. However, ANA is **nonspecific** for SLE and is found in many other diseases.

b. **RF** is often elevated in SLE, but like ANA, is **nonspecific.**

c. **Anti–double-stranded DNA (anti-dsDNA) antibodies** are much more **specific** (found only in SLE), and their levels **can be used as markers for active disease,** especially nephritis.

d. **Anti-Smith (anti-Sm) antibodies** are less prevalent in patients with SLE but when present are **very specific.** Unlike anti-dsDNA, anti-Sm antibody levels cannot be used as a measure of disease activity.

7. **Others**

a. **Antiphospholipid antibodies** (e.g., positive lupus anticoagulant or anticardiolipin antibodies) present in patients with SLE reflect an increased risk of **thrombotic events.**

b. **Decreased complement (C3 and C4)** is seen especially with active disease, and represents immune complex–mediated complement activation.

Table 16-5. Diagnostic Criteria for Systemic Lupus Erythematosus*

Mnemonic "SOAP BRAIN MD"
Serositis (pleuritis or pericardial inflammation)
Oral or nasal mucocutaneous ulcerations
Arthritis, nonerosive
Photosensitivity
Blood cytopenias (leukopenia, hemolytic anemia, or thrombocytopenia)
Renal disease (hematuria, proteinuria, hypertension)
ANA-positive
Immunoserology abnormalities (antibodies to double-stranded DNA, Smith antigen, false-positive RPR or VDRL assays)
Neurologic symptoms (encephalopathy, seizures, or psychosis)
Malar rash (butterfly rash)
Discoid lupus

---

*Four of eleven criteria provide a sensitivity and specificity of 96%.
RPR = rapid plasma reagin; *VDRL* = Venereal Disease Research Laboratories; *ANA* = antinuclear antibody.

G. **Management.** Therapy is based on a multidisciplinary, team approach that attempts (1) to minimize and prevent inflammation and end-organ dysfunction and (2) to treat complications.

1. **Control of inflammation**

   a. **NSAIDs** are useful only in the treatment of **minor** inflammatory symptoms, such as myalgias and arthralgias.

   b. **Immunosuppressive medications**

      (1) **Glucocorticoids** are the **mainstay of therapy** for children with SLE. Depending on disease severity and extent, treatment ranges from low-dose oral to high-dose intravenously pulsed steroids.

      (2) **Cyclophosphamide,** intravenously pulsed, is useful for children with severe lupus nephritis. Adverse effects of this cytotoxic agent include infertility and gonadal failure, secondary malignancies, and hemorrhagic cystitis.

      (3) **Other agents** include azathioprine, methotrexate, and cyclosporine.

2. **Treatment of complications**

   a. Patients with **thrombosis** and antiphospholipid antibodies should be anticoagulated with low-molecular weight heparin or warfarin.

   b. Patients with **renal failure** may require dialysis, fluid and electrolyte management, and ultimately renal transplant.

3. **Psychosocial and family support**

H. **Prognosis.** Before the advent of effective therapy, the outlook for patients with SLE was historically poor and uniformly fatal. However, with current treatment, the **survival rate is now 90%** at 5–10 years after initial diagnosis. The major causes of mortality are infection (because of immunosuppression), renal failure or nephritis, and CNS complications.

V. Dermatomyositis

A. **Definition.** This inflammatory condition of muscle results in progressive muscle weakness with characteristic skin findings.

B. **Epidemiology**

1. Affected individuals are usually **5–14 years** of age. The mean age of onset is 6 years of age.

2. **Females** are more likely to be affected (female-to-male ratio is 2:1).

C. **Clinical Features**

1. **Constitutional symptoms** are common and include fatigue, anorexia, malaise, low-grade fevers, and weight loss.

2. **Characteristic cutaneous findings,** particularly over **sun-exposed areas,** include:

   a. **Periorbital violaceous heliotrope rash,** which may also cross the nasal bridge

   b. **Gottron's papules,** in which the skin over the metacarpal and proximal interphalangeal joints (knuckles) may become erythematous and hypertrophic

3. **Proximal muscle weakness** (mostly of the hip girdle and legs) is insidious in onset and occurs weeks to months after the eruption of skin findings. It is characterized by a positive **Gowers' sign**, which is difficulty standing from the sitting position and having to "climb" up the thighs for support.

4. Other manifestations include:
   a. **Neck flexor muscle weakness**
   b. **Calcinosis** (calcium deposition in muscle, fascia, and subcutaneous tissue), which may occur in approximately 40% of children
   c. **Nail bed telangiectasias**
   d. **Constipation** from GI smooth muscle dysfunction
   e. **Dysphagia**
   f. **Cardiac involvement** with conduction abnormalities and dilated cardiomyopathy

D. **Diagnosis**
   1. **Classic clinical presentation** of proximal muscle weakness with associated characteristic rashes
   2. **Abnormal electromyography** findings
   3. **Abnormal muscle biopsy** findings
   4. **Increased muscle enzymes** (creatine phosphokinase, aspartate aminotransferase, alanine aminotransferase, lactate dehydrogenase, and aldolase)

E. **Management**
   1. **Corticosteroids** are the **mainstay of therapy.**
   2. Other immunosuppressive agents, including methotrexate, cyclophosphamide, and cyclosporine, may be required for severe muscle disease.
   3. **Vitamin D and calcium supplementation** may be necessary to help repair osteopenia and decrease frequency of fractures.

F. **Complications**
   1. **Aspiration pneumonia** is a frequent complication as a result of a diminished gag reflex.
   2. **Intestinal perforation** may result from GI vasculitis.
   3. **Osteopenia** secondary to steroid therapy and muscle weakness may result in frequent fractures.

G. **Prognosis**
   1. **Prognosis is better in children** than in adults.
   2. There is **no association with malignancy in pediatric dermatomyositis.** (In adult disease, malignancy develops in 25% of patients.)
   3. Mortality rate is approximately 3%.

VI. Rheumatic Fever

A. **Definition.** Rheumatic fever is a delayed, nonsuppurative, autoimmune complication of upper respiratory infection with group A β-hemolytic streptococcus (*Streptococcus pyogenes*) that is characterized by inflammation of the connective tissues. Rheumatic fever predominantly affects the heart, blood vessels, joints, CNS, and skin.

B. **Epidemiology**

1. Rheumatic fever is now **rare in the United States** and Western Europe but was a worldwide problem during the 1960s. It is currently still common in developing nations.

2. It is **most common in children 5–15 years of age,** reflecting the age group most susceptible to streptococcal throat infections.

3. It has no gender predilection.

4. The major risk factor is **pharyngitis** caused by certain strains of **group A β-hemolytic streptococcus (GABHS).** The streptococcal strains that cause streptococcal skin infection (i.e., impetigo) **do not** cause rheumatic fever.

C. **Etiology.** The **cause of rheumatic fever is unknown,** but the disease appears to be autoimmune in nature.

D. **Clinical Features**

1. **Major features**
   a. **Cardiac involvement** is found in **50% of patients.** It is the **hallmark** and **most important complication** of rheumatic fever. The inflammatory process may involve all layers of the heart, including the endocardium, myocardium, and pericardium.
      (1) **Endocarditis** is the **most common cardiac finding** and typically causes insufficiency of the **left-sided valves** (mitral and aortic). It rarely affects the pulmonic or tricuspid valves.
      (2) **Myocarditis** is usually manifested by **tachycardia out of proportion to the extent of the fever.** Other severe manifestations include cardiac dilatation and heart failure.
      (3) **Pericarditis** and pericardial effusions are less common.
   b. **Polyarthritis** is classically **migratory, asymmetric,** and exquisitely painful. It occurs in 70% of patients and most commonly involves the elbows, knees, ankles, and wrists. **It does not result in chronic joint disease.**
   c. **Sydenham's chorea** occurs later than the other rheumatic fever manifestations, often beginning subtly, months after GABHS pharyngitis. It reflects involvement of the basal ganglia and caudate nuclei. Chorea may start as hand clumsiness and progress to choreoathetoid movements with emotional lability.
   d. **Skin involvement**
      (1) **Erythema marginatum** is a nonpruritic rash that starts as pink to red macules, which may coalesce and spread centripetally with central clearing over the trunk and proximal limbs.

    (2) Subcutaneous nodules, although rarely seen, are associated with severe cardiac involvement. These small, mobile, and painless nodules occur on the bony prominences of the extensor surfaces of the extremities.

  2. Minor features include fever, arthralgias, leukocytosis, increased ESR, and prolonged PR interval on electrocardiogram.

E. Diagnosis. The **Jones criteria for rheumatic fever are shown in Table 16-6.** Diagnosis requires **evidence of recent streptococcal infection and either two major criteria, or one major plus two minor criteria.**

F. Laboratory Findings

  1. Nonspecific inflammatory markers

    a. Elevated ESR and C-reactive protein

    b. Elevated white blood cell (WBC) count

  2. Serologic markers

    a. **Antistreptolysin-O** titers are abnormally elevated in 70–80% of patients with rheumatic fever and are evidence of a recent GABHS infection.

    b. **Anti-DNase** and **anti-hyaluronidase** antibodies may also be used to document GABHS infection.

  3. Echocardiography typically shows evidence of carditis, such as decreased ventricular function, valvular insufficiency, or pericardial effusion.

G. Management

  1. Eradication of GABHS infection

    a. Benzathine **penicillin** intramuscular injection (one dose) or

    b. Penicillin orally for 10 days

  2. Control of inflammation

    a. **NSAIDs** are useful for control of joint pain and swelling, but if given before definitive diagnosis, they may obscure the diagnosis by halting

Table 16-6. The Jones Criteria for Diagnosis of Rheumatic Fever*

Major criteria:
  Migratory polyarthritis
  Carditis
  Sydenham's chorea
  Erythema marginatum
  Subcutaneous nodules
Minor criteria:
  Fever
  Arthralgia
  Previous rheumatic fever
  Leukocytosis
  Elevated erythrocyte sedimentation rate
  Elevated C-reactive protein
  Prolonged PR interval on electrocardiogram

*The diagnosis requires evidence of previous streptococcal infection **and** either (1) two major criteria or (2) one major plus two minor criteria.

the development of migratory arthritis. Therefore, their use is **recommended only after the diagnosis of rheumatic fever is certain.**

b. **Corticosteroids** are often used in patients with severe cardiac involvement, such as congestive heart failure and severe valvular dysfunction.

3. **Supportive therapy**

a. **Congestive heart failure** is treated with diuretics, dietary salt restriction, digoxin, and bed rest.

b. **Sydenham's chorea,** if severe, may be treated with haloperidol.

4. **Long-term management** includes continuous antimicrobial prophylaxis to prevent recurrent episodes of rheumatic fever.

H. **Prognosis**

1. There are no chronic sequelae of the joint, skin, and CNS manifestations of rheumatic fever.

2. Cardiac inflammation often leads to severe valvular dysfunction, which may require intervention immediately or many years after the event. Valvular insufficiency or stenosis is usually delayed (usually more than 3 years after rheumatic fever) and, if severe, may require valve replacement or valvuloplasty.

VII. Lyme Disease

A. **Definition.** This reactive inflammatory disorder of the skin, heart, CNS, and connective tissues is caused by spirochetal infection with ***Borrelia burgdorferi*** and transmitted via a tick bite.

B. **Epidemiology. High-risk areas** reflect the natural habitat of ticks of the *Ixodes* species, which are the vectors for Lyme disease transmission. These ticks are especially prevalent in woodlands and fields in the New England states and parts of the Pacific coast and Midwestern United States.

C. **Etiology**

1. **Vector.** In the United States, most human infections occur during feeding by an infected **deer tick,** *Ixodes scapularis*. Transmission from *Ixodes pacificus*, which is the tick most prevalent in the Western United States, is less common.

2. **Organism.** *B. burgdorferi* is passed into the bloodstream of the human host while the tick engorges itself with blood. The **infected tick** must be attached for more than 36–48 hours before the risk of *B. burgdorferi* transmission becomes substantial.

D. **Clinical features.** Clinical features are initially caused by the invasion of *B. burgdorferi* into local and distant tissues, and in later stages by a systemic inflammatory response against the spirochete. The untreated clinical course of Lyme disease is, therefore, divided into **two stages, early and late disease.**

1. **Early disease** (1–4 months after transmission)

    a. Early localized disease is the first stage of Lyme disease and re-
sults from local cutaneous invasion and subsequent inflammation.

        (1) Erythema migrans is the classic rash of Lyme disease and is
typically the first manifestation. It occurs in two thirds of patients
and is described as **annular and "targetlike"** with variable degrees of central clearing. Erythema migrans may be asymptomatic, pruritic, or painful, and if untreated may expand (thus the
term *migrans*) to more than 12 inches in diameter.

        (2) Constitutional symptoms may begin to occur during this stage
and include fever, headache, myalgias, fatigue, arthralgias, and
lymphadenopathy.

    b. Early disseminated disease is the second stage of Lyme disease
and typically occurs within 1–4 months after the tick bite. In addition
to cutaneous findings, it is characterized by involvement of other organ systems.

        (1) Skin. Up to 25% of children may develop **multiple secondary
erythema migrans** lesions, which tend to be smaller than the
initial lesion.

        (2) Constitutional symptoms (see section VII.D.1.a.(2)) may ini-
tially appear during and continue through this stage.

        (3) Neurologic

            (a) Aseptic meningitis may occur at this stage, but is rare (1%).

            (b) Facial nerve palsy is seen in approximately 3% of children.
Lyme disease must therefore be considered in a child with
unilateral or bilateral palsy of the seventh cranial nerve.

            (c) Encephalitis

        (4) Carditis is rare but usually presents as **heart block** or myo-
carditis.

  2. Late disease (5–12 months after transmission) occurs in approximately
7% of children, and its hallmark is **arthritis,** with other manifestations
occurring less frequently.

E. Diagnosis

  1. The diagnosis is strongly suggested in the presence of epidemiologic
risk factors and a classic erythema migrans rash.

  2. Laboratory diagnosis is important in establishing a definitive diagnosis
because erythema migrans is not always present and the clinical features
and routine laboratory test results for Lyme disease may be nonspecific.

    a. Serologic testing involves the measurement of antibodies to *B.
burgdorferi* in the patient's serum and is the recommended laboratory
approach. The Centers for Disease Control and Prevention currently
recommends a two-step procedure:

        (1) Enzyme-linked immunosorbent assay (ELISA), which has a
relatively high sensitivity

        (2) Western blot, if the ELISA is positive or equivocal to confirm the
diagnosis.

    b. Other laboratory tests (e.g., polymerase chain reaction, cultures
from body fluids or tissue) are occasionally used but currently offer no
advantage over the recommended serologic method.

F. **Management. Treatment** is aimed at eradicating *B. burgdorferi,* with the caveat that symptoms caused by immune-mediated inflammation may not resolve immediately.

1. **Early localized disease, or late disease with arthritis only,** is typically treated with either doxycycline (for children $\geq$ 9 years of age) or amoxicillin.

2. **Carditis** and **meningitis** require intravenous ceftriaxone or penicillin.

G. **Prognosis.** Children who are treated, even with arthritis or neurologic manifestations, have an excellent prognosis. Recurrent symptoms or chronic sequelae are rare.

VIII. Other Rheumatologic Conditions of Childhood. Disorders that are rare in children and adolescents are marked with an asterisk (*).

A. **Seronegative spondyloarthropathies.** This group of disorders involves the joints or axial skeleton and is characterized by the absence of RF, ANA, or other disease-specific serologic markers.

1. **Reactive arthritis.** Inflammation of the joints is triggered by a microorganism, typically an enteric or sexually transmitted pathogen. An example is **Reiter's disease,** with its triad of arthritis, urethritis, and conjunctivitis, which is classically triggered by *Chlamydia trachomatis.*

2. **Psoriatic arthritis.** This arthritis of the small and large joints is seen in patients with psoriatic skin disease. It is associated with the psoriatic findings of scaly skin plaques, nail pitting, and onycholysis (separation of the nail from the nailbed).

3. **Ankylosing spondylitis.** This **male-predominant, HLA-B27**–related syndrome of arthritis affects the joints of the lower extremities and axial skeleton. It is characterized by enthesitis, which is inflammation of the tendinous insertions on the bone. Males with late-onset **pauciarticular JRA are at high risk** for developing this syndrome as adults.

4. **Arthritis of inflammatory bowel disease (IBD).** This arthritis is associated with ulcerative colitis or Crohn's disease. Some patients with IBD and joint symptoms may be **HLA-B27** positive and have involvement of the axial skeleton in a **pattern indistinguishable from ankylosing spondylitis.**

B. **Other vasculitides.** Like previously described vasculitic diseases (e.g., Kawasaki disease, SLE, Henoch-Schönlein purpura), these disorders are characterized by constitutional symptoms and inflammation of blood vessels.

1. **Takayasu's arteritis**. This disease is a large-vessel vasculitis. The classic patient is an Asian female adolescent or young adult, with constitutional symptoms and **aneurysmal dilation or thrombosis of the aorta, carotid, or subclavian arteries.**

2. ***Polyarteritis nodosa.** This vasculitis is characterized by aneurysms and thrombosis of the small and medium-sized vessels (e.g., brachial, femoral, or mesenteric arteries).

3. ***Wegener's granulomatosis.** This vasculitis is characterized by necrotizing **granulomas** in multiple organs, most commonly the respiratory tract and kidneys. Classic clinical features include constitutional symptoms, severe **sinusitis, hemoptysis,** and **glomerulonephritis.**

C. ***Sjögren's syndrome.** This syndrome is defined by a classic triad of findings, including **sicca syndrome** (dry mouth and eyes), **high titers of autoantibodies** (usually ANA or RF), and **connective tissue disease.**

D. ***Scleroderma**

1. **Systemic scleroderma.** This disorder is better termed **systemic sclerosis** because it is characterized by excessive fibrosis and subsequent dysfunction of multiple organ systems. This process affects the skin and vessels of the heart, kidneys, lungs, and GI tract. The cutaneous hallmark is **skin thickening with loss of dermal ridges,** resembling "tightened" skin.

2. **CREST syndrome** refers to a form of scleroderma with less extensive involvement, manifesting with **c**alcinosis, **R**aynaud's phenomenon, **e**sophageal involvement, **s**clerosis of the skin, and **t**elangiectasias.

Review Test

1. A 10-year-old girl presents for evaluation of fatigue, diminished appetite, and weakness. On physical examination, a periorbital violaceous heliotrope rash is evident. Which of the following statements is most accurate regarding the probable diagnosis?

(A) Children with this diagnosis typically present with distal muscle weakness with an ascending pattern.
(B) This patient has a 25% likelihood of developing a subsequent malignancy.
(C) Steroids are contraindicated.
(D) The clinical course may be complicated by calcium deposition in the muscle, fascia, and subcutaneous tissue.
(E) This patient's disease is more common in males than in females.

2. A 4-year-old boy presents to the emergency department for evaluation after 1 day of diffuse abdominal pain and multiple petechial bruises on his bilateral thighs. He has no known history of prior bleeding or easy bruisability but does have a 4-day history of upper respiratory tract infection (URI) symptoms and low-grade fevers. Physical examination is remarkable for a nontoxic, alert, and afebrile child. There is a petechial eruption on the lateral thighs, along with some edema of the hands and bilateral ankles. The abdomen is not distended, and bowel sounds are present. However, the abdomen is mildly tender to palpation in the periumbilical region without rebound tenderness. Laboratory studies reveal a white blood cell count of 14,000 cells/mm^3, hemoglobin of 11.8 g/dL, and platelet count of 260,000 platelets/μL. Hospital admission for which of the following treatments would be the most appropriate course of management at this time?

(A) Intravenous immune globulin therapy for a presumed diagnosis of Kawasaki disease
(B) Intravenous immune globulin therapy for a presumed diagnosis of immune thrombocytopenic purpura
(C) Further evaluation by Child Protective Services for possible nonaccidental injury
(D) Observation and possible steroid therapy for a presumed diagnosis of Henoch-Schönlein purpura
(E) Parenteral antibiotic therapy for a presumed diagnosis of meningococcemia pending blood culture results

3. A 3-year-old boy presents to the emergency department for evaluation of acute right upper quadrant abdominal pain. Further history reveals a 1-week history of spiking fevers and sore throat. Physical examination reveals an irritable but consolable child with a temperature of 39.9°C (103.8°F). Other pertinent findings include bilateral conjunctivitis; red, cracked lips; swollen indurated fingers with erythematous palms; and an erythematous macular rash on the trunk. Which of the following is the most likely cause of the acute abdominal pain?

(A) Henoch-Schönlein purpura
(B) Hydrops of the gallbladder
(C) Intussusception
(D) Referred pain from arthritis involving the spine
(E) Constipation from gastrointestinal smooth muscle dysfunction

4. A 3-year-old girl is brought to your office by her parents, who report that she has had 2 months of intermittent high-spiking fevers to 103°F (39°C), which occur nightly and return quickly to normal. The parents report that their daughter's activity and appetite are diminished. She is often reluctant to walk because of swelling of her ankles and knees. Six months ago her weight was at the 50th percentile, and now her weight is at the 25th percentile for age. On examination, you note a fever of 102.6°F (39.2°C) and a pink-red maculopapular rash on the trunk. Diffuse lymphadenopathy is present, and the liver is palpable 4 cm below the right costal margin. Which of the following statements regarding this patient's likely diagnosis is most accurate?

(A) Measuring the erythrocyte sedimentation rate will confirm the diagnosis.
(B) Admission to the hospital and immediate treatment with intravenous immune globulin are necessary.
(C) Antinuclear antibodies are likely to be positive.
(D) The rash on the trunk is nonpruritic and is likely evanescent.
(E) The patient has a 10% chance of developing severe chronic arthritis.

5. A 10-year-old boy develops a headache, fever, and rash approximately 2 weeks after camping with his family. The rash is annular and "targetlike" with central clearing. Which of the following is most accurate regarding the most likely diagnosis?

(A) This patient has a high likelihood of developing carditis.

(B) An infected tick must be attached to the skin for at least 36–48 hours before there is a significant risk of developing this condition.

(C) The prognosis for a child with this disease is poor, even with treatment.

(D) Treatment should be immediately initiated with an intravenous first-generation cephalosporin.

(E) Serologic testing for this condition is unreliable, and the diagnosis must be confirmed by culture of body fluids or tissue.

6. A 7-year-old boy with complaints of shortness of breath, nonpruritic rash, and very painful migratory arthritis presents to your clinic for evaluation. Two weeks ago, he had a sore throat and fever. On physical examination, a truncal macular rash is evident, and a grade 3/6 loud holosystolic murmur is audible at the apex and axilla. Which of the following statements is most accurate regarding this patient's likely diagnosis?

(A) Management may include corticosteroid therapy.

(B) Antistreptolysin-O titers would be expected to be abnormally high in 25% of patients with this condition.

(C) Laboratory evaluation is likely to demonstrate an elevated erythrocyte sedimentation rate and leukopenia.

(D) Chorea is also likely to be found on examination of this patient.

(E) Development of chronic and debilitating arthritis is likely.

7. A 12-year-old boy presents with severe arthritis of the hips and sacroiliac joints. Laboratory studies reveal that the patient is HLA-B27 positive. Which of the following is the most likely diagnosis?

(A) Early-onset pauciarticular juvenile rheumatoid arthritis (JRA)

(B) Late-onset pauciarticular JRA

(C) Rheumatoid factor–negative polyarticular JRA

(D) Rheumatoid factor–positive polyarticular JRA

(E) Systemic-onset JRA

8. A 3-year-old girl is referred to you for evaluation of fever. Her fever has lasted 6 days, and her parents have noticed eye redness, a truncal rash, and swollen lips. Your physical examination confirms these findings, along with an enlarged left cervical lymph node measuring 3 cm in diameter. On the basis of your findings, you suspect Kawasaki disease. Which of the following findings on physical examination or laboratory analysis would best correlate at this time with the finding of coronary artery aneurysms on echocardiogram?

(A) Her current signs of fever, truncal rash, and swollen lips

(B) Elevated erythrocyte sedimentation rate

(C) Elevated platelet count of 840,000 platelets/μL

(D) Cervical adenopathy

(E) Laboratory evidence of aseptic meningitis

The response options for statements 9–14 are the same. You will be required to select one answer for each statement in the set.

(A) Henoch-Schönlein purpura
(B) Psoriatic arthritis
(C) Still's disease
(D) Reiter's disease
(E) Arthritis of inflammatory bowel disease
(F) Systemic lupus erythematosus
(G) Kawasaki disease
(H) Dermatomyositis
(I) Pauciarticular juvenile rheumatoid arthritis
(J) Rheumatic fever
(K) Lyme disease

For each patient, select the most likely diagnosis.

9. An HLA-B27–positive 14-year-old girl with abdominal pain and chronic diarrhea.

10. A 6-year-old boy with erythematous and hypertrophic papules over the metacarpal and proximal interphalangeal joints and "dark rings" around the eyes.

11. A sexually active 16-year-old girl with arthritis and conjunctivitis.

12. A 3-year-old boy with fever, bilateral knee swelling, and a "salmon-colored" rash on the trunk and proximal extremities.

13. A 14-year-old girl with arthritis, alopecia, leukopenia, and a "bad sunburn" on her face.

14. A 5-year-old girl with arthritis, abdominal pain, and a petechial eruption on her buttocks.

Answers and Explanations

1. The answer is D [V.C]. The constellation of clinical signs and symptoms that include fatigue, muscle weakness, and a heliotrope rash in a girl between 5 and 14 years of age is suggestive of dermatomyositis. Calcinosis, or calcium deposition, in muscle, fascia, and subcutaneous tissue occurs in up to 40% of children with this disorder. Dermatomyositis typically presents with proximal muscle weakness, characterized by a positive Gowers' sign (difficulty standing from the sitting position and, as a result, having to "climb" up the thighs for support). Females are twice as likely as males to develop dermatomyositis. In childhood dermatomyositis, unlike in adult dermatomyositis, there is no association with malignancy. Steroids are the mainstay of therapy.

2. The answer is D [I.A, I.C.1–2, I.E] Henoch-Schönlein purpura is an IgA-mediated vasculitis that involves the skin, joints, gastrointestinal tract, and kidneys. Despite the presence of petechiae, the platelet count is normal (i.e., a nonthrombocytopenic purpura). Steroids are indicated for patients who present with severe abdominal pain or with arthritis. The diagnosis of Kawasaki disease is unlikely given the absence of fever for a minimum of 5 days and the absence of at least four of the five diagnostic criteria. The patient's normal platelet count is inconsistent with the diagnosis of immune thrombocytopenic purpura. Although nonaccidental trauma must always be considered, there is no other bruising of concern on examination, and the clinical presentation is most compatible with the diagnosis of Henoch-Schönlein purpura. The diagnosis of meningococcemia is also unlikely because this patient is nontoxic, alert, and afebrile.

3. The answer is B [II.C, II.D.4]. This patient meets the diagnostic criteria for Kawasaki disease based on the duration of fever and the presence of four of five diagnostic criteria, including conjunctivitis, oropharyngeal changes, a truncal rash, and swelling of the distal extremities. Approximately 10% of patients with Kawasaki disease may develop hydrops of the gallbladder, which presents with acute right upper quadrant pain. Sore throat, conjunctivitis, and red cracked lips are not associated with constipation, arthritis, or intussusception. Dermatomyositis may present with constipation from smooth muscle dysfunction and constitutional symptoms, but abdominal pain is not a feature of the disorder. Although edema of the hands and abdominal pain can be seen in Henoch-Schönlein purpura, fevers and mucous membrane findings are not usually present.

4. The answer is D [III.D.3]. This patient has features consistent with systemic-onset juvenile rheumatoid arthritis (JRA). Intermittent high-spiking fevers, joint pain and swelling, lymphadenopathy, and hepatosplenomegaly are common features. The classic rash of systemic-onset JRA is described as salmon-colored and maculopapular, located on the trunk and proximal extremities. It is nonpruritic and evanescent (comes and goes) and tends to be more prominent during febrile episodes. Diagnosis is on the basis of characteristic clinical features and does not rely on specific laboratory tests. Although the erythrocyte sedimentation rate is often elevated, it is nonspecific because it is also elevated in many other inflammatory conditions, such as infectious disorders, some malignancies, and other rheumatologic conditions. Moderate to severe symptoms can be treated with anti-inflammatory (e.g., aspirin) or immunomodulatory medications (e.g., glucocorticoids), but intravenous immune globulin is not recommended for use in JRA. Children with systemic-onset JRA have a 50% chance of having a severe, erosive arthritis. Antinuclear antibodies (ANA) in patients with systemic-onset JRA are negative, in contrast to most patients with early-onset pauciarticular JRA and 50% of patients with polyarticular JRA in whom ANA is positive.

5. The answer is B [VII.C.2, VII.D.1–2, VII.F.1]. The scenario of constitutional symptoms in the face of a classic rash suggestive of erythema migrans, shortly after a camping trip, supports the diagnosis of Lyme disease. To transmit Lyme disease, an infected tick must be attached to the skin for at least 36 hours. Early in the disease, patients may present with fever, headache, myalgias, arthralgias, and lymphadenopathy, along with an annular, or "targetlike," skin eruption with central clearing. Treatment of early disease includes oral doxycycline for children ≥ 9 years of age or oral amoxicillin. Subsequent neurologic complications are not common but may include aseptic meningitis, facial cranial nerve palsy, and encephalitis. Cardiac complications are quite rare and may include heart block and myocarditis. The prognosis for a child with any stage of Lyme disease, if treated, is excellent. Arthritis, the hallmark of late disease, occurs 5–12 months after the initial clinical presentation. It occurs in approximately 7% of children with Lyme disease. Serologic testing (enzyme-linked immunosorbent assay and Western blot analysis) is recommended for confirmation of disease.

6. The answer is A [VI.A, VI.B.4, VI.D, VI.E, VI.G, Table 16-6]. This patient's clinical presentation should raise suspicion for acute rheumatic fever. The diagnosis of acute rheumatic fever requires evidence of previous group A β-hemolytic streptococcal infection, in addition to either two major Jones criteria or one major and one minor Jones criteria. The major Jones criteria include erythema marginatum, carditis, migratory polyarthritis, subcutaneous nodules, and Sydenham's chorea. Unlike the other major criteria, the onset of chorea is usually several months after the other manifestations. Minor Jones criteria include fever, arthralgias, elevated erythrocyte sedimentation rate, and leukocytosis (not leukopenia). The great majority of patients (70–80%) with acute rheumatic fever have elevated antistreptolysin-O titers. Acute management includes eradication of streptococcal infection with penicillin and control of inflammation with nonsteroidal anti-inflammatory agents or corticosteroids. This patient's shortness of breath may be caused by congestive heart failure or a pericardial effusion. There are usually no chronic joint sequelae from acute rheumatic fever.

7. The answer is B [III.D and Table 16-3]. Unlike all other types and subtypes of JRA, late-onset pauciarticular JRA is male predominant and almost always presents in children older than 8 years of age. Typically, patients with late-onset pauciarticular JRA, similar to patients with ankylosing spondylitis, are HLA-B27–positive and have involvement of the hips and sacroiliac joints. In contrast, patients with early-onset pauciarticular JRA are usually female, present between 1 and 5 years of age, have a high risk of developing chronic uveitis, and do not have involvement of the sacroiliac joints. Patients with polyarticular JRA (whether rheumatoid factor–positive or –negative) are also usually female and have involvement of multiple large and small joints but not typically the sacroiliac joints. Patients with systemic-onset JRA may be either male or female and also have involvement of large and small joints, with sacroiliac joints less commonly affected. Other presenting features of systemic-onset JRA include fever, a characteristic transient skin rash (salmon-colored), hepatosplenomegaly, and lymphadenopathy.

8. The answer is C [II.C–F]. Coronary artery aneurysms in Kawasaki disease are more likely to occur during the subacute phase of the disease, which begins 1–2 weeks after the onset of fever. The subacute phase is also characterized by decreasing erythrocyte sedimentation rate (ESR) and by marked thrombocytosis. High spiking fevers, rash, swollen lips, cervical adenopathy, brawny edema of the distal extremities, and elevations of the ESR and C-reactive protein are all characteristic of the acute phase of Kawasaki disease. Aseptic meningitis is a well-described complication of Kawasaki disease, but there is no known increased incidence of aneurysm formation in patients with aseptic meningitis.

9–14. The answers are E, H, D, C, F, and A, respectively [VIII.A.4, V.C.2, VIII.A.1, III.D.3, IV.C–E, Table 16-5, and I.C]. Abdominal pain and chronic diarrhea may be caused by inflammatory bowel disease. Arthritis may be associated with either ulcerative colitis or Crohn's disease. Some patients with inflammatory bowel disease are also HLA-B27 positive and have involvement of the axial skeleton that is clinically indistinguishable from ankylosing spondylitis. The diagnosis of dermatomyositis should be suspected in a child with proximal muscle weakness, a violaceous heliotrope rash around the eyes, and erythematous, hypertrophic papules over the knuckles (Gottron's papules). Reiter's disease is an example of a reactive arthritis triggered by an enteric or sexually transmitted pathogen (classically, *Chlamydia trachomatis*). Reiter's disease presents with arthritis, conjunctivitis, and urethritis. The diagnosis of systemic-onset juvenile rheumatoid arthritis (Still's disease) should be considered in a child presenting with fever of unknown origin, an evanescent salmon-colored rash, arthritis, organomegaly, and polyserositis. Systemic lupus erythematosus may be diagnosed when four of eleven diagnostic criteria are fulfilled, including photosensitivity and a malar rash. Adolescent females might also present with alopecia or Raynaud's phenomenon when their disease is active. Henoch-Schönlein purpura is a systemic IgA-mediated vasculitis that involves the skin, joints, gastrointestinal tract, and kidneys. It commonly presents with a nonthrombocytopenic purpuric or petechial eruption on the buttocks or thighs with abdominal pain, arthritis, and glomerulonephritis.

17

Orthopedics

Sharon L. Young, MD

I. Upper Extremity

A. **Brachial plexus injury** most commonly occurs as a result of **birth trauma** from excessive traction on the neonate's head, neck, or arm, which stretches the nerves of the brachial plexus. Congenital aplasia of the brachial plexus accounts for a very small percentage of cases.

1. **Erb's palsy** is an upper brachial plexus injury involving the **C5 and C6 nerve roots.** It is the **most common brachial plexus injury** and most often involves the right arm. **Clinical features** include a **flaccid arm and an asymmetric Moro reflex.** (See Chapter 2, Table 2-2 for a description of the Moro reflex.) The arm is held in internal rotation with the elbow extended, forearm pronated, and the wrist and fingers held in flexion. This positioning is often described as the **"waiter's tip."**

2. **Klumpke's palsy** is less common and is the result of a lower brachial plexus injury caused by upward traction on the arm. It involves the **C7 and C8 nerve roots. Clinical features** include a **claw hand** owing to unopposed finger flexion and decreased ability to extend the elbow and flex the wrist. Horner's syndrome (ipsilateral ptosis, miosis, and anhydrosis) may be present if the sympathetic fibers of the first thoracic nerve have also been damaged.

3. **Diagnosis** is on the basis of history and physical examination but may include a plain radiograph of the shoulder to evaluate for an associated clavicular fracture. Electromyography (EMG) and nerve conduction studies may be considered to assess for a neuropathy or myopathy.

4. **Management.** Treatment includes observation and range-of-motion physical therapy to prevent contractures. Improvement is often noted within 48 hours; however, should the arm not improve within 18 months, surgery may be necessary.

B. **Nursemaid's elbow** is a **subluxation of the radial head.** The usual mechanism of injury is an upward force on the arm, such as **pulling a toddler upward** by the hand to make the child stand. The radial head in children younger than 6 years of age has a slender shape, allowing it to slip out of the annular ligament, which normally keeps it in place.

1. **Clinical features**
   a. Sudden onset of pain, which is difficult to localize
   b. The **elbow is held flexed** and no swelling is present. The child is unwilling to use the affected arm, but hand function is normal.
2. **Diagnosis** usually is on the basis of the clinical presentation in patients younger than 6 years of age. No radiograph is needed; however, if a film is ordered, the technologist may accidentally reduce the subluxation in the process of positioning the arm for the radiograph.
3. **Management.** Treatment of the subluxation is to reduce it by simultaneously flexing the elbow and supinating the hand.
4. **Prognosis** is excellent. Usually, the child will start to use the arm within 15 minutes of the reduction, but use of the arm occasionally may be delayed for up to 24 hours. Subluxation may recur.

C. **Anterior shoulder dislocation** is the most common type of shoulder dislocation. It occurs with excessive external rotation, abduction, and extension of the shoulder, as may occur in gymnastics or wrestling.

1. **Diagnosis** is on the basis of radiographs (especially an axillary view) of the glenohumeral joint to visualize the dislocation.
2. **Management.** Treatment is immobilization after closed reduction. **Recurrence of dislocation approaches 90%** in the adolescent population. Therefore, some physicians recommend early surgery to restore stability.

II. Spine

A. **Disorders of the Cervical Spine**

1. **Torticollis** is defined as the tilting of the head to one side. It is either congenital or acquired.
   a. **Congenital torticollis** is very **common** and is usually the result of uterine constraint or birth trauma, either of which causes contracture of the sternocleidomastoid muscle. Congenital torticollis caused by cervical spine deformities is rare; however, an example is Klippel-Feil syndrome (see section II.A.3).
      (1) **Clinical features**
         (a) Head is tilted toward the affected side with the chin pointed away from the contracture. Decreased range of motion and stiffness are noted when stretching the head to the opposite side.
         (b) A soft tissue mass may sometimes be palpated within the sternocleidomastoid muscle representing bleeding into the muscle (this may occur from birth trauma).
         (c) Asymmetry of the head and ears may be noted in untreated torticollis.
      (2) **Diagnosis** is on the basis of physical examination. If the neck is very stiff, radiographs of the cervical spine can be used to assess for abnormalities of the cervical spine.

        (3) Management. Treatment includes stretching exercises to relieve the muscle contracture. If head asymmetry is noted, helmet therapy must be initiated by 4–6 months of age to correct the head shape as the head grows.

        (4) Complications include skull deformity and facial asymmetry (plagiocephaly, see Chapter 1, section II.B.2.d) if torticollis is not treated promptly.

        (5) Prognosis after 6 months of diligent muscle stretching is complete resolution in 90%.

    b. Acquired torticollis is torticollis arising later in childhood. It is rare compared with congenital torticollis. Causes may include cervical adenitis, peritonsillar or retropharyngeal abscess, cervical diskitis or osteomyelitis, neoplasms, strabismus and refractive errors, trauma, gastroesophageal reflux disease (Sandifer syndrome), and dystonic drug reactions.

  2. Atlantoaxial instability is caused by an unstable joint between the occiput and the first cervical vertebrae or between the first and second cervical vertebrae. The first and second cervical vertebrae may be abnormal in syndromes such as Down syndrome, skeletal dysplasias (see Chapter 5, section III.D), and Klippel-Feil syndrome (see section II.A.3).

    a. Clinical features. Physical examination is usually normal and patients are often asymptomatic. However, spinal cord injury may occur if a patient with instability sustains injury. A high index of suspicion for the above-mentioned syndromes is important to prevent injury.

    b. Diagnosis is made on the basis of lateral flexion-extension radiographs of the cervical spine.

    c. Management includes fusion of C1 and C2 if instability is severe.

    d. Complications include paralysis or even death if the instability is not detected before injury.

  3. Klippel-Feil syndrome is defined as failure of normal vertebral segmentation that results in relative fusion of the involved vertebrae. The fusion usually occurs in the cervical spine but can occur in the lumbosacral vertebrae or in groupings of vertebrae throughout the vertebral column. Associated abnormalities may include congenital torticollis, genitourinary anomalies, congenital heart disease, hearing loss, and **Sprengel's deformity** (congenital abnormality of the scapula in which the scapula is rotated laterally leading to shoulder asymmetry and diminished shoulder motion).

B. Scoliosis is defined as lateral curvature of the spine. This disorder occurs equally in males and females, but adolescent females require treatment eight times more frequently.

  1. Etiology

    a. Most cases of scoliosis (80%) are **idiopathic.**

    b. Other causes include leg length discrepancy, neuromuscular disorders, connective tissue disorders, vertebral anomalies, and genetic syndromes.

  2. Clinical features. Asymmetry of the shoulder height, scapular position, and the waistline may be present. As the patient bends forward, a hump, representing posterior displacement of the curved spine, may be seen (Adam's forward bending test; Fig. 17-1). Pain is absent and, if present, is a sign of an underlying disorder that should be investigated.

3. **Diagnosis** is on the basis of clinical findings and radiologic confirmation. Standing posterior-anterior (PA) and lateral radiographs of the spine are needed to confirm the curvature and are used to calculate the **Cobb angle.** The Cobb angle, which measures the degree of scoliosis, is measured by drawing a line along the superior aspect of the most angulated vertebrae at the top of the curvature and drawing another line along the inferior aspect of the lowest most angulated vertebrae of the curvature. The angle at the intersection of these lines is the Cobb angle.

4. **Management.** Treatment may include observation, bracing, and surgery. **Bracing prevents progression** of curvature. Surgery is required for very severe curves or to stop curve progression. **Progression of scoliosis occurs only during growth** or if the spinal curvature is greater than 50°. It is important to remember that almost all growth in females ceases within 6 months of menarche.

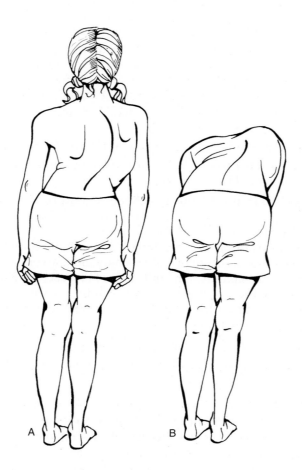

Figure 17-1. Scoliosis. **A.** Curve is visible when standing. **B.** Rib hump is visible when child performs Adam's forward bending test.

a. **Before and during growth spurt:**

   (1) For 10–20° of scoliosis, a follow-up scoliosis film is obtained 4–6 months later to assess for progression. Five degrees of progression is considered significant and warrants referral to an orthopedic surgeon.

   (2) For 20–40° of scoliosis, bracing is indicated.

   (3) For > 40° of scoliosis, surgery is indicated.

b. **After growth has concluded,** surgery is considered if scoliosis is > 50°.

5. **Complications,** such as respiratory or cardiovascular compromise, may occur if scoliosis is > 60–65°.

C. **Kyphosis** is defined as **anterior-posterior (AP) curvature of the thoracic spine.** A hunched back in the thoracic region is present.

   1. Flexibility in the rounded area should be assessed by having the patient extend his or her back while prone. Most adolescents with kyphosis have **flexible kyphosis** in which they can voluntarily correct the rounded area.

   2. **Scheuermann's kyphosis** is a stiff idiopathic kyphosis in which three consecutive vertebrae are wedged. It develops in previously normal adolescents.

D. **Back pain** is an infrequent pediatric complaint. Therefore, **any complaint of back pain that interferes with play should be evaluated for significant disease.** The differential diagnosis is extensive and includes fractures, osteomyelitis, rheumatologic diseases, neoplasms, and pyelonephritis. Some common causes include:

   1. **Back strain** is defined as muscular soreness from overuse or bad body mechanics. **Back strain is the most common cause of back pain in children.**

      a. **Clinical features.** Diffuse muscular pain is present without neurologic deficits. Physical examination is normal.

      b. **Management.** Treatment includes rest and analgesics.

   2. **Spondylolysis** is a **stress fracture in the pars interarticularis** (i.e., bone that connects the superior and inferior articular facets of a vertebral body) secondary to **repetitive hyperextension of the spine,** as occurs in gymnastics, tennis, and diving. It typically involves the lumbar region, particularly L5. Pain is localized and **increases with hyperextension.**

      a. **Diagnosis** is on the basis of AP, lateral, and oblique views of the lumbar spine. Because spondylolysis is a stress fracture, plain films may not detect the fracture. Therefore, a bone scan or a single photon-emission computed tomographic (SPECT) scan may be used for diagnosis if the fracture is acute.

      b. **Management.** Treatment includes rest and analgesics for pain. Casting or bracing for immobilization may be necessary if pain persists. Surgery is sometimes required.

      c. **Complications** include spondylolisthesis, which is discussed below.

   3. **Spondylolisthesis** occurs when the body of the vertebra involved in the spondylolysis slips anteriorly (i.e., subluxation of the vertebra). The sub-

luxed vertebra can impinge on nerve roots. Diagnosis and treatment is the same as for spondylolysis. Indications for surgery include nerve impingement, persistent pain, or progression of the subluxation.

4. **Diskitis** is defined as **infection (*Staphylococcus aureus* is the most commonly identified causal organism) or inflammation** (idiopathic, trauma, or rheumatic disease are causes) **of the intervertebral disk.**

   a. **Clinical features.** Diskitis typically begins with signs and symptoms of an upper respiratory illness or minor trauma, which are followed by back pain with **tenderness over the involved disk.** Fever is sometimes present. Children refuse to flex the spine, and young children may refuse to ambulate.

   b. **Diagnosis.** Clinical features are the basis of diagnosis. Erythrocyte sedimentation rate (ESR) is elevated. Magnetic resonance imaging (MRI) and bone scan can confirm the diagnosis.

   c. **Management.** Treatment includes bed rest. Use of antistaphylococcal antibiotics may be considered for patients thought to have infection.

5. **Herniated intervertebral disk** is much more common in adults but may occur in adolescents. The lumbar region is most commonly affected. Unlike in adults, herniation in adolescents is caused by repetitive activity and rarely by trauma. Treatment is conservative initially with bed rest. Surgery to remove the disk is necessary only if symptoms persist or if the neurologic examination is abnormal.

III. Hip

A. **Developmental Dysplasia of the Hip (DDH)** occurs when the acetabulum is abnormally flat, leading to the easy dislocation of the head of the femur. The spectrum of disease severity ranges from hip joint laxity to frankly dislocated hips. DDH was formerly termed **congenital hip dysplasia;** however, the name was changed because the hip in DDH may be normal at birth yet develop an abnormal acetabulum months later.

   1. **Epidemiology**
      a. DDH is more common in **girls** than in boys (6:1 ratio).
      b. Sixty percent of cases involve the left hip, twenty percent involve the right hip, and twenty percent involve both hips.
      c. Risk factors include female sex, first born, **breech presentation,** family history of DDH, and oligohydramnios.

   2. **Clinical features.** DDH is asymptomatic in infants. Physical examination shows the following findings:
      a. **Positive Barlow maneuver.** (The Barlow maneuver attempts to dislocate a dislocatable hip.) With the hips at 90° flexion, place the thumb on the medial side of the thigh and the middle finger on the greater trochanter and apply gentle pressure posteriorly and laterally to dislocate the hip. A "clunk" is felt as the hip dislocates.
      b. **Positive Ortolani maneuver.** (The Ortolani maneuver attempts to reduce a dislocated hip.) In the same position described above, abduct the hip, applying gentle pressure upward with the middle finger to

slide the head of the femur back into the acetabulum. In a positive Ortolani maneuver, the hip can be felt slipping into the acetabulum as it is being reduced.

    c. Abnormal **Galeazzi sign,** which assesses asymmetry of femur position. The Galeazzi sign is performed by placing the hips in flexion at 90°. If the hip is dislocated, the affected femur is shifted posteriorly compared with the normal limb. If both hips are dislocated, the Galeazzi sign is normal.

    d. Asymmetric abduction of the hips and asymmetric thigh or buttock folds. The older the infant, the more difficult it is to diagnose DDH using the Barlow or Ortolani maneuvers. Decreased ability to abduct the affected hip and asymmetric buttock folds are particularly useful in the diagnosis of DDH in older infants.

3. Diagnosis. Physical examination alone may be the basis of diagnosis. However, if the examination is equivocal, imaging may be helpful.

    a. Ultrasound is used to assess for DDH in young infants because the femoral head does not ossify until 4–6 months of age.

    b. AP radiographs of the pelvis may be used to assess for DDH if the infant is older than 6 months of age.

4. Management. Treatment depends on the age of the patient at the time of diagnosis. The **earlier the diagnosis, the less likely surgical intervention will be necessary.**

    a. The **Pavlik harness** holds the head of the femur against the acetabulum to stimulate formation of the normal cup shape of the acetabulum. It is typically used for 2–3 months if the diagnosis is made by 6 weeks of age. It is successful in 90–95% of cases.

    b. Surgery may be required if the diagnosis is made beyond 6 weeks of age, the hips are bilaterally dislocated, the hips are not reducible on physical examination, or the Pavlik harness fails to stabilize the hip. Surgery generally involves closed reduction of the hip. However, if closed reduction fails, open reduction may be necessary. After surgery, the infant is in a cast for 2–3 months.

5. Complications

    a. Avascular necrosis of the femoral head

    b. Limb length discrepancy, painful abnormal gait, and osteoarthritis if DDH is not treated

B. Limp is a common symptom during childhood. The differential diagnosis is extensive and is listed in **Table 17-1.** The more common causes include the following:

1. Septic arthritis is a bacterial infection of the joint, which can be caused by hematogenous spread, contiguous spread, or direct inoculation. **Septic arthritis of the hip is an orthopedic emergency.**

    a. Epidemiology

        (1) The age ranges from birth to 4 years of age; the peak is 1 to 3 years of age.

        (2) The **hip is most commonly affected in younger children,** whereas the knee is more commonly affected in older children.

Table 17-1. Differential Diagnosis for a Painful Limp

Mnemonic: "The joint STARTSS HOTT"	**Other causes of limp:**
S Septic arthritis	**D** Developmental hip dysplasia
T Transient synovitis	**D** Diskitis
A Acute rheumatic fever	**L** Legg-Calvé-Perthes
R Rheumatoid arthritis	**L** Limb length discrepancy
T Trauma	**L** Lyme disease
Fracture	
Strain or sprain	
S Sickle cell disease	
Pain crisis (vasoocclusive crisis)	
Osteomyelitis	
S Slipped capital femoral epiphysis	
H Henoch-Schönlein purpura	
O Osteomyelitis	
T Tuberculosis	
T Tumor	
Osteosarcoma	
Leukemia	

b. ***Staphylococcus aureus*** and ***Streptococcus pyogenes*** are the most common organisms. *Neisseria gonorrhoeae* may cause septic arthritis in adolescents.

c. Clinical features

(1) Fever and irritability are common.

(2) Limp, refusal to walk, and pain with movement of the joint may occur. The patient refuses to move the joint, and any attempt to move the joint results in significant pain. If the hip is affected, it is usually held in **flexion, abduction, and external rotation** to relieve the pressure within the joint capsule.

(3) Erythema, swelling, and asymmetry of soft tissue folds may be present.

d. Diagnosis

(1) Laboratory studies include an **elevated white blood cell (WBC) count, elevated ESR, and elevated C-reactive protein.**

(a) Blood culture is positive in 30–50% of cases.

(b) Analysis of the synovial fluid for cell count, Gram stain, and culture is useful. Synovial fluid demonstrating a WBC count $> 50,000–100,000$ cells/mm^3 is suggestive of septic arthritis. However, culture of the synovial fluid is positive in only 60% of cases.

(2) Imaging may be useful.

(a) Ultrasound is the best imaging screen and demonstrates fluid in the joint capsule.

        (b) Plain radiographs may reveal a widened joint space but are often normal.

    e. Management

        (1) Surgical decompression by joint aspiration is necessary to avoid avascular necrosis and to diagnose infection.

        (2) Empiric intravenous antibiotics to cover Gram-positive organisms should be started after cultures are obtained. Duration of antibiotic treatment is 4–6 weeks.

    f. Complications. The femoral head is vulnerable to ischemic injury. Ischemia may lead to **avascular necrosis and cartilaginous damage.**

2. Transient synovitis (also known as **toxic synovitis**) is a common self-limited, postinfectious response of the hip joint. Upper respiratory infection or diarrhea often precede transient synovitis. Transient synovitis is a **diagnosis of exclusion.** It is important to rule out septic arthritis, especially if a patient appears toxic or irritable, because the consequences of misdiagnosed septic arthritis can be serious.

    a. Epidemiology

        (1) Transient synovitis is the most common cause of a painful limp in toddlers.

        (2) Its peak age of presentation is 2–7 years.

        (3) It is more common in males.

    b. Clinical features

        (1) Low-grade fever, limp, and mild irritability may be present. Patients usually appear relatively well.

        (2) Hip pain may be acute or insidious in onset. Although patients may be more willing to move their legs than patients with septic arthritis, they may also hold their legs in a flexed, abducted, and externally rotated position, similar to the position seen in septic arthritis.

    c. Diagnosis is often on the basis of the history and physical examination.

        (1) The WBC count and ESR are normal or only slightly elevated.

        (2) There may be an effusion in the hip, and if fluid is present, it should be aspirated and analyzed to rule out septic arthritis.

    d. Management. Treatment includes nonsteroidal anti-inflammatory drugs (NSAIDs), bed rest, and observation.

    e. Prognosis is excellent. Pain usually improves within 3 days with analgesics and rest. Complete resolution of symptoms usually occurs by 3 weeks. Recurrence is unusual unless vigorous activities are resumed too soon.

3. Legg-Calvé-Perthes (Perthes) **disease** is **idiopathic avascular necrosis of the femoral head.**

    a. Epidemiology

        (1) The age of onset is 4–9 years.

        (2) The disease is more common in Caucasians and Asians.

(3) The disease is more common in boys and has a male-to-female ratio of 4:1.

(4) Patients are typically active, thin boys who are small for their age.

b. **Clinical features.** Children have a slightly painful limp with decreased internal rotation and abduction of the hip. This can be assessed on examination by log-rolling the leg internally. Pain may be referred to the knee and to the groin.

c. **Diagnosis** is on the basis of AP and frog-leg lateral radiographs of the pelvis, which show increased density in the affected femoral head or a crescentic subchondral fracture in the femoral head, termed the **"crescent sign."**

d. **Management.** Treatment involves containment, or ensuring that the femoral head is positioned within the acetabulum to facilitate its remolding and reossifying.

(1) Physical therapy and **restriction of vigorous exercise** are effective. If pain persists, analgesia, traction, casting, or crutches may be used.

(2) Surgery is indicated if there is more than 50% damage to the femoral head or if there is movement of the femoral head out of the acetabulum.

e. **Prognosis** is best in younger patients. If children develop the disease when they are younger than 9 years of age, complete resolution within 2 years is the norm. The majority of patients who are older than 9 years of age when they develop the disease develop osteoarthritis in the affected hip as adults.

4. **Slipped capital femoral epiphysis (SCFE)** is slipping of the femoral head off the femoral neck.

a. **Epidemiology**

(1) Age of onset is usually during adolescence.

(2) The male-to-female ratio is 2–3:1.

(3) The typical patient is an **obese adolescent boy.**

b. **Clinical features.** Patients have a painful limp with pain in the groin, hip, or knee. The degree of pain varies from severe (acute slip) to mild (chronic slip). Internal rotation, flexion, and abduction are usually decreased in the affected hip. SCFE is bilateral in 30% of cases, and patients with **hypothyroidism** are especially more likely to develop bilateral disease.

c. **Diagnosis.** AP and frog-leg lateral radiographs of the pelvis confirm the slipped epiphysis. A line drawn flanking the superior edge of the femoral neck (**Klein line**) crosses 10–20% of the epiphysis in a normal hip. However, in SCFE, the Klein line will not cross the epiphysis at all.

d. **Management.** Treatment involves pinning the epiphysis to prevent further slippage. The femoral head is not placed back into a normal position with the femoral neck because the force required may cause avascular necrosis.

e. **Complications**

(1) Avascular necrosis and collapse or deformity of the femoral head

(2) Chondrolysis (degeneration of articular cartilage of the hip)

    (3) Limb length discrepancy, which may cause limp and pain

    (4) Osteoarthritis

5. Osteomyelitis is an infection of the bone.

  a. Epidemiology

    (1) The peak ages of onset are less than 1 year and between 9 and 11 years.

    (2) The male-to-female ratio is 2:1.

  b. Etiology

    (1) *S. aureus* and *S. pyogenes* are the most common organisms. *Salmonella* should be considered in patients with **sickle cell anemia.** *Pseudomonas aeruginosa* infection of a bone in the foot can occur if a child steps on a nail while wearing sneakers.

    (2) Although contiguous spread and direct inoculation can cause osteomyelitis, children most commonly acquire infection by **hematogenous seeding.**

  c. Clinical features

    (1) Fever and irritability

    (2) Bone pain, erythema, swelling, and induration, which may develop in the area over the osteomyelitis

    (3) Painful limp

  d. Diagnosis

    (1) Laboratory studies include an **elevated WBC count, ESR, and C-reactive protein.**

      (a) Blood culture is positive in 50% of cases.

      (b) Blood culture in combination with a culture of the aspirated bone can identify the organism in 70% of cases.

    (2) Imaging, using **bone scan or MRI,** detects osteomyelitis a few days after the onset of symptoms. A **plain radiograph is not a good initial study** because it will be normal early in the infection. After 10–14 days of infection, a plain radiograph begins to reveal elevation of the periosteum, suggesting osteomyelitis.

  e. Management

    (1) Antibiotics should be given for 6 weeks, although the length of treatment varies depending on the organism.

    (2) Decreasing ESR generally indicates response to intravenous antibiotics, at which time oral antibiotics usually can be used to complete the antibiotic course.

    (3) Surgery is necessary to drain and debride a subperiosteal abscess if fever and swelling persist despite 48 hours of intravenous antibiotics.

  f. Complications

    (1) Spread of infection may occur, either by contiguous spread infecting a joint or distant seeding causing pneumonia.

    (2) Chronic osteomyelitis results from a nidus of residual infection, such as a **sequestrum** (i.e., focus of necrotic bone) or an **involucrum** (i.e., formation of new bone or fibrosis surrounding the necrotic, infected bone). Symptoms of chronic osteomyelitis are usually insidious, so the diagnosis is often delayed and complications are common. Both surgery and antibiotics are needed.

(3) Pathologic fracture at the site of the infection may occur as a result of healing and remodeling of bone, bone necrosis, or an involucrum. Activity should be restricted during antibiotic therapy to prevent a fracture, especially if the diagnosis of osteomyelitis was initially delayed.

(4) Angular deformity or limb length discrepancy if the growth plate is involved in the infection

IV. Lower Extremity

A. Torsional Abnormalities

1. **In-toeing** is a common parental concern. **Most in-toeing is normal** and corrects with growth. The following are the most common causes of in-toeing:

   a. **Metatarsus adductus** is **medial curvature of the mid-foot** (metatarsals).

      (1) Epidemiology and etiology

      (a) Metatarsus adductus occurs in children younger than 1 year of age.

      (b) It is usually caused by intrauterine constraint.

      (2) Clinical features include a C-shaped foot that can be straightened to varying degrees by gentle manipulation. Dorsiflexion is intact, but if the ankle cannot dorsiflex, clubfoot should be considered.

      (3) Diagnosis is by physical examination. Radiographs are not needed.

      (4) Management

      (a) Flexible foot that can overcorrect with passive motion needs observation only.

      (b) Flexible foot that can correct with passive motion, but not overcorrect, will benefit from exercises to stretch the foot.

      (c) Stiff foot that cannot be straightened warrants evaluation by a pediatric orthopedic specialist. Casting of the foot for 3–6 weeks may be necessary.

      (5) Prognosis is excellent. Resolution occurs in almost all patients.

   b. **Talipes equinovarus (clubfoot)** is a fixed foot in inversion with no flexibility. Bilateral involvement occurs in 50% of cases.

      (1) Epidemiology

      (a) Incidence is 1 in 1,000; it is increased to 6 in 1,000 in Pacific Islanders.

      (b) The male-to-female ratio is 2:1.

      (2) Etiology is multifactorial, but genetics is thought to play a strong role because of the increased incidence of clubfoot within families. Talipes equinovarus is associated with DDH, myelomeningocele, myotonic dystrophy, and some skeletal dysplasias.

(3) Clinical features. The ankle is held in plantarflexion and inversion. The forefoot is curved medially (metatarsus adductus). The deformity is rigid with very little range of motion in the ankle.

(4) Diagnosis is generally on the basis of physical examination.

(5) Management. Treatment involves casting within the first week of life. If the deformity is severe or if there is no improvement after 3 months of casting, surgical correction may be necessary.

(6) Prognosis is good, with 30–50% of patients improving with casting alone. Surgical correction is successful in 85% of patients.

   c. Internal tibial torsion is a medial rotation of the tibia, causing the foot to point inward.

      (1) Epidemiology and etiology

         (a) Internal tibial torsion is the **most common cause of in-toeing in children younger than 2 years of age.**

         (b) It is caused by in utero positioning.

      (2) Clinical features include a **foot that points medially** when the knee is flexed to 90°. The patella faces forward. Bilateral torsion is more common, but unilateral torsion also occurs. Torsion is present at birth but is often noted between 1 and 3 years of age when the child starts to stand.

      (3) Management involves observation only.

      (4) Prognosis is excellent with improvement by 3 years of age and resolution by 5 years of age.

   d. Femoral anteversion (or medial femoral torsion) is an inward angulation of the femur.

      (1) Epidemiology. Femoral anteversion is the **most common cause of in-toeing in children older than 2 years of age.** The female-to-male ratio is 2:1.

      (2) Clinical features

         (a) Feet and patella point medially.

         (b) Hips are able to internally rotate more than normal. External rotation is more limited than normal.

         (c) Child prefers to **sit in a "W" position** (opposite of sitting crossed-legged on the floor).

      (3) Management is observation only.

      (4) Prognosis is excellent with resolution by 8 years of age.

2. Out-toeing. The **major cause of out-toeing is a calcaneovalgus foot,** which is a flexible foot held in a lateral position.

   a. Epidemiology and etiology. Out-toeing occurs because of uterine constraint and is most common in firstborn infants.

   b. Clinical features include a flexible foot with the toes pointed outward. Plantar flexion is restricted. The foot is instead excessively dorsiflexed, and the dorsum of the foot can easily be placed into contact with the anterior leg.

   c. Management includes stretching the foot. Rarely, casting may be needed.

   d. Prognosis is excellent; the condition is self-limited.

3. **Angulation of the knee**

a. **Bowed legs (genu varum)** is symmetric bowing of the legs in children younger than 2 years of age. Bowed legs are a normal variation until 2 years of age, when the legs straighten.

(1) **Clinical features**

(a) **"Cowboy" stance.** When the child stands erect with the feet together, the knees bow laterally and the patella point forward.

(b) **Normal gait,** with the body weight held in midline throughout the gait cycle. If the weight seems to shift from side to side, then Blount's disease must be considered (see section IV.A.3.b).

(2) **Diagnosis** is on the basis of physical examination. Genu varum is present at birth but is usually not noticed until the child begins to walk. A standing AP radiograph of the lower extremities is indicated only if bowing is unilateral, is severe, or persists after 2 years of age to assess for pathologic bowing as may occur with rickets, growth plate injury, Blount's disease, or skeletal dysplasias.

(3) **Management** is observation. Progression of bowing may be monitored by measuring the intercondylar distance when the patient stands erect with the feet together. Bracing or corrective shoes are not necessary.

(4) **Prognosis** is excellent with resolution by 2 years of age.

b. **Blount's disease (tibia vara)** is a progressive angulation at the proximal tibia.

(1) **Epidemiology and etiology**

(a) It is more common in obese African American boys who are early walkers.

(b) It is thought to be a result of overload injury to the medial tibial growth plate causing inhibited growth only on the medial side.

(2) **Clinical features**

(a) **Angulation just below the knee**

(b) **Lateral thrust with gait** (i.e., the shifting of weight away from midline while walking)

(3) **Diagnosis.** Blount's disease should be **suspected in any child with progressive bowing, unilateral bowing, or persistent bowing after 2 years of age.** Diagnosis is on the basis of a standing AP radiograph of the lower extremities. A metaphyseal-diaphyseal (M-D) angle $> 11°$ is consistent with Blount's disease.

(4) **Management**

(a) **Bracing** for 1 year if the M-D angle is greater than 16° or if the patient is 2–3 years of age

(b) **Surgical osteotomy** if there is no improvement with bracing, if the patient is older than 4 years of age, if there is recurrence of angulation, or if the deformity is very severe

(5) **Prognosis**

(a) **Osteoarthritis** is common if angulation is not corrected.

        (b) **Recurrence of angulation** is common in obese children if treatment is started after 4 years of age or if the epiphysis is fragmented from injury.

    c. **Knock-knees (genu valgum)** is idiopathic angulation of the knees toward the midline.

      (1) **Epidemiology and etiology**

        (a) Age of onset is 3–5 years.

        (b) Most cases are physiologic as a result of overcorrection of normal genu varum.

      (2) **Clinical features**

        (a) **Separation of the ankles** when standing erect with knees together

        (b) **Swinging of legs laterally with walking or running**

      (3) **Diagnosis** is on the basis of physical examination.

      (4) **Management** is **observation** for the majority of patients. **Surgical intervention** is indicated only if genu valgum persists beyond 10 years of age or causes knee pain.

      (5) **Prognosis** is excellent as the condition spontaneously resolves in the majority of patients. Osteoarthritis may occur if the angulation persists beyond adolescence.

B. **Osgood-Schlatter disease** is an inflammation or microfracture of the tibial tuberosity caused by overuse injury.

  1. **Epidemiology.** Osgood-Schlatter disease is the most common **apophysitis,** which is an inflammation of a tuberosity.

    a. Age of onset is most commonly 10–17 years.

    b. Osgood-Schlatter disease usually occurs in children who participate in sports involving repetitive jumping, such as basketball or soccer. The disease is more common in boys.

  2. **Clinical features** include **swelling of the tibial tuberosity** and knee pain with point **tenderness over the tibial tubercle.** Pain occurs with extension of the knee against resistance. The pain worsens with running, jumping, and kneeling.

  3. **Diagnosis** is on the basis of history and physical examination. Radiographs are not necessary.

  4. **Management** includes rest, stretching of the quadriceps and hamstrings, and analgesics.

C. **Patellofemoral syndrome (formerly patellar chondromalacia)** is a slight malalignment of the patella that causes knee pain.

  1. **Epidemiology.** Patellofemoral syndrome is common in adolescent girls.

  2. **Clinical features**

    a. **Knee pain** directly under or around the patella

    b. Pain is worse with activity or with walking up and down stairs. It is relieved with rest, although pain may be noted shortly after sitting down.

    c. Physical examination of the knee may show the patella in a lateral position.

3. **Diagnosis** is on the basis of history and physical examination. A "sunrise view" radiograph of the knee may show the patella in a lateral position.

4. **Management** includes rest, stretching, and strengthening of the medial quadriceps.

D. **Growing Pains** are idiopathic bilateral leg pains that occur in the late afternoon or evening but **do not interfere with play during the day.**

1. **Epidemiology.** Growing pains are **very common** and occur in children 4–12 years of age.

2. **Clinical features.** Children may awaken at night crying in pain; however, the physical examination is normal.

3. **Management.** Treatment includes analgesics and reassurance.

V. Common Fractures

A. **Describing fractures** is critical because it may dictate the management of a fracture.

1. **Open or closed fracture** describes whether a break in the skin overlies a fracture. In a closed fracture, the skin is intact. In an open fracture, the skin is broken and antibiotics are required because of the risks of local infection and osteomyelitis.

2. **Spatial relationship of the fractured ends** describes the orientation of the fractured ends.
   a. **Nondisplaced or nonangulated** describes fracture ends that are well approximated and in normal position.
   b. **Displaced** describes fractured ends that are shifted.
   c. **Angulated** describes fractured ends that form an angle.
   d. **Overriding** describes a fracture whose ends override without cortical contact.

3. **Types of fractures (Fig. 17-2)**
   a. **Compression fracture (torus or buckle fracture)** occurs if the soft bony cortex buckles under a compressive force. This type of fracture commonly occurs in the metaphysis and requires only splinting for 3–4 weeks.
   b. **Incomplete fracture (greenstick fracture)** occurs if only one side of the cortex is fractured with the other side intact. The intact side is the site of compression injury and may be bent, whereas the fractured side receives the tension and fractures. Because angulation can increase even within a cast, reduction may include fracturing the other side of the cortex.
   c. **Complete fractures**
      (1) **Transverse** describes a fracture that is horizontal across the bone.
      (2) **Oblique** describes a diagonal fracture across the bone.
      (3) **Spiral** describes an oblique fracture encircling the bone. Spiral fractures may occur with twisting injury and therefore may be associated with **child abuse.**
      (4) **Comminuted** describes a fracture that is composed of multiple fracture fragments.

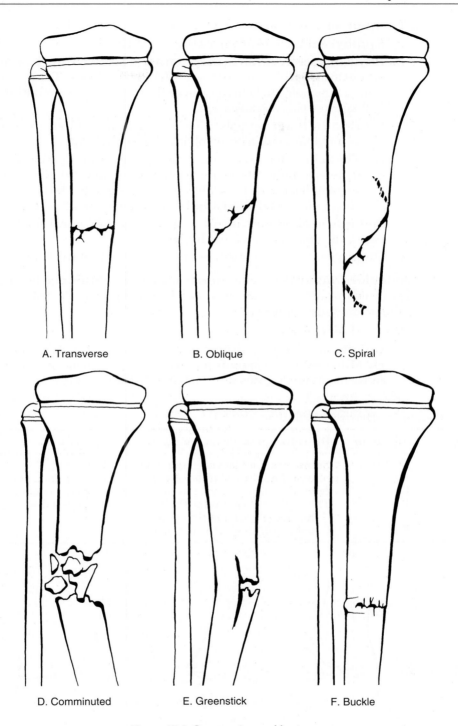

A. Transverse   B. Oblique   C. Spiral

D. Comminuted   E. Greenstick   F. Buckle

Figure 17-2. Common types of fractures.

4. **Location of the fracture**
    a. **Epiphyseal** fracture involves the end of the bone.
    b. **Physeal** fracture involves the growth plate. The **Salter-Harris classification** describes fractures involving the physis. **Table 17-2** contains a mnemonic to help remember the classification, and **Figure 17-3** illustrates this classification.
        (1) Because the growth plate has not calcified, children are especially vulnerable to injuries involving the growth plate.
        (2) The Salter-Harris classification is an important prognostic factor in determining subsequent growth of the limb. For example, subsequent bone growth is affected in some **grade II–III** Salter-Harris fractures and all **grade IV–V** Salter-Harris fractures.
    c. **Metaphyseal** fracture involves the ends of the central shaft (i.e., between the epiphysis and diaphysis).
    d. **Diaphyseal** fracture involves the central shaft of the bone.

B. **Clavicular fractures** are **common fractures in childhood** and are usually caused by falling onto the shoulder. **Birth injury** is the major cause of clavicular fractures in neonates.

1. **Clinical features**
    a. **Infants** may be **asymptomatic** or may present with an **asymmetric Moro reflex or pseudoparalysis** (refusal to move extremity because of pain). Crepitus may be felt over the fracture.

Figure 17-2. Salter-Harris Classification

Grade	Acronym	Description of Fracture
I	S	*Same:* Fracture is within the physis
II	A	*Above:* Fracture is in the physis and above into the metaphysis
III	L	*Low:* Fracture is in the physis and below into the epiphysis
IV	T	*Through and through:* Fracture is in the physis through both the metaphysis and the epiphysis
V	R	*Crush:* Crushing of the physis

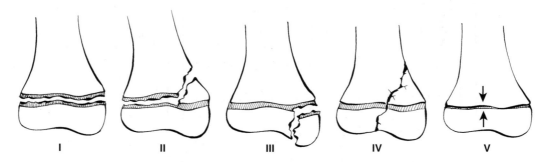

Figure 17-3. Salter-Harris classification of fractures. Grade I is a fracture within the physis. Grade II is a fracture within the physis and into the metaphysis. Grade III is a fracture within the physis and into the epiphysis. Grade IV is a fracture through the metaphysis, physis, and epiphysis. Grade V is a crush fracture of the physis. (Redrawn with permission from Tolo VT, Wood B. Pediatric Orthopaedics in Primary Care. Baltimore: Williams and Wilkins, 1993:3.)

    b. Children typically hold the affected limb with the opposite hand, and the child's head is often tilted toward the affected side. Point tenderness and deformity may be noted over the fracture.

  2. Diagnosis is on the basis of plain radiographs showing the fracture. Most fractures caused by trauma involve the middle and lateral aspects of the clavicle.

  3. Management. Treatment includes placement in a sling for 4–6 weeks to assist in immobilizing the limb. A "figure-of-eight bandage" can be used to draw the shoulder back but is cumbersome. Neonates with clavicle fractures often do not require any treatment.

  4. Complications. Injury to nerves and vessels is rare. However, brachial plexus injuries can coexist with clavicular fractures in neonates as a result of birth injury.

C. Supracondylar fracture occurs when a child falls onto an outstretched arm or elbow. Children younger than 10 years of age are most at risk for this type of fracture because the mechanical force of the impact is transmitted to the supracondylar area. **A supracondylar fracture is an orthopedic emergency if the fracture is displaced and angulated because of the risk of neurovascular injury and compartment syndrome.**

  1. Clinical features

    a. Point tenderness, swelling, and deformity of the elbow may be seen.

    b. It is important to assess the pulse, sensation, and movement of the fingers to **detect neurovascular injury.** If the fractured fragment is angulated or displaced, it can cause injury by stretching the radial or median nerves or the brachial artery.

    c. Pain with passive extension of the fingers is suggestive of compartment syndrome.

  2. Diagnosis is on the basis of AP and lateral radiographs. A triangular fat pad shadow posterior to the humerus may be observed if a fracture is present (i.e., **"posterior fat pad sign"**).

  3. Management. Passive movement of the elbow (i.e., when the examiner moves the arm) may increase the risk of further neurovascular injury. Therefore, **if a supracondylar fracture is suspected, never passively move the arm.**

    a. Nondisplaced and nonangulated fractures require casting.

    b. Displaced or angulated fractures require surgical reduction and pinning.

  4. Complications

    a. Compartment syndrome occurs when the pressure within the anterior fascial compartment is greater than 30–45 mm Hg, leading to ischemic injury and Volkmann's contracture (flexion deformity of the fingers and the wrist). The **"5 Ps" of compartment syndrome** (pallor, pulselessness, paralysis, pain, and paresthesias) are late signs. A more sensitive indication of impending compartment syndrome is **pain with passive extension of the fingers.**

    b. Injury to the **radial, median, or ulnar nerve** may cause temporary palsy but usually resolves.

    c. **Cubitus varus** is a decreased or absent carrying angle as a result of poor positioning of the distal fragment.

D. Forearm Fractures

    1. Common types of forearm fractures

        a. **Colles fracture** is a fracture of the distal radius.

        b. **Monteggia fracture** is a fracture of the proximal ulna with dislocation of the radial head.

        c. **Galeazzi fracture** is a fracture of the radius with distal radioulnar joint dislocation.

    2. Diagnosis is on the basis of AP and lateral radiographs.

    3. Management. Treatment includes open or closed reduction and splinting. A cast replaces the splint in 4–7 days after the swelling has resolved. Forearm fractures heal within 6–8 weeks.

E. Femur fractures require a great deal of mechanical force. Therefore, it is important to assess for other injuries in the joint above and below the fracture.

    1. Clinical features include erythema, swelling, deformities, and point tenderness.

    2. Diagnosis is on the basis of AP and lateral radiographs that include the joint above and below the area of injury.

    3. Management. Treatment includes casting for 8 weeks. Some femur fractures require traction for callus formation before casting, whereas others may be internally or externally fixated.

F. Toddler's fracture is a **spiral fracture of the tibia.** This type of fracture may occur after very mild or no identified trauma. The fibula remains intact.

    1. Epidemiology. Toddler's fractures usually occur between 9 months and 3 years of age. Typically, they occur when a child trips and falls while running or playing.

    2. Clinical features. The child refuses to bear weight but is willing to crawl. Erythema, swelling, and mild point tenderness may be found over the distal tibia on examination.

    3. Diagnosis. Oblique views of the tibia may show the fracture line, although sometimes plain radiographs do not visualize the fracture.

    4. Management. Treatment involves a long leg cast for 3–4 weeks.

G. Fractures typical of child abuse. Certain fractures should raise suspicion for abuse and must be investigated. (See also Chapter 20, section VI.B.2.d) A **"skeletal survey"** (radiographic studies of all bones) is the screening tool used to assess for current and previous bony injuries. The following fractures should make the clinician suspect abuse:

    1. Metaphyseal fractures (corner or bucket handle fractures)

    2. Posterior or first rib fractures

3. **Multiple fractures at various ages of healing**

4. **Complex skull fractures**

5. **Scapular, sternal, and vertebral spinous process fractures**

6. Any fracture whose **mechanism does not fit the history provided or the child's developmental abilities** (e.g., spiral fracture of the lower extremities in a nonambulatory child)

Review Test

1. A healthy, developmentally normal 15-month-old boy is brought to the emergency department because he is irritable and refuses to walk after falling down on carpet this afternoon. His parents report that he was running when he fell, but the fall did not seem to be very forceful. A radiograph of the right tibia reveals a nondisplaced spiral fracture. The fibula is intact. Which of the following is most appropriate in the management of this patient?

(A) Casting only
(B) Immediately filing a report with Child Protective Services for suspected abuse
(C) Consulting orthopedics for operative management of the fracture
(D) Ordering a skeletal survey and awaiting the results before calling Child Protective Services
(E) Beginning intravenous antibiotics

2. A 15-year-old girl comes to your office complaining of knee pain. She is on the high school basketball team, and she began having knee pain after 4 weeks of preseason training. On examination, she has mild tenderness and swelling over her left anterior tibial tuberosity; the examination is otherwise normal. Which of the following is the most appropriate management step?

(A) Casting for suspected fracture
(B) Sunrise radiograph of the knee to confirm patellofemoral syndrome
(C) Hip ultrasound for possible transient synovitis
(D) Explanation to the patient that these are growing pains and do not require treatment
(E) Temporary restriction from athletics, muscle stretching, and pain control

3. The parents of a 6-month-old boy are concerned because his feet "turn in." They noticed his "pigeon" toes since he was a few months old. On examination, the infant's mid-foot curves inward but can be straightened by gentle manipulation, even beyond midline. Which of the following is the most appropriate treatment?

(A) Reassurance only
(B) Referral for corrective orthotic shoes
(C) Prescription of special shoes that are connected by a bar to point the toes outward
(D) Referral for casting
(E) Referral to pediatric orthopedic surgery for operative repair

4. A 15-month-old boy is brought to the emergency department because of a 1-day history of high fever to 103°F (39.4°C) and refusal to walk. He previously was able to walk without difficulty. No known trauma has occurred. On examination, the child is fussy but consolable, and manipulation of his left hip elicits moderate discomfort. Range of motion in the left hip, however, is normal. Laboratory studies reveal a white blood cell count of 28,000 cells/mm^3 and an erythrocyte sedimentation rate of 42 mm/hr. Which of the following is the next most appropriate management step?

(A) Order an ultrasound of the hip.
(B) Order magnetic resonance imaging of the hip.
(C) Admit the patient to the hospital and immediately begin intravenous antibiotics.
(D) Order plain radiographs of the spine and pelvis.
(E) Discharge the patient home with reassurance and close follow-up.

5. A 15-year-old girl is brought to your office because the school nurse noticed possible scoliosis on a screening examination. She is a previously healthy girl. Menarche occurred at 13 years of age. On examination when she stands upright, the iliac crests appear level, but there is an obvious curvature of the back and the left shoulder is 1.5 cm lower than the right shoulder. When she bends forward at the waist, there is a rib hump in the right thoracic region. You order a standing spine radiograph, which reveals scoliosis with a Cobb angle of 30°. Which of the following is the most appropriate treatment at this point?

(A) Referral for surgery
(B) Referral for bracing
(C) Referral for shoe orthotics
(D) Referral for physical therapy for anticipated back pain associated with scoliosis
(E) Reassurance that her curve will not worsen significantly because the majority of her growth has concluded

6. An 8-year-old boy is brought to the emergency department after being hit by a car after he ran into the street. Lower extremity radiographs reveal a physeal fracture of the proximal tibia that extends into the medial metaphysis. Which of the following is the Salter-Harris grade of this fracture?

(A) Grade I
(B) Grade II
(C) Grade III
(D) Grade IV
(E) Grade V

7. A 7-year-old girl is jumping up and down on a bed when she falls onto her outstretched right hand. She has severe elbow pain and is brought to the emergency department. On examination, she is crying and holding her right arm at her side. Because of the mechanism of injury, you suspect a supracondylar fracture. A radiograph confirms your suspected diagnosis and demonstrates a displaced and angulated supracondylar fracture. Which of the following statements regarding her fracture is most likely correct?

(A) Pain with passive flexion of the fingers is an early sign that she may have compartment syndrome.
(B) Passive movement of the right elbow should be performed by the examiner to assess for neurovascular involvement.
(C) Even though the fracture is displaced, casting within the emergency department with outpatient orthopedic follow-up is an appropriate management step for this type of fracture.
(D) Child Protective Services should be consulted because this fracture is unusual in a child of her age and is suggestive of child abuse.
(E) Orthopedics should be contacted immediately because this is an orthopedic emergency.

8. A 12-year-old obese boy is brought to your office for pain in the right hip and thigh during the past 24 hours. He is also limping. Six months ago he was diagnosed with slipped capital femoral epiphysis (SCFE) of the left hip and underwent surgical repair. You suspect he may have SCFE involving the right hip. Which of the following tests would be appropriate to assess for other pathology associated with bilateral SCFE?

(A) Antinuclear antibody
(B) Rheumatoid factor
(C) Thyroid studies
(D) Calcium level
(E) Magnesium level

9. During a 2-week health maintenance evaluation, you notice that a 15-day-old male infant seems to favor looking to the right side only. On examination, range of motion in the neck is also diminished, and there is stiffness of the left sternocleidomastoid muscle. Within the body of the muscle, you appreciate a soft 1 × 2 cm mass. Which of the following statements regarding the most likely diagnosis is correct?

(A) The symptoms are most likely caused by a congenital cervical spine abnormality.
(B) Urgent ophthalmologic referral should be made for possible lack of vision in the left eye given the patient's right gaze preference.
(C) Plagiocephaly is a potential complication.
(D) Neurosurgical consultation should be obtained to rule out atlantoaxial instability.
(E) Otolaryngology consultation should be obtained to biopsy the mass within the sternocleidomastoid muscle.

10. A 7-year-old girl presents with low back pain of 4 days' duration. Although she had a cold 3 weeks ago, she now has no cough, dysuria, or abdominal pain. No history of trauma is noted. On examination, she hunches her shoulders forward and begins to cry as you extend her low back. There is tenderness over the space between L2 and L3, and the range of motion of the spine is limited. A plain radiograph of her spine is normal. Which of the following is the most likely diagnosis?

(A) Spondylolysis
(B) Spondylolisthesis
(C) Scheuermann's kyphosis
(D) Diskitis
(E) Herniated intervertebral disk

11. A 17-year-old boy is evaluated in the emergency department after falling down an embankment while hiking. His left mid-thigh is swollen and tender with deep lacerations. Lower extremity radiographs reveal a left femur that is fractured at the middle portion of the shaft, with the ends overlapping side by side, without angulation. Which of the following best describes this fracture?

(A) Closed, nondisplaced, nonangulated, transverse, diaphyseal fracture of the femur
(B) Closed, overriding, angulated, transverse, diaphyseal fracture of the femur
(C) Open, displaced, angulated, transverse, diaphyseal fracture of the femur
(D) Open, nondisplaced, nonangulated, transverse, diaphyseal fracture of the femur
(E) Open, overriding, nonangulated, transverse, diaphyseal fracture of the femur

12. A 12-year-old girl with Down syndrome is in your office for a sports physical examination before participation in the Special Olympics. She would like to be on the gymnastics team. On examination, the typical facial and body features of Down syndrome are noted, and the musculoskeletal examination is normal. Which of the following is an appropriate management step at this point?

(A) On the basis of a normal musculoskeletal examination, approve her to participate in gymnastics.
(B) Order lateral flexion-extension radiographs of her cervical spine.
(C) Order a complete skeletal survey to fully evaluate her bones to assess for osteopenia and a risk of fracture.
(D) Order pulmonary function testing.
(E) Restrict her from participating in gymnastics because of the risk of injury in a patient with Down syndrome.

Answers and Explanations

1. The answer is A [V.F]. The patient's age, the mechanism of injury, and the radiographic findings are classic characteristics of a toddler's fracture. A toddler's fracture is a spiral fracture of the tibia without concomitant fracture of the fibula. It occurs after little or no trauma. Casting only is appropriate for a nondisplaced toddler's fracture. Although it is always necessary to be vigilant for child abuse, a toddler's fracture alone in an ambulatory child should not raise suspicion of abuse, and therefore neither a skeletal survey nor immediate referral to Child Protective Services is indicated. Operative management is not needed in a nondisplaced spiral fracture. This toddler's fracture is not an open fracture and therefore antibiotics are not required.

2. The answer is E [IV.B]. This patient has swelling and tenderness over the tibial tuberosity, which is consistent with Osgood-Schlatter disease. Osgood-Schlatter disease is an overuse injury that is characterized by inflammation or microfracture of the tibial tuberosity. It is the most common apophysitis (i.e., inflammation of a bony outgrowth) in childhood. Treatment includes rest, quadriceps and hamstring stretching, and pain control. A fracture is unlikely because the patient has the ability to ambulate, and casting is unnecessary. Patellofemoral syndrome is a misalignment of the patella that results in pain around the patella or directly under the knee. The tibial tuberosity is not involved. Transient synovitis is unlikely because of the absence of hip pain. It is also uncommon during adolescence. Growing pains occur in younger children during growth spurts, not in adolescents. Growing pains, which are bilateral, occur mainly at night and do not interfere with daily activities.

3. The answer is A [IV.A.1.a]. This child has metatarsus adductus, which is a medial curvature of the mid-foot usually caused by intrauterine constraint. In a child whose foot can be manipulated beyond straight (beyond midline), no intervention is necessary and reassurance alone is sufficient. In contrast, a child with a flexible curved foot that cannot be straightened beyond a straight position would benefit from exercises to stretch the foot. Neither corrective shoes nor shoes with a bar are indicated for metatarsus adductus. Casting is reserved for feet that do not correct with manipulation. Surgical repair is not indicated for metatarsus adductus.

4. The answer is A [III.B.1.c.2, III.B.1.d–e]. Although transient synovitis is a consideration because this boy is nontoxic and is able to move his hip without severe pain, the presence of high fever, along with an abnormal erythrocyte sedimentation rate and white blood cell count, mandates evaluation for septic arthritis. The most appropriate next test is an ultrasound to assess for fluid in the joint. If fluid is present, it must be aspirated and analyzed. Magnetic resonance imaging can also detect joint fluid, but it is expensive and time-consuming and often requires sedation in a young child to help decrease motion artifact. Intravenous antibiotics and admission to the hospital are required for the treatment of septic arthritis, but antibiotics should be started only after cultures are obtained so that the infecting organism can be identified. A plain radiograph of the pelvis may show a widened joint space but is often normal in septic arthritis. Reassurance without further evaluation would risk missing the diagnosis of septic arthritis, which can potentially lead to avascular necrosis.

5. The answer is E [II.B.3–4]. Because the growth spurt in females precedes menarche, almost all growth ceases within 6 months after the onset of menstrual cycles. Menarche occurred 2 years before evaluation of this patient, and therefore no treatment for scoliosis is necessary because growth has likely concluded. Surgery is indicated after the growth spurt if the Cobb angle is > 50°. Scoliosis alone should cause no pain unless the curve is very great. Bracing is not indicated because it only prevents progression of scoliosis during the growth period. Neither shoe orthotics nor physical therapy is useful in scoliosis.

6. The answer is B [V.A.4.b; Table 17-2; Figure 17-3]. A physeal fracture that extends into the metaphysis is a grade II Salter-Harris fracture. A grade I fracture is within the physis. A grade III fracture is in the physis and into the epiphysis. A grade IV fracture is in the physis and through both the metaphysis and epiphysis. A grade V fracture describes a crushing of the physis.

7. The answer is E [V.C]. A supracondylar fracture occurs most commonly in a child younger than 10 years of age who falls on an elbow or on an outstretched hand. The displaced and angulated supracondylar fracture in this patient is an orthopedic emergency because of the risks of compartment syndrome and neurovascular injury. Passive extension of the digits of the hand is a sensitive indicator of compartment syndrome. Passive movement of the elbow (examiner moves the extremity) can result in neurovascular injury and should not be performed if a supracondylar fracture is suspected. A fracture that is displaced will very likely require surgical reduction and pinning, rather than casting alone. Abuse should always be considered in any childhood injury. However, a supracondylar fracture is a typical fracture in a child of this age, and this injury fits with the purported mechanism.

8. The answer is C [III.B.4.b]. Slipped capital femoral epiphysis (SCFE) is a slipping of the femoral head off the femoral neck. It is most common in males and is associated with obesity. Thirty percent of patients have bilateral involvement, and patients with hypothyroidism are especially at risk for bilateral disease. Therefore, it would be appropriate to obtain thyroid studies. Systemic lupus erythematosus and juvenile rheumatoid arthritis can cause hip pain, but they are not associated with bilateral SCFE; thus, neither antinuclear antibody nor rheumatoid factor would be helpful. Neither calcium nor magnesium abnormalities play a role in SCFE.

9. The answer is C [II.A.1.a]. This patient most likely has congenital torticollis, a tilting of the head to one side as a result of intrauterine constraint or birth trauma. Congenital torticollis is commonly associated with asymmetry of the head and face (plagiocephaly). The treatment of congenital torticollis, including head positioning during sleep and physical therapy, should be started as soon as the diagnosis is made to prevent this complication. A congenital cervical spine abnormality (e.g., Klippel-Feil syndrome) may cause congenital torticollis, but this is uncommon. Vision problems should always be considered in a child with a gaze abnormality, but the presence of a stiff neck muscle makes it unlikely that a problem with vision is the cause of the torticollis. Atlantoaxial instability is an unstable joint high in the cervical spine and does not manifest as congenital torticollis. The mass within the sternocleidomastoid muscle represents bleeding into the muscle body and does not require biopsy by otolaryngology.

10. The answer is D [II.D.4]. Besides muscle strain, the most common orthopedic causes of back pain in children are diskitis, spondylolisthesis, and Scheuermann's kyphosis. This patient's history and examination are most consistent with diskitis, an infection or inflammation of the intervertebral disk. Diskitis often occurs after minor trauma or an upper respiratory illness, and presentation includes local tenderness, decreased range of motion of the spine, and occasionally fever. Spondylolysis is stress fracture in the pars interarticularis, which may be diagnosed by spine radiographs. It is caused by repetitive spine hyperextension, as may occur in gymnastics, diving, and tennis, and would, therefore, be less likely in a child of this age. Spondylolisthesis is a subluxation of a vertebra, and, like spondylolysis, it would be unusual in a child of this age. Radiographs would also reveal this subluxation. Scheuermann's kyphosis causes a painful "hunched back" that can be diagnosed radiographically by finding three consecutive wedged vertebrae. A herniated intervertebral disk is much more common in adults although it may occasionally occur in adolescents.

11. The answer is E [V.A]. An accurate description of a fracture is important when determining a need for surgical intervention or consultation with an orthopedic specialist. A description should include whether there is a break in the skin (open versus closed), the spatial relation of the fractured ends (displaced versus angulated), the type of fracture, and the location of the fracture. In this patient, the fracture has resulted in a break in the skin (open fracture), and the ends of the fracture override (overriding ends). The fracture is nonangulated and cuts all the way across the bone (transverse) in the mid-thigh (diaphyseal fracture).

12. The answer is B [II.A.2]. Children with Down syndrome are at risk for atlantoaxial instability, an unstable joint between the occiput and first cervical vertebrae or between the first and second cervical vertebrae. Children with atlantoaxial instability may be asymptomatic, and physical examination may be normal. Therefore, before participation in athletics, lateral flexion-extension cervical spine radiographs should be performed to rule out any instability. If instability is absent, full sports participation is allowed. Neither pulmonary function testing nor a skeletal survey is indicated.

18

Ophthalmology

Kenneth Wright, M.D., and Robert Rhee, M.D.

I. Ocular Examination and Vision Screening

A. The **purpose** of ocular examination and vision screening is **early detection and treatment** of pediatric ocular disease. **Delay in diagnosis may result in irreversible vision loss**, and even death.

B. Vision screening principles can be remembered using the **acronym I-ARM** (Inspection, Acuity assessment, Red reflex testing, Motility assessment).

    1. Inspection includes evaluation for pupil and eyelid symmetry, face or head tilt, conjunctival redness, and squinting.

    2. Acuity assessment

        a. Neonates and infants: evaluation of eye fixation and pupillary responses

        b. Children: use of eye charts or cards

    3. Red reflex assessment, in which a direct ophthalmoscope is directed at the patient's eyes from a distance of 2 feet (**Bruckner test**), is the **single best screening examination** for infants and children. Table 18-1 presents information about the differential diagnosis of an abnormal red reflex.

    4. Motility assessment of each eye involves having the child follow a target in all directions. At the same time, alignment is assessed by evaluating for the symmetry of light reflecting off both corneas (**Hirschberg test**).

II. Normal Visual Development and Amblyopia

A. Visual Development

    1. Visual acuity is poor at birth, in the range of 20/200, as a result of immaturity of the visual centers in the brain responsible for vision processing.

    2. Visual acuity rapidly **improves during the first 3–4 months of life** as a clear in-focus retinal image stimulates functional and structural development of the visual centers of the brain.

515

Table 18-1. Differential Diagnosis of an Abnormal Red Reflex

Disorder	Red Reflex Finding
Cataract	Dark, dull, or white reflex
Vitreous hemorrhage	Dark or dull reflex
Retinoblastoma	Yellow or white reflex
Anisometropia	Unequal red reflex
Strabismus	Brighter red reflex in deviated eye
	Corneal light reflex will be uncentered
Glaucoma	Dull reflex

3. **Normal visual development** is dependent on both of the following:
   a. **Proper eye alignment**
   b. **Equal visual stimulation of each retina** with clearly focused images

4. **Abnormal visual development** results from the following:
   a. **Improper eye alignment,** such as uncorrected strabismus (see section IX)
   b. Any pathologic condition that **blocks retinal stimulation,** such as a congenital cataract (see section VIII.B)

5. **Visual development is most critical during the first 3–4 months of life.** Any pathologic condition that disrupts alignment or retinal stimulation during this period may result in poor vision as a result of amblyopia (see section II.B).

6. **Binocular vision** requires the integration of retinal images from both eyes into a single, three-dimensional perception (binocular fusion). Binocular cortical connections are present at birth, but appropriate visual input from each eye is necessary to refine and maintain these binocular neural connections.

7. **Normal depth perception (stereopsis),** similar to normal visual development, may also be impaired because of the following:
   a. **Improper eye alignment**
   b. Any pathologic condition that **unilaterally blurs the retinal image,** such as a congenital cataract.

B. **Amblyopia**

1. **Definition.** Amblyopia is poor vision caused by abnormal visual stimulation that results in abnormal visual development.

2. **Epidemiology.** Amblyopia is the **most common cause of decreased vision during childhood** and occurs in approximately 2% of the general population.

3. **Etiology.** Any pathologic condition that causes abnormal retinal stimulation can cause amblyopia.
   a. **Eye misalignment (strabismus:** see section IX). If a child has a strong preference for one eye and constant suppression of the nonpreferred eye, amblyopia will develop in the nonpreferred eye.
   b. **Any pathologic condition that causes a blurred visual image.** Opacification of the lens (cataract), severe uncorrected refractive er-

ror, significant differences in refractive errors between the eyes (**ani-sometropia**), and vitreous opacities (hemorrhage) all lead to poor visual stimulation and therefore abnormal visual development.

    4. Clinical features. Severity of amblyopia depends on when the abnormal stimulus began, the length of exposure to the abnormal stimulus, and the severity of the blurred image.

        a. The earlier the onset, the longer the duration of the abnormal stimulus, and the more blurry the image, the **more severe the vision loss.**

        b. Children are **most susceptible to amblyopia** during the **first 3–4 months of life,** the period of critical visual development.

    5. Diagnosis

        a. In infants and preverbal children, the bilateral red reflex test (see section I.B.3) is the best screening test.

        b. In older children, formal acuity testing is the best screening test.

    6. Management. Early detection and **early intervention** are **critical** to the treatment of amblyopia.

        a. Ensure that there is a clear retinal image by correcting any refractive errors with eyeglasses or by surgically removing any visually significant lens opacities.

        b. Patching the normal eye forces the use of the amblyopic eye, which in turn stimulates visual development.

        c. The earlier the intervention, the better the prognosis.

III. Conjunctivitis and Red Eye.
Conjunctivitis is a nonspecific finding that refers to conjunctival inflammation. It may be the result of infectious or noninfectious causes. The causes of conjunctivitis vary with patient age.

    A. Neonatal Conjunctivitis (ophthalmia neonatorum)

        1. Definition. Conjunctivitis occurring during the **first month of life**

        2. Etiology. Causes of neonatal conjunctivitis may include infections or chemical irritation.

            a. Infection is **acquired from the vaginal canal** during birth or from hand-to-eye contamination from infected individuals. Infectious agents include *Neisseria gonorrhoeae, Chlamydia trachomatis,* and herpes simplex virus.

            b. Chemical conjunctivitis. Chemical irritation (chemical conjunctivitis) results from drops or ointment that are topically instilled into a newborn's eyes as prophylaxis against *Neisseria gonorrhoeae.* Chemical conjunctivitis is most often secondary to **1% silver nitrate. Other medications** used to prevent *N. gonorrhoeae,* such as 1% tetracycline and 0.5% erythromycin, tend to be **less irritating** to the conjunctiva.

                (1) Chemical conjunctivitis is the most common cause of red, watery eyes in the **first 24 hours of life.**

                (2) This **self-limited** condition lasts for less than 24 hours.

        3. Clinical features, diagnosis, and management (Table 18-2)

Table 18-2. Etiology, Clinical Features, Diagnosis, and Management of Neonatal Conjunctivitis

Etiology	Onset and Clinical Features	Conjunctival Studies	Management
Chemical	**Within first 24 hours** **Watery** discharge	Negative Gram stain Few PMNs	No treatment necessary
Neisseria gonorrhoeae	**2–4 days of life** **Purulent** discharge Eyelid swelling Can lead to corneal ulcer	Gram-negative intracellular diplococci Positive gonococcal culture	Intravenous cefotaxime and topical erythromycin Treat parents
Chlamydia trachomatis	**4–10 days of life** **Serous or purulent** discharge Variable lid swelling	Cytoplasmic inclusion bodies Positive DFA or culture	**Oral** erythromycin Treat parents
Herpes simplex virus	**6 days–2 weeks of life** Usually **unilateral** **Serous** discharge	Multinucleated giant cells on Gram stain Positive HSV culture	Intravenous acyclovir and topical trifluorothymidine

PMNs = polymorphonuclear neutrophils; *DFA* = direct fluorescent antibody assay; *HSV* = herpes simplex virus.

4. **Differential diagnosis** of a red, teary eye in newborns also includes the following:

   a. **Congenital glaucoma** (see section VI) characterized by clear tears, enlarged cornea, and corneal edema

   b. **Dacryocystitis** (infection of the nasolacrimal sac)

   c. **Endophthalmitis** (infection within the eye itself), a rare but devastating infection that often results in blindness

B. **Red eye in older infants and children**

   1. **Etiology**. The differential diagnosis of red eye in infants and children is extensive (Figure 18-1). The most common causes include **viral, bacterial, and allergic conjunctivitis**, as well as **blepharitis** (eyelid inflammation).

   2. **Evaluation**

      a. **History,** which often establishes the cause

         (1) **Infectious causes** are suggested by history of contact with others who have conjunctivitis.

         (2) **Allergic conjunctivitis** is suggested by severe itchiness and is usually seasonal.

         (3) **Conjunctivitis associated with contact lens use** may be secondary to **allergy** to the contact lens solution, to a **corneal abrasion,** or to a **vision-threatening bacterial corneal ulcer.**

         (4) **Unilateral conjunctivitis** may be associated with a **foreign body, corneal ulcer, or herpes simplex keratitis.**

      b. **Ocular examination (I-ARM** acronym; see section I.B)

      c. **Fluorescein staining** of the corneal epithelium to evaluate for an abrasion of the corneal tissue. Positive staining is most commonly associated with **trauma** but may also be associated with a **bacterial corneal ulcer** or **herpes simplex keratitis.**

   3. **Specific causes of conjunctivitis.** The **distinguishing clinical features** of the common causes of pediatric red eye are presented in **Table 18-3.**

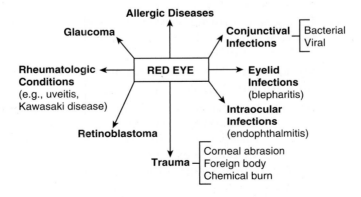

Figure 18-1. Differential diagnosis of red eye in older infants and children.

Table 18-3. Distinguishing Clinical Features of Conjunctivitis

Clinical Feature	Bacterial	Viral	Allergic	Blepharitis
Discharge	Purulent	Watery	Watery or mucoid	Minimal
Itching	Minimal	Minimal	Severe	Minimal (irritation rather than itching)
Preauricular lymphadenopathy	Absent	Common	Absent	Absent
Laboratory findings	Bacteria and PMNs on Gram stain	No bacteria on Gram stain	Eosinophils on conjunctival scraping	Positive culture for *Staphylococcus aureus*

PMNs = Polymorphonuclear neutrophils.

a. **Bacterial conjunctivitis**

(1) **Etiology.** Causes most commonly include **nontypeable *Haemophilus influenzae*, *Streptococcus pneumoniae*, *Moraxella catarrhalis*, and *Staphylococcus aureus*.**

(2) **Clinical features.** Purulent discharge, conjunctival erythema, and lid swelling are usually present. Bilateral involvement is common. Some patients have associated otitis media.

(3) **Diagnosis. History and clinical presentation** are the basis of diagnosis.

(a) **Conjunctival cultures** and **Gram stain** are not performed routinely for mild to moderate infections, and patients are usually treated empirically.

(b) However, **conjunctival cultures** and **Gram stain** should be obtained in **severe** cases.

(4) **Management**

(a) **Topical antibiotics** are effective and include sulfacetamide, polymyxin B and trimethoprim sulfate, gentamicin, tobramycin, and erythromycin.

(b) Indications for referral to an ophthalmologist include severe eye involvement, conjunctivitis associated with contact lenses, suspected corneal ulcer, or lack of improvement with topical antibiotics.

b. **Viral conjunctivitis**

(1) **Pharyngoconjunctival fever** is characterized by an upper respiratory infection that includes pharyngitis and fever and **bilateral conjunctivitis.**

(a) **Etiology.** The cause is **adenovirus,** types 3 and 7.

(b) **Clinical features**

(i) **Symptoms and signs: severe watery conjunctival discharge,** hyperemic conjunctiva, chemosis (conjunctival edema), preauricular lymphadenopathy, and, typically, a foreign body sensation caused by corneal involvement.

(ii) **Highly contagious** and lasts for 2–3 weeks

(c) **Management.** Treatment is supportive and includes cool compresses and topical nonsteroidal anti-inflammatory drug

(NSAID) drops. Antibiotics may be necessary if bacterial superinfection occurs.

(2) Epidemic keratoconjunctivitis is clinically similar to pharyngoconjunctival fever, but symptoms are confined to the eyes.

   (a) Etiology. The cause is **adenovirus,** types 8, 19, and 37.

   (b) Clinical features

      (i) **Symptoms and signs: petechial conjunctival hemorrhage,** preauricular lymphadenopathy, and a **pseudomembrane** along the conjunctiva.

      (ii) **Photophobia** from corneal inflammation (**keratitis**) caused by a hypersensitivity reaction to the virus (occurs in **one third** of patients)

      (iii) Lack of fever or pharyngitis

      (iv) Highly contagious

   (c) Management. Treatment is **supportive,** including cool compresses and topical NSAID drops. Children with corneal involvement should be referred to an ophthalmologist.

(3) Primary ocular herpes simplex virus

   (a) Etiology. The cause is **herpes simplex virus type 1 (HSV-1)** and typically represents the initial exposure to HSV-1 virus.

   (b) Clinical features

      (i) **Skin eruption** with **multiple vesicular lesions**

      (ii) **Corneal ulcer** (rare)

   (c) Diagnosis. History, clinical presentation, and positive viral culture or direct fluorescent antibody staining of vesicular fluid are the basis of diagnosis.

   (d) Management

      (i) **Systemic or topical acyclovir** may speed recovery if administered within 1–2 days of onset.

      (ii) **Topical antibiotics** applied to the skin may prevent **secondary bacterial infection.**

c. Allergic conjunctivitis

   (1) Epidemiology. Allergic conjunctivitis is most typically seasonal, often accompanying seasonal allergic rhinitis. It affects 10% of the population.

   (2) Etiology. The cause is a **type 1 hypersensitivity reaction.**

   (3) Clinical features. Marked itching and watery discharge are present.

   (4) Diagnosis. History and clinical presentation are the basis of diagnosis.

   (5) Management

      (a) Removal of environmental allergens

      (b) Topical mast cell stabilizing drops, such as **cromolyn**

      (c) Topical antihistamines

d. Hemorrhagic conjunctivitis is a dramatic presentation of pediatric red eye in which the child presents with both conjunctivitis and subconjunctival hemorrhage. Causes include infection with *Haemophilus influenzae*, **adenovirus, and picornavirus.**

   e. **Blepharitis**

     (1) **Definition.** Blepharitis is **eyelid inflammation.**

     (2) **Epidemiology.** Blepharitis is one of the most common causes of red eye.

     (3) **Etiology.** The usual cause is *Staphylococcus aureus* infection.

     (4) **Clinical features.** Burning, **crusting, and scales** at the eyelash base; thickened and hyperemic eyelid margins; broken or absent eyelashes; and a history of awakening in the morning with eyelashes stuck together are characteristic.

     (5) **Diagnosis.** History and clinical presentation are the basis of diagnosis.

     (6) **Management.** Treatment includes **eyelid hygiene,** in which eyelids are scrubbed twice daily with baby shampoo. Topical erythromycin ointment is also applied.

IV. Abnormal Tearing

  A. **Nasolacrimal Duct (NLD) Obstruction**

   1. **Definition.** NLD obstruction is failure of complete canalization of the lacrimal system that results in obstruction to tear outflow. Obstruction typically occurs distally, at **Hasner's valve.**

   2. **Epidemiology.** NLD occurs in 1–5% of children.

   3. **Etiology.** The cause of incomplete canalization is unknown.

   4. **Clinical features**

    a. **Watery eye** with increased tear lake

    b. **Matted eyelashes**

    c. **Mucus** in the medial canthal area

    d. **Bilateral** involvement (**one third** of patients)

   5. **Management**

    a. **Observation** only is needed for most children.

     (1) **One half** of cases resolve spontaneously within **6 months.**

     (2) **Nasolacrimal massage** may help open the distal obstruction.

     (3) **Topical antibiotics** are administered if infection is present.

    b. **NLD probing,** in which a small steel wire is passed through the nasolacrimal system through Hasner's valve into the nose, will cure NLD obstruction in most cases. It is typically performed between 6 and 12 months of age.

  B. **Amniotocele (dacryocele)**

   1. **Definition.** Amniotocele is swelling of the nasolacrimal sac.

   2. **Etiology.** The cause is accumulation of fluid as a result of NLD obstruction.

   3. **Clinical features**

    a. **Bluish swelling** in the medial canthal area may be apparent and represents fluid sequestered within the distended nasolacrimal sac.

      b. **Infection** may occur, manifesting as warmth, erythema, tenderness, and increased induration.

    4. Management

      a. **Local massage,** if there is no evidence of infection

      b. **Intravenous antibiotics** and **urgent NLD probing,** if infection is present

V. Ocular Trauma

A. Retinal Hemorrhages

    1. Etiology

      a. Retinal hemorrhages are **highly suggestive of child abuse.** (Physical characteristics of child abuse are described further in Chapter 20, section VI.)

      b. **Nonabuse causes** of retinal hemorrhages include birth trauma, leukemia, increased intracranial pressure, malignant hypertension, bacterial endocarditis, immune thrombocytopenic purpura, and, rarely, cardiopulmonary resuscitation.

    2. Clinical features. Retinal hemorrhages appear as hemorrhagic dots and blots, or hemorrhage within the preretinal vitreous on a dilated funduscopic examination, ideally performed by an ophthalmologist.

B. Corneal Abrasion

    1. Definition. Corneal abrasion is damage to and loss of corneal epithelium.

    2. Etiology. The cause is trauma, including injury from contact lens use.

    3. Clinical features

      a. **Severe pain,** tearing, and photophobia

      b. **Foreign body sensation**

    4. Diagnosis. Identification of the abrasion on **fluorescein staining** of the cornea is the basis of diagnosis.

    5. Management. Healing usually occurs within 24–48 hours.

      a. **Placement** of a protective shield or patch for 24–48 hours may be recommended in severe cases.

      b. **Instillation** of a topical antibiotic prevents bacterial superinfection.

      c. **Ophthalmologic consultation** to evaluate for a bacterial corneal ulcer is necessary if the abrasion is associated with contact lens use.

C. Hyphema

    1. Definition. Hyphema is **blood within the anterior chamber.**

    2. Etiology

      a. **Blunt trauma** is the **most frequent cause.** Blunt trauma compresses the globe, and when the globe subsequently re-expands, the iris vasculature tears, resulting in bleeding.

      b. **Nontraumatic causes** include iris neovascularization (associated with diabetes mellitus, intraocular tumors, retinal vascular diseases) and iris tumors (e.g., **juvenile xanthogranuloma**).

3. **Clinical features**
   a. **Impaired vision.** As blood settles, a **blood-aqueous** fluid level may be seen. A large hyphema may obscure the pupil and iris, thereby impairing vision.
   b. **Complications**
      (1) **Rebleeding 3–5 days** after initial injury
      (2) **Glaucoma**
      (3) **Staining of the cornea with blood**
      (4) **Optic nerve damage** in children with sickle cell disease
4. **Management.** Treatment includes ophthalmologic consultation and bed rest for at least 5 days.

D. **Orbital Floor Fracture ("blow-out" fracture)**
   1. **Etiology. Blunt trauma** to the eye or orbital rim fractures the orbital floor, which is normally thin and easy to fracture.
   2. **Clinical features**
      a. **Orbital fat** and the **inferior rectus muscle** can become entrapped within the fracture, leading to **diplopia** as a result of restricted vertical eye movement, to **strabismus,** and to **enophthalmos** (backward displacement of the globe into the orbit).
      b. **Numbness of the cheek and upper teeth** below the orbital fracture may occur as a result of **infraorbital nerve injury.**
   3. **Management**
      a. **Empiric oral antibiotics** are administered to prevent infectious contamination of the orbit from organisms from the maxillary sinus.
      b. **Surgical repair** is indicated if diplopia persists 2–4 weeks after injury or if enophthalmos is significant.

VI. Congenital Glaucoma

A. **Definition.** Congenital glaucoma is **increased intraocular pressure** occurring at or soon after birth.
   1. **Normal intraocular pressure** in infants is **10–15 mm Hg.** Infants with **congenital glaucoma** have intraocular pressures **exceeding 30 mm Hg.**
   2. **Congenital glaucoma** is very different from adult glaucoma.
      a. **Adult glaucoma** is characterized by increased intraocular pressure that damages the optic nerve but does not change the size of the eye.
      b. **Congenital glaucoma** not only results in optic nerve injury but also expands the size of the eye because the eye wall is much more elastic during infancy. Congenital glaucoma results in corneal edema, corneal clouding, and amblyopia.

B. **Etiology**
   1. **Outflow of aqueous humor** is reduced because of maldevelopment of the trabecular meshwork.

    2. Most cases are inherited in an **autosomal dominant** fashion.

    3. Other causes include infection (e.g., congenital rubella syndrome), ocular abnormalities (e.g., aniridia [absence of the iris]), or genetic syndromes, (e.g., Sturge-Weber syndrome, neurofibromatosis, Marfan syndrome).

C. Clinical Features

    1. Tearing, photophobia, **enlarged cornea, corneal clouding,** and a **dull red reflex** are common.

    2. Glaucoma may be initially **misdiagnosed as NLD obstruction** because of the presence of tearing.

    3. Bilateral involvement is present in **70% of patients.**

D. Management

    1. Surgery to open outflow channels is **almost always required.**

    2. Topical or systemic medications, such as β-adrenergic and carbonic anhydrase inhibitors, may help lower intraocular pressure.

E. Prognosis. Congenital glaucoma, if not detected and surgically treated early, leads to blindness.

VII. Retinopathy of Prematurity (ROP)

A. Definition. ROP is the **proliferation of vessels** seen in premature infants exposed to oxygen.

B. Etiology

    1. The **precise cause** of ROP is **unknown.** However, **high concentrations of oxygen play a major role** in the development of ROP.

    2. Other risk factors include low birth weight ($< 1,500$ grams), young gestational age, blood transfusions, hyaline membrane disease (surfactant deficiency syndrome), and intracranial hemorrhage.

C. Late complications. Myopia, astigmatism, amblyopia, strabismus, and blindness may develop.

D. Management

    1. Ophthalmologic examinations are performed every 1–2 weeks in patients with ROP to monitor for progression.

    2. If disease is severe, retinal cryotherapy and laser therapy may be effective.

E. Screening and Prevention

    1. Early detection is essential.

    2. Minimizing the **amount of oxygen delivered** and effective treatment of hyaline membrane disease are the two most important factors for prevention of ROP.

    3. Infants born at a gestational age of 28 weeks or less or with a birth weight of less than 1,500 g should have a **dilated ophthalmoscopic examination** at 4–6 weeks of age.

VIII. Leukocoria. Leukocoria is a white pupil and refers to an opacity at or behind the pupil. It may be caused by a cataract, by an opacity within the vitreous, or by retinal disease, such as retinoblastoma.

A. **Congenital Cataract**

1. **Definition.** Congenital cataract is a crystalline opacity of the lens present at birth.

2. **Etiology.** The **majority of cataracts are idiopathic.** Other causes include the following:

a. **Genetic syndromes**, such as Down, Noonan, Marfan, Alport, and Smith-Lemli-Opitz syndromes

b. **Nonsyndromic genetic inheritance**

c. **Metabolic derangements**, such as hypoglycemia, **galactosemia,** and diabetes mellitus

d. **Intrauterine infections,** such as cytomegalovirus and rubella

e. **Trauma**

3. **Management.** Treatment includes evaluation for underlying disease and **early surgery to prevent amblyopia.**

4. **Prognosis.** Congenital cataracts treated within the first weeks of life have a good prognosis, whereas surgery performed after 2–3 months of age is associated with poor visual outcome.

B. **Retinoblastoma**

1. **Definition.** Retinoblastoma is a **malignant tumor** of the sensory retina.

2. **Epidemiology**

a. Retinoblastoma is the most common ocular malignancy in childhood.

b. **The average age at presentation is 13–18 months. More than 90% of cases are diagnosed before 5 years of age,** which makes retinoblastoma a tumor of toddlers and preschool children.

3. **Etiology**

a. **Mutation or deletion** of a growth suppressor gene on **both alleles on the long arm of chromosome 13.** Because the development of retinoblastoma requires two deletions or mutations (one on each allele), the cause has been termed the "two-hit" model.

b. **Mutations** may be **sporadic** or inherited in an **autosomal recessive** fashion.

4. **Clinical features**

a. **Leukocoria** and **strabismus** are the **two most common presenting signs.**

b. Glaucoma, vitreous hemorrhage, retinal detachment, and hyphema are less common presenting signs.

c. **Calcification within the tumor,** identified on imaging studies of the eye, is a **hallmark** of retinoblastoma.

5. **Diagnosis.** Visual inspection with an ophthalmoscope is the basis of diagnosis. Ocular ultrasound or computed tomographic scan

of the orbit can further evaluate the tumor and assess for tumor extension.

6. **Management**
   a. **Early diagnosis is critical. Retinoblastoma should be suspected in any child with leukocoria.**
   b. **Large tumors** involving the macula have a poor prognosis and are generally treated by removal of the entire eye (i.e., enucleation).
   c. **Smaller tumors** may be treated with external beam radiation; however, radiation may induce formation of secondary tumors.
   d. **Very small peripheral tumors** may be treated with cryotherapy or laser photocoagulation.

7. **Prognosis.** Outcome is excellent if retinoblastoma is identified early. The **cure rate** is 90% if the tumor does not extend beyond the sclera or into the orbit. Retinoblastoma is uniformly lethal if untreated.

IX. Strabismus

A. **Definition.** Strabismus is **misalignment** of the eyes.
   1. **Esotropia** refers to the eye turned nasally.
   2. **Exotropia** refers to the eye turned laterally.
   3. **Vertical** strabismus refers to the eye turned up or down.
   4. **Pseudostrabismus** is a prominence of the epicanthal folds that results in the **false appearance of strabismus,** even though the eyes are actually appropriately aligned.

B. **Etiology.** The cause of most childhood strabismus is usually **unknown.** However, brain tumors, farsightedness (hypermetropia), or neurologic processes causing paresis of cranial nerves III, IV, or VI may also cause strabismus.

C. **Clinical Features**
   1. **If strabismus occurs before 5–7 years of age,** the child suppresses the image in the deviated eye. If this suppression is prolonged, amblyopia may result.
   2. **If strabismus occurs later than 5–7 years of age** (i.e., **acquired strabismus**), the mature visual system is unable to suppress the image in the deviated eye, and **diplopia** results.
   3. **Acquired strabismus, decreased eye movement, ptosis, decreased vision, and abnormal red reflex are all red flags that suggest a dangerous underlying cause,** such as a tumor or neurologic process.

D. **Management.** Treatment depends on the underlying cause.
   1. Ocular patching to prevent amblyopia is important.
   2. Strabismus associated with farsightedness is initially treated with corrective lenses.
   3. Surgery is often required to correct any misalignment that does not respond to patching or glasses.

Review Test

1. A 1-month-old male infant is brought to the office for a routine health maintenance visit. The infant has been feeding well, and the parents have no concerns. Physical examination is unremarkable except for a lens opacity in the right eye. Which of the following statements regarding this finding is most correct?

(A) Because of this infant's age, he is not susceptible to amblyopia.
(B) Immediate referral for cataract surgery is indicated.
(C) The opacity was probably not present at birth but has developed after birth.
(D) Surgery can be safely delayed until 6 months of age.
(E) Red reflex testing is normal and does not identify this finding.

2. A 3-year-old girl with a normal past medical history presents with a 5-day history of bilateral mucoid conjunctival discharge and conjunctival hyperemia. The girl is rubbing her eyes, and her mother believes that her daughter's eyes are very itchy. Which of the following statements regarding the most likely diagnosis is correct?

(A) The girl's symptoms are secondary to a type 2 hypersensitivity reaction.
(B) Topical antihistamines would be effective.
(C) *Staphylococcus aureus* is the likely pathogen.
(D) Coexisting rhinitis would be unusual.
(E) Topical polymyxin B and trimethoprim sulfate is an effective treatment.

3. A 14-year-old boy who wears contact lenses presents with conjunctival hyperemia and severe photophobia of the right eye. Which of the following statements regarding his diagnosis and management is most correct?

(A) Immediate ophthalmologic evaluation is necessary.
(B) Viral conjunctivitis is likely and supportive care should be provided.
(C) Eosinophils are seen on conjunctival scraping.
(D) Fluorescein staining is normal.
(E) Topical erythromycin should be prescribed and the patient should follow up if no improvement is seen in 1 week.

4. A 5-year-old boy presents with a history of fever, bilateral watery conjunctival discharge, sore throat, and a foreign body sensation in his eyes. Physical examination is notable for bilateral conjunctival hyperemia with watery discharge and bilateral preauricular lymphadenopathy. Which of the following statements regarding the most likely diagnosis is correct?

(A) Topical nonsteroidal anti-inflammatory drugs are contraindicated in the management of this illness.
(B) Corneal involvement is unlikely.
(C) Cool compresses should be used.
(D) Bilateral eye involvement is uncommon.
(E) This highly contagious illness is most often caused by *Staphylococcus aureus*.

5. A 2-year-old is brought to the office with a 3-month history of "uneven eyes." Physical examination shows right eye exotropia and leukocoria. Computed tomography of the orbit reveals a large retinoblastoma that involves the macula. Which of the following statements regarding the diagnosis is most correct?

(A) This tumor occurs sporadically and is not inherited.
(B) Computed tomography reveals calcifications within the tumor.
(C) Strabismus is uncommon at presentation.
(D) Radiation therapy is effective and has few complications.
(E) The age at diagnosis is unusual.

6. A 10-year-old girl is brought to the emergency department after sustaining a baseball injury to the right eye. Which of the following signs or symptoms is most consistent with the suspected diagnosis of a fracture of the orbital floor?

(A) Glaucoma
(B) Exophthalmos
(C) Diplopia
(D) Numbness of the lower teeth and chin
(E) Hyphema

The response options for statements 7–10 are the same. You will be required to select one answer for each statement in the set.

(A) Chemical conjunctivitis
(B) Conjunctivitis caused by *Neisseria gonorrhoeae*
(C) Conjunctivitis caused by *Chlamydia trachomatis*
(D) Conjunctivitis caused by herpes simplex virus

For each patient, select the most likely diagnosis.

7. A 7-day-old male infant with purulent conjunctival discharge and mild lid swelling.

8. A 12-hour-old male infant with bilateral watery conjunctival discharge.

9. A 10-day-old female infant with unilateral serous conjunctival discharge and multinucleated giant cells on Gram stain.

10. A 2-day-old female infant with purulent eye discharge and eyelid swelling.

Answers and Explanations

1. The answer is B [VIII.A, I.A]. Presentation with a lens opacity is consistent with a congenital cataract, a potentially very serious opacity of the lens. Immediate referral to a pediatric ophthalmologist is warranted. Surgery must occur within the first several weeks of life to ensure a good prognosis. If an opacity is not removed promptly in a young infant, the retina and nervous connections are not appropriately stimulated, and amblyopia (poor vision caused by abnormal retinal stimulation) may develop. Children are most susceptible to amblyopia during the first 3–4 months of life. Congenital cataracts are present at birth. The majority of cataracts are idiopathic, although known causes include trauma, metabolic abnormalities, genetic syndromes, and non-syndromic genetic inheritance. The Bruckner test, which is used in the assessment of the bilateral red reflex, is usually abnormal in the presence of a cataract.

2. The answer is B [III.B.2.a.(2), III.B.3.c]. Itching is the hallmark of allergic conjunctivitis, the likely cause of this patient's symptoms. Symptoms and signs of allergic conjunctivitis also include conjunctival erythema and watery or mucoid discharge. Management includes topical antihistamines, topical mast cell stabilizers, and environmental modification (removing from the environment any known or suspected allergens such as stuffed animals, pets, or carpet). Allergic conjunctivitis is a type 1 hypersensitivity reaction and is commonly seasonal. Uncomplicated allergic conjunctivitis is not associated with bacterial infection. Other signs and symptoms of allergy are commonly found, including allergic rhinitis. Topical antibiotics are ineffective for allergic conjunctivitis.

3. The answer is A [III.B.2.a.(3), V.B.5.c]. Conjunctivitis associated with contact lens use suggests three major possibilities, including an allergy to the contact lens solution, a corneal abrasion, or a vision-threatening bacterial corneal ulcer. A possible corneal ulcer requires urgent ophthalmologic consultation. Viral conjunctivitis is unlikely because of the acuity of the presentation, the unilateral findings, and severe photophobia. Eosinophils on conjunctival scraping are found in allergic conjunctivitis. A corneal ulcer usually appears on fluorescein staining. Because a corneal ulcer is a possibility, prescribing antibiotics with follow-up in a week would risk missing the early diagnosis of this serious condition.

4. The answer is C [III.B.3.b.(1)]. This patient's signs and symptoms are consistent with pharyngoconjunctival fever, a highly contagious illness that lasts for 2–3 weeks and is best managed with supportive care, including topical nonsteroidal anti-inflammatory drugs and cool compresses. Corneal involvement does occur and usually manifests as a foreign body sensation within the eye. Pharyngoconjunctival fever is commonly bilateral. It is a highly contagious illness caused by infection with adenovirus. The presence of preauricular adenopathy and watery discharge is inconsistent with bacterial conjunctivitis.

5. The answer is B [VIII.B]. Retinoblastoma is diagnosed on the basis of visual inspection and imaging studies, such as computed tomography or ocular ultrasound. Calcification within the tumor is a hallmark of retinoblastoma. Retinoblastoma is inherited sporadically or in an autosomal recessive fashion. The two most common presenting features are leukocoria (white light reflex) and strabismus. Management of large tumors often includes enucleation, although small retinoblastomas may be managed with external beam radiation. The side effects of radiation therapy include induction of secondary tumors. The majority of children with retinoblastoma are younger than 5 years of age.

6. The answer is C [V.D.2]. Orbital floor fracture, or a "blow-out" fracture, is generally secondary to blunt trauma to the orbit and can lead to entrapment of orbital fat and the inferior rectus muscle within the fracture. Glaucoma is typically not a complication of an orbital floor fracture. Entrapment leads to enophthalmos (i.e., retracted globe), restricted vertical movement of the eye, and strabismus with resultant double vision (diplopia). Because the infraorbital nerve may be injured, numbness of the cheek and upper teeth may result. Hyphema, or blood within the anterior chamber, also occurs secondary to blunt trauma. Hyphema should certainly increase

530

your index of suspicion for other injuries associated with blunt trauma, but hyphemas frequently occur without concurrent injuries to the orbital floor.

7–10. The correct answers are C, A, D, and B, respectively [III.A.1–3 and Table 18-2]. Neonatal conjunctivitis is defined as conjunctivitis occurring within the first month of life. *Chlamydia trachomatis* causes serous or purulent conjunctivitis with variable lid swelling in infants between 4 and 10 days of age (question 7). Conjunctivitis within the first 24 hours (question 8) is characteristic of chemical irrigation from neonatal prophylaxis drops or ointment, such as 1% silver nitrate. Herpes simplex virus presents with vesicles, corneal ulcers, and multinucleated giant cells on Gram stain of conjunctival cells (question 9). *Neisseria gonorrhoeae* causes purulent conjunctivitis with lid swelling in infants between 2 and 4 days of age (question 10).

19

Dermatology

Harry W. Saperstein, M.D., and Lloyd J. Brown, M.D.

I. General Concepts

A. **Skin examination** should be conducted in good light and should be complete, including evaluation of the scalp, hair, nails, eyes, mouth, palms, and soles. Examination should be both visual and tactile.

B. **Description** of skin disease requires identification of primary lesions and any secondary characteristics. Configuration and distribution of lesions should also be noted.

1. **Primary lesions**
    a. **Macules** are flat and nonpalpable and represent a cutaneous color change. A **patch** is a large macule.
    b. **Papules** are epidermal or superficial dermal lesions that are elevated **above the skin surface.** A **plaque** describes large or coalesced papules.
    c. **Nodules** are dermal lesions that are generally **below the skin surface,** although they may have an epidermal component that rises above the skin surface. A **tumor** is a large nodule.
    d. **Vesicles** are fluid-filled papules. A **bulla** is a large vesicle.
    e. **Pustules** are purulent-filled papules.
    f. **Cysts** are nodules filled with expressible material.
    g. **Wheals** are cutaneous elevations caused by dermal edema.

2. **Secondary characteristics** include:
    a. **Scaling:** desquamation of the stratum corneum
    b. **Crusting:** dried exudate and debris
    c. **Pigmentation changes**
    d. **Excoriations:** linear erosions into the epidermis caused by fingernail scratches
    e. **Scars:** thickened fibrotic dermis
    f. **Ulcers:** absence of epidermis and some of the dermis
    g. **Atrophy:** thinning of the epidermis or dermis
    h. **Fissures:** linear cracks into the dermis

3. Configuration and distribution

a. Configuration of lesions may be described as **linear, annular** (i.e., in circles), **arcuate** (i.e., in half-circles), **grouped,** or **discrete** (i.e., distinct and separate).

b. Distributions include generalized, acral (hands, feet, buttocks), confined to a dermatome, or other specific locations.

C. Diagnostic Procedures

1. Woods light can identify pigmentary changes and some dermatophytes.

2. Scrapings

a. Fungus. Ten percent potassium hydroxide (KOH) can be added to a scraping of a scale or exudate to identify fungal hyphae.

b. Scabies. Examination under a microscope of a scraping of an unscratched lesion or burrow for mites, eggs, or feces may be diagnostic of scabies.

c. Herpes simplex virus (HSV). The base of a vesicle can be scraped for laboratory identification of the herpes virus.

3. Cultures may be obtained for bacteria, virus, and fungus.

4. Invasive techniques

a. Incision and drainage may be performed for diagnosis, to obtain cultures, or for therapy.

b. Biopsy

(1) Shave or tangential biopsy for epidermal and superficial dermal lesions

(2) Punch biopsy for epidermal, dermal, and superficial subcutaneous lesions

(3) Excision biopsy for complete lesion removal

5. Immunofluorescent staining of biopsied lesions may be useful in autoimmune vasculitic disorders.

D. Management

1. General concepts

a. Absorption of topical agents through the skin of a child is equal to the absorption through the skin of an adult, except in a premature infant in whom absorption is greater because of a thinner stratum corneum.

b. Therapeutic efficacy of a topical agent is related to both the active ingredient and the **vehicle** (e.g., cream, lotion, ointment).

2. Hydration of the skin is critical. Dry, irritated skin is a poor barrier and easily damaged. Moisturizers include:

a. Ointments contain little or no water and have **maximal water-retaining properties,** making them useful for very dry skin.

b. Creams contain 20–50% water and are useful for skin of average dryness.

c. Lotions contain more water than creams and are useful for minimally dry skin or for large surface areas.

d. Solutions and **alcohol-based gels** are most useful for areas with hair (e.g., scalp).

3. **Thickened skin** (hyperkeratosis) requires **keratolytics,** such as salicylic acid, urea, α-hydroxy acids, and retinoic acid.

4. **Destructive therapies** (e.g., for warts, molluscum contagiosum) include high-dose salicylic acid, podophyllin, 5-fluorouracil, cryotherapy, electrotherapy, and laser therapy.

5. **Anti-infective agents** include topical antibiotics, antifungals, antivirals, and antiparasitic agents.

6. **Anti-inflammatory agents**

   a. **Topical corticosteroids** are categorized on the basis of their vehicle and potency. Effectiveness and potential side effects mirror steroid potency. **The weakest steroid that will achieve the treatment goal should be used first.** In general, only low-potency corticosteroids should be used on the face or groin because the epidermis is thinner in these areas, resulting in an increased risk of side effects.

      (1) **Systemic side effects.** Systemic steroid levels can be achieved if very potent steroids are used on damaged or thin skin for longer than 2 weeks. Effects include **adrenal suppression,** depressed growth, cataracts, glaucoma, and Cushing syndrome (see also Chapter 6, section IV.E.2.b).

      (2) **Local side effects** are **more common** and may occur after only a few days of treatment.

         (a) **Acne** (acne rosacea)

         (b) **Hirsutism**

         (c) **Folliculitis**

         (d) **Striae** (especially in axilla or groin)

         (e) **Hyper- or hypopigmentation**

         (f) **Atrophy**

         (g) **Ecchymoses and telangiectasias**

         (h) **Tachyphylaxis** (insensitivity to the medication)

   b. **Other anti-inflammatory agents**

      (1) **Tacrolimus ointment,** an immunomodulator, for atopic dermatitis

      (2) **One to five percent sulfur,** formulated with other medications, for acne

      (3) **Tar,** used for eczema and psoriasis

II. Newborn Skin Diseases (see Chapter 4, section I.B)

III. Inflammatory Disorders

A. **Contact Dermatitis**

   1. **Definition.** Contact dermatitis is inflammation of the epidermis and superficial dermis secondary to direct contact with the skin by a sensitizing substance.

   2. **Categories**

    a. Allergic contact dermatitis
- **(1) Etiology.** Allergic contact dermatitis occurs as a direct **T-cell–mediated** response to an exogenous applied allergen. There must be an initial sensitization and then a rechallenge (which may be very small and is not dose-dependent) to elicit a reaction. **Common causes** include poison ivy, oak, or sumac; nickel-containing jewelry and belt buckles; topical lotions and creams; and perfumes and soaps.
- **(2) Clinical features.** Erythematous papules and vesicles occur in the area that came into contact with the allergen.
- **(3) Management.** Treatment involves topical corticosteroids and avoidance of the offending allergen.

    b. Primary irritant contact dermatitis
- **(1) Etiology.** Primary irritant contact dermatitis is caused by caustic substances that irritate the skin, rather than an allergic reaction. No prior sensitization is needed. The reaction is dose-dependent. The **most common type is diaper dermatitis,** a multifactorial disorder caused by prolonged contact with urine and fecal matter, friction, maceration, and proteases contained in the feces. Secondary infection with *Candida albicans* may occur.
- **(2) Clinical features** of diaper dermatitis include erythema with papules on the upper thighs, buttocks, and genitourinary area **without involvement of the inguinal creases.** Involvement of the inguinal creases, more-intense confluent erythema, and satellite lesions all suggest candidal superinfection.
- **(3) Management** of diaper dermatitis includes keeping the skin free from urine and stool, skin moisturizers, barrier creams and ointments (e.g., zinc oxide), and frequent diaper changes. Low-potency corticosteroids may be used for severe inflammation. Candidal infection may be treated with antifungal medication (e.g., nystatin, clotrimazole).

B. Atopic Dermatitis (see Chapter 15, section III)

C. Seborrheic Dermatitis
1. **Epidemiology.** Seborrheic dermatitis predominantly affects two age groups, infants and adolescents.
2. **Etiology.** The cause is **unknown** but may in part be the result of a hypersensitivity reaction to a saprophytic yeast (*Pityrosporum ovale*) that lives in areas that overproduce sebum.
3. **Clinical features.** Eruption of red scales and crusts in areas with high numbers of **sebaceous glands,** such as the scalp, face (including the eyebrows, nose, and beard area), chest, and groin. Skin lesions may be **greasy.**
   - **a. Infants** may have dermatitis limited to the scalp, termed seborrheic capitis, or **cradle cap.** This may also involve the face, upper chest, and flexor creases of the extremities.
   - **b. Adolescents** may have dermatitis in the nasolabial folds, pinna, and scalp.

    4. Management

      a. Low-potency topical corticosteroids

      b. Sulfur, zinc, or salicylic acid-based shampoos may be applied, followed by light scrubbing with a brush to remove crusts. Loose scales may also be removed with mineral oil.

      c. Topical antifungal medication to eradicate *Pityrosporum ovale*

D. Pityriasis Rosea

    1. Epidemiology. Pityriasis rosea is uncommon before 5 years of age but is extremely common during late childhood and adolescence.

    2. Etiology. The cause is unknown, although it clinically appears similar to a hypersensitivity reaction to a virus.

    3. Clinical features

      a. Papulosquamous disorder that begins with a solitary, large 2- to 5-cm scaly, erythematous lesion (**herald patch**) that is usually located on the trunk or extremities. The herald patch is present for 1–30 days.

      b. Approximately 1–2 weeks after the appearance of the herald patch, **oval erythematous macules and papules** erupt for 3–6 weeks from the chin to the mid-thigh, following skin lines in a "**Christmas tree**" distribution on the trunk.

      c. Lesions are pruritic in 50% of cases.

    4. Management. Treatment may include topical or systemic antihistamines. Exposure to ultraviolet light may shorten the disease course.

E. Psoriasis

    1. Epidemiology. Psoriasis occurs in 3% of children in the United States. Although it is more common in adults, 30% of patients develop signs and symptoms during childhood.

    2. Etiology. Childhood-onset psoriasis is often a **genetic disease** with **autosomal dominant inheritance.** It is caused by immune dysregulation, causing epidermal proliferation.

    3. Clinical features

      a. Distribution of skin lesions and severity are variable. If severe, psoriasis may be disfiguring.

      b. Lesions are characterized by **scaling papules and plaques** often found on the scalp (nongreasy scaling without hair loss), ears, elbows, knees, lumbosacral area, and groin. Some lesions have a classic **silvery scale.**

      c. Lesions often demonstrate the **Koebner phenomenon** in which new lesions develop at sites of skin trauma.

      d. Nail involvement is common and may include pits, distal thickening, lifting of the nail bed, and nail destruction.

      e. Arthritis during childhood is uncommon.

    4. Management. Treatment may include moderate- or high-potency corticosteroids, ultraviolet light therapy, analogs of vitamin D, 3% salicylic acid in mineral oil for scalp involvement, retinoids, and anthralin (downregulates epidermal growth factor).

F. Miliaria Rubra (Heat Rash)

1. **Etiology.** Heat rash is caused by **disrupted sweat ducts** near the upper dermis (often caused by occlusion or friction) that result in sweat being released onto the skin. The sweat on the skin produces an inflammatory response. Therefore the more sweat produced and the more occlusion, the more likely heat rash will develop.

2. **Clinical features.** Small erythematous pruritic papules or vesicles occur in areas of occlusion or in areas that have been rubbed, such as the inguinal region, axilla, chest, and neck.

3. **Management.** Treatment is avoidance of occlusive clothing to decrease sweating. Medications are unnecessary.

IV. Hypersensitivity Disorders

A. **Urticaria** (see Chapter 15, section VI).

B. **Serum sickness** may initially appear as urticaria but has systemic signs and symptoms such as fever, arthralgias, and adenopathy and evidence of organ injury. Medications, such as cephalosporins, are common causes.

C. **Erythema Multiforme**

1. **Definition.** Erythema multiforme is a hypersensitivity reaction to many possible stimuli, including drugs, viruses, bacteria, fungi, protozoa, and systemic disease.

2. **Categories.** There are three major categories: **erythema multiforme minor, erythema multiforme major, and Stevens-Johnson syndrome.** The **classic skin lesion** present in all cases is a **target lesion,** a **fixed,** dull red, oval macule with a dusky center that may contain a papule or vesicle. **Table 19-1** summarizes the **causes, clinical features, management, and prognosis** of each type of erythema multiforme.

D. **Toxic Epidermal Necrolysis** is a severe reaction to **drugs** (e.g., anticonvulsants, antibiotics, anti-inflammatory drugs) that results in **widespread epidermal necrosis.** Clinical features include sloughing of the epidermis (usually > 30% skin loss) and severe mucous membrane involvement. No target lesions are usually seen. **Nikolsky sign** (skin peels away with lateral pressure) is often present. Mortality is high (10–30%) as a result of the high incidence of sepsis, dehydration, and electrolyte abnormalities.

V. Infections of the Skin

A. **Fungal (Dermatophyte) Infections**

1. **Epidemiology.** Fungal infections are common during childhood and are most associated with humidity and with urban and crowded living conditions.

2. **Categories.** Fungal infections can involve the hair, skin, or nails.
   a. **Tinea capitis** is a fungal infection of the **hair.**

Table 19-1. Characteristic Features of the Types of Erythema Multiforme

	Erythema Multiforme Minor	Erythema Multiforme Major	Stevens-Johnson Syndrome
Major cause	Herpes simplex virus	*Mycoplasma pneumoniae;* Drugs	Drugs
Skin findings	Symmetric target lesions; acral distribution	Typical symmetric target lesions; acral and truncal distribution	Widespread **atypical, asymmetric** target lesions, blisters, and necrosis
Mucous membrane findings	Occurs in 25%; only one surface involved (often mouth)	At least two mucosal surfaces involved (often mouth and eyes)	At least two mucosal surfaces involved (often mouth and eyes)
Systemic findings	Prodrome of low-grade fever, arthralgias, myalgias	Prodrome of low-grade fever, arthralgias, myalgias	Prodrome of high fever, cough, malaise, headache, arthralgias
Management	Supportive care	Supportive care	Supportive care
	Acyclovir may prevent recurrence	Erythromycin or azithromycin if *M. pneumoniae* is suspected	Stop any offending drug Ophthalmology consultation
		Stop offending drug	Consider steroids, IVIG, burn unit
Prognosis	Good; possible recurrence	Good	High morbidity and mortality (5%)

IVIG = intravenous immune globulin.

(1) Etiology. Tinea capitis is most commonly caused by *Trichophyton tonsurans* (95%), acquired from human-to-human contact, and *Microsporum canis* (5%), acquired from cats and dogs.

(2) Clinical features

(a) Patchy hair loss in which the hairs break off at the scalp (**black dot ringworm**) or in which the broken hairs are thickened and white (seen in *M. canis* infection).

(b) Infected areas may have **scales** and **pustules.**

(c) Kerion (large red boggy nodule) may be present and is a hypersensitivity reaction to the dermatophyte.

(d) Occipital and posterior cervical lymphadenopathy are very suggestive of tinea capitis.

(3) Diagnosis. The basis of diagnosis is microscopic evaluation of hairs with 10% KOH to identify fungal hyphae, or fungal culture. Hairs fluoresce under Woods light if *M. canis* is the infecting organism.

(4) Management. Treatment includes **systemic oral antifungal therapy** (e.g., griseofulvin) for 6–8 weeks. **Topical antifungal agents are ineffective.** Topical 2.5% or 5% selenium sulfide shampoo may reduce infectivity.

b. Fungal infection of the skin may include **tinea corporis** (infection on the body), **tinea pedis** (infection on the foot), and **tinea cruris** (infection in the groin).

(1) Etiology. Pathogens include *M. canis, T. tonsurans,* and other *Trichophyton* species.

(2) Clinical features

(a) Tinea corporis ("ringworm") presents as oval or circular **scaly erythematous patches with partial central clearing.**

(b) Tinea pedis (athlete's foot) presents most commonly in **postpubertal adolescents** with scaling and erythema between the toes or on the plantar aspect of the foot. Vesicles may also be seen.

(c) Tinea cruris presents as scales and erythema in the groin and inguinal creases.

(3) Diagnosis. Clinical features are often the basis of diagnosis. KOH examination of skin scrapings for fungal hyphae or fungal culture can confirm the diagnosis.

(4) Management. Treatment includes topical antifungal medications (e.g., clotrimazole, terbinafine, ketoconazole).

c. Tinea unguium (onychomycosis) is a fungal infection of the nails characterized by thickening and yellow discoloration of one or several nails (usually toenails). Topical management is challenging; treatment requires prolonged therapy and is often unsuccessful. Systemic medications, such as griseofulvin, terbinafine, and ketoconazole, have been used with varying success.

d. Tinea versicolor is a superficial fungal disorder most common in adolescents and young adults. It is caused by *Pityrosporum orbiculare,* a yeast that invades the stratum corneum.

(1) **Clinical features** vary and include fine, scaly oval macules on the trunk, proximal arms, and face. Macules may be hypo- or hyperpigmented and become more prominent with sun exposure. Infection may also be asymptomatic.

(2) **Diagnosis** is by identification of fungal hyphae or circular spores on KOH examination of a scraping of a lesion ("spaghetti and meatballs" appearance), or by yellow or orange fluorescence under Woods light evaluation.

(3) **Management.** Treatment includes overnight application of 2.5% selenium sulfide weekly for 3–4 weeks, ketoconazole shampoo or cream, or systemic antifungal medications.

B. Bacterial infections, including **impetigo, cellulitis, erysipelas, scarlet fever, toxic shock syndrome, and staphylococcal scalded skin syndrome,** are discussed in Chapter 7, section IX.

C. Viral Infections

1. **Viral exanthem** refers to a skin rash associated with a viral infection. Any virus may cause an exanthem, and the rash may take many forms. An **enanthem** (describes involvement of the oral mucosa) may also be present.

   a. **Morbilliform:** measles-like

   b. **Scarlatiniform** (scarlet fever–like): papular, vesicular, and petechial

2. **Measles and rubella** (see Chapter 7, sections XIII.C and D)

3. **Erythema infectiosum (fifth disease)**

   a. **Epidemiology.** Fifth disease is most common in school-age children, although cases can occur at any age.

   b. **Etiology**

      (1) The cause is **parvovirus B19.** Fifth disease is transmitted by respiratory secretions.

      (2) Parvovirus B19 infection may also cause **aplastic crisis** (especially in patients with hemoglobinopathies), **prolonged anemia** in immunosuppressed patients, and **fetal hydrops** or **miscarriage** in pregnant women.

   c. **Clinical features**

      (1) Fifth disease begins with upper respiratory symptoms (cough, fever, rhinorrhea) that are followed 1–2 weeks later by a bright red macular rash on the cheeks ("**slapped-cheek**" appearance) that lasts several days. Patients are generally **no longer contagious when the characteristic facial rash appears.**

      (2) **Lacy, reticular rash** on the trunk and extremities follows the facial rash and generally lasts 3–5 days. In some patients, exercise, heat, or sunlight can induce the lacy rash to recur.

      (3) **Arthralgias** may be present, although they are more common in adults.

   d. **Management.** Treatment is **supportive.** However, intravenous immune globulin may be used treat chronic anemia in immunosuppressed patients.

4. **Roseola infantum (exanthem subitum)**
   a. **Epidemiology.** Roseola is most common in children younger than 2 years of age.
   b. **Etiology.** Roseola is most commonly caused by **human herpes virus 6 and 7.** Other causes include adenovirus, parvovirus B19, and echovirus 16.
   c. **Clinical features.** Roseola begins with 3–5 days of **high fever.** Once the fever resolves, a pink papular eruption occurs on the trunk that generally fades in 24–48 hours.
   d. **Management.** Treatment is **supportive.**

5. **Gianotti-Crosti syndrome (papular acrodermatitis)** most often occurs in children younger than 3 years of age. Gianotti-Crosti is associated with **hepatitis B** infection, Epstein-Barr virus, cytomegalovirus, and coxsackievirus. Clinical features include red or flesh-colored flat-topped papules in the **acral areas** (extremities, buttocks, and cheeks). Skin lesions may last for weeks and may recur. Upper respiratory symptoms may precede the eruption. Treatment is supportive.

6. **Varicella (chickenpox)**
   a. **Epidemiology.** The incidence of varicella has decreased as a result of routine early childhood immunization in many states. Varicella may occur at any age in unimmunized children and adolescents.
   b. **Clinical features**
      (1) Intensely pruritic erythematous macules develop acutely after a **7- to 21-day incubation period.** The macules develop central vesicles within 1–2 days. The classic lesion is described as a "**dew drop on a rose petal,**" or a vesicle on a red background.
      (2) **Crops of lesions** appear during the course of 2–5 days, and the lesions soon crust. Hundreds of vesicles may be present.
      (3) **Fever is common.**
   c. **Management.** Treatment includes antipyretics, cleansing with antibacterial soaps to prevent bacterial superinfection, antihistamines for itching, and monitoring and treating any complications. Acyclovir is generally administered intravenously for patients with varicella pneumonia and encephalitis, orally for those at high risk for complications and topically in the eyes for those with ophthalmic involvement.
   d. **Complications** (Table 19-2)

7. **Herpes simplex virus infection (HSV-1 and HSV-2)**
   a. **Pathophysiology**
      (1) **Neonatal** infection is generally acquired during passage through the birth canal of a mother with primary HSV infection. Two thirds of neonatal infections are caused by HSV-2 and one third are caused by HSV-1.
      (2) **Gingivostomatitis** is the most common HSV infection during infancy and childhood and is almost always caused by HSV-1.
   b. **Clinical features**
      (1) **Characteristic lesions are grouped vesicles on an erythematous base.**

Table 19-2. Complications of Varicella Infection

Bacterial superinfection (often *Staphylococcus aureus*)
Necrotizing fasciitis (group A streptococcus)
Scarring
Reye syndrome (associated with ingestion of salicylates)
Pneumonia
Encephalitis
Acute cerebellar ataxia
Hepatitis
Herpes zoster
Infection during pregnancy:
    Teratogenic effects (congenital varicella syndrome: zigzag scarring of the skin, shortened or malformed extremities, central nervous system damage, and eye abnormalities such as cataracts or chorioretinitis)
    Severe varicella infection in a neonate may develop if mother acquires varicella within one week of delivery

---

    (2) HSV gingivostomatitis presents most often in young infants with grouped vesicles and ulcers on the lips, in the corners of the mouth, and on the tongue. Pain on swallowing, drooling, and fever may be present. Infection lasts 1–2 weeks.

    (3) Neonatal HSV commonly presents in the first week of life with variable signs and symptoms. Neonates may have only a few vesicles at the site (often the scalp) that was in contact with the infecting maternal lesion, or may present with signs and symptoms of sepsis, including apnea, lethargy, irritability, and seizures. **Serious sequelae** include **meningoencephalitis,** hepatitis, sepsis, shock, and death.

    (4) Herpetic whitlow describes HSV-1 infection of the thumb or fingers that is usually secondary to thumb- or finger-sucking by a child with an oral HSV lesion.

    (5) HSV resides in the **dorsal root ganglion** after initial infection and therefore **recurrent HSV infection** may occur. Recurrent HSV lesions are more mild and less symptomatic than primary infection and generally occur on the lip. Fever, sunlight, emotional stress, and trauma may all reactivate the latent virus.

  c. Diagnosis. HSV may be diagnosed by identification of epidermal giant cells on microscopic evaluation of a **Tzanck preparation,** by detection of HSV antigen on direct fluorescent antibody testing, or by culture of the base of the lesion. Polymerase chain reaction (PCR) technology is commonly used to identify HSV in the cerebrospinal fluid.

  d. Management

    (1) Neonatal HSV infection is a **medical emergency** and requires immediate hospitalization and treatment with intravenous acyclovir.

    (2) Cutaneous and oral HSV may be treated with **oral acyclovir,** although treatment must be started promptly to alter the disease course. Oral acyclovir, when given daily, may also prevent recurrent infection.

8. **Hand-foot-mouth disease and herpangina**
   a. **Etiology.** Hand-foot-mouth disease and herpangina are caused by infection with **coxsackievirus types A16 (most common)**, A2, A5, and A10.
   b. **Clinical features** include vesicles, papules, or pustules on the palms, soles, or fingertips and shallow ulcers or erosions on the soft palate or tongue. If only oral lesions are present, the disorder is termed **herpangina.** Fever may occur with both forms.
   c. **Management.** Treatment is supportive.

9. **Warts**
   a. **Etiology.** The cause is **human papillomavirus.**
   b. **Clinical features.** Warts may occur on any skin surface and appear as irregularly shaped discrete flesh-colored papules that may be smooth or rough. Warts often increase in size, are contagious, and may spread to adjacent skin. **Condylomata acuminata** is the term used to describe multiple external warts in the genital area (see Chapter 3, section VII.B.7).
   c. **Management.** Most warts resolve spontaneously within 1–2 years. Treatment to remove warts may include liquid nitrogen, salicylic acid, cantharidin, podophyllin, and surgical excision. Recurrence after any treatment is high.

10. **Molluscum contagiosum**
   a. **Etiology.** The cause is a **poxvirus.**
   b. **Clinical features**
      (1) Small asymptomatic **flesh-colored papules with central umbilication** are characteristic.
      (2) Lesions may be present anywhere on skin with hair follicles, although the face, proximal extremities, and trunk are most commonly involved.
      (3) Lesions are **contagious.**
      (4) **HIV infection** may be associated with extensive eruptions of molluscum.
   c. **Management.** Treatment is often observation with expected resolution without therapy. Removal can be accomplished by curettage or application of podophyllin, trichloroacetic acid, liquid nitrogen, salicylic acid, or cantharidin.

D. **Ectoparasites**
   1. **Louse infestation** may involve the scalp (**head lice**), body (**body lice**), or groin (**pubic lice**).
      a. **Etiology.** Causative organisms include *Pediculus humanus,* the cause of head and body lice, and *Phthirus pubis,* the cause of pubic lice. The louse is a small six-legged insect that attaches to the skin and ingests blood.
      b. **Epidemiology.** Louse infestations are associated with crowded living conditions and sharing of hats, clothes, combs, and hairbrushes.
      c. **Clinical features**
         (1) **Head lice** are associated with **itching.** The **nits** (eggs) may be

seen as oval white bodies attached to the hair shaft. The louse may be found on the scalp.

(2) Body lice are associated with papules and pustules on the trunk with excoriations.

(3) Pubic lice are associated with lice or nits in the groin and black-crusted papules or blue macules (macula cerulea).

d. **Management**

(1) Head lice are treated with 1% permethrin shampoo and a comb to remove the nits. Five percent permethrin and malathion are sometimes used for resistant lice.

(2) Body and pubic lice are treated with a 12-hour application of 1% γ-benzene hexachloride lotion.

2. **Scabies**

a. **Etiology.** Scabies is caused by the mite ***Sarcoptes scabiei.***

b. **Clinical features.** Pruritic papules or vesicles are most commonly located on the abdomen, dorsum of the hands, groin, axilla, flexor surfaces of the wrists, and interdigital spaces. Infants may have facial and neck involvement. **Itching is severe,** and S-shaped **burrows** may be seen.

c. **Diagnosis.** Microscopic examination of a scraping from an unscratched burrow demonstrating the mite, eggs, or mite feces is diagnostic.

d. **Management.** Treatment includes an overnight application of 5% permethrin lotion, or 1% lindane (adolescents and adults only). Scabies is highly contagious, and therefore all household contacts should be treated. Itching may persist for up to 30 days after treatment. All bed sheets, pillowcases, and clothing should be washed in hot water.

VI. Pigmentary Disorders

A. **Hypopigmentation.** Causes include the following:

1. **Postinflammatory hypopigmentation** may follow any skin inflammation (e.g., atopic dermatitis) and generally resolves over months to years.

2. **Pityriasis alba** is thought to be related to atopic dermatitis. It is characterized by hypopigmented, dry, scaly patches, most commonly on the cheeks. Treatment includes moisturizers and mild corticosteroids.

3. **Vitiligo** is a **complete loss of skin pigment** in patchy areas and is caused by melanocyte destruction. Partial repigmentation may sometimes occur. There is no effective treatment, although psoralen combined with ultraviolet light may be helpful.

4. **Oculocutaneous albinism** is caused by a genetic defect in melanin synthesis. Clinical features include white skin and hair, blue eyes, and other eye findings, such as photophobia and nystagmus. There is no treatment.

B. **Neurocutaneous Disorders. Table 19-3** summarizes the clinical features of **tuberous sclerosis and neurofibromatosis.**

Table 19-3. Clinical Features of Neurocutaneous Syndromes

	Tuberous Sclerosis	Neurofibromatosis Type 1 (NF-1)*
Inheritance	Autosomal dominant	Autosomal dominant
Skin findings	**Ash-leaf spots** (hypopigmented macules seen best under Woods light) Angiofibromas on nose or face (**adenoma sebaceum**) **Shagreen patch** (thickened orange peel appearance) Ungual fibromas	**Café-au-lait spots** Axillary or inguinal freckling Plexiform neurofibroma or skin neurofibromas
CNS findings	Seizures (95%), including **infantile spasms** Intracranial calcifications Cortical or subependymal tubers	Optic glioma (usually present by age 3) Intracranial calcifications CNS neurofibromas **Lisch nodules** (iris hamartoma)
Systemic findings	Renal cysts Cardiac rhabdomyomas (**number one cause of neonatal cardiac tumors**) Retinal astrocytoma or hamartoma Mental retardation	Osseous lesions (present by age 1): sphenoid dysplasia or thinning of long bone cortex Scoliosis Hypertension Learning problems

CNS = central nervous system.

Note: Diagnosis of neurofibromatosis type 1 requires two of the following seven clinical findings: six or more café-au-lait spots (≥ 5 mm in children or 15 mm in adults); two or more neurofibromas or one plexiform neurofibroma; freckling in axilla or groin; optic glioma; two or more Lisch nodules; characteristic osseous lesion; first-degree relative with neurofibromatosis type 1.

*Neurofibromatosis type 2 accounts for 10% of all cases of neurofibromatosis and is characterized by bilateral acoustic neuromas. Skin findings of café-au-lait spots and neurofibromas are less common findings as compared with neurofibromatosis type 1.

C. **Nevocellular nevi** are pigmented lesions that may be congenital or acquired.

    1. **Congenital nevi.** These black, brown, tan, or flesh-colored papules or plaques are first detected between birth and 6 months of age. They occur in 1–2% of neonates. **All congenital nevi may have an increased risk of malignancy,** but **giant nevi** (> 20 cm in diameter) have a 6–7% lifetime risk of development of malignant melanoma. Management of giant nevi often includes excision, if possible, and careful observation of all other congenital nevi.

    2. **Acquired nevi** (moles). Peak ages of development are 2–3 years and 11–18 years. Moles are characterized as well-demarcated brown or black papules that increase in size and number during puberty or pregnancy and after sunburn. Most acquired nevi in childhood are **junctional nevi.** The risk of malignant transformation is lower than for congenital nevi. Management is careful observation.

VII. Disorders of the Hair

A. **Alopecia Areata**

    1. **Etiology.** The cause is thought to be autoimmune lymphocyte-mediated injury to the hair follicle.

    2. **Epidemiology.** Alopecia areata affects 1 in 1,000 persons.

    3. **Clinical features**

        a. **Complete hair loss** occurs in one to three sharply demarcated scalp areas without any scalp inflammation. The hair loss is described as occurring suddenly, and the underlying skin is smooth and soft.

        b. Pitting of the nails occurs in 40% of patients.

        c. Subtypes of alopecia areata include **alopecia totalis** (loss of all scalp hair) and **alopecia universalis** (loss of all body and scalp hair).

    4. **Management.** Most patients have regrowth of hair within 1 year without any treatment. Accelerated hair growth may occur with topical or injected corticosteroids and topical minoxidil. Wigs and counseling may be necessary because of the psychological consequences of the significant hair loss.

B. **Tinea capitis** is a common cause of hair loss (see section V.A.2).

C. **Traumatic alopecia** is also a common cause of childhood hair loss and may be one of two types:

    1. **Trichotillomania** is hair loss that occurs as a result of **conscious or unconscious pulling or twisting of hair**. Clinical features include irregularly bordered areas of hair loss in which hairs are broken off at different lengths. Scalp may show perifollicular petechiae and excoriations. Eyelashes and eyebrows may also be involved. The cause is unknown, although it may be associated with anxiety. Management includes stress relief, a search for precipitating events, and application of oils to make the hairs more difficult to pull out.

    2. **Traction alopecia** is hair loss caused by constant traction or friction and may be the result of tight hair braids or curlers, vigorous scalp massage, or constant rubbing. Clinical features include patchy areas of alope-

cia with thinned, small hairs, but with few broken hairs. Management is to stop the inciting trauma.

D. Telogen effluvium is the second most common type of alopecia, after male pattern baldness. It is caused by any **acutely stressful event** (e.g., pregnancy, surgery, acute illness, trauma) that converts hairs from a growing phase (**anagen**) to a final resting phase (**telogen**). Clinical features include complaints of **generalized excessive hair loss** (hair loss > 100 hairs per day; normal hair loss is 50–100 hairs per day) 2–3 months after the precipitating event. Hair loss continues for 3–4 months, and then spontaneous regrowth occurs.

E. Other conditions that cause hair loss include hypothyroidism, diabetes mellitus, hypopituitarism, nutrition disorders (e.g., hypervitaminosis A, zinc deficiency, marasmus), medications (e.g., warfarin, heparin, chemotherapy, cyclophosphamide), ectodermal dysplasia, and hair shaft structural defects.

VIII. Acne Vulgaris. Acne is the **most common skin disease,** and its sequelae may include scarring and disfigurement and adverse effects on psychosocial development, such as depression and other emotional problems.

A. Pathophysiology. Acne is caused by a combination of the following processes:

1. Excessive shedding and cohesion of cells that line the sebaceous follicles located on the chest, back, and face

2. Production of **sebum** by sebaceous glands under the influence of androgens. Obstruction of sebum outflow from the follicle leads to the formation of **comedones.**

3. **Inflammation as a result of the proliferation of the bacteria, *Propionibacterium acnes.***

B. Clinical Features

1. Acne begins 1–2 years before puberty.

2. **Noninflammatory acne** is characterized by **open comedones** (blackheads) and **closed comedones** (whiteheads).

3. **Inflammatory acne** is characterized by erythematous papules, pustules, nodules, and cysts.

4. Most patients have a combination of inflammatory and noninflammatory acne.

C. Management. Treatment is individualized based on the disease severity and on the location and type of lesions.

1. Topical benzoyl peroxide, tretinoin (Retin-A), and salicylic acid are effective for noninflammatory acne and mild inflammatory acne.

2. Antibiotics (oral or topical) and benzoyl peroxide are effective for inflammatory acne.

3. **Systemic isotretinoin (Accutane)** is highly effective for all types of acne, including nodular and cystic acne. Women must be tested for pregnancy before treatment and must use effective birth control during treatment to prevent pregnancy because of the risk of **teratogenic effects** associated with its use.

Review Test

1. A 1-week-old female infant has several vesicles on her scalp. She also has a 1-day history of fever to 100.8°F (38.2°C) and irritability. She is breastfed and is eating slightly less vigorously than usual. The mother's pregnancy was uncomplicated. Which of the following statements regarding the presumptive diagnosis is correct?

(A) Herpes simplex virus type 1 is the most likely causative pathogen.
(B) The infection was likely acquired after birth.
(C) A Tzanck smear of the base of one of the vesicles may demonstrate epidermal giant cells.
(D) Oral acyclovir should be started immediately.
(E) Oral antibiotics to cover staphylococcal and streptococcal infection should be started promptly.

2. A 9-year-old girl is brought the office by her parents. She has a 1-month history of two large well-demarcated areas of hair loss in the parietal scalp. On examination, no inflammation of the skin is apparent, and the underlying skin is smooth and soft. Which of the following statements regarding the likely diagnosis is correct?

(A) The fingernails are likely to be normal.
(B) Stress is not a likely cause of the disorder.
(C) Oral griseofulvin should be prescribed after cultures.
(D) Zinc should be prescribed for suspected zinc deficiency.
(E) The hair loss is likely to be permanent.

3. A 6-year-old boy presents with a 1-month history of patchy alopecia in the occipital region of the scalp. Examination reveals a well-circumscribed area of hair loss in which all the hairs appear to be broken off at the scalp surface. Occipital lymph nodes are prominent. Which of the following statements regarding the likely diagnosis is correct?

(A) This infection is contagious, and brushes, combs, and hats should not be shared.
(B) Topical management with clotrimazole is the initial appropriate treatment.
(C) Exposure to dogs or cats is the likely cause of infection.
(D) Hairs will likely fluoresce under Woods light examination.
(E) Oral antifungal therapy should be administered for 2 weeks.

4. A 5-year-old boy presents with a 6-week history of scaling, nongreasy papules and plaques in the occipital region of the scalp and in the inguinal region. The lesions have a "silvery scale" appearance. Which of the following statements regarding the likely disorder is correct?

(A) Low-potency corticosteroids are indicated.
(B) It would be unusual for other family members to also have this disorder.
(C) New lesions would be expected to develop at any site of skin trauma.
(D) Hair loss is associated with scalp involvement.
(E) Arthritis is expected.

5. A 10-year-old girl presents with a history of malaise and a headache that was followed 4 days later with a body rash. Examination reveals a 3-cm scaly erythematous plaque on the upper arm and oval, red macules and papules on the back that follow skin lines. Which of the following management steps is most appropriate?

(A) Low-potency topical corticosteroids
(B) Moderate- to high-potency topical corticosteroids
(C) Topical clotrimazole
(D) Oral antibiotics
(E) Reassurance only

6. A 4-month-old male infant is brought to the office by his parents for a routine health maintenance examination. On examination, you note significant hyperpigmentation in the inguinal area. Medical history is remarkable for suspected diaper dermatitis treated with zinc oxide and high-potency corticosteroids for 3 weeks. Which of the following statements regarding this patient and his clinical findings is most correct?

(A) Topical antifungal therapy should now be prescribed to treat suspected fungal superinfection.

(B) Zinc oxide should be immediately discontinued.

(C) Atrophy of skin in the inguinal area may also be present.

(D) The hyperpigmentation is not associated with any systemic problems.

(E) Ultraviolet light therapy should be prescribed.

7. A 4-year-old boy with a history of atopic dermatitis presents for evaluation of his skin. Examination shows that the skin on his upper and lower extremities is very dry and irritated. You would like to suggest a moisturizer in addition to topical corticosteroids. Which of the following types of moisturizers is most appropriate?

(A) Lotion
(B) Cream
(C) Ointment
(D) Solution
(E) Gel

8. A 13-year-old boy is brought to the office by his parents because of concerns regarding his acne. Examination reveals scattered open and closed comedones on the forehead and nose. Which of the following statements regarding this condition is correct?

(A) Topical benzoyl peroxide is an appropriate first-line treatment.

(B) Oral isotretinoin is an appropriate first-line treatment.

(C) Oral clindamycin is an appropriate first-line treatment.

(D) Sebum plays little role in the pathophysiology at this stage.

(E) Reassurance only should be given because the patient's skin findings are currently of little consequence.

For statements 9–13, the response options are the same. You will be required to select one answer for each statement in the set.

(A) Papule
(B) Macule
(C) Pustule
(D) Nodule
(E) Vesicle
(F) Cyst
(G) Wheal
(H) Target lesion
(I) Plaque

Match the disorder with its most characteristic skin lesion.

9. A 3-year-old boy with herpes simplex virus infection involving the upper and lower lips.

10. A 7-year-old boy with suspected vitiligo involving both hands.

11. A 15-month-old girl with molluscum contagiosum on the cheeks and forehead.

12. A 6-year-old boy with erythema multiforme major.

13. A 10-year-old girl with suspected Gianotti-Crosti syndrome.

For statements 14 and 15, the response options are the same. You will be required to select one answer for each statement in the set.

(A) Neurofibromatosis type 1
(B) Neurofibromatosis type 2
(C) Tuberous sclerosis

For each patient, select the most likely associated neurocutaneous syndrome.

14. A 3-year-old boy with seizures and Lisch nodules on ophthalmologic examination.

15. A 12-month-old infant with infantile spasms.

Answers and Explanations

1. The answer is C [V.C.7.c–d]. This patient's clinical presentation is most consistent with neonatal herpes simplex virus (HSV) infection. Diagnosis is by identification of (1) the virus by culture or (2) the viral antigen by rapid testing techniques. Infection may also be diagnosed by identification of epidermal giant cells on a Tzanck preparation. Two thirds of herpes simplex infections acquired during the neonatal period are caused by HSV-2, and this infection is most often acquired during passage through the birth canal of a mother infected with the virus. Neonatal HSV is a medical emergency that requires prompt admission and management with intravenous acyclovir. Oral antibiotics are not useful.

2. The answer is B [VII.A]. This patient's presentation with well-demarcated hair loss without scalp inflammation is likely caused by alopecia areata. The cause of alopecia areata is thought to be an autoimmune lymphocyte-mediated injury to the hair follicle. Stress is not likely to cause this form of alopecia. Associated findings include nail pitting in 40% of patients. The clinical presentation is neither consistent with tinea capitis nor zinc deficiency; therefore, neither griseofulvin nor zinc is indicated. Regrowth of hair within 1 year occurs in the majority of patients.

3. The answer is A [V.A.2.a]. Clinical features of alopecia with hairs broken off at the scalp and occipital lymphadenopathy suggest tinea capitis, a fungal infection of the hair. The most common causal pathogen is *Trichophyton tonsurans,* acquired from human-to-human contact, including by sharing hats, brushes, and combs. Topical antifungal therapy is ineffective for tinea capitis. Dogs and cats are a source of infection with *Microsporum canis,* which currently causes only 5% of tinea capitis infections. Infection with *M. canis* is characterized by thickened, white broken hairs, and only hairs infected with *M. canis* fluoresce under Woods light. Treatment of tinea capitis involves 6–8 weeks of oral antifungal therapy.

4. The answer is C [III.E.3]. Skin lesions with a silvery scale appearance suggest psoriasis. Lesions of psoriasis may also demonstrate the Koebner phenomenon, in which new lesions develop at sites of skin injury. Corticosteroids must be moderate or high potency to be effective as treatment agents. Psoriasis is inherited in an autosomal dominant fashion, and therefore other family members may also have the disorder. Involvement of the scalp is common; however, associated alopecia is uncommon. Arthritis is uncommon during childhood.

5. The answer is E [III.D.3–4]. This patient's clinical presentation and examination findings are consistent with pityriasis rosea. Pityriasis rosea may be a hypersensitivity reaction to a viral infection, although its true cause is unknown. Pityriasis rosea resolves without medications, although antihistamines may relieve any associated itching.

6. The answer is C [I.D.6.a]. The hyperpigmentation in the inguinal region is most likely a side effect of the high-potency corticosteroid therapy. Only low-potency corticosteroids should be applied to the groin because of the thinness of the epidermis of the groin; absorption of corticosteroids is greater in this area. Systemic side effects may occur, including growth suppression, Cushing syndrome, and adrenal suppression. Local side effects include pigmentation changes, atrophy, acne, folliculitis, and telangiectasias. Neither antifungal medications nor ultraviolet light is indicated. Discontinuation of zinc oxide will not affect this patient's skin findings.

7. The answer is C [I.D.2]. Adequate hydration of the skin is crucial in many dermatologic conditions, especially atopic dermatitis. Ointments are especially useful for very dry skin because they have maximal water-retaining properties and would be the best choice for this patient. Lotions are helpful for minimal dryness, and creams are useful for average dryness. Both solutions and gels are most useful for surfaces with hair.

8. The answer is A [VIII.C]. This patient's skin findings are consistent with acne. The open and closed comedones are characteristic of noninflammatory acne, and a topical agent is most appropriate. Benzoyl peroxide is very effective for both noninflammatory and inflammatory acne and is the most appropriate initial treatment for this patient. Neither oral antibiotics nor isotretinoin is a first-line treatment for noninflammatory acne. Oral antibiotics are most useful in inflammatory acne. Systemic isotretinoin is helpful in all types of acne; however, it is most beneficial in severe cystic or nodular acne. Obstruction to sebum outflow from the follicle leads to comedone development and therefore is important in the pathophysiology. Acne should never be dismissed as of no consequence, even in the early stages, because it may be associated with future scarring and may have effects on a child's psychosocial development.

9–13. The answers are E, B, A, H, and A, respectively [V.C.7.b, VI.A.3, V.C.10.b.(1), IV.C.2, V.C.5, Table 19-1]. Herpes simplex virus is characterized by grouped vesicles on an erythematous base. Vitiligo is a depigmentation disorder characterized by hypopigmented macules. Molluscum contagiosum is characterized by flesh-colored papules with central umbilication. Erythema multiforme major is characterized by target lesions. Red or flesh-colored papules are characteristic of Gianotti-Crosti syndrome.

14–15. The answers are A and C, respectively [Table 19-3]. The 3-year-old boy has neurofibromatosis type 1, which is characterized by café-au-lait spots, axillary freckling, and neurofibromas in the skin and other organs. Seizures may occur because of central nervous system involvement that may include intracranial calcifications, neurofibromas, and optic glioma. Characteristic eye findings include Lisch nodules or iris hamartomas. The 12-month-old infant has tuberous sclerosis, which is associated with characteristic skin findings including ash-leaf spots, angiofibromas, and Shagreen patch. Almost all children with tuberous sclerosis have seizures, including infantile spasms, because of central nervous system involvement.

20

Emergency Medicine

Calvin G. Lowe, M.D.

I. Infant and Child Cardiopulmonary Resuscitation (CPR)

A. **General Concepts**

1. The **most common cause of cardiac arrest in a child** is a **lack of oxygen supply** to the heart secondary to a pulmonary problem (e.g., choking, suffocation, airway or lung disease, near drowning), respiratory arrest, or shock. Cardiac arrest can often be prevented if assisted breathing is initiated promptly.

2. **Heart disease is an uncommon cause of cardiac arrest** in infants and children.

3. **Chances for survival increase dramatically** if CPR and advanced life support are begun quickly.

B. **Essentials of CPR are the ABCs: A̲irway, B̲reathing, and C̲irculation.**

1. **Airway**

   a. **First priority** in resuscitation is to **open the victim's airway.**

   b. The **victim's tongue** is the most common cause of airway obstruction.

   c. The **airway** may be opened by the **head-tilt method,** which lifts the tongue from the back of the throat, or by the **jaw-thrust method** if the child has suspected **neck or cervical spine injury.** (Cervical spine injury should be suspected in face, head, or neck trauma.)

2. **Breathing**

   a. **After the airway is opened,** assessment for breathing is performed by the **look, listen, and feel method,** in which the rescuer **looks** for a rise and fall in the chest, **listens** for exhaled air, and **feels** for exhaled airflow.

   b. **Rescue breathing** must be performed if spontaneous breathing is absent.

3. **Circulation**

   a. **Need for chest compressions** should be determined after two rescue breaths.

    b. Pulse is assessed in the **brachial artery** for **infants** and in the **carotid artery** for children.

    c. Chest compressions are administered for asystole or bradycardia.

II. Shock

A. General Concepts

    1. Definition. Shock is a clinical state characterized by **inadequate delivery of oxygen and metabolic substrates to meet the metabolic demands of tissues.**

    2. Shock may be present with **normal or decreased blood pressure.**

B. Classification. Shock may be classified by the degree of compensation and by the cause.

    1. Shock may be **compensated, decompensated, or irreversible.**

        a. Compensated shock is characterized by **normal blood pressure** and cardiac output with **adequate tissue perfusion** but **maldistributed blood flow** to essential organs.

        b. Decompensated shock is characterized by **hypotension,** low cardiac output, and **inadequate tissue perfusion.**

        c. Irreversible shock is characterized by **cell death** and is **refractory** to medical treatment.

    2. Shock may also be classified on the basis of the cause.

        a. Hypovolemic shock is the **most common cause** of shock in children and is caused by any condition that results in decreased circulating blood volume, such as **hemorrhage** or **dehydration** (e.g., from acute gastroenteritis). The amount of volume loss determines the success of compensatory mechanisms, such as **endogenous catecholamines,** in maintaining blood pressure and cardiac output. Volume losses greater than 25% result in decompensated shock.

        b. Septic shock occurs secondary to an inflammatory response to invading microorganisms and their toxins and results in abnormal blood distribution. There are two clinical stages:

            (1) Hyperdynamic stage is characterized by normal or high cardiac output with **bounding pulses,** warm extremities, and a wide pulse pressure.

            (2) Decompensated stage follows the hyperdynamic stage if aggressive treatment has not been initiated. It is characterized clinically by impaired mental status, cool extremities, and diminished pulses.

        c. Distributive shock is associated with distal pooling of blood or fluid extravasation, and is typically caused by anaphylactic or neurogenic shock, or as a result of medications or toxins.

            (1) Anaphylactic shock is characterized by acute angioedema of the upper airway, bronchospasm, pulmonary edema, urticaria, and hypotension because of extravasation of intravascular fluid from permeable capillaries (see Chapter 15, section I).

            (2) Neurogenic shock, typically secondary to spinal cord transection or injury, is characterized by a total loss of distal sympathetic cardiovascular tone with hypotension resulting from pooling of blood within the vascular bed.

    d. Cardiogenic shock occurs when cardiac output is limited because of primary cardiac dysfunction. Causes include dysrhythmias (e.g., supraventricular tachycardia), congenital heart disease (e.g., any lesion that impairs left ventricular outflow), and cardiac dysfunction after cardiac surgery. Clinical features are the signs and symptoms of congestive heart failure (CHF; see Chapter 8, section I.D).

C. Diagnosis

1. **Recognition of shock may be difficult** because of the presence of compensatory mechanisms that prevent hypotension until 25% of intravascular volume is lost. **Therefore, the index of suspicion for shock must be high.**

2. **Historic features** that may suggest the presence of shock include:
   - a. **Severe vomiting and diarrhea**
   - b. **Trauma with hemorrhage**
   - c. **Febrile illness,** especially in an immunocompromised patient
   - d. **Symptoms of CHF**
   - e. **Exposure to a known allergic antigen**
   - f. **Spinal cord injury**

3. **Physical examination**
   - a. **Blood pressure may be normal** in the initial stages of hypovolemic and septic shock.
   - b. **Tachycardia almost always accompanies shock** and occurs before blood pressure changes in children.
   - c. **Tachypnea** may be present as a compensatory mechanism for severe metabolic acidosis.
   - d. **Mental status changes** may indicate poor cerebral perfusion.
   - e. **Capillary refill** may be prolonged with cool and mottled extremities.
   - f. **Peripheral pulses** may be **bounding** in early septic shock.

4. **Laboratory studies** should include:
   - a. **Complete blood count (CBC)** to assess for blood loss and infection.
   - b. **Electrolytes** to assess for metabolic acidosis and electrolyte abnormalities.
   - c. **Blood urea nitrogen and creatinine** to evaluate renal function and perfusion.
   - d. **Calcium and glucose** to assess for frequently encountered metabolic derangements.
   - e. **Coagulation factors** to evaluate for disseminated intravascular coagulation (DIC), which may accompany shock.
   - f. **Toxicology screens** to evaluate for a poisoning, which could cause shock.

D. Management

1. **Initial resuscitation** involves the **ABCs,** including:
   - a. **Supplemental oxygen**
   - b. **Early endotracheal intubation** to secure the airway and decrease the patient's energy expenditure

   c. **Vascular access** with appropriate **fluid resuscitation.** Fluids should initially include a 20 mL/kg bolus of normal saline or lactated Ringer's solution.

2. **To restore intravascular volume, intravenous crystalloid or colloid** solutions should generally be used before administration of inotropic and vasopressor agents.

3. **Inotropic and vasopressor medications** (e.g., dobutamine, dopamine, epinephrine) are indicated if the blood pressure increase in response to fluids is inadequate.

4. **Metabolic derangements,** such as metabolic acidosis, hypocalcemia, or hypoglycemia, should be treated.

5. **Other considerations** include administration of **broad-spectrum antibiotics** for septic shock, **blood products** for hemorrhage, and **fresh-frozen plasma** for DIC.

III. Trauma

A. **General Concepts**

1. **Trauma is the leading cause of death** in children older than 1 year of age.

2. **Motor vehicle accidents are the leading cause of trauma.**

3. **Anatomic and physiologic differences** between a child and an adult account for the child's unique response to trauma.

   a. **Head injuries** are **common** because a child's head comprises a **larger percentage of total body mass.**

   b. The **neck** of a child is **shorter** and supports a relatively **greater weight.**

   c. The **rib cage** of a child is more pliable, leading to greater energy transmitted to internal organs, such as the **spleen** and **liver.**

   d. The **growth plates** in the bones of a growing child result in a relatively **weak epiphyseal-metaphyseal junction.** Ligaments are stronger than the growth plate, and therefore with injury the **growth plate is at the highest risk of injury.**

B. **Primary Survey.** This rapid initial assessment of the patient should be performed within 5–10 minutes of arrival in the emergency department. The primary survey can be recalled using the mnemonic **ABCDEs:** <u>**A**</u>**irway** maintenance, <u>**B**</u>**reathing** and ventilation with 100% oxygen, <u>**C**</u>**irculation** and control of hemorrhage, <u>**D**</u>**isability** assessment using the **Glasgow coma score (GCS;** the GCS is used to assess the extent of neurologic impairment based on physical examination [Table 20-1]), and <u>**E**</u>**xposure/**<u>**En**</u>**vironmental** control in which the patient is undressed completely to facilitate examination and then warmed to prevent hypothermia.

C. **Adjuncts to the primary survey**

1. **Electrocardiographic (ECG) monitoring** is mandatory for all patients.

   a. **Dysrhythmias** may indicate cardiac injury.

Table 20-1. Glasgow Coma Scale (GCS)*

Verbal Patient	GCS Score	Nonverbal Patient (Child)
Eye opening		
Spontaneously	4	Spontaneously
Response to voice	3	Response to voice
Response to pain	2	Response to pain
No response	1	No response
Best motor response		
Obeys commands	6	Normal movements
Localizes pain	5	Localizes pain
Flexion withdrawal	4	Flexion withdrawal
Decorticate posturing	3	Flexion abnormal
Decerebrate posturing	2	Extension abnormal
No response	1	No response
Best verbal response		
Oriented/appropriate	5	Cries normally, smiles, and coos
Disoriented conversation	4	Cries
Inappropriate words	3	Inappropriate crying and screaming
Incomprehensible words	2	Grunts
No response	1	No response

*This scale is used to assess the level of neurologic impairment on the basis of a patient's physical examination (eye opening, motor response, and verbal response). A GCS of 13–15 indicates mild head injury; GCS of 9–12 indicates moderate head injury; GCS < 8 indicates severe head injury.

      b. Pulseless electrical activity may indicate cardiac tamponade, tension pneumothorax, or profound hypovolemia.

  2. A **urinary catheter** and **nasogastric tube** should be placed to monitor urine output and to reduce abdominal distension.

  3. Diagnostic studies typically include **radiographs of the cervical spine, chest, and pelvis and computed tomographic (CT) scans of the head and abdomen.**

 D. Secondary Survey. This head-to-toe evaluation includes a complete history and thorough physical examination.

 E. Specific injuries in the pediatric trauma patient

  1. Head trauma

    a. Seizures are **common** after head trauma but are **self-limited.**

    b. Infants are at risk for bleeding in the **subgaleal** and **epidural spaces** because of **open fontanelles and cranial sutures.** However, these open structures also allow infants to be more tolerant of expanding intracranial masses.

    c. Intracranial bleeding may occur in the epidural space, subdural space, or within the brain parenchyma itself after even mild head trauma without skull fracture or loss of consciousness.

      (1) Epidural hematoma is bleeding between the inner table of the skull and the dura. It is associated with tearing of the **middle meningeal artery.**

        (a) Clinical features are the signs and symptoms of increased intracranial pressure (ICP; see section III.E.1.d).

   (b) Diagnosis is by **head CT,** which shows a **lenticular density** representing blood within the epidural space.

   (c) Management is immediate surgical drainage.

   (d) Prognosis is generally good if surgery can be performed rapidly.

  (2) Subdural hematoma is blood beneath the dura. It is associated with tearing of the bridging **meningeal veins** by direct trauma or shaking. It is **more common than epidural hematoma** and is seen most commonly in infancy.

   (a) Clinical features include seizures and signs and symptoms of increased ICP (see section III.E.1.d). Subdural hematomas are bilateral in 75% of cases, and symptoms develop more slowly than with an epidural bleed.

   (b) Diagnosis is by **head CT,** which shows a **crescentic density** representing blood in the subdural space.

   (c) Management includes neurosurgical consultation and usually surgical drainage.

   (d) Prognosis may be **poor** if the underlying brain is also injured.

  (3) Intracerebral hematoma is bleeding within the brain parenchyma. Frontal and temporal lobes are most often affected, usually on the opposite side of the impact injury (**contrecoup injury**). Management is surgical drainage if the hematoma is accessible.

 d. Increased ICP (see Chapter 12, section II.D)

  (1) Clinical features

   (a) Headache is the **first symptom.**

   (b) Pupillary changes and **altered mental status** are the **first signs.**

   (c) Table 20-2 lists the clinical features of increased ICP.

  (2) Complications. Increased ICP may lead to cerebral herniation, most commonly **transtentorial or uncal herniation** in which the temporal lobe or uncus is displaced into the infratentorial compartment. Clinical features of herniation include:

   (a) Bradycardia, which is an **early sign of herniation in children younger than 4 years of age**

Table 20-2. Symptoms and Signs of Elevated Intracranial Pressure

Symptom	Sign
Headache	Papilledema
Vomiting	Cranial nerve palsies
Stiff neck	Stiff neck
Double vision	Head tilt
Transient loss of vision	Retinal hemorrhage
Episodic severe headache	Macewen's sign*
Gait disturbance	Obtundation
Dulled intellect	Unconsciousness
Irritability	Progressive hemiparesis

*Macewen's sign is hyperresonance of the skull on percussion.

       (b) Fixed and dilated ipsilateral pupil

       (c) Contralateral hemiparesis

       (d) Pupils will eventually become bilaterally fixed and dilated. Bilateral hemiparesis will also eventually occur.

       (e) Cushing's triad, a late sign, is characterized by **bradycardia, hypertension,** and **irregular breathing**.

      (3) Management. The goal of treatment is to prevent secondary brain injury and includes:

       (a) Mild hyperventilation with **100% oxygen** to lower $PaCO_2$ to 30–35 mm Hg, which in turn mildly vasoconstricts cerebral vessels. Aggressive hyperventilation can lead to worsening cerebral ischemia.

       (b) Elevation of the head to 30°–45°, which encourages venous drainage.

       (c) Diuretics (e.g., mannitol)

       (d) Neurosurgical consultation

  2. Spinal cord injury. Injury to the spinal cord may occur in children. Even in the presence of serious injury, radiographs of the cord may be normal (**spinal cord injury without radiographic abnormality [SCIWORA]**). SCIWORA occurs more commonly in children than in adults.

  3. Chest trauma

    a. A child's **soft and pliable chest wall** allows transmission of forces to the lung parenchyma.

    b. Tension pneumothorax may occur and is **life-threatening.**

      (1) Clinical features include **distended neck veins, decreased breath sounds,** hyperresonance to percussion, **displaced trachea,** pulseless electrical activity, and shock.

      (2) Management is emergent chest decompression by needle thoracotomy. **Waiting for radiographic confirmation of the diagnosis can lead to a patient's death.**

  4. Abdominal trauma is common because of underdeveloped abdominal musculature.

    a. Duodenal hematoma often occurs secondary to injury to the right upper quadrant, commonly from a **bicycle handle bar.** Clinical features include abdominal pain and vomiting. Bowel obstruction is found on radiographic evaluation.

    b. Lap belt injuries from a motor vehicle accident include a **chance fracture** (flexion disruption of the lumbar spine), liver and spleen lacerations, and bowel perforation.

    c. Spleen, liver, and kidneys are often injured by blunt trauma.

IV. Burns

  A. Epidemiology. Burns are the **second most common cause of accidental death in children**.

    1. Scalding injuries from hot liquids are the **most common type of burn.**

2. **Not all burns are accidental, and child abuse should be considered** (see section VI.B.2.c).

B. **Classification** of burns is on the basis of **degree** (depth of skin injured) and **body surface area** (BSA).

1. **First-degree burns** involve only the **epidermis** and are characterized by **red, blanching, painful skin** that heals without scarring (e.g., sunburn).

2. **Second-degree burns** (partial-thickness burns) involve the **entire epidermis and part of the dermis.**

   a. **Superficial partial-thickness burns** involve the entire epidermis and outer portion of the dermis. Burns are moist, painful, and red. They **blister** but usually do not scar.

   b. **Deep partial-thickness burns** involve destruction of the entire epidermis and lower portion of the dermis. Burns are **pale white.** They may **blister** and they heal **with scarring.**

3. **Third-degree burns or full-thickness burns** involve the **complete destruction of the epidermis, dermis, and part of the subcutaneous tissue.** Burns are **dry, white, and leathery** to the touch, and skin grafts are needed. Because nerve endings are burned, the victim is usually **insensitive to pain.**

4. **BSA** burned is expressed in a percentage. The Lund-Browder classification may be used to help measure the burned area. Although the "rule of 9s" is used to measure percent BSA burned in adolescents and adults (each arm = 9%, each leg = 18%, anterior trunk = 18%, posterior trunk = 18%, head and neck = 9%), this rule overestimates burns in a child because of a child's relatively larger head and smaller legs. A more approximate estimate of percent BSA burned uses the size of the patient's palm to measure the burned area; the palm is approximately equivalent to 1% BSA.

C. Management

1. **Initial resuscitation** should include the **ABCs.**

   a. **Endotracheal intubation** should be performed in any victim suspected of **inhaling** hot gases, which may burn the upper airway and lead to progressive edema and airway obstruction.

   b. **Assess oxygenation** by pulse oximetry; administer 100% oxygen and assess for carbon monoxide inhalation (see section VIII.D.6).

   c. **Intravenous access** should be obtained through nonburned skin.

2. **Fluid resuscitation** is **critical,** because large volumes of fluid may be lost from burned skin and leaky capillaries.

3. **Skin care** depends on the degree of burn.

   a. **First-degree burns** require only moisturizers and analgesics.

   b. **Second-degree burns** require appropriate analgesics (e.g., opiates) and debridement of dead skin to prevent infection. Bullae (large blisters), if intact, are generally not removed because the skin of the bullae forms a barrier to infection and prevents fluid loss. Bullae that have ruptured should be removed.

    c. **Third-degree burns** require skin grafting and hydrotherapy. **Escharotomy** (i.e., surgical removal of a constricting scar) may be needed if the burn restricts blood flow or chest expansion.

    d. **Antibiotics,** usually topical 1% silver sulfadiazine, are applied to second- and third-degree burns to decrease the risk of infection.

  4. **Hospitalization** is required for partial-thickness burns > 10% BSA, full-thickness burns > 2% BSA, burns to specific areas of the body (e.g., face, perineum, hands, feet, burns overlying a joint, or circumferential burns), suspected inhalation injury, and suspected nonaccidental trauma (i.e., inflicted burn).

V. Near Drowning

  A. **Definition.** A **near drowner** is a victim who survives, sometimes only temporarily, after asphyxia while submerged in a liquid.

  B. **Epidemiology. Submersion-related injuries** are the **fifth leading cause of death** in the United States. There is a bimodal age distribution in childhood.

    1. **Older infants and toddlers** who may wander into unfenced pools or tip over into water containers (e.g., toilets and buckets)

    2. **Adolescents,** most commonly males, whose submersion injury is typically associated with alcohol or drug ingestion

  C. **Pathophysiology**

    1. **Victims** may suffer asphyxia from aspirating liquid (wet drowner) or from laryngospasm (dry drowner).

    2. **Both fresh and salt water drowning** result in denaturing of surfactant, alveolar instability and collapse, and pulmonary edema.

    3. The end result is decreased pulmonary compliance, increased airway resistance, increased pulmonary artery pressures, and impaired gas exchange.

  D. **Clinical Features**

    1. **Respirations** may be absent or irregular, and the victim may cough up **pink, frothy material.**

      a. **Physical examination** may reveal rales, rhonchi, and wheezes.

      b. **Pneumonia** from **aspiration of fluid containing mouth flora** may develop **after 24 hours.**

      c. **Slow deterioration** of pulmonary function (e.g., hypoxemia and hypercarbia) may occur during the first 12–24 hours.

    2. **Neurologic** insult (hypoxic central nervous system [CNS] injury) is directly related to the length and severity of the hypoxia. The victim may appear alert initially or may be agitated, combative, or comatose.

    3. **Cardiovascular** abnormalities include dysrhythmias and myocardial ischemia.

    4. **Hematologic** abnormalities include hemolysis and DIC.

    5. **Renal failure** may occur.

E. **Management.** Treatment is the **same regardless of whether the near drowning occurred in salt or fresh water.**

1. **Initial resuscitation** includes the **ABCs,** cervical spine immobilization (because of the possibility of coexistent head trauma), and removal of wet clothing to reduce heat loss.

2. **Intubation and mechanical ventilation** with high positive end-expiratory pressures (PEEP) are indicated for patients with respiratory failure.

3. **Rewarming** of body core with warm saline gastric lavage, bladder washings, or peritoneal lavage should be performed if needed. In severely hypothermic patients, resuscitation should continue until patient is rewarmed to 32°C (89.6°F).

4. **Attention** should be paid to fluid and electrolyte imbalance.

F. **Prognosis.** In general, children have a better outcome from near drowning because their primitive dive reflex shunts blood to vital organs, such as the heart, brain, and liver. However, prognosis is poor for the following victims:

1. **Children younger than 3 years of age**

2. **Submersion time > 5 minutes**

3. **Resuscitation delay > 10 minutes**

4. **Cardiopulmonary resuscitation required**

5. **Abnormal neurologic examination or seizures**

6. **Arterial blood pH < 7**

VI. Child Abuse

A. **General Concepts**

1. In most states, health-care personnel have a **legal obligation to report suspected child abuse or neglect** to appropriate protective service or law enforcement agencies.

2. The **index for suspicion of abuse should be high,** especially in situations in which injuries found on examination are unaccounted for or are inconsistent with the caregiver's history or the child's developmental abilities.

3. Child abuse includes **physical abuse, psychological abuse, neglect, and sexual assault.**

B. **Physical Abuse**

1. **Epidemiology**

a. **Any child is at risk for abuse. The risk of abuse is greatest,** however, in children with the following characteristics:

(1) **Age younger than 4 years,** especially younger than 1 year

(2) **Mental retardation,** developmental delay, severe handicaps, hyperactivity, or challenging temperament (including colic or frequent tantrums)

       (3) **History** of premature birth, low birth weight, neonatal separation from parents, or multiple births

       (4) **Chronic illness**

  b. Child abusers come from all socioeconomic, cultural, and ethnic groups. **Risk factors** for an **abusive caregiver** include the following:

       (1) **Low self-esteem, social isolation, depression, or history of substance abuse**

       (2) **History of abuse as a child**

       (3) **History of mental illness**

       (4) **History of violent temperament**

       (5) **Family dynamics** that include single parenthood, unemployment, poverty, marital conflicts, domestic violence, poor parent-child relationships, and unrealistic expectations of the child

2. Clinical features

  a. Bruises

       (1) **Bruises on fleshy or protected areas,** such as the face, neck, back, chest, abdomen, buttocks, and genitalia, are often consistent with **inflicted injury.** In contrast, bruises on exposed areas, such as the shins, knees, elbows, and forehead, are typically from noninflicted trauma.

       (2) **Bruises** may be **aged on the basis of color (Table 20-3).**

       (3) **Patterns** of bruising may help determine the type of object used to inflict the trauma (e.g., distinctive marks are left by belt loops, buckles, hangers, and hands).

  b. Human bites may be found anywhere on the body, including the genitalia and buttocks of infants.

  c. Burns often have distinguishable patterns.

       (1) **Accidental burns** have an **irregular, splashlike** configuration. In contrast, **nonaccidental burns** typically have a **clear line of demarcation** (e.g., "stocking" or "glovelike" pattern, suggesting submersion injury).

       (2) **Objects** used to burn may be **branded** to the skin (e.g., irons and cigarettes).

  d. Fractures that are inconsistent with the history or with the child's developmental ability may be secondary to abuse (see Chapter 17, section V.G). The following fractures are considered highly suggestive of abuse:

Table 20-3. Age of Bruise on the Basis of Color Pattern

Color	Age of Bruise
Red-blue	0–3 days
Blue-purple	3–5 days
Green	5–8 days
Yellow-brown	8–14 days

(1) **Metaphyseal fractures ("bucket handle" or corner fractures),** which are caused by torsional force on the limb (i.e., pulling and twisting) or by violent shaking.

(2) **Fractures** of the **posterior or first ribs, sternum, scapula, and vertebral spinous process.**

(3) **Multiple fractures in different stages of healing.**

e. **Head injuries,** caused by trauma, asphyxiation, or shaking, are the **leading cause** of death and morbidity from child abuse. **Shaken baby syndrome** may occur in a child younger than 2 years of age who is violently shaken. (This syndrome is termed "shaken impact syndrome" if the child is thrown after the shaking.) Retinal hemorrhages, subdural hematomas, metaphyseal fractures, and significant brain injury are characteristic.

f. **Visceral injuries** are the **second leading cause** of death from child abuse and include rupture and injury of the intestinal tract, liver, and spleen.

3. **Diagnosis**

a. **History is critical** in differentiating inflicted from noninflicted trauma. **Child development should correlate with the nature of the injury.** Delays in seeking medical attention, implausible histories, and histories that change or are inconsistent among caregivers are suspicious for abuse.

b. **Physical examination** should focus both on acute injuries and on identifying old lesions that may be secondary to abuse. If shaken baby syndrome is suspected, a dilated ophthalmoscopic evaluation for retinal hemorrhages should be performed (see Chapter 18, section V.A).

c. **Accessory tests** should include a **skeletal survey** to evaluate for old or healing fractures, and head or abdominal CT scans to evaluate for acute injuries.

4. **Management. Child protective services or law enforcement agencies must be notified if there is a suspicion of abuse.** Hospitalization may be required if medically appropriate, or until a safe location for the child has been identified.

C. **Sexual Abuse**

1. **General concepts**

a. Unlike physical abuse, there are typically **no overt physical signs of trauma.**

b. **Perpetrators** are often **known to the child** before the abuse.

2. **Epidemiology.** Eighty percent of sexual abuse occurs in **females.**

3. **Diagnosis**

a. **History is critical** to confirm abuse.

(1) **Obtaining a history of abuse from a young child is difficult.** Ideally, the history should be obtained with open-ended questions from an interviewer trained in sexual abuse evaluation.

(2) **Sexually abused children** typically present with multiple **nonspecific complaints,** including abdominal and urogenital symptoms.

(3) **Sexual behavior** in young children raises red flags for abuse.

b. **Physical examination** should be performed after rapport with the patient has been established.

    (1) **Signs of trauma** should be noted.

    (2) **Genital and perianal examination** should be performed last and should include inspection of the hymen, vagina, and perianal areas (penis, scrotum, and perianal area in males) with notation of any discharge, injury, or bleeding.

    (3) **Physical examination is normal in most victims.**

c. **Laboratory studies** to collect forensic evidence should be performed if the abuse occurred within 72 hours of presentation and should include cultures or serologic testing for sexually transmitted diseases (STDs), including human immunodeficiency virus (HIV). If appropriate, testing for pregnancy and assessment of vaginal fluid for spermatozoa should also be performed.

d. **Management**

    (1) **Safety of the child** should be the **highest priority** in determining placement.

    (2) **Child protective services** or social services must be notified and should arrange follow-up and support.

    (3) **Pregnancy** may be prevented with high-dose oral contraceptives (morning-after pills).

    (4) **Antibiotics** are often prescribed to empirically treat STDs.

VII. Sudden Infant Death Syndrome (SIDS)

A. **Definition.** SIDS is the **death of an infant younger than 1 year of age whose death remains unexplained after a thorough case investigation** that includes autopsy, death scene evaluation, and review of the clinical history.

B. **Epidemiology**

    1. **SIDS** is the **most common cause of death in children younger than 1 year of age.**

    2. **Incidence** is approximately 2 in 1,000 live births. Peak incidence is at 2–4 months of age.

    3. The **typical victim** is found dead in the morning in bed after being put to sleep at night.

    4. **Risk factors** associated with SIDS may be found in **Chapter 9, section IV.E.2.b.**

C. **Management**

    1. **Resuscitation** should be attempted on all patients because of the difficulty in ascertaining the period of time the infant has been apneic and pulseless.

    2. **If resuscitation is unsuccessful,** the child's body is referred to the medical examiner for autopsy. Postmortem examination may demonstrate **intrathoracic petechiae** (the most common autopsy finding in 80% of cases, but one whose cause is unknown), pulmonary congestion or edema, small airway inflammation, and evidence of hypoxia.

VIII. Poisonings

A. **General Concepts**

1. **Epidemiology**

   a. **Sixty percent of all poisonings** occur in children younger than 6 years of age.

   b. **Ninety percent of poisonings are accidental.** The majority of poisonings occur at **home** when the child's caregiver is **distracted.**

   c. Most poisons are ingested, although poisons may also be inhaled, spilled on the skin or into the eyes, or injected intravenously.

   d. **Mortality is < 1%.**

2. **Etiology.** The most common toxic exposures involve **commonly used** household products.

   a. **Cosmetics** and **personal-care products (most common toxic exposure)**

   b. **Cleaning agents**

   c. **Cough and cold preparations**

   d. **Vitamins, including iron**

   e. **Analgesics (e.g., acetaminophen, nonsteroidal anti-inflammatory drugs [NSAIDs], aspirin)**

   f. **Plants (6–7% of all ingestions)**

   g. **Alcohols** (e.g., **ethanol**) and **hydrocarbons** (e.g., gasoline, paint thinner, furniture polish)

   h. **Carbon monoxide (see section VIII.D.6)**

   i. **Prescription medications**

B. **Evaluation**

1. **Consider poisoning** in patients presenting with **nonspecific signs and symptoms,** such as seizures, severe vomiting and diarrhea, dysrhythmias, altered mental status or abnormal behaviors, shock, trauma, or unexplained metabolic acidosis.

2. **History** obtained from caregivers typically identifies the poison.

   a. **Information about the toxin** should include the type or name of toxin, toxin concentration (if known), and the route of exposure.

      (1) **Potential poison dose** is calculated for the **worst-case scenario.** Toxicity is typically on the basis of the amount ingested per kilogram of body weight.

      (2) **Consider multiple agents** in adolescents.

   b. **Information about the environment** should include location of victim when discovered and medications, plants, vitamins, herbs, and chemicals in the home. Time of occurrence, if known, is very important.

3. **Physical examination** should be comprehensive and may provide additional clues to the identity of the toxin. **Figure 20-1** shows the link between some typical physical findings and associated toxins.

4. **Laboratory studies**

   a. **Screening laboratory tests** include serum glucose, serum and urine toxicology screens, and electrolytes.

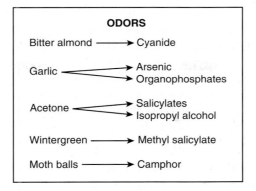

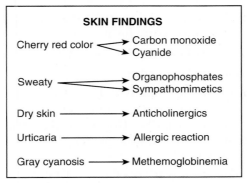

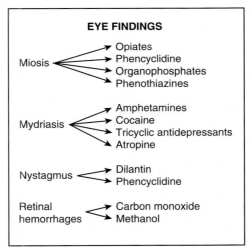

FEVER

Cocaine, tricyclic antidepressants, phencyclidine, salicylates, thyroxine, anticholinergics, amphetamines, theophylline

Figure 20-1. Selected physical examination findings and their associated toxins.

(1) **Anion gap** $[Na^+ - (Cl^- + HCO_3^-)]$ should be calculated.

(2) **Causes of an increased anion gap (> 16)** may be recalled using the mnemonic **AMUDPILES** (**a**lcohol, **m**ethanol, **u**remia, **d**iabetic ketoacidosis, **p**araldehyde, **i**ron and **i**soniazid, **l**actic acidosis, **e**thylene glycol, **s**alicylates).

b. **Radiographic imaging** of the abdomen may reveal radiopaque substances. These may be recalled using the mnemonic **CHIPE** (**c**hloral hydrate and **c**alcium, **h**eavy metals, **i**odine and **i**ron, **p**henothiazines, **e**nteric-coated tablets).

C. General Management Principles

1. The **ABCs** are the initial management priority.

2. If the patient has **altered mental status,** administer **dextrose** for hypoglycemia and **naloxone** for possible opiate overdose.

3. A **poison control center** may be consulted to assist with management.

4. **Gastric decontamination**

a. **Syrup of ipecac** rapidly induces **emesis** by direct gastric irritation and CNS chemoreceptor stimulation.

(1) It is **theoretically effective only within the first 30 minutes after ingestion,** after which time toxic substances are beyond the stomach.

(2) It is **contraindicated** in victims with decreased level of consciousness, caustic or hydrocarbon ingestions, and in children younger than 6 months of age.

(3) **Evidence** suggests that **ipecac does not improve clinical outcome, and its use is out of favor.**

b. **Gastric lavage** is performed with a **large bore orogastric tube** placed into the stomach to evacuate the stomach contents.

(1) **Indications** include **life-threatening** ingestions presenting within **1 hour** after ingestion and ingestion of toxins that delay gastric emptying (e.g., salicylates).

(2) **Contraindications** include caustic, hydrocarbon, and nontoxic ingestions, and delayed presentation.

(3) Evidence of improvement in clinical outcome with its use is lacking.

c. **Activated charcoal** has a **very large absorptive surface area** that **binds toxins** and minimizes their absorption.

(1) **Activated charcoal** should be **considered** for all poisonings. However, it is **ineffective** for some poisons such as **iron**, lithium, alcohols, ethylene glycol, iodine, potassium, and arsenic. In addition, activated charcoal interferes with visualization during endoscopy and therefore should not be used for caustic ingestions.

(2) **Evidence** suggests that activated charcoal **improves clinical outcome,** especially if given within 1 hour after an ingestion.

d. **Whole-bowel irrigation** (WBI) is rapid, complete emptying of the intestinal tract accomplished using **polyethylene glycol** (an osmotic agent) and an **electrolyte solution** (to prevent electrolyte imbalance).

Preliminary studies show that WBI may be effective for ingestions of iron and other heavy metals and sustained-release medications.

   e. **Antidotes** exist for a relatively small number of compounds **(Table 20-4)**.

D. Specific Poisonings

  1. **Acetaminophen.** This drug is one of the most common medications ingested by children and adolescents.

    a. **Pathophysiology**

      (1) **Hepatic damage,** the major sequelae of toxicity, is directly related to the depletion of **glutathione,** a cofactor used during the metabolism of acetaminophen by the cytochrome P-450 system.

      (2) **Toxic intermediates** produced when glutathione is depleted bind directly to hepatocytes, causing hepatocellular necrosis.

    b. **Clinical features.** There are **four stages** of acetaminophen poisoning **(Table 20-5)**.

    c. **Management**

      (1) **Gastric lavage,** if ingestion appears to be life-threatening

      (2) **Activated charcoal**

      (3) **Obtain serum acetaminophen level 2–4 hours** after ingestion. Level should be plotted on the **Matthew-Rumack nomogram** to determine the potential for hepatitis.

      (4) If the nomogram predicts hepatitis, the antidote, ***N*-acetylcysteine (NAC),** a glutathione precursor, is indicated.

        (a) **NAC** is given orally as a 140 mg/kg loading dose and is followed with 70 mg/kg every 4 hours for 17 doses. Intravenous NAC may also be used.

        (b) **NAC is hepatoprotective** if given **within 8 hours** of ingestion. It may still be helpful up to 72 hours after ingestion.

  2. **Salicylates.** Salicylate poisoning has decreased as acetaminophen's usage has increased; however, salicylates remain an ingredient in many compounds, such as Pepto-Bismol, Ben-Gay, and oil of wintergreen.

    a. **Pathophysiology**

      (1) **Salicylates directly stimulate respiratory centers.** This causes hyperventilation that may overcompensate for metabolic acidosis produced by the salicylate (it is a weak acid), resulting in a **respiratory alkalosis.**

      (2) **Salicylates uncouple oxidative phosphorylation,** producing lactic **acidosis** and enhancing ketosis.

    b. **Clinical features.** Common signs and symptoms include fever, diaphoresis, and flushed appearance; tinnitus; vomiting; headache; lethargy, restlessness, coma, and seizures; hyperpnea; and dehydration.

    c. **Laboratory findings**

      (1) **Respiratory alkalosis with an anion gap metabolic acidosis is the most common acid–base disturbance.**

      (2) Hyperglycemia, followed later by hypoglycemia

      (3) Hypokalemia

Table 20-4. Selected Toxins and Their Antidotes

Toxin	Antidote
Acetaminophen	NAC
Anticholinergic agents	Physostigmine
Benzodiazepines	Flumazenil
Black widow spider envenomation	Antivenin *Latrodectus mactans*
Carbon monoxide	Oxygen
Coral snake envenomation (Eastern U.S. or Texas coral snake)	Antivenin *Micrurus fulvius*
Cyanide	Cyanide antidote kit (contains amyl nitrite, sodium nitrite, sodium thiosulfate) Hydroxocobalamin (vitamin B_{12})
Digitalis glycosides	Digoxin-specific Fab antibodies
Heavy metals (mercury, manganese, copper, gold, nickel, zinc, lead, arsenic)	D-Penicillamine (for lead, mercury, arsenic, copper) Dimercaprol (British anti-lewisite [BAL] in oil) for all the heavy metals and lewisite (chemical weapon) DMSA (for lead and possibly mercury, arsenic, other metals) EDTA, calcium (for lead, nickel, zinc, manganese)
Inducers of dystonia	Diphenhydramine Benztropine
Inducers of methemoglobinemia	Methylene blue
Iron	Deferoxamine
Isoniazid	Pyridoxine (vitamin B_6)
Methanol; ethylene glycol	Ethanol, fomepizole
Narcotics	Naloxone
Organophosphates; carbamate pesticides	Atropine Pralidoxime ([2-PAM] for organophosphates)
Pit viper snake bite (rattlesnake, water moccasin, copperhead envenomation)	Antivenin, *Crotalidae* polyvalent *Crotalidae* polyvalent Fab antibodies
β-Blockers; calcium-channel blockers	Glucagon
Sulfonylurea oral hypoglycemic agents	Octreotide Glucagon

EDTA = ethylenediaminetetraacetic acid; *DMSA* = dimercaptosuccinic acid; *NAC* = *N*-acetylcysteine.

Table 20-5. Stages of Acetaminophen Toxicity

Stage	Time After Ingestion	Signs and Symptoms
1	30 minutes–24 hours	**Asymptomatic,** or vomiting and diarrhea
2	24–72 hours	**Gastrointestinal symptoms resolve;** at 36 hours, hepatic transaminases begin to increase
3	72–96 hours	**Hepatic necrosis,** jaundice, hypoglycemia, lactic acidosis, hepatic encephalopathy, coagulopathy, and renal failure
4	4 days–2 weeks	Resolution of symptoms, progressive liver damage requiring liver transplantation, or death

d. **Management**
   (1) **Gastric lavage** may be useful, because salicylates may delay gastric emptying.
   (2) **Activated charcoal** is effective and may be **readministered every 4 hours** in severe poisonings.
   (3) **Obtain serum salicylate level** at least **6 hours** after ingestion. The level should then be plotted on the **Done nomogram** to assess for potential toxicity.
   (4) **Alkalinization of urine with sodium bicarbonate to a urine pH > 7** and large-volume intravenous fluids enhance renal excretion of salicylates.
   (5) **Dialysis** may be required for life-threatening ingestions.

3. **Iron**
   a. **Epidemiology**
      (1) Iron is one of the most common and potentially fatal childhood poisonings. As little as 20 mg/kg of iron is toxic.
      (2) Adult-strength ferrous sulfate tablets and **iron in prenatal vitamins** are the most common sources of accidental iron ingestion.
   b. **Pathophysiology**
      (1) **Direct damage to the gastrointestinal tract** leading to hemorrhage
      (2) **Hepatic injury and necrosis**
      (3) **Third spacing and pooling of blood** in the vasculature leading to hypotension
      (4) **Interference** with oxidative phosphorylation
   c. **Clinical features.** There are four stages of iron toxicity (**Table 20-6**).
   d. **Management**
      (1) **Gastric lavage** should be performed.
      (2) **Activated charcoal does not bind to iron.**
      (3) **Hypovolemia,** blood loss, and shock should be anticipated and treated.
      (4) **WBI** should be considered for life-threatening ingestion.
      (5) **Serum iron level should be obtained 2–6 hours after ingestion.**
      (6) **Intravenous deferoxamine,** an iron-binding ligand, should be given if:
         (a) **Serum iron levels > 500 µg/dL,** or if **> 300 µg/dL** and acidosis, hyperglycemia, or leukocytosis are present
         (b) **Severe gastrointestinal symptoms** are present
         (c) **More than 100 mg/kg of iron** is ingested
      (7) Before the serum iron level is known, a test dose of **deferoxamine** may be administered. If the patient's urine then turns a red or pink (**vin rose**) color (the color of chelated iron), the challenge is considered positive, indicating a clinically significant iron ingestion. Intravenous deferoxamine should then be continued.

4. **Lead**
   a. **Epidemiology. Sources of lead** include ingestion of lead-based paint chips, water carried by outdated lead pipes, improperly glazed

Table 20-6. Stages of Iron Toxicity

Stage	Time After Ingestion	Signs and Symptoms
1	1–6 hours	Abdominal pain, vomiting, diarrhea, GI bleeding Shock from bleeding and vasodilation Fever and leukocytosis
2	6–12 hours	Resolution of stage 1 symptoms
3	12–36 hours	Metabolic acidosis Circulatory collapse Hepatic and renal failure DIC Neurologic deterioration
4	2–6 weeks	Late sequelae includes pyloric or intestinal scarring with stenosis

DIC = disseminated intravascular coagulation; *GI* = gastrointestinal.

or foreign-made ceramic food or water containers, and pica (compulsive eating of nonnutrient substances such as dirt, paint, and clay). (See Chapter 1, section IV.J.)

   b. **Clinical features.** Lead poisoning is typically a **chronic ingestion;** however, children may also present with **acute lead intoxication.**

   (1) **Abdominal complaints** include colicky pain, constipation, anorexia, and vomiting.

   (2) **CNS complaints** include listlessness, irritability, seizures, and decreased consciousness with encephalopathy.

   (3) **Peripheral blood smear** may show **microcytic anemia, basophilic stippling,** and red blood cell precursors.

   (4) Radiopacities may be seen on **abdominal radiographs,** and **dense metaphyseal bands** may be present show on radiographs of the knees and wrists (**lead lines**).

   c. **Diagnosis.** An **elevated lead level** or elevated **erythrocyte protoporphyrin** is the basis of diagnosis.

   d. **Management.** Treatment for significant toxicity includes dimercaprol, British anti-lewisite (BAL), or calcium disodium ethylenediaminetetraacetic acid (EDTA).

5. **Caustic agents.** These are **acids or alkalis with corrosive potential.**

   a. **Pathophysiology**

   (1) **Acids** (e.g., toilet bowl cleaner) cause **coagulation necrosis** that produces **superficial damage** to the mouth, esophagus, and stomach. More severe injury results from compounds that have a pH < 2.

   (2) **Alkalis** (e.g., oven and drain cleaners, bleach, laundry detergent) cause **liquefaction necrosis** that produces **deep and penetrating damage,** most commonly to the mouth and esophagus. More severe injury results from compounds that have a pH > 12.

   b. **Clinical features**

   (1) **Immediate burning** sensation with intense **dysphagia, salivation,** retrosternal chest pain, and vomiting

   (2) **Obstructive airway edema** (especially with acid ingestion)

      (3) Gastric perforation and peritonitis may follow acid ingestion.

      (4) Esophageal perforation with mediastinitis may follow alkali ingestion.

   c. Management. Treatment initially includes the ABCs.

      (1) No attempt should be made to neutralize the caustic agent, because the combination of acid and alkali will generate an exothermic reaction and worsen any burn.

      (2) Ipecac, gastric lavage, and activated charcoal are all contraindicated. Activated charcoal interferes with endoscopy.

      (3) Endoscopy is performed to assess the degree of damage.

      (4) Household bleach has less corrosive potential and generally does not require treatment.

6. Carbon monoxide poisoning

   a. Epidemiology. Carbon monoxide (CO) is a byproduct of incomplete combustion of carbon-containing material. Excessive exposure may occur from fires, tobacco, faulty home heaters, car exhaust, and industrial pollution. **CO is odorless, tasteless,** and **colorless.**

   b. Pathophysiology. CO interferes with oxygen delivery and utilization.

      (1) CO displaces oxygen from the hemoglobin molecule, forming **carboxyhemoglobin (CO-Hb),** which can no longer carry oxygen. The bond between CO and hemoglobin is more than 200 times stronger than the bond between oxygen and hemoglobin.

      (2) The **oxygen-hemoglobin dissociation curve** is shifted to the **left.** This leads to tighter binding of the remaining oxygen bound to hemoglobin and impaired release of oxygen to tissues.

      (3) CO also interferes with cellular oxidative metabolism.

   c. Clinical features depend on the CO-Hb level.

      (1) Low levels are associated with **nonspecific symptoms** such as **headache, flulike illness,** dyspnea with exertion, and dizziness.

      (2) High levels are associated with **visual and auditory changes,** vomiting, **confusion** and later syncope, slurred speech, cyanosis, myocardial ischemia, coma, and death.

      (3) Classic physical examination findings, although uncommon, include **cherry red skin** (venous blood carries more oxygen than normal as a result of impaired release of oxygen to tissues) and **retinal hemorrhages.** Tachycardia and tachypnea may be present.

      (4) Young children (< 8 years of age) have more symptoms at lower CO-Hb levels. Young children are also more likely to have gastrointestinal symptoms (e.g., vomiting and diarrhea) instead of neurologic symptoms.

      (5) Delayed permanent neuropsychiatric syndrome, consisting of memory loss, personality changes, deafness, and seizures, may occur in some victims up to 4 weeks after CO exposure.

   d. Diagnosis is made by measuring the **CO-Hb level.** It is important to remember that CO-Hb levels are not always indicative of the degree of CO exposure and may even be low in victims with significant intoxication. Other abnormal findings include anion-gap metabolic acidosis, low oxygen saturation (however, PaO_2 may be normal), and evidence of myocardial ischemia on ECG or elevated cardiac enzymes.

    e. **Management**

        (1) One hundred percent oxygen is administered to displace CO from hemoglobin.

        (2) If available, **hyperbaric oxygen** more rapidly displaces CO from hemoglobin as compared to oxygen alone, and also improves oxygen delivery to tissues.

        (3) Hospitalization is indicated for CO-Hb levels > 25%, CO-Hb levels > 10% during pregnancy, history or presence of neurologic symptoms, or presence of metabolic acidosis or ECG changes.

IX. Mammalian Bites

A. Epidemiology

    1. Dogs (80% of bites), cats, rodents, other wild or domesticated animals, and humans (2–3% of bites) may all cause a bite injury.

    2. Most bites occur in **boys** during the spring and summer months.

B. Dog Bites

    1. Clinical features

        a. Bites range in severity from scratches, punctures, and lacerations to severe soft tissue injury. Note that the jaw pressure of a dog may exceed 200–450 pounds per square inch.

        b. Young children are typically bitten on the **head and neck,** whereas older children are bitten predominantly on the extremities.

        c. Secondary infections may result from anaerobic and aerobic organisms, such as *Staphylococcus aureus, Pasteurella multocida, and* Streptococcus species.

    2. Management. Treatment includes meticulous and prompt local wound care.

        a. Copious wound irrigation

        b. Wounds on the face, large wounds, and wounds less than 12 hours old should be sutured. Facial wounds < 24 hours old can be sutured because the face has increased vascularity.

        c. Wounds at high risk for infection include those on the hand, wrist, and foot, and small puncture wounds.

        d. Antibiotics, such as amoxicillin-clavulanic acid, should be administered.

        e. Tetanus prophylaxis should be given if needed.

C. Cat Bites

    1. Clinical features

        a. Puncture wounds to the upper extremity are most common.

        b. Victims have a high risk of infection due to *P. multocida.*

        c. Cat scratch disease (regional lymphadenitis) may also develop (see Chapter 7, section XVII.B).

    2. Management. Treatment is similar to the management of dog bites. Because the injury is typically a puncture wound, adequate irrigation is often difficult.

D. Human Bites

1. **Clinical features**

    a. **Wound** is typically located on the trunk or face in young children. If the wound occurred during a fistfight, it is typically located at the **metacarpophalangeal (MP) joint.** Wounds to the MP joint are extremely serious, because infection may penetrate the avascular fascial layers resulting in deep infection and tendonitis.

    b. **Infection rate is high.**

        (1) **Mixed bacterial infection** is often present. Pathogens include *Streptococcus viridans, S. aureus,* and anaerobic bacteria such as *Bacteroides, Peptostreptococcus,* and *Eikenella corrodens.*

        (2) **Other systemic infections**, such as hepatitis B, HIV, and syphilis may also be transmitted.

2. **Management.** Treatment includes copious wound irrigation, closure of large lacerations, and antibiotics (e.g., amoxicillin-clavulanic acid).

X. Biologic Poisonings (Venoms)

A. Black Widow Spider (*Lactrodectus* species)

1. **General concepts**

    a. The black widow spider is characterized by a **red or orange hourglass marking** on the ventral surface.

    b. Only the **female spider** is dangerous, and **bites only if provoked.**

    c. The **web** is located in dark recesses, such as closets, woodpiles, and attics.

2. **Clinical features** result from the venom, a potent **neurotoxin.**

    a. The **bite causes few local symptoms,** except for burning or a sharp pinprick sensation.

    b. **Pathognomonic signs and symptoms** include **severe hypertension and muscle cramps.**

    c. **Nonspecific symptoms,** such as headache, dizziness, nausea, vomiting, anxiety, and sweating, may also occur.

3. **Management**

    a. **Local wound care,** including wound irrigation and tetanus prophylaxis (if needed), is important.

    b. **Benzodiazepines** and narcotics may relieve muscle cramps.

    c. *Latrodectus* **antivenin** is given for signs and symptoms suggesting severe envenomation.

B. Brown Recluse Spider (*Loxosceles* species)

1. **General concepts**

    a. The brown recluse spider (also called the **fiddle-back spider**) is characterized by a **brown violin-shaped** marking on the dorsum of the thorax.

    b. The spider **bites only if provoked.**

    c. The **web** is located in dark recesses.

2. **Clinical features** result from the venom, a **cytotoxic** compound containing **tissue-destructive enzymes.**

   a. The **bite** results in little initial pain. However 1–8 hours later, a painful itchy papule that increases in size and discolors during the course of 3–4 days develops at the site of the bite.

   b. Some patients develop a **necrotic and ulcerated deep lesion** at the bite site.

   c. **Systemic reactions** may occur 24–48 hours after the bite with fever, chills, weakness, vomiting, joint pain, DIC, hemolysis, and renal failure from myoglobinuria.

3. **Management.** Treatment includes local wound care and tetanus prophylaxis, if needed. Treatment of a necrotic ulcer is controversial but may include steroids, skin grafting, dapsone, and hyperbaric oxygen. There is no antivenin.

C. **Pit viper snakes (family *Crotalidae*)** account for more than **95%** of all snakebites. **Rattlesnake, cottonmouth, and copperhead snakes** are members of the *Crotalidae* family.

1. **Pathophysiology**

   a. **Bite location** and **amount of venom injected** determine the severity of envenomation. Head and trunk bites are most severe.

   b. **Venom** is a complex mixture of **proteolytic enzymes.**

2. **Clinical features**

   a. **Local findings** include puncture marks and progressive severe swelling and ecchymosis.

   b. **Systemic effects** include **paresthesias** of the scalp, periorbital fasciculations, **weakness,** diaphoresis, dizziness, nausea, and a **metallic taste** in the mouth.

   c. **Coagulopathy, thrombocytopenia, hypotension, and shock** may also develop.

3. **Management.** Treatment involves local wound care, tetanus prophylaxis if needed, immobilization of the bitten extremity, and **immediate transport** to the nearest emergency department.

   a. **Incision and suction are not recommended.**

   b. **Tourniquets,** ice, and direct pressure on the wound may cause **more injury.**

   c. *Crotalidae* polyvalent antivenin should be considered for **all bites.**

      (1) **Children** require **more antivenin** because they receive proportionally more venom per kilogram body weight.

      (2) **Antivenin** is **most effective** if given within **4–6 hours** of the bite.

      (3) **Complications** of antivenin are common and include **serum sickness and anaphylaxis.**

   d. **Crotalidae polyvalent immune Fab** is also available for envenomation and is safe, more potent, and very effective.

D. **Coral snakes (family *Elapidae*)** account for **1–2%** of all snakebites. Coral snakes may be identified by their stripe pattern using the mnemonic **"red next to yellow, kill a fellow; red next to black, venom lack."**

1. **Clinical features** result from the **neurotoxic** venom and include mild local swelling and tenderness, and **severe systemic symptoms,** such as paresthesias, vomiting, weakness, diplopia, fasciculations, confusion, and respiratory depression.

2. **Management** should be aggressive and includes **antivenin** (available only for the Eastern U.S. and Texas coral snake), local wound care, and supportive care.

Review Test

1. You are urgently summoned to the waiting room of the emergency department by a clerk after she witnessed a 3-year-old boy collapse. You are concerned that he may be in cardiac arrest. Which of the following is the correct order of steps for the initial management of a child found in full cardiopulmonary arrest?

(A) Open the airway, check for a pulse, administer rescue breaths, start chest compressions.
(B) Check for a pulse, open the airway, start chest compressions, administer rescue breaths.
(C) Check for a pulse, start chest compressions, open the airway, administer rescue breaths.
(D) Open the airway, administer rescue breaths, start chest compressions, check for a pulse.
(E) Open the airway, administer rescue breaths, check for a pulse, start chest compressions.

2. A 2-year-old boy sustains severe head trauma in a three-story fall. Which of the following statements regarding head injury in a patient of this age is correct?

(A) Epidural hematoma has a crescentic density on head computed tomography.
(B) The prognosis is better if he has a subdural hematoma rather than an epidural hematoma.
(C) Cushing's triad is an early sign of increased intracranial pressure.
(D) The occipital lobe is the most common site of intracerebral hematoma.
(E) Bradycardia is an early sign of herniation.

3. A 1-year-old girl has been involved in a motor vehicle accident, and you suspect she has sustained head injury. On examination, she is unconscious but she opens her eyes to pain and also has abnormal flexion of her extremities to pain. She does not cry but rather grunts with stimulation. What is her Glasgow coma score?

(A) 4
(B) 5
(C) 6
(D) 7
(E) 8

4. A 19-month-old boy has a burn on his right hand that occurred 3 hours ago. On examination, the burn appears to be in a "stocking glove" distribution. The involved area is moist, painful, and red and contains two moderate-sized intact blisters. Which of the following statements regarding this burn is correct?

(A) This patient has suffered a superficial partial-thickness burn.
(B) This burn will most likely scar.
(C) Child abuse is unlikely based on the burn's characteristics.
(D) Blisters should be ruptured and debrided.
(E) Hospitalization is not needed.

5. A 2-year-old girl is found submerged in a lake. She is suspected to have been under the water for more than 15 minutes. Paramedics find her apneic and pulseless. On arrival at the hospital, her core body temperature is 82.4°F (28°C). Which of the following statements regarding the management, expected clinical findings, and prognosis in this patient is correct?

(A) Management is dependent on whether the lake contains fresh or salt water.
(B) Because the child was found apneic and pulseless, resuscitative efforts should not be attempted.
(C) Cervical spine immobilization is unnecessary.
(D) Pulmonary function would be expected to improve during the next 18 hours.
(E) The prognosis is poor.

6. A 17-year-old girl is brought by her parents to the emergency department after a possible suicide attempt. She discloses that she swallowed 100 aspirin tablets 4 hours ago. Which of the following acid–base relationships would most likely be found on an arterial blood gas study of this patient?

(A) Metabolic alkalosis and respiratory acidosis
(B) Metabolic alkalosis and respiratory alkalosis
(C) Metabolic acidosis and respiratory acidosis
(D) Metabolic acidosis and respiratory alkalosis
(E) Respiratory alkalosis only

7. A 2-year-old girl is brought to the emergency department by her parents. She swallowed an unknown amount of industrial-strength drain cleaner from her father's plumbing van 30 minutes ago. Which of the following statements regarding the clinical findings and management of this incident is correct?

(A) Ipecac should be administered immediately.
(B) Activated charcoal should be administered.
(C) Nasogastric tube for lavage should be avoided.
(D) Lower intestinal perforation is a possible complication.
(E) The drain cleaner should be neutralized with acetic acid.

8. A 14-year-old boy is involved in a fistfight with another teenager at school. He is brought to the emergency department 2 hours later with a laceration on the dorsum of his right hand over the knuckle secondary to a human bite. Which of the following statements regarding this human bite is correct?

(A) If infection develops, it is usually secondary to both anaerobes and aerobes.
(B) If irrigated appropriately, human bites are unlikely to become infected.
(C) This wound most likely involves an interphalangeal joint.
(D) Antibiotics should not be prescribed until an infection develops because of the risk of selection of resistant organisms.
(E) If infection develops, it is most likely caused by *Pasteurella multocida.*

9. A 5-year-old girl is brought to a rural emergency department after being bitten on the leg by a rattlesnake. The bite occurred 30 minutes ago. No antivenin is available at the hospital, and transfer to another hospital is pending. Which of the following should be done immediately?

(A) Local wound care, leg immobilization, and supportive care only.
(B) Incise the wound and apply suction to remove the venom.
(C) Apply direct pressure to the wound.
(D) Apply a tight tourniquet proximal to the wound to prevent venom from spreading.
(E) Rub ice over the fang marks.

The response items for statements 10 and 11 are the same. You will be required to select one answer for each statement in the set.

(A) Black widow spider
(B) Brown recluse spider

For each of the following patients, select the most likely spider bite.

10. A 5-year-old girl with severe muscle cramps and hypertension.

11. A 10-year-old boy with fever, chills, vomiting, and disseminated intravascular coagulation 24 hours after a suspected bite. Five days later, a necrotic, ulcerated skin lesion is evident.

The response items for statements 12–14 are the same. You will be required to select one answer for each statement in the set.

(A) Distributive shock
(B) Septic shock
(C) Cardiogenic shock
(D) Hypovolemic shock
(E) Neurogenic shock

For each patient, select the most likely type of shock.

12. A 10-month-old female infant presents with hypotension. An electrocardiogram reveals supraventricular tachycardia.

13. A 10-year-old boy presents with a 2-day history of high fever, chills, vomiting, diarrhea, and weakness. Examination reveals hypotension with bounding pulses and warm extremities.

14. A 5-year-old boy presents with acute onset of wheezing, urticaria, stridor, and hypotension.

15. A 2-year-old girl is brought to the emergency department after ingesting her mother's prenatal vitamins 60 minutes ago. Which of the following statements regarding the clinical findings, diagnosis, and management of this type of poisoning is correct?

(A) Activated charcoal is effective.
(B) Basophilic stippling is seen on peripheral blood smear.
(C) Ipecac should be administered.
(D) An abdominal radiograph may reveal the ingested poison.
(E) Shock is uncommon.

Answers and Explanations

1. The answer is E [I.B]. The ABCs (<u>a</u>irway, <u>b</u>reathing, <u>c</u>irculation) should begin every resuscitation of a child. The airway should be opened first by either a chin lift–head tilt maneuver, or by a jaw-thrust maneuver if the patient has suspected neck or cervical spine injury. After looking, listening, and feeling for respirations, rescue breaths are given to an apneic infant or child. The pulse is next assessed to determine whether cardiac function is present. If the patient is bradycardic or asystolic, chest compressions are then administered.

2. The answer is E [III.E.1.d]. In children younger than 4 years of age, bradycardia is often the initial sign of cerebral herniation. Epidural hematomas have a lenticular appearance on head computed tomography, whereas subdural hematomas generally have a crescentic appearance. Patients with subdural hematomas generally have a worse prognosis compared with those with epidural hematomas because of the bleeding directly on the surface of the brain parenchyma. Cushing's triad (hypertension, bradycardia, and an irregular breathing pattern) is a late finding of increased intracranial pressure. The frontal and temporal lobes are the most common sites of intracerebral bleeding.

3. The answer is D [Table 20-1]. The Glasgow coma score (GCS) is used to assess the level of neurologic impairment on the basis of the patient's physical examination. It includes assessment of three components: eye opening, motor response, and verbal response. This scoring system has been modified for the nonverbal pediatric patient. This patient has a GCS score of 7; she opens her eyes to pain (2), has abnormal extremity flexion to pain (3), and grunts with stimulation (2). A GCS of less than 8 signifies severe head injury.

4. The answer is A [VI.B.2.c, IV.B.2.a, IV.C]. This patient's burn is classified as a superficial partial-thickness burn on the basis of the presence of pain, blisters, and erythema. Superficial partial-thickness burns involve the epidermis and outer dermis and do not scar. Child abuse must be considered for well-demarcated burns (e.g., "stocking glove" distribution) that suggest submersion injury. If intact, blisters should not be ruptured because the risk of infection and loss of fluid from the skin would increase. All patients with burns to the hands, feet, perineum, face, and skin overlying joints should be hospitalized for treatment.

5. The answer is E [V.D–F]. A poor prognosis is associated with age younger than 3 years, submersion times greater than 5 minutes, and the need for cardiopulmonary resuscitation, all of which are present in this patient. In general, however, the outcome of drowning in children is better than in adults because children have a primitive dive reflex that preferentially shunts blood to vital organs such as the brain, heart, and liver. Management is the same regardless of the type of water in which the patient was submerged. Despite the apnea and asystole, this patient should be resuscitated, and efforts at resuscitation should continue until the core body temperature reaches at least 89.6°F (32°C). Head and neck trauma should always be suspected, and therefore cervical spine immobilization is important. Pulmonary function tends to deteriorate during the 12–24 hours after submersion injury.

6. The answer is D [VIII.D.2.d]. Salicylates are weak acids and cause an anion-gap metabolic acidosis. However, salicylates also directly stimulate the respiratory centers in the brainstem. The stimulation of the respiratory center causes hyperventilation, which overcompensates the metabolic acidosis, producing a respiratory alkalosis. Therefore, the most common acid–base finding in a patient who has ingested a toxic amount of salicylates is a metabolic acidosis and a respiratory alkalosis.

7. The answer is C [VIII.D.5.b–c]. Drain cleaners are alkalis, which typically cause severe deep burns to the mouth and esophagus by liquefaction necrosis. Because the esophagus may be injured, a nasogastric tube for suction or lavage is contraindicated. Ipecac is also contraindicated in caustic ingestions. Activated charcoal should be avoided as well because it interferes with endoscopy. Neither acids nor alkalis cause lower intestinal perforation. Neutralization with an acid produces an exothermic reaction that results in further injury.

8. The answer is A [IX.D]. Human bites have a very high infection rate, despite appropriate wound cleaning. Infection is typically a mixed infection consisting of both aerobes and anaerobes. The hand, specifically the metacarpophalangeal joint, is most commonly bitten in a fistfight. Antibiotics should always be prescribed. Infection with *Pasteurella multocida* occurs in cat and dog bites, not human bites. Other infections such as syphilis, HIV, and hepatitis B also may be transmitted by human bites.

9. The answer is A [X.C.3]. Management of a rattlesnake bite involves the immediate administration of snake antivenin. If antivenin is unavailable, the victim should be transported to a facility that has antivenin. Local wound care (including tetanus prophylaxis if needed) and immobilization of the affected extremity are all that are needed until antivenin becomes available. Incision and suction are not recommended, and direct pressure, tourniquets, and ice may aggravate the injury.

10–11. The answers are A and B, respectively [X.A, X.B]. The black widow spider (*Lactrodectus* species) generally produces few local symptoms; however, muscle cramps and systemic hypertension are pathognomonic. The brown recluse spider (*Loxosceles* species) produces significant local signs and symptoms in some patients, including a deep necrotic ulcerated skin lesion. In some patients, systemic symptoms, such as disseminated intravascular coagulation, vomiting, fever, chills, hemolysis, and joint pain, may occur 24–48 hours after the bite.

12–14. The answers are C, B, and A, respectively [II.B.2.d, II.B.2.b, II.B.2.c]. The 10-month-old female infant with supraventricular tachycardia has cardiogenic shock, which is generally caused by cardiac dysrhythmias. The 10-year-old boy has signs and symptoms of infection. Shock associated with infection may include septic shock and hypovolemic shock. However, bounding pulses and warm extremities are found only in the initial hyperdynamic stage of septic shock. The 5-year-old boy has signs and symptoms of anaphylaxis. Shock associated with anaphylaxis is distributive shock, which may also be secondary to spinal cord injury and drug poisoning.

15. The answer is D [VIII.B.4.b, VIII.D.3.d, Table 20-6]. Prenatal vitamins contain iron, an important cause of childhood poisoning. Iron tablets are radiopaque and may be seen on imaging studies of the abdomen. There are four clinical stages of iron ingestion, including the first stage in which gastrointestinal bleeding can occur along with shock and vasodilation. Management of suspected iron ingestion includes gastric lavage, whole-bowel irrigation if poisoning is severe, and treatment with the iron chelator, deferoxamine. Activated charcoal is not effective for iron ingestion. Ipecac is not helpful. Basophilic stippling is seen in lead intoxication.

Comprehensive Examination

1. At a routine health maintenance visit, the parents of a well-appearing 2-week-old female infant have no concerns other than jaundice they have noted since the infant was 1 week of age. The patient is alert and feeding well. Laboratory evaluation reveals a total bilirubin level of 14.2 mg/dL and a direct bilirubin level of 6.2 mg/dL. Which of the following studies is most likely to be diagnostic of this patient's condition?

(A) Hepatic ultrasound
(B) Complete blood count and blood culture
(C) Coombs testing
(D) Levels of thyroxine and thyroid-stimulating hormone (TSH)
(E) Osmotic fragility test

2. The parents of a 15-month-old boy bring him to the office for a routine health maintenance visit. Which of the following is a contraindication to administering the diphtheria, tetanus, and acellular pertussis (DTaP) vaccine at this time?

(A) Signs and symptoms of an upper respiratory illness with a fever to 101°F (38.3°C)
(B) A history of intravenous immune globulin infusion for immune thrombocytopenic purpura at 9 months of age
(C) A 4-year-old sibling in the household receiving chemotherapy
(D) A history of moderate swelling at the injection site after the 6-month DTaP vaccination
(E) Uncontrolled epilepsy

3. A 6-year-old girl with a 3-week history of malaise, decreased appetite, and intermittent tactile fevers is brought to see you by her parents for evaluation of a "purplish rash" around her eyes. On further questioning, you learn that the child also has less energy, which the parents attribute to the "flu." Joint swelling, abdominal pain, oral ulcers, cough, nausea, vomiting, and diarrhea are absent. Physical examination reveals an afebrile, tired-appearing child with a periorbital violaceous rash that crosses the nasal bridge. There is no evidence of arthritis, although the patient has an erythematous hypertrophic rash over the knuckles. Which of the following laboratory or diagnostic studies is most consistent with the most likely diagnosis?

(A) Abnormal electromyography findings
(B) Increased serum immunoglobulin levels against Epstein-Barr virus
(C) Positive antinuclear antibody
(D) Positive urine culture for cytomegalovirus
(E) Low creatine kinase levels

4. A 13-year-old previously healthy boy is injured when his scooter collides with a parked car. On arrival at the emergency department, he is unconscious, and you suspect head injury. On examination, he does not open his eyes to voice or to pain. He has decerebrate posturing of the extremities to pain, and he moans with stimulation (you are unable to understand any of his words). Which of the following is this patient's Glasgow coma score (GCS)?

(A) 4
(B) 5
(C) 6
(D) 7
(E) 8

5. A 5-year-old boy has a 2-week history of persistent daily fevers and a 1-week history of pain in his right arm. Physical examination reveals a very pale child with a markedly enlarged liver and spleen and generalized lymphadenopathy. His right arm is nontender to palpation with normal range of motion. On the basis of his clinical presentation and examination, you suspect acute lymphocytic leukemia (ALL). Which of the following statements about the presenting features of ALL is most accurate?

(A) The age at presentation is unusual.
(B) Bone pain is a common presenting symptom.
(C) The disease is more common in females.
(D) Pallor is an uncommon sign at presentation.
(E) White blood cell count is almost always high ($> 50,000$ cells/mm^3).

6. A 7-year-old boy presents to the emergency department with swelling in his knee. His parents state that the swelling developed very rapidly over 30 minutes after their son bumped his knee into a door. On physical examination, you note that his knee is very swollen with what appears to be blood. Based on his presentation, you consider an evaluation for hemophilia A. Which of the following statements regarding this diagnostic possibility is correct?

(A) Activated partial thromboplastin time (aPTT) is prolonged.
(B) Males and females are equally affected.
(C) Management includes replacement of factor IX.
(D) Bleeding time is prolonged.
(E) The cause is a deficiency of a vitamin K-dependent coagulation factor.

7. A 3-year-old boy has a 2-week history of viral upper respiratory symptoms and a 2-day history of swelling around his eyes. Physical examination reveals normal vital signs and moderate periorbital edema, mild scrotal edema, and mild edema of the feet. Urinalysis reveals 3+ proteinuria. Which of the following statements regarding the likely diagnosis is most accurate?

(A) Serum cholesterol level is low.
(B) He is predisposed to hemorrhage.
(C) Should the patient become febrile, management involves administration of empiric antibiotics to cover encapsulated organisms.
(D) Referral for a diagnostic renal biopsy is warranted.
(E) The patient is not likely to respond to corticosteroid therapy and will likely require treatment with cyclophosphamide or cyclosporin.

8. A 16-year-old girl presents with a 1-week history of gray-white vaginal discharge with a strong "fishy" odor. On physical examination, you confirm the fishy odor and note minimal vulvar inflammation. Which of the following is correct regarding her likely condition?

(A) Treatment of her sexual partners is necessary.
(B) Wet-mount saline preparation will demonstrate motile protozoa.
(C) The infection is caused by a change in the normal vaginal flora.
(D) Topical antiyeast medication should be prescribed.
(E) Oral doxycycline and intramuscular ceftriaxone should be administered after obtaining appropriate cultures.

9. A 7-year-old girl is brought to the emergency department with a 5-day history of fever, malaise, and anorexia. Her past medical history is significant for aortic stenosis. Physical examination reveals a loud systolic ejection murmur at the cardiac base that radiates to the carotids and a systolic ejection click. Splenomegaly and a petechial eruption on the patient's palms and soles are also present. Laboratory studies reveal a white blood cell count of 19,000 cells/mm^3 and an erythrocyte sedimentation rate of 78 mm/hr. Which of the following statements regarding the most likely diagnosis is correct?

(A) Abnormal rheumatoid factor is unusual.
(B) Transthoracic echocardiogram is the most sensitive test for detecting vegetations.
(C) Gram-negative rods are the most common causative agents.
(D) Ophthalmologic evaluation is useful in diagnosis.
(E) Antibiotics should be administered promptly without waiting for blood cultures to be drawn.

10. A 6-month-old male infant is referred to you for evaluation of failure to thrive. The parents report that their child has always been a "poor feeder," and they deny any vomiting, diarrhea, or frequent infections. Physical examination reveals generalized weakness with particularly poor head control owing to weakness of the neck flexor muscles. One of the diagnostic possibilities is juvenile myasthenia gravis. Which of the following statements regarding juvenile myasthenia gravis is most accurate?

(A) Most patients with this condition have fasciculations.
(B) This condition is most likely related to ingestion of honey.
(C) Bilateral ptosis is the most common presenting sign of this condition.
(D) Deep tendon reflexes are diminished.
(E) The Tensilon test demonstrates increased weakness.

11. A 6-year-old girl has a history of daily fevers to 102°F (38.9°C) for the past 2 weeks. Preliminary workup and physical examination have not revealed a diagnosis. Which of the following statements regarding this patient's fever of unknown origin (FUO) is correct?

(A) The FUO is likely caused by a rare illness.
(B) The FUO is most likely caused by a rheumatologic disorder.
(C) Hospitalization is not indicated unless the patient becomes more ill.
(D) The FUO is likely to resolve without a diagnosis having been made.
(E) The FUO is likely caused by an unusual presentation of a common infection.

12. You are called to evaluate a 1-day-old infant born at 32 weeks gestation who develops respiratory distress at 12 hours of life. Which of the following diagnoses is the most likely cause of this infant's respiratory distress?

(A) Meconium aspiration syndrome
(B) Bronchopulmonary dysplasia
(C) Respiratory distress syndrome
(D) Neonatal sepsis
(E) Intraventricular hemorrhage

13. A 7-month-old male infant is born at 29 weeks gestation. While hospitalized in the neonatal intensive care unit, he develops necrotizing enterocolitis and undergoes a resection of the majority of his small intestine. He is now dependent on total parenteral nutrition for his calories and growth. Which of the following is a complication associated with the treatment of his disorder?

(A) Gastrointestinal bleeding
(B) Gallstones
(C) Chronic constipation
(D) Pancreatic insufficiency
(E) Inflammatory bowel disease

14. A 9-year-old girl is brought to the emergency department after falling off her bicycle. She complains of pain in her right leg. Radiography reveals a tibial fracture that extends from the epiphysis, through the physis, and into the metaphysis. Which of the following is the Salter-Harris grade of this fracture?

(A) Grade I
(B) Grade II
(C) Grade III
(D) Grade IV
(E) Grade V

15. A 6-month-old male infant has an asymmetrically shaped head. A computed tomography scan of the skull reveals premature closure of a cranial suture. Which of the following is the most likely cause of this condition?

(A) Perinatal asphyxia
(B) Genetic syndrome
(C) Positional, from sleeping on the back
(D) Unknown
(E) Congenital muscular torticollis

The response options for statements 16 and 17 are the same. You will be required to select one answer for each statement in the set.

(A) Strawberry hemangioma
(B) Nevus flammeus
(C) Erythema toxicum neonatorum
(D) Pustular melanosis
(E) Milia
(F) Cutis marmorata
(G) Acrocyanosis
(H) Neonatal acne

For each patient, select the skin lesion described or associated with the clinical presentation.

16. A 6-month-old male infant has seizures. Computed tomography of the head reveals intracranial calcifications.

17. A 5-day-old female infant has papules and pustules on her trunk. Microscopic evaluation of the fluid within a lesion reveals eosinophils.

18. A 16-year-old boy with homocystinuria is on a methionine-restricted diet. He is also taking folic acid and pyridoxine. Which of the following medications should you add to his medical regimen?

(A) Propranolol
(B) Vitamin C
(C) D-Penicillamine
(D) Aspirin
(E) Zinc

The response options for statements 19–21 are the same. You will be required to select one answer for each statement in the set.
(A) Turner syndrome
(B) Prader-Willi syndrome
(C) Kallmann syndrome
(D) Laurence-Moon-Biedl syndrome
(E) McCune-Albright syndrome

For each patient, select the most likely diagnosis.

19. A 3-year-old girl has bilateral femur fractures and Tanner stage 2 breast development.

20. A 15-year-old girl has delayed puberty and a decreased sense of smell.

21. A 6-month-old infant has hypotonia, small hands and feet, and small gonads. Weight and height are at the fifth percentile.

22. An 18-month-old boy is brought to your clinic by authorities for an examination. Neighbors called the police after they noticed the child had multiple bruises and appeared malnourished and unkempt. The police are concerned about possible child abuse. Which of the following findings, by itself, is most suggestive of child abuse?

(A) Bruises on the knees, shins, and elbows in different stages of healing
(B) Metaphyseal ("corner") fracture of the distal left humerus
(C) Burns to the right arm that have an irregular, splashlike configuration
(D) Nondisplaced spiral fracture of the left tibia
(E) Displaced supracondylar fracture of the right elbow

23. An 11-month-old boy is brought to your office by his mother. She is concerned because her son coughs and wheezes day and night for 2 weeks after every cold, and he seems to have a cold every month. He uses no medication for these symptoms. He is otherwise well with normal growth and development. The patient's father smokes cigarettes, but always away from his son. Which of the following statements about this patient's condition is correct?

(A) Asthma is very unlikely because of his young age.
(B) A trial of prophylactic inhaled cromolyn sodium may be beneficial.
(C) Smoking cigarettes in a separate room should not affect the patient's symptoms.
(D) An albuterol inhaler should be prescribed for prevention of his symptoms.
(E) Inspiratory and expiratory radiographs should be performed to rule out a foreign body.

24. A 9-month-old boy is brought to the emergency department in cardiac arrest. His parents found him unconscious, and cardiopulmonary resuscitation was initiated immediately. Which of the following is the most common cause of cardiac arrest in a child?

(A) Poisoning
(B) Cardiac dysrhythmia secondary to heart disease
(C) Seizures
(D) Hypoxia
(E) Trauma

25. During a routine health maintenance examination, an obese 13-year-old girl is noted to have acanthosis nigricans. Your counseling of the patient includes a discussion of the association between acanthosis nigricans and type 2 diabetes mellitus. Which of the following is also associated with type 2 diabetes mellitus?

(A) HLA haplotypes DR3 and DR4
(B) Environmental triggers, such as coxsackievirus
(C) Islet cell antibodies
(D) Peripheral tissue resistance to insulin
(E) Insulin antibodies

26. A 7-month-old male infant is brought to your office with a 1-month-long history of fussiness, intermittent vomiting, and nonbloody, foul-smelling stools. He has not gained weight since his 6-month health maintenance examination. His diet consists of formula and wheat cereal that was introduced at 6 months of age. Which of the following is the most likely diagnosis?

(A) Lactase deficiency
(B) Celiac disease
(C) Crohn's disease
(D) Gastroesophageal reflux disease
(E) Cow's milk protein intolerance

27. You are called urgently to the newborn nursery to evaluate a "blue" infant. On administration of 100% oxygen, there is significant increase in the patient's PaO_2. Which of the following is the most likely diagnosis?

(A) Neonatal pneumonia
(B) Tetralogy of Fallot
(C) Respiratory distress syndrome
(D) Truncus arteriosus
(E) Meconium aspiration syndrome

28. A 3-year-old girl is diagnosed with cervical adenitis and is discharged home with a 7-day course of amoxicillin–clavulanic acid. Five days into therapy, she presents for reevaluation with no decrease in the size of the enlarged cervical node. The child's fevers have also been persistent. Physical examination is remarkable for a febrile toddler with conjunctivitis, pharyngitis, right anterior cervical adenopathy (the node is 2 cm in diameter), and an erythematous macular rash on the chest and back. Which of the following courses of management would be most appropriate at this time?

(A) Send the patient home on oral penicillin with a presumptive diagnosis of scarlet fever.
(B) Perform a tuberculin skin test and discharge the patient on oral dicloxacillin, with follow-up in 48 hours.
(C) Admit the patient for a rule-out sepsis workup that includes evaluation of blood, urine, and cerebrospinal fluid for bacterial infection.
(D) Admit the patient for high-dose intravenous immune globulin therapy.
(E) Admit the patient for high-dose corticosteroid therapy.

The response items for statements 29 and 30 are the same. You will be required to select one answer for each statement in the set.

(A) Dilated cardiomyopathy
(B) Hypertrophic cardiomyopathy
(C) Restrictive cardiomyopathy

For each patient, select the associated cardiomyopathy.

29. A newborn girl is born at full term by cesarean section weighing 9 pounds 8 ounces. Her mother developed diabetes during pregnancy. The girl is admitted to the neonatal intensive care unit because of tachypnea. On examination, a harsh systolic ejection murmur is heard.

30. A 12-year-old boy presents to the emergency department after an episode of chest pain that occurred during baseball practice. Electrocardiography reveals evidence of myocardial infarction. Because of this unusual presentation, you suspect he may have anomalous origin of the left coronary artery from the pulmonary artery.

31. A 3-year-old girl is brought to the office with a 2-week history of melena. Physical examination and vital signs are normal. A complete blood count reveals a hemoglobin of 6 g/dL. Which of the following is the next most appropriate step to evaluate the cause of her anemia and bleeding?

(A) Computed tomography of the abdomen
(B) Meckel's scan
(C) Colonoscopy
(D) Chest and abdominal radiography
(E) Upper endoscopy

32. A 3-year-old boy is brought to the office for evaluation of a rash. The parents report that 1 week earlier he had the "stomach flu," characterized by fever, abdominal pain, and foul-smelling loose stools with occasional blood streaks. The gastrointestinal symptoms resolved spontaneously. For the past 2 days, he has been less active than usual and somewhat irritable with a decreased appetite. On physical examination, the patient is irritable but consolable, with mild periorbital edema, pale mucous membranes, and a petechial eruption on the abdomen. Laboratory studies reveal a leukocyte count of 12,000 cells/mm³, a hemoglobin count of 7.5 g/dL, and a platelet count of 34,000/μL. The serum creatinine is 1.4 mg/dL. Which of the following statements regarding this patient's most likely diagnosis is most accurate?

(A) The thrombocytopenia is most likely caused by antibody-mediated destruction.
(B) Antibiotic therapy is not indicated.
(C) The anemia is most likely secondary to blood losses associated with his prior episodes of bloody diarrhea.
(D) The prognosis is poor.
(E) The most common pathogen associated with this condition in North America is *Shigella dysenteriae* type 1.

33. The parents of an 18-month-old girl return to see you for a follow-up of their child's anemia. You prescribed iron (5 mg/kg per day) when you discovered that the girl had a microcytic, hypochromic anemia with a hemoglobin (Hgb) of 10.1 g/dL on routine anemia screening. Today, her Hgb is 10 g/dL despite iron therapy for the past 3 months. She is asymptomatic. Which of the following is an appropriate course of management at this time?

(A) Represcribe iron and suggest that it be given daily with orange juice.
(B) Represcribe iron and suggest that it be given daily with whole cow's milk.
(C) Consider referral for a red blood cell transfusion if the Hgb does not respond to iron within the next month.
(D) Order an Hgb electrophoresis and iron level to rule out other causes of anemia before restarting iron.
(E) Prescribe folic acid.

34. The parents of a 3-month-old female infant are concerned about their child's vomiting. For the past 6 weeks, their daughter has spit up after each feed. She takes both breast milk and a cow's milk–based formula and spits up after either is given. She does not seem bothered by the spitting up, and her parents deny that she has diarrhea, fever, cough, apnea, cyanosis, or discomfort. She weighed 7 pounds 4 ounces at birth and now weighs 11 pounds 1 ounce. Physical examination is normal. Which of the following is the most appropriate next step in management?

(A) Provide education and reassurance that her spitting up is common and normal and will resolve without treatment.
(B) Order a pH probe study to document gastroesophageal reflux.
(C) Change her diet to a hydrolyzed amino acid formula.
(D) Prescribe an H₂-blocker as a therapeutic trial.
(E) Order a barium upper gastrointestinal study to evaluate the esophagus, stomach, and duodenum.

35. The mother of a 2-year-old girl calls you urgently, concerned that her child fell in the backyard and traumatically avulsed her maxillary incisor. Which of the following is the most appropriate management at this time?

(A) The mother should wrap the tooth in a clean, dry towel and bring the tooth to the dentist within 24 hours.
(B) The mother should store the avulsed tooth in milk and seek emergency dental care immediately.
(C) The mother should scrub the tooth, rinse it with water, and replace it in the socket.
(D) The mother should replace the tooth in the socket and seek emergency dental care immediately.
(E) No intervention is required.

36. A 3-year-old boy is brought to the office with a 1-week history of upper respiratory symptoms and the acute onset of a limp. Physical examination is notable for a petechial eruption on the thighs. Laboratory analysis reveals a normal platelet count. Which of the following statements regarding the most likely diagnosis is most accurate?

(A) This patient has a multiorgan system vasculitis associated with increased serum IgE levels.
(B) Recurrences of this condition are rare.
(C) Steroids are contraindicated for the treatment of this condition.
(D) The rash in this condition typically begins on the palms and soles.
(E) The renal manifestations of this condition may not become clinically apparent for up to 3 months after the initial presentation.

37. A 4-year-old previously healthy boy is brought to the emergency department after being bitten by a dog 18 hours ago. He has two small puncture wounds on his left wrist. Which of the following regarding the dog bite in this patient is correct?

(A) Wound irrigation is the most appropriate initial treatment.
(B) The wound should be sutured.
(C) Infection, if it develops, is most commonly caused by *Bartonella henselae*.
(D) Antibiotics should be withheld until infection is clinically present.
(E) Tetanus immunization is not needed for dog bites.

The response items for statements 38–41 are the same. You will be required to select one answer for each statement in the set.

(A) Topical tobramycin drops
(B) Topical acyclovir drops
(C) Baby shampoo scrubs of the eyelids
(D) Topical mast cell stabilizer drops
(E) Oral erythromycin
(F) Oral acyclovir
(G) Intravenous penicillin

For each patient, select the most appropriate initial management.

38. A 7-day-old boy with bilateral conjunctival discharge.

39. An 8-year-old girl with burning, crusting, and scales at the eyelash base.

40. A 9-month-old girl with purulent conjunctival discharge.

41. A 3-year-old boy with conjunctival redness, itching, and watery discharge.

42. A 6-year-old boy is brought to the office with complaints of sore throat, mild fatigue, and headache for 2 days. On physical examination, he is febrile to 101°F (38.3°C) and is well-hydrated, comfortable, and without distress. White exudates on his tonsils and anterior cervical lymphadenopathy are present. Which of the following is the most important initial management step?

(A) Initiate antibiotic therapy for "strep throat."
(B) Order a Monospot test.
(C) Obtain a throat culture.
(D) Recommend supportive care with acetaminophen and throat lozenges.
(E) Obtain a lateral neck radiograph.

43. You are called to the emergency department to evaluate a 3-year-old girl referred for evaluation of a 2-day history of fever, emesis, and progressive lethargy. Computed tomography of the head demonstrates marked dilation of the ventricular system consistent with communicating hydrocephalus. Which of the following is the most likely cause of this condition?

(A) Brain atrophy
(B) Chiari type II malformation
(C) Bacterial meningitis
(D) Aqueductal stenosis
(E) Dandy-Walker malformation

The response options for statements 44 and 45 are the same. You will be required to select one answer for each statement in the set.

(A) Vitamin A deficiency
(B) Vitamin B_1 deficiency (thiamine)
(C) Vitamin B_6 deficiency (pyridoxine)
(D) Vitamin B_{12} deficiency (cobalamin)
(E) Vitamin C deficiency
(F) Vitamin D deficiency
(G) Vitamin K deficiency

For each patient, select the most likely vitamin deficiency.

44. A 2-year-old boy is a "picky" eater and has anemia, swollen gums, and a deep abrasion to the right leg that has taken almost 3 weeks to heal.

45. A 4-year-old girl has dry eyes and difficulty seeing in the dark.

46. A 17-year-old boy presents with dysuria and increased urinary frequency. He has had several sexual partners and indicates that he uses condoms "most of the time." Which of the following statements regarding the likely diagnosis is correct?

(A) Trimethoprim-sulfamethoxazole should be given for a presumed urinary tract infection.
(B) Evidence of greater than five white blood cells per high-power field on a Gram stain of his urethral secretions is sufficient for a presumptive diagnosis.
(C) This diagnosis is more common in females.
(D) The causative agents almost always cause symptoms that lead to the diagnosis.
(E) Obtaining a culture from a urethral swab is the only method that provides a definitive diagnosis.

47. A 7-year-old boy is brought to the office with a 3-day history of painful swelling anterior to his left ear. On physical examination, a small amount of pus can be expressed from Stensen's duct. Which of the following statements regarding the most likely diagnosis is correct?

(A) Placement of a skin test for tuberculosis should be considered.
(B) Supportive care for probable mumps infection is indicated.
(C) Epstein-Barr virus or cytomegalovirus infection is the most likely cause of the infection.
(D) Surgery should be immediately consulted to drain the infection.
(E) Antibiotics to cover *Streptococcus pneumoniae* are indicated.

48. The parents of a 6-week-old male infant bring him to the office for an evaluation because of concerns about their infant's color. They note that he turns "purple" whenever he cries and is very fussy. He is otherwise well. He feeds vigorously, and his weight is 1 pound 3 ounces above his birth weight. He is pink and happy when not crying. On physical examination, a systolic murmur is heard at the upper left sternal border. Which of the following is the most likely diagnosis?

(A) Transposition of the great arteries
(B) Tetralogy of Fallot
(C) Tricuspid atresia without a ventricular septal defect
(D) Total anomalous pulmonary venous connection
(E) Truncus arteriosus

The response items for statements 49–53 are the same. You will be required to select one answer for each statement in the set.

(A) Seborrheic dermatitis
(B) Contact dermatitis
(C) Tinea corporis
(D) Pityriasis rosea
(E) Miliaria rubra
(F) Psoriasis
(G) Fifth disease

For each patient, select the most likely diagnosis.

49. An 8-year-old boy has oval scaly erythematous patches on the upper extremity with partial central clearing.

50. A 15-year-old boy has red greasy scales and crusts in the nasolabial skin folds.

51. A 13-year-old girl has scaling papules and plaques. When she injures her skin, new lesions develop at the site of the trauma.

52. A 6-month-old girl has small erythematous pruritic papules on the chest and neck in the summertime.

53. A 3-year-old boy has erythematous papules in a "Christmas tree" distribution on the trunk.

54. An 18-month-old boy with a history of myelomeningocele repair at birth and subsequent ventriculoperitoneal shunt placement is brought to the office for a routine health maintenance visit. Medical history is also significant for an extensive stay in the neonatal intensive care unit, which was complicated by sepsis. Since the neonatal period, he has been relatively well, although his mother notes occasional rashes described as "red welts." Considering this patient's medical history, this patient is most likely to be allergic to which of the following?

(A) Penicillin
(B) Cow's milk protein
(C) Dust mites
(D) Latex
(E) Wool

55. At birth, a newborn has thrombocytopenia, enlarged liver and spleen, hearing loss, heart murmur, and bilateral cataracts. His mother recalls a brief viral illness during her first trimester of pregnancy. Congenital infection with which of the following organisms is the most likely cause of this infant's symptoms?

(A) Toxoplasmosis
(B) Rubella
(C) Varicella
(D) Herpes simplex virus
(E) Cytomegalovirus

56. An infant is brought to the office for a routine health maintenance visit. The infant can sit with support, vocalize with mixed vowel and consonant sounds, and has just learned to transfer objects from hand to hand. The most likely age is:

(A) 4 months
(B) 6 months
(C) 8 months
(D) 9 months
(E) 10 months

57. A 4-year-old girl is brought to the office with a persistent cough. Her mother is concerned because she has had a wet-sounding cough for the past 4–5 months without improvement. Past medical history is significant for three episodes of pneumonia in the past 18 months, each episode treated with antibiotics. Her mother is also concerned that she has been underweight for the past 12 months. On physical examination, the patient is afebrile, and her respiratory rate is 24 breaths/min. Her weight and height are both less than the fifth percentile. Lung examination reveals diffuse crackles and wheezes. Which of the following tests would reveal her most likely underlying diagnosis?

(A) Chest radiograph
(B) Sputum culture
(C) Sweat chloride assessment
(D) Bilateral decubitus radiographs
(E) Cold agglutinins

The response options for statements 58–60 are the same. You will be required to select one answer for each statement in the set.

(A) Viral meningitis
(B) Bacterial meningitis
(C) Tuberculous meningitis
(D) Partially treated bacterial meningitis
(E) Brain abscess
(F) Fungal meningitis

For each patient, select the most likely diagnosis.

58. A 14-month-old boy has fever and irritability. Cerebrospinal fluid (CSF) analysis reveals 7,500 white blood cells (WBCs) per cubic millimeter with a polymorphonuclear leukocyte predominance, a low glucose, and a high protein.

59. A 5-year-old girl has had fevers for 2 weeks and is now confused and sleepy. CSF analysis reveals 200 WBCs/mm^3 with a lymphocyte predominance, a very low glucose, a very elevated protein, and a negative Gram stain.

60. A 9-year-old boy presents with headache, photophobia, and 1 day of fever. CSF analysis reveals 350 WBCs/mm^3 with a polymorphonuclear leukocyte predominance, a normal glucose, a normal protein, and a negative Gram stain.

61. A 6-week-old boy is brought to the office in September with a 2-day history of cough and increased work of breathing. Past medical history is significant for vaginal delivery without complications at 38 weeks. At 10 days of age, he was treated with erythromycin ointment for conjunctivitis. On physical examination, the patient is afebrile. He is coughing rapidly and has a respiratory rate of 54 breaths/min. Diffuse wheezes are present throughout the lung fields along with mild subcostal retractions. Which of the following is the most likely cause of the patient's signs and symptoms?

(A) *Mycoplasma pneumoniae*
(B) *Chlamydia trachomatis*
(C) Respiratory syncytial virus
(D) *Streptococcus pneumoniae*
(E) Asthma

62. A 13-year-old boy has a 3-hour history of severe pain in his right scrotum. On physical examination, his right testicle is diffusely tender and swollen. The right cremasteric reflex is absent. Which of the following statements regarding this patient's likely diagnosis is correct?

(A) Radionuclide imaging will demonstrate increased uptake to the right testicle.
(B) Definitive diagnosis can be made on the basis of relief of pain when the right testicle is elevated.
(C) Management includes oral doxycycline and oral cefixime for presumptive epididymitis.
(D) Surgery consultation within the next 12 hours is indicated for possible surgical intervention.
(E) Surgical intervention will involve both testicles.

63. A 7-year-old boy is brought to the office with a 6-month history of daytime enuresis. Which of the following findings would be most important in prompting you to order imaging studies?

(A) Positive family history of enuresis in the patient's father, who wet the bed until he was 12 years of age
(B) Onset of symptoms when the parents separated
(C) Abnormal anal wink reflex
(D) Constipation without encopresis
(E) Frequent voiding of small amounts of urine

The response items for statements 64–66 are the same. You will be required to select one answer for each statement in the set.

(A) Acute dactylitis
(B) Sequestration crisis
(C) Acute chest syndrome
(D) Hyperhemolytic crisis
(E) Aplastic crisis

For each patient with sickle cell disease, select the type of sickle cell crisis.

64. A 3-year-old boy has pallor, jaundice, and fatigue. He has an increased reticulocyte count, increased bilirubin level, and decreased hemoglobin (Hgb).

65. A 4-year-old girl has pallor and fatigue. Her reticulocyte count and Hgb levels are decreased.

66. A 2-year-old boy has pallor, fatigue, tachycardia, and hypotension. His reticulocyte count is high, and his Hgb level is low.

67. A 4-month-old female infant is brought to the office for a routine health maintenance visit. Which of the following motor skills accurately describes the expected developmental abilities of this infant?

(A) When the infant is pulled from a supine to a sitting position, her head lags behind her shoulders.
(B) In the prone position, the infant can raise her head slightly but cannot push up with her arms.
(C) In the prone position, the infant can push up using her arms and hold her head up.
(D) When pulled from a supine to a sitting position, the infant anticipates the movement and leads with her head.
(E) In the prone position, the infant can roll to a supine position and can then get into a sitting position.

68. A 15-month-old boy is brought to the office for a routine health maintenance visit. His parents are concerned that he has not yet started to walk. Other motor milestones and verbal milestones are on target. On examination, you note normal strength and movement of all extremities; however, his thigh folds are asymmetric, and there appears to be a limb length discrepancy of 1 inch. Which of the following is the most likely diagnosis?

(A) Transient synovitis
(B) Developmental hip dysplasia
(C) Legg-Calvé-Perthes disease
(D) Femoral anteversion
(E) Slipped capital femoral epiphysis

The response items for statements 69–71 are the same. You will be required to select one answer for each statement in the set.

(A) Wilms' tumor
(B) Neuroblastoma
(C) Lymphoma
(D) Pheochromocytoma
(E) Rhabdomyosarcoma

For each patient, select the most likely malignancy.

69. A 3-year-old girl presents with the acute onset of an unsteady gait. On physical examination, she has random jerking eye movements in all directions, myoclonus, and ataxia with ambulation.

70. A 18-month-old girl presents for a routine health maintenance evaluation. On physical examination, she has a left-sided abdominal mass, absence of her bilateral irides, and hypertrophy of her right thigh and right leg.

71. A 5-month-old girl diagnosed with an abdominal malignancy has a localized tumor with metastases to her bone marrow and right femur. Without treatment, her tumor regresses.

72. A 23-day-old male infant has a 2-day history of streaks of blood and mucus with each stool. His parents report no fever, vomiting, or ill contacts. Which of the following is the most likely cause of his symptoms?

(A) Juvenile polyp
(B) Meckel's diverticulum
(C) Infectious enterocolitis
(D) Allergic colitis (protein intolerance)
(E) Inflammatory bowel disease

The response options for statements 73 and 74 are the same. You will be required to select one answer for each statement in the set.

(A) Head ultrasound
(B) Audiologic evaluation
(C) Ophthalmologic evaluation
(D) Thyroid screen
(E) Flexion and extension cervical spine radiographs

For each patient, select the most appropriate screening test to be used to evaluate for a complication of the condition.

73. A short 16-year-old girl with delayed puberty, a webbed neck, and shield chest.

74. A 4-year-old boy with fragile bones, easy bruisability, and blue sclerae.

75. You are called to the emergency department to evaluate a severely ill 5-year-old child who collapsed while at kindergarten. On physical examination, you find a comatose child whose respirations are irregular with no particular pattern. This patient's respiratory pattern is most suggestive of which of the following?

(A) Cerebellar injury
(B) Cerebral stroke
(C) Narcotic ingestion
(D) Impending brain death

76. A 3-year-old boy recently adopted from an international adoption agency is referred to you for evaluation of short stature. The details of the patient's past medical history are unknown. Physical examination reveals an alert child whose weight is at the third percentile and whose height is well below the third percentile for age (50th percentile for a 16-month-old child). The patient's upper-to-lower body segment ratio is high (i.e., above the expected ratio for age). Which of the following causes might explain this patient's short stature?

(A) Malnutrition
(B) Child neglect
(C) Growth hormone deficiency
(D) Fetal alcohol syndrome
(E) Rickets

77. A previously healthy 4-year-old boy is admitted to the hospital for a 5-day history of fever and severe right leg pain. There is no history of trauma. On examination, the boy is nontoxic; however, his right tibia above the ankle is warm, erythematous, and indurated. You suspect he may have osteomyelitis. Which of the following statements regarding this diagnosis is correct?

(A) A plain radiograph demonstrates periosteal elevation and should be the initial diagnostic study.
(B) The infection was most likely acquired by hematogenous seeding.
(C) The most likely pathogen is *Salmonella typhi.*
(D) Blood culture is positive in almost all patients with osteomyelitis.
(E) An oral first-generation cephalosporin should be started for outpatient treatment of osteomyelitis because the child is nontoxic.

78. You are performing an initial physical examination on a term newborn in the delivery room. The presence of which of the following leads you to suspect an underlying congenital anomaly?

(A) Umbilical hernia
(B) Hypospadias
(C) Single umbilical artery
(D) Nevus simplex on the right upper eyelid
(E) Diastasis recti

79. A 17-year-old boy presents to your office for a routine health maintenance evaluation. He has been well with the exception of some fatigue for the past few months and vague, nonspecific discomfort in his abdomen. On physical examination, the spleen is significantly enlarged, extending down to the left lower quadrant of his abdomen. On the basis of his symptoms and the splenomegaly, chronic myelogenous leukemia is in your differential diagnosis. Which of following statements regarding the most likely type of chronic myelogenous leukemia in this patient is correct?

(A) Further examination will likely reveal an eczematous-like facial rash and petechiae.
(B) The Philadelphia chromosome is present on cytogenetic analysis of leukemic cells.
(C) Radiation therapy is effective.
(D) The illness is very likely to be fatal within months.
(E) The white blood cell count will likely be < 30,000 cells/mm^3.

80. A 6-year-old girl who lives in Vermont develops fever, headache, muscle and joint aches, and several enlarged lymph nodes. On physical examination, an erythematous ringlike skin rash with a clear center is evident on her trunk. Which of the following would be the most appropriate treatment at this time?

(A) Oral doxycycline
(B) Oral amoxicillin
(C) Intravenous penicillin
(D) Intravenous ceftriaxone
(E) No antibiotic treatment

81. An 18-month-old female infant is brought to the office with a 3-day history of nasal congestion and rhinorrhea. Today she developed a fever to 101°F (38.3°C) and a barky cough. She is eating well and has remained active. On initial evaluation in the emergency department, she has a normal respiratory rate with no respiratory distress, is playful, and has no stridor. However, when you begin your examination, she begins to cry and immediately you hear inspiratory stridor. As she calms down, the stridor resolves completely. The remainder of the examination is normal. Which of the following should be your management approach?

(A) Cool mist and supportive care only
(B) A 10-day course of oral corticosteroids
(C) Nebulized albuterol
(D) Nebulized racemic epinephrine
(E) Nebulized ribavirin

82. A 3-year-old boy has a focal seizure involving his left arm and left leg. Computed tomography (CT) of the head reveals a calcified cyst within the brain parenchyma. Which of the following statements regarding the most likely diagnosis is correct?

(A) Surgical excision of the cyst is indicated.
(B) Anticonvulsant therapy alone is indicated.
(C) Ingestion of contaminated poultry is the likely cause.
(D) Ova and parasite stool examination is a reliable and sensitive diagnostic technique.
(E) The cyst noted on CT scan is evidence of active infection.

83. A 13-year-old girl who resided outside of the United States for 6 months visited a physician for knee and ankle pain. She was diagnosed with systemic lupus erythematosus (SLE). She now has returned to the United States, and she is brought to your office for a second opinion. She currently has no symptoms other than mild joint pains. A negative or normal result of which of the following tests makes the diagnosis of SLE most dubious?

(A) Erythrocyte sedimentation rate
(B) Anti–double-stranded DNA antibody
(C) Anti-Smith antibody
(D) Antinuclear antibody
(E) Rheumatoid factor

The response items for statements 84–88 are the same. You will be required to select one answer for each statement in the set.

(A) Naloxone
(B) Oxygen
(C) Deferoxamine
(D) Ethanol
(E) Atropine
(F) Pyridoxine
(G) Diphenhydramine
(H) *N*-acetylcysteine
(I) Flumazenil
(J) Glucagon
(K) D-Penicillamine
(L) Pralidoxime

For each poisoning, select the appropriate antidote.

84. A 15-month-old boy has severe vomiting and bloody stools 3 hours after swallowing 30 prenatal vitamin tablets.

85. A 15-year-old girl has vomiting and abdominal pain 2 hours after swallowing 18 extra-strength acetaminophen tablets.

86. A 6-year-old boy presents in the winter with acute onset of headache, vomiting, confusion, blurry vision, and slurred speech. On examination, his skin is cherry red in color.

87. An 8-year-old boy who is developmentally delayed presents with seizures. His mother found an empty bottle of isoniazid recently prescribed for tuberculosis infection in his bedroom.

88. A 4-year-old girl develops dystonia while being treated with an antiemetic (a phenothiazine) for acute gastroenteritis.

89. A 15-year-old sexually active girl presents with a 6-month history of frequent painful irregular menstrual periods. She describes her periods as occurring every 2–3 weeks and each lasting 10–12 days. The amount of bleeding is very heavy. Which of the following statements regarding her condition is correct?

(A) The term menometrorrhagia describes the vaginal bleeding.
(B) Management involves hormonal contraception; pelvic examination is not necessary.
(C) The bleeding is likely secondary to excessive progesterone production.
(D) Laboratory testing is not indicated because her diagnosis is a clinical diagnosis.
(E) Dilation and curettage are indicated.

90. A 5-year-old boy is brought to the emergency department. His parents state that he is unable to walk. On physical examination, the patient is afebrile with normal vital signs. He is very irritable and scared. Neurologic examination shows significant symmetric weakness and diminished deep tendon reflexes in the lower extremities. Strength and deep tendon reflexes of the upper extremities are preserved. Sensation is normal in both the upper and lower extremities. Which of the following features is most consistent with the most likely diagnosis?

(A) Symmetric descending paralysis
(B) Elevated cerebrospinal fluid protein with low cell counts
(C) Normal nerve conduction studies
(D) Abnormal spinal magnetic resonance imaging
(E) Concurrent diarrheal infection with *Clostridium botulinum*

91. A 3-year-old boy is brought to your office for evaluation of a limp. For the past 2 days he has been limping and crying intermittently, saying that he is in pain and pointing to his left thigh. The patient has been afebrile, and his parents deny any trauma. Medical history further reveals an upper respiratory infection 2 weeks ago that resolved rapidly. On physical examination, the boy appears healthy but anxious, and he refuses to walk. His temperature is 97.6°F (36.4°C). When lying on the examination table, he holds his left hip in external rotation and abduction. Movement of his left hip results in mild pain. Laboratory evaluation reveals a white blood cell count of 11,000 cells/mm^3 and an erythrocyte sedimentation rate of 18 mm/hr. Which of the following is the most likely diagnosis?

(A) Septic arthritis of the hip
(B) Osteomyelitis of the hip
(C) Slipped capital femoral epiphysis
(D) Transient synovitis
(E) Toddler's fracture

92. During a routine health maintenance visit, the mother of a 3-year-old boy expresses concern that her son has had "too many infections." On further questioning, you discover he had pneumonia at 6 months of age and at 20 months of age, and "many, many ear infections" since infancy. Most recently, he was treated with a 2-week course of antibiotics for suspected sinusitis. Despite these infections, the child has been growing and developing normally. Which of the following laboratory studies would confirm the most likely diagnosis?

(A) Complete blood count
(B) Anergy skin test
(C) Quantitative serum IgA level
(D) Assessment of T-cell response to mitogens
(E) Total hemolytic complement

93. The parents of a 4-year-old boy are concerned about their son's bowed legs. The bowing has been apparent ever since he began to walk. However, they are a bit concerned now because the bowing in his right leg has become more pronounced, while his left leg appears to be improving. On physical examination, the right leg is bowed laterally to a greater degree than his left leg, and when he walks, his body shifts laterally away from midline. Which of the following is the most appropriate management of this patient?

(A) Standing anterior-posterior radiograph of the lower extremities
(B) Referral for physical therapy to strengthen the muscles of the lower extremities
(C) Parental reassurance that the condition is genu varum and will resolve without treatment
(D) Parental reassurance that the condition is genu valgum and will resolve without treatment
(E) Referral to a podiatrist for orthotic shoes

94. A 9-year-old girl has a 2-week history of restlessness, episodes of excessive crying, and increased difficulty writing her name. Magnetic resonance imaging of her head is normal. Which of the following is the most likely diagnosis?

(A) Migraine
(B) Complex partial epilepsy
(C) Sydenham chorea
(D) Hydrocephalus with increased intracranial pressure
(E) Tourette syndrome

95. A 12-year-old boy returns from a camping trip in the Arkansas mountains. He has fever and severe headache. As you are examining him, a petechial rash suddenly appears on his hands and feet. Which of the following statements regarding the most likely cause of his illness is correct?

(A) The illness is caused by infection with a spirochete.
(B) Definitive serologic evidence of infection should be obtained before the initiation of therapy.
(C) Thrombocytopenia and anemia may be present.
(D) Prophylactic antibiotics are indicated to prevent this infection.
(E) Incidence of infection is highest in infants and very young children.

96. A 10-year-old boy presents with fever, hypotension, diarrhea, and diffuse erythroderma of the skin. Nikolsky sign is absent. Laboratory studies reveal thrombocytopenia and an elevated creatine kinase. Cultures of his blood, urine, and cerebrospinal fluid are negative. Which of the following is the most likely cause of the infection?

(A) Group A β-hemolytic streptococcus
(B) *Borrelia burgdorferi*
(C) *Staphylococcus aureus*
(D) Kawasaki disease
(E) *Escherichia coli* 0157:H7

The response options for statements 97–100 are the same. You will be required to select one answer for each statement in the set.

(A) High serum ceruloplasmin
(B) Low serum copper
(C) High serum copper
(D) Low serum zinc
(E) Low serum calcium
(F) High serum calcium
(G) Low serum glucose
(H) High serum ammonia

For each patient, select the likely laboratory finding.

97. A 12-year-old boy with ataxia, seizures, abnormal behavior, elevated transaminases, and yellowish discoloration of the peripheral cornea.

98. A 6-year-old boy with myoclonic seizures, mental retardation, and hair that is easily breakable and unmanageable.

99. A 12-month-old boy with vesicles and scales in the diaper area, failure to thrive, and chronic diarrhea.

100. A 2-year-old boy with interrupted aortic arch, recurrent fungal infections, a small chin, and short palpebral fissures.

Answers and Explanations

1. The correct answer is A [Chapter 4, Section X.E.3, Figures 4-2 and 4-3]. The differential diagnosis of direct (conjugated) hyperbilirubinemia includes obstructive jaundice secondary to a choledochal cyst, obstructive jaundice secondary to biliary atresia, neonatal hepatitis, cystic fibrosis, and inborn errors of metabolism. Hepatic ultrasound is able to diagnose choledochal cyst and is also useful in the evaluation of biliary atresia. Sepsis (diagnosed with a blood culture) should be considered in the differential diagnosis of both direct and indirect hyperbilirubinemia; however, it is very unlikely in an otherwise well-appearing infant who is alert and feeding well. ABO incompatibility (diagnosed with Coombs testing), hypothyroidism (diagnosed with thyroid hormone studies), and hemolytic disorders such as hereditary spherocytosis (diagnosed with an osmotic fragility test) all are causes of indirect (unconjugated) hyperbilirubinemia.

2. The correct answer is E [Chapter 1, Section III.E]. There are three major contraindications to administering the DTaP vaccine. These contraindications include a severe allergic reaction (i.e., anaphylaxis) after a previous vaccine dose or to a vaccine component, encephalopathy within 7 days of administration of a previous dose of DTaP, and a progressive neurologic disorder, which includes progressive encephalopathy and uncontrolled epilepsy. A mild respiratory illness with a low-grade fever is not a contraindication to administering the DTaP vaccine, nor is a history of moderate swelling at the injection site after a previous dose. Administration of intravenous immune globulin within the preceding 3–11 months is a precaution to immunization with live virus vaccines, such as measles, mumps, and rubella (MMR) and varicella. Immunocompromised status or the presence of an immunocompromised sibling in the household is not a contraindication to administration of DTaP.

3. The correct answer is A [Chapter 16, Section V.D]. This child's presentation is most consistent with dermatomyositis. Characteristic cutaneous manifestations include a periorbital heliotrope rash that may cross the nasal bridge and an erythematous and hypertrophic rash over the metacarpal and proximal interphalangeal joints (Gottron's papules). Characteristic laboratory and diagnostic studies include abnormal electromyography findings, abnormal muscle biopsy findings, and increased muscle enzymes, including creatine kinase. A positive antinuclear antibody is not specific and would be more suggestive of systemic lupus erythematosus (SLE) or juvenile rheumatoid arthritis (JRA), although this patient fails to meet four of the eleven diagnostic criteria required for the diagnosis of SLE and has no arthritis, which is characteristic of JRA. Although both Epstein-Barr virus infection and cytomegalovirus infection may present with chronic fatigue, neither infection would present with the characteristic rashes described in this patient.

4. The correct answer is B [Chapter 20, Table 20-1]. The GCS is used to assess a patient's level of neurologic impairment. It is based on the physical examination and includes assessment for motor response, verbal response, and eye opening. In a young child, a modified scoring system can be used, which has been adapted for the nonverbal patient. The patient described has a GCS score of 5 because he does not open his eyes to pain or to voice (scored 1), has decerebrate posturing (scored 2), and moans with stimulation with incomprehensible words (scored 2). Because his GCS is < 8, he has likely suffered severe head injury.

5. The correct answer is B [Chapter 14, Section II.A]. The most common presenting symptoms of ALL are fever and bone or joint pain, as in this boy. The peak incidence of ALL is between 2 and 6 years of age, and ALL is more common in males. Pallor, hepatosplenomegaly, and lymphadenopathy are among the most common presenting findings on physical examination. The white blood cell count varies on presentation and is elevated in only one third of patients.

6. The correct answer is A [Chapter 13, Section IV.B.2]. Hemophilia A, a deficiency of factor VIII, is an X-linked inherited disorder that occurs only in males. Typical features include deep soft-tissue bleeding and hemarthroses. Laboratory findings include a prolonged aPTT in all but very mild cases, but prothrombin time and bleeding time are normal. Management includes replacement of factor VIII, which is not a vitamin K-dependent coagulation factor.

7. The correct answer is C [Chapter 11, Section V]. This patient's presentation is consistent with nephrotic syndrome, which is characterized by heavy proteinuria, hypoalbuminemia, hypercholesterolemia, and edema. Most children present with edema, which can range from mild periorbital edema, to scrotal or labial edema, to widespread edema; this edema often follows an upper respiratory infection. Patients with nephrotic syndrome are at an increased risk for infection with encapsulated organisms, such as *Streptococcus pneumoniae*. Because of this risk, if a patient with active nephrotic syndrome becomes febrile, evaluation should include a blood culture, urine culture, and chest radiograph, and broad-spectrum empiric intravenous antibiotics should be initiated immediately. Patients with nephrotic syndrome are predisposed to thrombosis (stroke, renal vein thrombosis, deep vein thrombosis, and sagittal sinus thrombosis) secondary to hypercoagulability. Renal biopsy is rarely indicated in a child with nephrotic syndrome, unless the creatinine clearance is impaired or initial management with corticosteroids is ineffective. Most patients with nephrotic syndrome respond to corticosteroid therapy.

8. The correct answer is C [Chapter 3, Section VII.B.1.b]. Bacterial vaginosis is the most common cause of vaginitis in adolescents. It results from a change in the patient's normal vaginal flora secondary to a reduction in lactobacilli. It presents with gray-white, malodorous discharge, a fishy odor, and little vaginal or vulvar inflammation. Wet-mount saline preparation demonstrates the presence of "clue cells." Bacterial vaginosis is not thought to be transmitted sexually, so partners do not need treatment. Neither antibiotics nor antiyeast medications are indicated.

9. The correct answer is D [Chapter 8, Section V.C and Table 8-6]. This clinical presentation is consistent with bacterial endocarditis. Ophthalmologic examination is warranted to evaluate for Roth spots and retinal hemorrhages, which can help confirm the diagnosis. Diagnosis is often made on confirmation of vegetations by echocardiography. Transesophageal echocardiography is more sensitive than transthoracic echocardiography in detecting vegetations. Rheumatoid factor and other acute-phase reactants, as well as the white blood cell count and the erythrocyte sedimentation rate, are often elevated. Gram-positive cocci, including *Streptococcus* and *Staphylococcus* species, are the most common infecting organisms. Gram-negative organisms are uncommon causes of endocarditis. Management includes appropriate intravenous antibiotics, but antibiotics can be safely withheld until at least three blood cultures are obtained in an attempt to identify the infecting organism and to use appropriate antibiotic therapy.

10. The correct answer is C [Chapter 12, Section X.E]. Myasthenia gravis is an immune-mediated condition caused by antibodies that form against the acetylcholine receptor at neuromuscular junctions. Most patients first come to medical attention with eye problems, especially bilateral ptosis. One of the hallmarks of patients with myasthenia gravis is that their weakness progresses as the day progresses. Fasciculations (i.e., spontaneous, small twitches of muscle fibers caused by denervation) are commonly seen in Guillain-Barré syndrome but not in myasthenia gravis. Botulism is associated with honey ingestion and would more likely present acutely with constipation followed by weakness. Deep tendon reflexes are normal in myasthenia gravis. The Tensilon test is a useful test that can confirm the diagnosis of myasthenia gravis. It is performed by intravenously injecting edrophonium chloride, a rapidly acting cholinesterase inhibitor, which produces transient improvement of ptosis.

11. The correct answer is E [Chapter 7, Table 7-2 and Sections III.B–C]. The majority of children with FUO (defined as unexplained fever lasting longer than 8 days to 3 weeks) have a common infection with an unusual presentation. Infectious diseases are the most common causes of FUO, whereas rheumatologic causes (e.g., Kawasaki disease, systemic juvenile rheumatoid arthritis) are the second most common cause of FUO. Hospitalization is often indicated to facilitate the evaluation and to document the fever and identify any coexisting signs and symptoms. A cause is identified in approximately 75% of patients after an extensive workup; no cause is identified in 25% of children despite a thorough evaluation.

12. The correct answer is C [Chapter 4, Section VI.C.1]. The most frequent cause of respiratory distress in preterm infants is respiratory distress syndrome (RDS) (also known as hyaline membrane disease or surfactant deficiency syndrome), which occurs in as many as 50% of newborns born before 30 weeks gestation (0.5% of all neonates). Meconium aspiration syndrome, neonatal sepsis, and intraventricular hemorrhage may all present with respiratory distress, but these conditions occur less frequently than RDS. Bronchopulmonary dysplasia is a chronic complication of RDS and does not occur in the immediate newborn period.

13. The correct answer is B [Chapter 10, Section II.D.6]. The patient's disorder, short bowel syndrome, occurs after surgical resection of small bowel, or damage to the small intestine from Crohn's disease or from radiation. The loss of small bowel reduces the absorptive capacity of the gut, leading to malabsorption and electrolyte abnormalities. Total parenteral nutrition (TPN) is commonly used to maintain adequate nutrition; however, TPN causes cholestatic liver disease and, in many patients, gallstones. Other complications of this disorder include bacterial overgrowth within the remaining intestine, nutritional deficiencies, poor bone mineralization, renal stones, and secretory diarrhea. Patients on TPN or with short bowel syndrome generally do not have gastrointestinal bleeding, constipation, pancreatic insufficiency, or inflammatory bowel disease.

14. The correct answer is D [Chapter 17, Section V.A.4.b, Table 17-2, Figure 17-2]. A physeal fracture that extends through the physis and into both the epiphysis and metaphysis is a grade IV Salter-Harris fracture. A grade I fracture is within the physis. A grade II fracture is within the physis and extends into the metaphysis. A grade III fracture is in the physis and extends into the epiphysis. A grade V fracture describes a crush injury of the physis.

15. The correct answer is D [Chapter 1, Section II.B.2.c.(2)]. The patient described has craniosynostosis, a premature closure of a cranial suture. Eighty to ninety percent of cases of craniosynostosis are sporadic in occurrence with an unknown cause. Ten to twenty percent of cases are familial or are a component of a genetic syndrome (e.g., Apert syndrome, Crouzon syndrome). Sleeping on the back and congenital muscular torticollis may cause plagiocephaly, which is skull asymmetry without premature suture closure. Perinatal asphyxia causes microcephaly as a result of inadequate brain growth, rather than premature suture closure.

16 and 17. The correct answers are 16 (B) and 17 (C) [Chapter 4, Section I.B]. Sturge-Weber syndrome is a neurocutaneous syndrome characterized by a nevus flammeus ("port wine stain") in the area innervated by the ophthalmic branch of the trigeminal nerve (V-I). It is associated with seizures, intracranial and intraspinal malformations, and intracranial calcifications (question 16). Erythema toxicum neonatorum is a benign rash of infancy characterized by erythematous macules, papules, and pustules on the trunk and extremities. The lesions are filled with eosinophils, and no treatment is required (question 17).

18. The correct answer is D [Chapter 5, Section V.A.3]. Patients with homocystinuria are hypercoagulable. The tendency toward thromboembolism leads to significant morbidity, including deep vein thrombosis, myocardial infarction, and stroke. Daily aspirin greatly decreases the risk of thromboembolic events. Propranolol, a β-blocker, is useful for patients at risk for aortic dissection, such as patients with Marfan syndrome. Vitamin C may be useful in transient tyrosinemia of the newborn as it can assist in tyrosine elimination. D-Penicillamine increases the clearance of copper and is useful in Wilson' disease. Zinc is useful for children who have problems with healing, such as patients with acrodermatitis enteropathica. Propranolol, vitamin C, D-penicillamine, and zinc do not play useful roles in the management of patients with homocystinuria.

19 through 21. The correct answers are 19 (E), 20 (C), and 21 (B) [Chapter 6, Sections II.B.2.d.(3)(c)(i), II.C.3.f; Chapter 5, Sections III.A.2, III.C.1]. McCune-Albright syndrome (question 19) is characterized by endocrine dysfunction (peripheral precocious precocity, hyperthyroidism), irregularly bordered hyperpigmented macules ("coast of Maine" spots), and fibrous dysplasia of the bones that may lead to fractures. Kallmann syndrome (question 20), a form of hypogonadotropic hypogonadism, is associated with anosmia (absent sense of smell). Prader-Willi syndrome (question 21) is characterized by hypotonia, hypogonadism, and small hands and feet, with growth problems in the first year of life (secondary to feeding problems), followed by hyperphagia and obesity later in childhood. Turner syndrome is characterized by ovarian dysgenesis, short stature, webbing of the neck, and left-sided congenital heart disease, with an increased incidence of hypothyroidism. Laurence-Moon-Biedl syndrome is characterized by hypogonadism, retinitis pigmentosa, obesity, and polysyndactyly.

22. The correct answer is B [Chapter 20, Section VI.B.2; Chapter 17, Sections V.C, V.F]. Findings consistent with child abuse include specific types of fractures, such as metaphyseal ("corner" or "bucket handle") fractures. These fractures occur as a result of torsional force placed on an extremity (i.e., pulling and twisting) or from violent shaking. Other fractures highly suggestive of abuse include posterior and first rib fractures, fractures of the sternum, scapula, and vertebral spinous processes, and fractures in different stages of healing. Bruises on exposed areas, such as the knees, shins, elbows, and forehead, are common during childhood and are typical of accidental injury. Burns that have an irregular splashlike configuration are generally accidental. Toddler's fracture (i.e., spiral fracture of the distal tibia) can occur with little trauma, such as a fall when running, and alone are not suggestive of abuse. Supracondylar fractures are common during childhood and usually occur when a child falls on an outstretched arm, and alone are not suggestive of abuse.

23. The correct answer is B [Chapter 9, Section IV.A.7 and Table 9-4]. Asthma is the most likely diagnosis because of the symptoms of recurrent cough and wheezing. This patient likely has mild persistent asthma, given the frequency and persistence of symptoms. Because asthma is an inflammatory disorder, antiinflammatory medications, such as cromolyn sodium or low-dose inhaled corticosteroids, are recommended for persistent asthma symptoms. In as many as 50% of patients with asthma, symptoms may develop during the first year of life. Smoking should not be allowed in any place that a child with asthma may visit, including the home and automobile. Passive smoke exposure is an airway irritant and a trigger of asthma. Although albuterol would be useful for the management of acute symptoms, it has no effective role in prevention, except for preventing symptoms of exercise-induced asthma. Foreign body aspiration is less likely in a child with both persistent and recurrent symptoms. In addition, inspiratory and expiratory films could not be obtained in an 11-month-old child; therefore, decubitus films would be indicated if foreign body aspiration was suspected.

24. The correct answer is D [Chapter 20, Section I.A.1]. The most common cause of cardiac arrest in a child is a lack of oxygen supply to the heart. Respiratory problems that result in a lack of oxygen supply include choking, airway disease, lung disease, suffocation, and brain injury. The end result of any of these processes is decreased oxygen tension within the blood (hypoxia). Cardiac arrest can often be prevented if assisted breathing is administered rapidly. Heart disease is an uncommon cause of cardiac arrest during childhood. Seizures, poisonings, and trauma are also less common causes of cardiac arrest than hypoxia.

25. The correct answer is D [Chapter 6, Section VII.B]. Peripheral tissue resistance to insulin is seen in type 2 diabetes mellitus (DM). All of the other choices listed are more commonly associated with type 1 DM. The evolution of type 1 DM is thought to have numerous causes. It begins with a genetic predisposition (HLA haplotypes DR3/DR4), a viral infection acting as an environmental triggering event, and lastly an autoimmune process that ultimately results in beta cell destruction. Autoimmune antibodies, such as islet cell and insulin antibodies, may be found in type 1 DM.

26. The correct answer is B [Chapter 10, Section II.C.2–3]. Patients with celiac disease may present with vomiting, bloating, foul-smelling stools, or failure to thrive. Infants also may be irritable. This infant developed his symptoms after the introduction of wheat cereal that contains gluten. Gluten is found in wheat, rye, barley, and oats (if the oats are harvested in fields that also grow wheat). Celiac disease is a gluten-sensitive enteropathy in which antibodies to gluten cross-react and damage the mucosa of the small intestine, which results in flat, atrophic villi. Lactase deficiency causes bloating and watery stools, but not failure to gain weight. Crohn's disease is uncommon during infancy. Gastroesophageal reflux disease may be associated with vomiting and irritability; however, stools are not foul-smelling. Cow's milk protein intolerance may be associated with diarrhea, irritability, and vomiting, but stool blood and mucus are often present, and symptoms often begin before 6 months of age.

27. The correct answer is B [Chapter 4, Section IV.D.2]. The 100% oxygen test helps distinguish whether cyanosis is caused by cardiac or respiratory disease. Patients with cyanotic congenital heart disease associated with reduced pulmonary blood flow, such as tetralogy of Fallot, do not respond with any increase of significance in the PaO_2 level when given 100% oxygen. In contrast, infants with cyanotic congenital heart disease associated with normal or increased pulmonary blood flow, such as truncus arteriosus, may have some increase in the PaO_2 level, but not as much of an increase as that seen in patients with primary pulmonary disease. Patients with primary lung disease, such as neonatal pneumonia, respiratory distress syndrome, or meconium aspiration syndrome, demonstrate a very significant increase in the PaO_2 levels when administered 100% oxygen.

28. The correct answer is D [Chapter 16, Section II.G]. This patient presents with diagnostic criteria consistent with Kawasaki disease, and treatment includes high-dose intravenous immune globulin together with high-dose aspirin therapy. Oral penicillin is not an appropriate course of management in this patient because there is no evidence of the fine sandpaper-like rash consistent with scarlet fever, a sequelae of group A β-hemolytic streptococcal infection. Oral dicloxacillin can be used for suspected acute bacterial cervical adenitis; however, the lack of improvement on amoxicillin–clavulanic acid and the other findings on physical examination make cervical adenitis alone less likely. Admission for an evaluation for invasive bacterial disease (rule-out sepsis workup) is not indicated because this patient is neither toxic-appearing nor has meningeal signs. The presentation is also not consistent with high fever without a source, which requires empiric broad-spectrum antibiotic coverage. Steroids are controversial and currently not routinely indicated for the treatment of Kawasaki disease.

29 and 30. The correct answers are 29 (B) and 30 (A) [Chapter 8, Section V.F]. Cardiomyopathy may be categorized as dilated, hypertrophic, or restrictive. Hypertrophic cardiomyopathy (question 29) may be inherited in an autosomal dominant manner or may occur in infants of diabetic mothers. Infants of diabetic mothers have transient septal hypertrophy and have a systolic ejection murmur because of obstruction of left ventricular outflow. Causes of dilated cardiomyopathy (question 30) include viral myocarditis, carnitine deficiency, anomalous origin of the left coronary artery and hypocalcemia. Anomalous origin of the left coronary artery from the pulmonary artery may present with evidence of myocardial infarction. As a result of infarction, cardiac function may be impaired, and an echocardiogram shows a dilated ventricle with poor ventricular function. Causes of restrictive cardiomyopathy include inherited infiltrative disorders (such as hemochromatosis and Gaucher disease) and amyloidosis.

31. The correct answer is E [Chapter 10, Section X.C.2]. Melena, a term used to describe dark and tarry stools, is most often caused by upper gastrointestinal (GI) bleeding proximal to the ligament of Treitz. The most common causes of melena in a 3-year-old girl include gastritis, ulcers, swallowed blood from epistaxis, mechanical injury to the mucosa from vomiting (Mallory-Weiss tear) or a foreign body, and varices. To best evaluate the cause of upper GI bleeding, upper intestinal endoscopy is used to visualize the source of bleeding and, if indicated, to perform biopsies and treat active bleeding. Computed tomography of the abdomen is not useful in the diagnosis of upper GI bleeding. A Meckel's scan and colonoscopy have more utility in the investigation of lower, rather than upper, GI bleeding. Plain film radiography is generally not useful in diagnosis unless a foreign body or intestinal perforation is suspected.

32. The correct answer is B [Chapter 11, Section VI]. This patient's clinical presentation of a prodrome of bloody diarrhea followed by the onset of anemia, thrombocytopenia, and acute renal failure is most consistent with hemolytic uremic syndrome (HUS). The most common subtype of HUS seen in childhood is shiga toxin-associated HUS resulting from an intestinal infection with a toxin-producing bacteria. The treatment of shiga toxin-associated HUS is supportive, and antibiotics are not indicated. Vascular endothelial injury by the shiga toxin is the key to the pathogenesis of injury in shiga toxin-associated HUS. The toxin binds to endothelial cells, causing endothelial cell injury, most especially in the renal vasculature, leading to platelet thrombi formation and renal ischemia. Although the patient's bloody diarrhea may have contributed to his anemia, patients with HUS have hemolytic anemia. The prognosis for children with shiga toxin-associated HUS is usually favorable but depends on the severity of the initial episode. In North America, the most common pathogen associated with shiga toxin-associated HUS is *Escherichia coli* 0157:H7.

33. The correct answer is D [Chapter 13, Section I.D.2.d.(2)]. Although iron-deficiency anemia is the most common cause of anemia during childhood, other causes of anemia should be considered in patients who do not respond to iron therapy for suspected iron-deficiency anemia. In this case, this patient may have β-thalassemia minor (trait), a heterozygous condition that causes mild asymptomatic anemia. Because she did not respond to iron, she should undergo further testing, including an Hgb electrophoresis, blood smear, lead level, and an iron level (which is normal or elevated in β-thalassemia minor). Continuing to treat her with iron may not be beneficial at this point. Red blood cell transfusion is not indicated for this Hgb level. Folic acid is not helpful or indicated; folic acid deficiency causes a macrocytic anemia.

34. The correct answer is A [Chapter 10, Section III.D]. This patient is presenting with symptoms of physiologic gastroesophageal reflux, a finding found in up to 60% of infants. Gastroesophageal reflux does not need workup, change in the diet, or medical treatment. The spitting up is benign and resolves with time. Given her normal weight gain and the absence of pain, she does not have gastroesophageal reflux disease (GERD). GERD merits further evaluation with a barium upper gastrointestinal study to evaluate the anatomy of the stomach, esophagus, and duodenum, and a pH probe to confirm the presence of reflux.

35. The correct answer is E [Chapter 1, Section VI.E]. Avulsed primary teeth do not require reimplantation. In the case of an avulsed secondary (permanent) tooth, extraoral time is the most important prognostic factor for successful reimplantation. A tooth that has been stored dry, even after only 30 minutes, has a very poor prognosis. Management of an avulsed secondary tooth includes gentle rinsing with saline or water, placement of the avulsed tooth into the tooth socket or into a liquid such as milk, and emergent referral to a dentist.

36. The correct answer is E [Chapter 16, I.C]. The constellation of a nonthrombocytopenic petechial eruption on the thighs and a limp (arthritis) in a toddler, along with upper respiratory symptoms, is most consistent with the diagnosis of Henoch-Schönlein purpura (HSP). The renal manifestations of HSP are variable, ranging from mild hematuria or proteinuria to end-stage renal disease in 1% of patients. Classically, the renal manifestations of HSP may not become clinically apparent for up to several months after the patient's initial presentation. HSP is a multiorgan system vasculitis associated with increased serum IgA levels. Recurrences of HSP are quite common, occurring in approximately 50% of patients. Steroids are the mainstay of therapy for severe abdominal pain. The rash of HSP characteristically appears on the thighs and buttocks, not the palms and soles.

37. The correct answer is A [Chapter 20, Section IX.B]. The most important initial treatment for any bite is local wound care, which includes copious and prompt wound irrigation. Dog bites may become infected, especially bites to the hand, wrist, and foot, and bites that are small puncture wounds, as in this patient. Large wounds, wounds to the face, and wounds less than 12 hours old should all be sutured. However, wounds greater than 12 hours old should be allowed to close on their own (except facial wounds, which may still be safely closed up to 24 hours later as a result of the high vascularity of the face). Aerobic and anaerobic organisms, including *Staphylococcus aureus* and *Pasteurella multocida,* are the usual pathogens causing infection. *Bartonella henselae* is not a usual pathogen in dog bites but rather is a cause of cat scratch disease. Antibiotics should be started empirically, without waiting for clinical signs of infection, because of the high risk of infection. Tetanus prophylaxis is necessary for unimmunized or underimmunized patients who sustain dog bites.

38 through 41. The correct answers are 38 (E), 39 (C), 40 (A), and 41 (D) [Chapter 18, Table 18-2 and Section III.B.3]. Diagnosis of a red eye can often be made on the basis of history and physical examination. Conjunctivitis that occurs between days 4–10 of life is most likely caused by *Chlamydia trachomatis* and is best treated with oral erythromycin (question 38). Oral therapy is used to kill *Chlamydia* organisms in both the conjunctiva and nasopharynx simultaneously. If *Chlamydia* organisms within the nasopharynx are not killed, pneumonia may develop between 1 and 3 months of age. Burning, crusting, and scales at the eyelash margin suggest blepharitis, a condition treated with baby shampoo scrubs of the eyelashes (question 39). Purulent conjunctivitis in a young child is typically bacterial in origin and would prompt administration of topical antibiotics, such as tobramycin (question 40). Itching is a hallmark of allergy and suggests allergic conjunctivitis. Allergic disease of the eyes is best treated with topical antihistamines or topical mast cell stabilizers (question 41).

42. The correct answer is C [Chapter 7, Section V.D.2–3]. Because the clinical features of viral pharyngitis and group A β-hemolytic streptococcal (GABHS) pharyngitis overlap, children presenting with pharyngitis should undergo laboratory testing to confirm GABHS infection before the institution of antibiotic therapy. Such testing may include rapid antigen testing or a throat culture (the gold standard). Although infectious mononucleosis should be considered in patients with pharyngitis, this patient's acute presentation is unlikely to be caused by infectious mononucleosis, and therefore a Monospot test is not indicated. Supportive care with analgesics and lozenges is helpful for pharyngitis, but it is not the most important initial management step. A lateral neck radiograph is not indicated given the absence of clinical features consistent with upper airway obstruction.

43. The correct answer is C [Chapter 12, Section II.B–C]. Communicating hydrocephalus is caused by decreased absorption of cerebrospinal fluid (CSF) or, less commonly, by increased CSF production. Meningitis causes inflammation and scarring of the arachnoid membrane, which prevents the normal absorption of CSF and results in communicating hydrocephalus. Brain atrophy does not cause hydrocephalus but rather a condition called *hydrocephalus ex vacuo*, in which the ventricles are enlarged because of loss of surrounding brain tissue. Chiari type II malformation produces a noncommunicating hydrocephalus caused by blockage of flow in the ventricular system. Aqueductal stenosis may cause noncommunicating hydrocephalus for the same reason. A Dandy-Walker malformation is characterized by an absent or hypoplastic cerebellar vermis and cystic enlargement of the fourth ventricle, which blocks the flow of CSF, thereby causing noncommunicating hydrocephalus.

44 and 45. The correct answers are 44 (E) and 45 (A) [Chapter 10, Table 10-1]. Scurvy (question 44) is caused by vitamin C deficiency and causes symptoms that include hematologic abnormalities, edema, poor wound healing as a result of impaired synthesis of collagen, and a characteristic spongy swelling of the gums. Vitamin A deficiency (question 45) presents with xerophthalmia (dry conjunctiva and cornea) and night blindness.

46. The correct answer is B [Chapter 3, Section VII.B.5]. This patient's presentation with dysuria and increased urinary frequency are consistent with urethritis. A urinary tract infection is possible, but it is less likely in a male. Because of his sexual activity and the intermittent nature of his condom use, a sexually transmitted disease is most likely. Urethritis may be the result of *Neisseria gonorrhoeae* or nongonococcal causes, such as *Chlamydia trachomatis*. Diagnosis may be made presumptively by finding greater than five white blood cells per high-power field on a Gram stain of the patient's urethral secretions or by finding evidence of pyuria on a first-morning voided urine. Urethritis is more common in males than in females. Unlike this patient, many patients have asymptomatic infection. Definitive diagnosis can be made either by culture of the urethral secretions (via a urethral swab) or by nonculture tests on urine or on discharge (direct fluorescent antibody staining, polymerase chain reaction, ligase chain reaction, enzyme-linked immunoassay, or nucleic acid hybridization).

47. The correct answer is A [Chapter 7, Sections VIII.B, VIII.C, VIII.E]. On the basis of this patient's clinical features, parotitis is the most likely diagnosis. Unilateral parotitis is generally caused by an infection with *Staphylococcus aureus, Streptococcus pyogenes,* or *Mycobacterium tuberculosis*. Therefore, placement of tuberculin skin should be considered for patients with unilateral parotid infection. Mumps, Epstein-Barr virus, and cytomegalovirus generally result in bilateral parotitis. Management of bacterial parotitis rarely requires surgical drainage unless there is an abscess.

48. The correct answer is B [Chapter 8, Section IV.B]. The clinical presentation is consistent with tetralogy of Fallot. Children with tetralogy of Fallot may be cyanotic or pink at rest. The degree of cyanosis depends on the amount of resistance to flow through the obstructed pulmonary outflow tract and on the systemic vascular resistance, both of which affect the degree of right-to-left shunting across the ventricular septal defect (VSD). Crying can be a cause of hypercyanotic, or "tet," spells in a child with tetralogy of Fallot. Crying increases the child's heart rate. The elevated heart rate increases right ventricular outflow tract resistance, which increases right-to-left shunting, causing increasing cyanosis. Patients with transposition of the great arteries, tricuspid atresia without a VSD, and total anomalous pulmonary venous connection are expected to be cyanotic at all times (including at rest). Patients with truncus arteriosus may be only mildly cyanotic but also commonly manifest signs and symptoms of congestive heart failure, with poor weight gain because of excessive pulmonary blood flow.

49 through 53. The correct answers are 49 (C), 50 (A), 51 (F), 52 (E), and 53 (D) [Chapter 19, Sections III.C.3.b, III.D.3, III.E.3.c, III.F.2, V.A.2.b.(2)(a)]. Tinea corporis (ringworm) is a fungal infection characterized by oval or circular patches with central clearing (question 49). Seborrheic dermatitis in an adolescent may present with greasy scales and crusts in the nasolabial folds, beard areas, chest, and scalp (question 50). Psoriasis is characterized by scaling papules and plaques, and lesions may demonstrate the Koebner phenomenon, in which new lesions appear at the site of skin trauma (question 51). Miliaria rubra, or heat rash, occurs in association with heat and occlusive clothing. The sweat irritates the skin, causing pruritic papules, often on the neck, chest, inguinal area, or axilla (question 52). Pityriasis rosea is characterized by a large single scaly erythematous lesion ("herald patch") that is followed by oval erythematous macules and papules that follow skin lines in a "Christmas tree" distribution (question 53).

54. The correct answer is D [Chapter 15, Section VI.C.1]. Latex allergy is seen in health-care workers and in patients with myelomeningocele more frequently than in the general population because of more frequent exposure to latex (patients with myelomeningocele often require intermittent bladder catheterization, which exposes them to latex repeatedly). Latex exposure can cause acute urticaria and anaphylaxis in patients with latex allergy. Patients with neural tube defects do not have increased risks of developing allergies to penicillin, cow's milk protein, dust mites, or wool.

55. The correct answer is B [Chapter 7, Section XIII.D.4.c]. This infant most likely has congenital rubella syndrome. Cataracts, congenital heart disease (most often patent ductus arteriosus), and sensorineural hearing loss are the hallmarks of this syndrome. Presenting features may also include thrombocytopenia and extramedullary hematopoiesis manifesting as a "blueberry muffin" appearance to the skin. Congenital toxoplasmosis presents with hydrocephalus, intracranial calcifications, and chorioretinitis. Congenital varicella is uncommon but may present with a dermatomal rash or scarring. Perinatally acquired herpes simplex virus infection presents with a vesicular rash or encephalitis, but not with structural defects. Congenital cytomegalovirus infection typically presents with microcephaly, hepatosplenomegaly, and cerebral calcifications and usually not with cataracts or congenital heart disease.

56. The correct answer is B [Chapter 2, Tables 2-3 and 2-4]. A 6-month-old infant should be able to sit with support and may be able to sit independently. Language development in a normal 6-month-old includes babbling, which is placing consonants and vowels together. Another 6- to 7-month milestone is transferring objects from hand to hand. At 4 months, infants are learning to bring their hands to midline and to mouth but would not be able to transfer objects. By 8 months, infants should be sitting without support. At 9 and 10 months, infants should be able to use jargon, which integrates babbling with the intonational patterns, and would have moved beyond sitting with support to crawling, creeping, and pulling up to stand.

57. The correct answer is C [Chapter 9, Section IV.B.5–6]. This patient's presentation with chronic cough, recurrent pneumonia, and failure to thrive is most consistent with cystic fibrosis. Patients with cystic fibrosis may also present with chronic diarrhea as a result of steatorrhea and may have a history of meconium ileus at birth. Diagnosis of cystic fibrosis may be confirmed by documenting an elevated sweat chloride level or by documenting mutations in the gene associated with cystic fibrosis. Although a chest radiograph may help identify pneumonia, chest radiographic findings are not specific for cystic fibrosis. Sputum culture is difficult to obtain in a young child, and even if it could be obtained, it would not diagnose her underlying disorder. Foreign body aspiration, diagnosed by decubitus radiographs, should be considered in patients with cough, choking, stridor, and hoarseness, but would not typically cause failure to thrive. *Mycoplasma pneumoniae* infection, suggested by elevated cold agglutinins, would not cause failure to thrive, recurrent pneumonia, or cough for 4–5 months.

58 through 60. The correct answers are 58 (B), 59 (C), and 60 (A) [Chapter 7, Table 7-3]. Bacterial meningitis (question 58) is characterized by high WBC count on CSF analysis, with a polymorphonuclear leukocyte (PMN) predominance, low glucose, and high protein. Tuberculous meningitis (question 59) is characterized by very high protein, low glucose, and a WBC generally < 500 cells/mm^3 with a lymphocyte predominance. Viral meningitis (question 60) may also have an early PMN predominance, but the CSF WBC is usually lower than in bacterial meningitis and the glucose is normal.

61. The correct answer is B [Chapter 9, Section III.E.4.c]. *Chlamydia trachomatis* is a common cause of afebrile pneumonia in a child 1–3 months of age. It presents with a staccato cough, respiratory distress, and a history of conjunctivitis (50%). On examination, patients often have tachypnea and wheezing. Infection with *Mycoplasma pneumoniae* is more common in older children and adolescents, and it typically presents with a chronic nonproductive cough and headache.

Respiratory syncytial virus is a common cause of pneumonia and bronchiolitis during the late fall and winter (November through April). It should be considered in any infant with wheezing; however, upper respiratory symptoms such as rhinorrhea and low-grade fever generally develop before cough and wheezing. Bacterial infection with *Streptococcus pneumoniae* can occur in young infants, although they would be expected to have fever. Asthma is a chronic disorder characterized by repeated episodes of wheezing and therefore is not present in a patient of this young age.

62. The correct answer is E [Chapter 3, Section IX.B.1]. This patient's presentation with sudden onset of scrotal pain, a tender and swollen testicle, and absent cremasteric reflex on the affected side is consistent with torsion of the spermatic cord, which is a urologic emergency. Emergent surgical consultation and intervention are necessary. Detorsion of the torsed spermatic cord must be performed within 6 hours to preserve testicular function, and at the time of the procedure the opposite testicle is also fixed to the scrotum because it has an increased incidence of torsion in the future. The diagnosis of torsion of the spermatic cord is a clinical diagnosis. Although not always necessary, confirmation of the torsion can be made by finding decreased uptake on radionuclide imaging or absent pulsations on Doppler ultrasound. Elevation of the torsed testicle can relieve pain in many instances; however, this is not a reliable test for diagnosis. This patient's presentation is inconsistent with epididymitis, because the entire testicle, not just the epididymis, is tender and swollen.

63. The correct answer is C [Chapter 2, Section V.B.5]. An abnormal anal wink reflex raises concern that there may be a neurologic reason for enuresis, and imaging studies of the spine and brain should therefore be considered. Family history is frequently positive in uncomplicated nocturnal enuresis. Psychosocial factors such as parental divorce or the birth of a sibling are frequently associated with uncomplicated secondary enuresis, which does not require imaging studies if the neurologic examination is normal. Constipation is a frequent comorbid factor that should be treated because it causes impingement on the bladder. Children with small bladder capacities often present with a history of frequent small voids and can sometimes be cured through bladder stretching exercises.

64 through 66. The correct answers are 64 (D), 65 (E), and 66 (B) [Chapter 13, Table 13-4]. Most patients with sickle cell disease have one or more crises during their lifetime. A hyperhemolytic crisis (question 64) is characterized by rapid hemolysis that leads to anemia. Patients present with fatigue, pallor, and jaundice. Laboratory evaluation reveals decreased Hgb, elevated bilirubin, and an elevated reticulocyte count. An aplastic crisis (question 65) is characterized by cessation of red blood cell (RBC) production, most commonly as a result of infection with Parvovirus B19. Patients present with pallor and fatigue. Laboratory evaluation reveals decreased Hgb and decreased reticulocyte count. Treatment is transfusion of RBCs. Sequestration crisis (question 66) is characterized by the acute accumulation of blood within the spleen or liver. Patients may present with pallor, fatigue, shortness of breath, and shock. Laboratory findings include a low Hgb and very elevated reticulocyte count. Urgent transfusion of RBCs is indicated.

67. The correct answer is C [Chapter 2, Table 2-1]. When a 4-month-old infant lies on its stomach, it can push up onto its elbows and look around with its head held up. When a 4-month-old infant is pulled from a supine to a sitting position, it should also be able to keep its head even with its body. A 2-month-old infant has head lag when pulled from a supine to a sitting position. A 2-month-old infant can pull the shoulders up slightly and move the head from side to side when placed in the prone position. A 6-month-old can lead with its head when pulled from a supine to a sitting position. Some 4-month-old infants can roll from a supine to a sitting position but are not likely to be able to get into a sitting position at this age.

68. The correct answer is B [Chapter 17, Section III.A]. This patient's physical examination is consistent with developmental hip dysplasia (DDH). Patients with DDH whose diagnosis is delayed may present with a limb length discrepancy. Examination may also reveal asymmetric thigh or buttock folds and diminished abduction of the affected hip. Transient synovitis, a postinfectious inflammatory response within the joint, also causes a limp, but a limb length discrepancy would not be present. Legg-Calvé-Perthes disease is idiopathic avascular necrosis of the femoral head that occurs most commonly in children 4–9 years of age. Femoral anteversion is an inward angulation of the femur that results in in-toeing, and it is not manifested by a limb length discrepancy or asymmetric skin folds. Slipped capital femoral epiphysis is slippage of the femoral head off the femoral neck and is most common during adolescence.

69 through 71. The correct answers are 69 (B), 70 (A), 71 (B) [Chapter 14, Section V.A–B and Figure 14-1]. Both Wilms' tumor and neuroblastoma are commonly manifested by an abdominal mass in the first 5 years of life. Clinical features of neuroblastoma vary based on the tumor location. Two percent of patients with neuroblastoma have acute cerebellar atrophy with ataxia, opsoclonus, and myoclonus (so-called "dancing eyes and dancing feet"; question 69). Clinical features of Wilms' tumor include hemihypertrophy, aniridia, and genitourinary malformations (question 70). The prognosis for neuroblastoma is very good for children younger than 1 year of age, and spontaneous regression is possible, even with metastatic disease (stage IV-S disease; question 71).

72. The correct answer is D [Chapter 10, Section X.D.1 and Table 10-5]. Age is an important factor in determining the cause of lower gastrointestinal (GI) bleeding. In neonates and infants, an allergy to protein antigens in their food source can cause intestinal inflammation with GI bleeding, which may be occult or frank. Mucus may also be present in the stool. Juvenile polyp is the most common cause of lower GI bleeding after the neonatal period. Meckel's diverticulum, especially and infectious enterocolitis are important causes of bleeding, especially after infancy. Inflammatory bowel disease typically occurs later in childhood.

73 and 74. The correct answers are 73 (D) and 74 (B) [Chapter 5, Sections III.C.1 and III.A.8]. Turner syndrome is characterized by short stature, a webbed neck with a low posterior hairline, a shield chest, and ovarian dysgenesis that manifests as delayed puberty. Complications of Turner syndrome include scoliosis, left-sided cardiac lesions, and hypothyroidism. Therefore, screening for hypothyroidism is indicated (question 73). Osteogenesis imperfecta type I is characterized by blue sclerae, fragile bones that result in frequent fractures, and easy bruisability. Patients are at risk for skeletal deformities and for early conductive hearing loss. Therefore, audiologic evaluation is indicated (question 74).

75. The correct answer is D [Chapter 12, Section IV.C.4.e]. Irregular respirations with no particular pattern are also termed ataxic respirations and result from severe brainstem injury. This respiratory pattern often suggests impending brain death. Cerebellar injury and cerebral strokes do not usually result in changes in the respiratory pattern. Acute drug overdose with narcotics or sedatives causes hypoventilation.

76. The correct answer is E [Chapter 6, Section I.D.2.b]. Pathologic short stature (child's height is greater than three standard deviations below the mean with abnormal growth velocity) may be characterized as proportionate or disproportionate. Disproportionate short stature is defined as short stature in patients who are very short-legged with an increased upper-to-lower (U/L) body segment ratio, suggesting either a skeletal dysplasia or rickets (the latter would also be expected to present with bowing). In contrast, malnutrition, child neglect, growth hormone deficiency, and fetal alcohol syndrome are all causes of proportionate short stature, in which the patient has a normal U/L body segment ratio.

77. The correct answer is B [Chapter 17, Section III.B.5]. Osteomyelitis is characterized clinically by fever, irritability, localized bone pain, and swelling and erythema of the infected site. Osteomyelitis during childhood is most commonly acquired by hematogenous seeding. Direct inoculation and contiguous spread are less common ways of acquiring this infection. A plain radiograph is not a good study to assess early osteomyelitis because it is usually normal early in the course of disease. The elevation of periosteum as a result of infection does not usually become evident on a plain radiograph until after 10–14 days. *Staphylococcus aureus* and *Streptococcus pyogenes* are the two most common causative pathogens. *Salmonella typhi* infection occurs most commonly in a child with underlying sickle cell disease. Blood culture is positive in only 50% of patients with osteomyelitis. All children with osteomyelitis require initial management with intravenous antibiotics.

78. The correct answer is C [Chapter 4, Section I.H.1]. The normal umbilical cord should contain two arteries and one vein. The presence of only one umbilical artery should prompt suspicion of an associated underlying congenital renal anomaly. Neither an umbilical hernia nor diastasis recti (the separation of the rectus abdominis muscles at the midline of the abdomen) is associated with underlying structural problems. Patients with hypospadias, in which the urethral meatus is located on the ventral surface of the penis, are not likely to have associated urinary malformations. This is in contrast to epispadias (in which the urethral meatus is located on the dorsal surface of the penis), in which associated problems, such as bladder extrophy, may be present. A nevus simplex (or "salmon patch") is the most common vascular lesion of infancy and is also not associated with underlying pathology. This is in contrast to a nevus flammeus, or "port wine stain" in the distribution of the ophthalmic branch of the trigeminal nerve, which may be associated with Sturge-Weber syndrome.

79. The correct answer is B [Chapter 14, Section II.C.2.a]. This patient's age and his presentation with splenomegaly are most consistent with adult-type chronic myelogenous leukemia (CML). Most patients with adult-type CML are older children and adolescents, and they may be diagnosed with splenomegaly noted as an incidental finding during a routine health maintenance visit. Adult-type CML is characterized by the presence of the Philadelphia chromosome. Juvenile monomyelocytic leukemia (JMML), another type of CML, often presents with fever, a chronic eczematous-type facial rash (not found in adult-type CML), lymphadenopathy, petechiae, and purpura. JMML occurs in young children and infants. Radiation therapy is ineffective in adult-type CML; chemotherapy and bone marrow transplantation are more useful. Adult-type CML follows a biphasic course, characterized by easy control of elevated white blood cell (WBC) counts for several years followed by an acute deterioration resembling acute leukemia. Adult-type CML is characterized by extremely high WBC counts, often >100,000 cells/mm³.

80. The correct answer is B [Chapter 16, Section VII.F]. This patient's clinical presentation, including the geographic location in which she lives, is consistent with Lyme disease. The management of Lyme disease is aimed at eradicating *Borrelia burgdorferi*, the spirochete that causes the infection. This patient has early localized disease and should be treated with amoxicillin. Doxycycline should be avoided in children younger than 9 years of age because of concerns regarding permanent tooth discoloration. Patients with complications of carditis or meningitis require intravenous penicillin or intravenous ceftriaxone.

81. The correct answer is A [Chapter 9, Sections III.B.4, III.B.6]. This patient presents with signs and symptoms consistent with croup (laryngotracheobronchitis). Given the lack of stridor at rest and the absence of respiratory distress, cool mist and supportive care alone are indicated. Patients with stridor at rest benefit from corticosteroid treatment to reduce airway inflammation. Patients with both stridor at rest and respiratory distress also benefit from nebulized racemic epinephrine to vasoconstrict subglottic tissues. Albuterol can be useful if wheezing is present but does not have efficacy on the edematous subglottic tissues. Ribavirin is not effective in croup.

82. The correct answer is B [Chapter 7, Section XVI.B]. This patient's presentation is typical of neurocysticercosis, a helminth infection caused by the ingestion of the eggs of *Taenia solium*, a pork tapeworm. Treatment includes anticonvulsant medications; surgical excision is not indicated. Ova and parasite evaluation detects the eggs of the organism in only 25% of cases. Diagnosis is often made by findings on CT or magnetic resonance imaging, which reveal cysts that may be calcified. Calcifications are evidence of old, quiescent infection.

83. The correct answer is D [Chapter 16, IV.F.6]. The antinuclear antibody (ANA), although not specific, is almost universally elevated in children with SLE (> 95%). If a patient has a negative ANA, it is very unlikely that he or she has SLE. Erythrocyte sedimentation rate and rheumatoid factor are often, but not always, elevated in SLE but are nonspecific. Anti–double-stranded DNA antibodies are relatively specific for SLE, and uniquely, their levels can be used to monitor progression of disease, especially renal disease. Antibodies to the Smith antigen are elevated in only 30% of patients with SLE, but they are strongly suggestive of SLE when present.

84 through 88. The correct answers are 84 (C), 85 (H), 86 (B), 87 (F), and 88 (G) [Chapter 20, Table 20-4; Sections VIII.D.1, VIII.D.3, VIII.D.6]. Antidotes exist for a relatively small number of toxins. Iron is commonly found in prenatal vitamins (question 84). The antidote for iron is deferoxamine, an iron chelator. The blood level of acetaminophen in the 15-year-old girl (question 85) should be plotted on the Matthew-Rumack nomogram. If it is elevated, she should be treated with *N*-acetylcysteine, the antidote for acetaminophen poisoning. Symptoms and signs of carbon monoxide toxicity include headache, vomiting, auditory and visual changes, slurred speech, and mental status changes (question 86). Cherry red skin is a characteristic, although uncommon, finding. The antidote is 100% oxygen, which displaces carbon monoxide from the hemoglobin molecule. Isoniazid can cause seizures (question 87), and the antidote is pyridoxine (vitamin B$_6$). Dystonia can occur from several types of medications, including phenothiazines (question 88), and antidotes for dystonia include diphenhydramine and benztropine.

89. The correct answer is A [Chapter 3, Section VIII.D]. Bleeding that is prolonged and that occurs at irregular intervals, as found in this patient, is termed menometrorrhagia. The bleeding may be secondary to dysfunctional uterine bleeding (DUB), which is the most common cause of vaginal bleeding during adolescence, but the presence of painful bleeding is inconsistent with DUB. Because she is having painful bleeding and because her bleeding is heavy, both a pelvic examination and laboratory studies to evaluate for pregnancy, anemia, and blood dyscrasias are indicated. Bleeding secondary to DUB occurs because of unopposed estrogen production. Dilation and curettage may be required for bleeding that does not stop with hormonal therapy, but it is not the first-line treatment.

90. The correct answer is B [Chapter 12, Section VII.D]. The patient's presentation is consistent with Guillain-Barré syndrome, an acute inflammatory demyelinating polyneuropathy and a well-described cause of symmetric ascending weakness in childhood. Albuminocytologic dissociation in the cerebrospinal fluid (CSF), usually present 1 week after the onset of symptoms, is an important hallmark of Guillain-Barré syndrome. Patients classically have increased CSF protein levels but normal cell counts. Demyelination results in slowing of the nerve conduction velocity. Magnetic resonance imaging of the spine would be expected to be normal. Guillain-Barré syndrome is associated with many infectious agents, most commonly a recent infection with *Campylobacter jejuni*.

91. The correct answer is D [Chapter 17, Section III.B.2]. The patient's presentation is most consistent with transient synovitis, a postinfectious inflammatory response in the hip joint that is a common cause of limp in toddlers. Transient synovitis commonly follows an upper respiratory infection or diarrheal illness, and is characterized by limp, irritability, low grade fever or absence of fever, and a normal or slightly elevated white blood cell (WBC) count and erythrocyte sedimentation rate (ESR). Examination may reveal hip flexion, external rotation, and abduction, similar to that seen in septic arthritis, although usually less pain is elicited on movement of the hip joint compared with septic arthritis, in which pain is very significant. Septic arthritis and osteomyelitis also have an elevated WBC count and ESR, and patients are usually more ill-appearing. Slipped capital femoral epiphysis is a slipping of the femoral head off the femoral neck and typically presents with a painful limp, although this is more common in adolescence. A toddler's fracture is a spiral fracture of the tibia, which may occur after only mild trauma. A patient with a toddler's fracture may suddenly refuse to walk or bear weight. However, examination of the hip would be normal, although mild erythema, swelling, and tenderness may be found over the tibial fracture site.

92. The correct answer is C [Chapter 15, Section X.A]. IgA deficiency is the most common immune deficiency and is associated with an increased incidence of sinusitis, otitis media, bronchitis, and pneumonia. Low quantitative IgA levels confirm the diagnosis. A complete blood count is usually part of the workup for immune deficiency but would not confirm IgA deficiency. Anergy skin testing and the assessment of T-cell response to mitogens evaluate the competency of T-cell–mediated immunity, and patients with cellular-mediated immunodeficiency are more likely to present with recurrent viral, fungal, or protozoan infections. A normal total hemolytic complement demonstrates that all components of the complement pathway are present and functional. Patients with terminal complement deficiency usually present with recurrent meningococcal and gonococcal infections.

93. The correct answer is A [Chapter 17, Section IV.A.3.b]. Blount's disease, a progressive angulation of the proximal tibia, should be suspected in any child with progressive bowing, unilateral bowing, or persistent bowing after 2 years of age. In this patient with progressive bowing more prominent in one leg, Blount's disease would be a concern. Blount's disease is diagnosed with a standing anterior-posterior radiograph of the lower extremities that reveals an exaggerated metaphyseal-diaphyseal angle. Physical therapy is not effective. Genu varum (bowed legs) is not likely, because the bowing is more prominent in one extremity and because it is still present after 2 years of age. Genu valgum (knock-knees) is characterized by knees angulated toward the midline. Orthotic shoes are not useful in Blount's disease.

94. The correct answer is C [Chapter 12, Section VIII.A]. Sydenham chorea is an autoimmune response of the central nervous system to group A β-hemolytic streptococcal infection. The major clinical features include chorea and emotional lability. The choreic movements of the arms and legs can interfere with daily activities such as eating, writing, and walking. Migraine does not present with motor difficulties. In complex partial epilepsy, motor, psychomotor, or sensory findings may occur, but consciousness is decreased during the seizure. Hydrocephalus with increased intracranial pressure most commonly presents with vomiting and early morning headache, rather than with emotional lability, restlessness, and clumsiness. Tourette syndrome presents with motor or phonic tics.

95. The correct answer is C [Chapter 7, Section XVII.A.2]. The patient's clinical features are consistent with Rocky Mountain spotted fever, which is caused by infection with *Rickettsia rickettsii*, a Gram-negative bacteria transmitted by the bite of a tick. Clinical features include fever, a petechial rash that begins on the hands and feet, myalgias, hypotension, and hepatosplenomegaly. Thrombocytopenia and anemia also occur. Treatment should be started empirically on the basis of the clinical and epidemiologic features rather than waiting for confirmation by serologic testing. Prophylactic antibiotics to prevent infection are not indicated. The incidence is highest in school-aged children.

96. The correct answer is C [Chapter 7, Section IX.A.6 and Table 7-5]. The patient's clinical presentation is most consistent with toxic shock syndrome (TSS). The most common organism associated with TSS is *Staphylococcus aureus,* although some cases may be associated with group A β-hemolytic streptococcus. This patient's signs and symptoms are inconsistent with Kawasaki disease, hemolytic uremic syndrome (caused by *Escherichia coli* 0157:H7), or Lyme disease (caused by *Borrelia burgdorferi).*

97 through 100. The correct answers are 97 (C), 98 (B), 99 (D), and 100 (E) [Chapter 5, Sections XI.A.2, XI.B, XI.C, III.A.5.a]. Patients with Wilson's disease (question 97) have a high serum copper level that leads to copper deposition in the brain, eyes, and liver because of a copper excretion defect. These patients present with neurologic findings such as behavioral changes, seizures and ataxia, hepatic dysfunction, and Kayser-Fleisher rings in the peripheral cornea that represent copper deposition in Descemet's membrane. Patients with Menkes kinky hair disease (question 98) present with myoclonic seizures, progressive neurologic degeneration, mental retardation, and pale kinky friable hair. Menkes kinky-hair disease is caused by a defect in copper transport, and patients have a low serum copper level. Patients with acrodermatitis enteropathica (question 99) present with a symmetric dry vesiculobullous scaly rash, failure to thrive, and chronic diarrhea. Acrodermatitis enteropathica is caused by zinc deficiency, and low serum zinc is found on laboratory evaluation. Patients with DiGeorge syndrome (question 100) have hypocalcemia (caused by parathyroid hypoplasia), cellular-mediated immunodeficiency, which may result in recurrent fungal infections (caused by thymic hypoplasia), and cardiac findings that may include aortic arch abnormalities. DiGeorge syndrome is caused by a defect in the structures derived from the third and fourth pharyngeal pouches.

Index

Page numbers in *italics* denote figures; those followed by "t" denote tables; those followed by "Q" denote questions; and those followed by "E" denote explanations.